A
FIRST COURSE
IN
LINEAR MODEL
THEORY

CHAPMAN & HALL/CRC
Texts in Statistical Science Series

Series Editors
C. Chatfield, *University of Bath, UK*
Tim Lindsey, *University of Liege, Belgium*
Martin Tanner, *Northwestern University, USA*
J. Zidek, *University of British Columbia, Canada*

A
FIRST COURSE
IN
LINEAR MODEL
THEORY

Nalini Ravishanker and Dipak K. Dey

Department of Statistics
University of Connecticut
Storrs, Connecticut

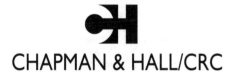

CHAPMAN & HALL/CRC

A CRC Press Company
Boca Raton   London   New York   Washington, D.C.

Library of Congress Cataloging-in-Publication Data

Ravishanker, Nalini.
    A first course in linear model theory / Nalini Ravishanker and Dipak K. Dey
        p.   cm. — (Texts in statistical science series)
    Includes bibliographical references and index.
    ISBN 1-58488-247-6 (alk. paper)
    1. Linear models (Statistics) I. Dey, Dipak. II. Title. III. Texts in statistical science.

QA276.R38 2001
519.5'35—dc21
                                            2001053726
                                                CIP

Visit the CRC Press Web site at www.crcpress.com

© 2002 by Chapman & Hall/CRC

No claim to original U.S. Government works
International Standard Book Number 1-58488-247-6
Library of Congress Card Number 2001053726
Printed in the United States of America   2 3 4 5 6 7 8 9 0
Printed on acid-free paper

To Ravi, Vivek and Varun.   N.R.

To Rita and Debosri   D.K.D.

Preface

Linear Model theory plays a fundamental role in the foundation of mathematical and applied statistics. It has a base in distribution theory and statistical inference, and finds application in many advanced areas in statistics including univariate and multivariate regression, analysis of designed experiments, longitudinal and time series analysis, spatial analysis, multivariate analysis, wavelet methods, etc. Most statistics departments offer at least one course on linear model theory at the graduate level. There are several excellent books on the subject, such as "Linear Statistical Inference and its Applications" by C.R. Rao, "Linear Models" by S.R. Searle, "Theory and Applications of the Linear Model" by F.A. Graybill, "Plane Answers to Complex Questions: The Theory of Linear Models" by R. Christiansen and "The Theory of Linear Models" by B. Jorgensen.

Our motivation has been to incorporate general principles of inference in linear models to the fundamental statistical education of students at the graduate level, while our treatment of contemporary topics in a systematic way will serve the needs of professionals in various industries. The three salient features of this book are: (1) developing standard theory of linear models with numerous applications in simple and multiple regression, as well as fixed, random and mixed-effects models, (2) introducing generalized linear models with examples, and (3) presenting some current topics including Bayesian linear models, general additive models, dynamic linear models and longitudinal models. The first two chapters introduce to the reader requisite linear and matrix algebra. This book is therefore a self-contained exposition of the theory of linear models, including motivational and practical aspects. We have tried to achieve a healthy compromise between theory and practice, by providing a sound theoretical basis, and indicating how the theory works in important special cases in practice. There are several examples throughout the text. In addition, we provide summaries of many numerical examples in different chapters, while a more comprehensive description of these is available in the first author's web site (http://www.stat.uconn.edu/~nalini). There are several exercises at the end of each chapter that should serve to reinforce the methods.

Our entire book is intended for a two semester graduate course in linear models. For a one semester course, we recommend essentially the first eight chapters, omitting a few subsections, if necessary, and supplementing a few selected topics from chapters 9-11, if time permits. For instance, section 5.5, section 6.4, sections 7.5.2-7.5.4, and sections 8.5, 8.7 and 8.8 may be omitted in a one semester course. The first two chapters, which present a review on vectors and matrices specifically as they pertain to linear model theory, may also be assigned as background reading if the students had previous exposure

x

to these topics. Our book requires some knowledge of statistics; in particular, a knowledge of elementary sampling distributions, basic estimation theory and hypothesis testing at an undergraduate level is definitely required. Occasionally, more advanced concepts of statistical inference are invoked in this book, for which suitable references are provided.

The plan of this book follows. The first two chapters develop basic concepts of linear and matrix algebra with a view towards application in linear models. Chapter 3 describes generalized inverses and solutions to systems of linear equations. We develop the notion of a general linear model in Chapter 4. An attractive feature of our book is that we unify full-rank and non full-rank models in the development of least squares inference and optimality via the Gauss-Markov theorem. Results for the full-rank (regression) case are provided as special cases. We also introduce via examples, balanced ANOVA models that are widely used in practice. Chapter 5 deals with multivariate normal and related distributions, as well as distributions of quadratic forms that are at the heart of inference. We also introduce the class of elliptical distributions that can serve as error distributions for linear models. Sampling from multivariate normal distributions is the topic of Chapter 6, together with assessment of and transformations to multivariate normality. This is followed by inference for the general linear model in Chapter 7. Inference under normal and elliptical errors is developed and illustrated on examples from regression and balanced ANOVA models. In Chapter 8, topics in multiple regression models such as model checking, variable selection, regression diagnostics, robust regression and nonparametric regression are presented. Chapter 9 is devoted to the study of unbalanced designs in fixed-effects ANOVA models, the analysis of covariance (ANACOVA) and some nonparametric test procedures. Random-effects models and mixed-effects models are discussed in detail in Chapter 10. Finally in Chapter 11, we introduce several special topics including Bayesian linear models, dynamic linear models, linear longitudinal models and generalized linear models (GLIM). The purpose of this chapter is to introduce to the reader some new frontiers of linear models theory; several references are provided so that the reader may explore further in these directions. Given the exploding nature of our subject area, it is impossible to be exhaustive in a text, and cover everything that should ideally be covered. We hope that our judgment in choice of material is appropriate and useful.

Most of our book was developed in the form of lecture notes for a sequence of two courses on linear models which both of us have taught for several years in the Department of Statistics at the University of Connecticut. The numerical examples in the text and in the web site were developed by NR over many years. In the text, we have acknowledged published work, wherever appropriate, for the use of data in our numerical examples, as well as for some of the exercise problems. We are indeed grateful for their use, and apologize for any inadvertent omission in this regard.

xi

In writing this text, discussions with many colleagues were invaluable. In particular, we thank Malay Ghosh, for several suggestions that vastly improved the structure and content of this book. We deeply appreciate his time and goodwill. We thank Chris Chatfield and Jim Lindsey for their review and for the suggestion about including numerical examples in the text. We are also very grateful for the support and encouragement of our statistical colleagues, in particular Joe Glaz, Bani Mallick, Alan Gelfand and Yazhen Wang. We thank Ming-Hui Chen for all his technical help with Latex.

Many graduate students helped in proof reading the typed manuscript; we are especially grateful to Junfeng Liu, Madhuja Mallick and Prashni Paliwal. We also thank Karen Houle, a graduate student in Statistics, who helped with "polishing-up" the numerical examples in NR's web site. We appreciate all the help we received from people at Chapman & Hall/CRC – Bob Stern, Helena Redshaw, Gail Renard and Sean Davey.

Ravi, what can I say, except thanks for the warm smiles and hot dinners! N.R. Rita and Debosri, without your sacrifice, the project wouldn't be completed on time. D.K.D.

Nalini Ravishanker and Dipak K. Dey
Department of Statistics
University of Connecticut
Storrs, CT

Contents

Chapter 1

A Review of Vector and Matrix Algebra

In this chapter, we introduce basic results dealing with vector spaces and matrices, which are essential for an understanding of univariate and multivariate linear statistical methods. We provide several numerical and geometrical illustrations of these concepts. The material presented in this chapter will be found in most textbooks that deal with matrix theory pertaining to linear models, including Graybill (1983), Harville (1997), Rao (1973a) and Searle (1982). Unless stated otherwise, all vectors and matrices are assumed to be real, i.e., they have real numbers as elements.

1.1   Notation

An $m \times n$ matrix $\mathbf{A}$ is a rectangular array of real numbers of the form

$$\mathbf{A} = \begin{pmatrix} a_{11} & a_{12} & \cdots & a_{1n} \\ a_{21} & a_{22} & \cdots & a_{2n} \\ \vdots & \vdots & \vdots & \vdots \\ a_{m1} & a_{m2} & \cdots & a_{mn} \end{pmatrix} = \{a_{ij}\}$$

with row dimension m, column dimension n, and (i,j)th element a_{ij}. For example,

$$\mathbf{A} = \begin{pmatrix} 5 & 4 & 1 \\ -3 & 2 & 6 \end{pmatrix}$$

is a 2×3 matrix. An n-dimensional column vector

$$\mathbf{a} = \begin{pmatrix} a_1 \\ a_2 \\ \vdots \\ a_n \end{pmatrix}$$

1

can be thought of as a matrix with n rows and one column. For example,

$$\mathbf{a} = \begin{pmatrix} 1 \\ -1 \end{pmatrix}, \quad \mathbf{b} = \begin{pmatrix} 3 \\ 1 \\ 5 \end{pmatrix}, \text{ and } \mathbf{c} = \begin{pmatrix} 0.25 \\ 0.50 \\ 0.75 \\ 1.00 \end{pmatrix}$$

are respectively 2-dimensional, 3-dimensional and 4- dimensional vectors. An n-dimensional column vector with each of its n elements equal to unity is called the unit vector, and is denoted by $\mathbf{1}_n$, while a column vector whose elements are all zero is called the null vector and is denoted by $\mathbf{0}_n$. For any integer $n \geq 1$, we can write an n-dimensional column vector as $\mathbf{a} = (a_1, \cdots, a_n)'$, i.e., as the *transpose* of the n-dimensional (row) vector with components $a_1, \cdots, a_n$.

An $m \times n$ matrix $\mathbf{A}$ with the same row and column dimensions, i.e., with $m = n$, is called a square matrix of order n. An $n \times n$ identity matrix is denoted by $\mathbf{I}_n$; each of its n diagonal elements is unity while each off-diagonal element is zero. An $m \times n$ unit matrix $\mathbf{J}_{mn}$ has each element equal to unity. An $n \times n$ unit matrix is denoted by $\mathbf{J}_n$. For example, we have

$$\mathbf{I}_3 = \begin{pmatrix} 1 & 0 & 0 \\ 0 & 1 & 0 \\ 0 & 0 & 1 \end{pmatrix} \text{ and } \mathbf{J}_3 = \begin{pmatrix} 1 & 1 & 1 \\ 1 & 1 & 1 \\ 1 & 1 & 1 \end{pmatrix}.$$

An $n \times n$ matrix whose elements are zero except on the diagonal, where the elements are nonzero, is called a diagonal matrix. We will denote a diagonal matrix by $\mathbf{D} = \mathrm{diag}(d_1, d_2, \cdots, d_n)$. Note that $\mathbf{I}_n$ is an $n \times n$ diagonal matrix, written as $\mathbf{I}_n = \mathrm{diag}(1, 1, \cdots, 1)$. An $m \times n$ matrix $\mathbf{C}$ all of whose elements are equal to the same constant c is called a constant matrix. If $c = 0$, the resulting matrix is the null matrix $\mathbf{0}$. An $n \times n$ matrix is said to be an upper triangular matrix if all the elements below and to the left of the main diagonal are zero. Similarly, if all the elements located above and to the right of the main diagonal are zero, then the $n \times n$ matrix is said to be lower triangular. For example,

$$\mathbf{U} = \begin{pmatrix} 5 & 4 & 3 \\ 0 & 2 & -6 \\ 0 & 0 & 5 \end{pmatrix} \text{ and } \mathbf{L} = \begin{pmatrix} 5 & 0 & 0 \\ 4 & 2 & 0 \\ 3 & -6 & 5 \end{pmatrix}$$

are respectively upper triangular and lower triangular matrices. A square matrix is triangular if it is either upper triangular or lower triangular. A triangular matrix is said to be a unit triangular matrix if $a_{ij} = 1$ whenever $i = j$. Unless explicitly stated, we assume that vectors and matrices are non null.

A submatrix of a matrix $\mathbf{A}$ is obtained by deleting certain rows and/or columns of $\mathbf{A}$. For example, let

$$\mathbf{A} = \begin{pmatrix} 1 & 3 & 5 & 7 \\ 5 & 4 & 1 & -9 \\ -3 & 2 & 6 & 4 \end{pmatrix} \text{ and } \mathbf{B} = \begin{pmatrix} 5 & 4 & 1 \\ -3 & 2 & 6 \end{pmatrix}.$$

The 2×3 submatrix $\mathbf{B}$ has been obtained by deleting Row 1 and Column 4 of the 3×4 matrix $\mathbf{A}$. Any matrix can be considered to be a submatrix of itself. An $r \times r$ principal submatrix $\mathbf{B}$ of an $n \times n$ matrix $\mathbf{A}$ is obtained by deleting the same rows and columns from $\mathbf{A}$. For $r = 1, 2, \cdots, n$, the $r \times r$ leading principal submatrix of $\mathbf{A}$ is obtained by deleting the last $(n - r)$ rows and columns from $\mathbf{A}$. The 2×2 leading principal submatrix of the matrix $\mathbf{A}$ shown above is

$$\mathbf{B} = \begin{pmatrix} 1 & 3 \\ 5 & 4 \end{pmatrix}.$$

It may be easily verified that a principal submatrix of a diagonal, upper triangular or lower triangular matrix is respectively diagonal, upper triangular or lower triangular.

Some elementary properties of vectors and matrices are given in the next section. Familiarity with this material is recommended before a further study of properties of special matrices that are described in the following two chapters.

1.2 Basic definitions and properties

An n-dimensional vector $\mathbf{a}$ is an ordered set of measurements, which can be represented geometrically as a directed line in n-dimensional space with component a_1 along the first axis, component a_2 along the second axis, $\cdots$, and component a_n along the nth axis. We can represent 2-dimensional and 3-dimensional vectors respectively as points in the plane and in 3-dimensional space.

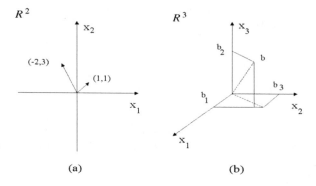

(a)   (b)

Figure 1.2.1. Geometric representation of two and three-dimensional vectors.

Any 2-dimensional vector $\mathbf{a} = (a_1, a_2)'$ can be graphically represented by the point with coordinates (a_1, a_2) in the Cartesian coordinate plane, or as the arrow starting from the origin $(0, 0)$, whose tip is the point with coordinates (a_1, a_2).

For $n = 2$, Figure 1.2.1 (a) shows the vectors $(1, 1)$ and $(-2, 3)$ as arrows starting from the origin. For $n = 3$, Figure 1.2.1 (b) shows a vector $\mathbf{b} = (b_1, b_2, b_3)'$ in $\mathcal{R}^3$.

Two vectors can be added (or subtracted) only if they have the same dimension, in which case the sum (or difference) of the two vectors is the vector of sums (or differences) of their elements, i.e.,

$$\mathbf{a} \pm \mathbf{b} = (a_1 \pm b_1, a_2 \pm b_2, \cdots, a_n \pm b_n)'.$$

The sum of two vectors emanating from the origin is the diagonal of the parallelogram which has the vectors $\mathbf{a}$ and $\mathbf{b}$ as adjacent sides. Vector addition is commutative and associative, i.e., $\mathbf{a} + \mathbf{b} = \mathbf{b} + \mathbf{a}$, and $\mathbf{a} + (\mathbf{b} + \mathbf{c}) = (\mathbf{a} + \mathbf{b}) + \mathbf{c}$.

The scalar multiple $c\mathbf{a}$ of a vector $\mathbf{a}$ is obtained by multiplying each element of $\mathbf{a}$ by the scalar c, i.e.,

$$c\mathbf{a} = (ca_1, \cdots, ca_n)'.$$

Scalar multiplication has the effect of expanding or contracting a given vector. Scalar multiplication of a vector obeys the distributive law for vectors, the distributive law for scalars, and the associative law, i.e., $c(\mathbf{a} + \mathbf{b}) = c\mathbf{a} + c\mathbf{b}$, $(c_1 + c_2)\mathbf{a} = c_1\mathbf{a} + c_2\mathbf{a}$, and $c_1(c_2\mathbf{a}) = (c_1 c_2)\mathbf{a}$. Also, $\mathbf{a} + \mathbf{0} = \mathbf{0} + \mathbf{a} = \mathbf{a}$, $1\mathbf{a} = \mathbf{a}$, and for every $\mathbf{a}$, there exists a corresponding vector α such that $\mathbf{a} + \alpha = \mathbf{0}$. A collection of n-dimensional vectors (with the associated field of scalars) satisfying the above properties is a linear vector space and is denoted by $\mathcal{V}_n$.

The product of two vectors can be formed only if one of them is a row vector and the other is a column vector and the result is called their inner product or dot product.

Definition 1.2.1. Inner product of vectors.   The inner product of two n-dimensional vectors $\mathbf{a}$ and $\mathbf{b}$ is denoted by $\mathbf{a} \bullet \mathbf{b}$ or $\mathbf{a}'\mathbf{b}$ and is the scalar

$$\mathbf{a}'\mathbf{b} = (a_1, a_2, \cdots, a_n) \begin{pmatrix} b_1 \\ b_2 \\ \vdots \\ b_n \end{pmatrix} = a_1 b_1 + a_2 b_2 + \cdots + a_n b_n = \sum_{i=1}^{n} a_i b_i.$$

The inner product of a vector $\mathbf{a}$ with itself is $\mathbf{a}'\mathbf{a}$. The positive square root of this quantity is called the *Euclidean norm*, or *length*, or *magnitude* of the vector, and is

$$\| \mathbf{a} \| = (a_1^2 + a_2^2 + \cdots + a_n^2)^{1/2} .$$

The Euclidean distance between two vectors $\mathbf{a}$ and $\mathbf{b}$ is defined by

$$d = \| \mathbf{a} - \mathbf{b} \|.$$

Geometrically, the length of a vector $\mathbf{a} = (a_1, a_2)$ in two dimensions may be viewed as the hypotenuse of a right triangle, whose other two sides are given by the vector components, a_1 and a_2. Scalar multiplication of a vector $\mathbf{a}$ changes its length,

$$\| ca \| = (c^2 a_1^2 + c^2 a_2^2 + \cdots + c^2 a_n^2)^{1/2} = |c|(a_1^2 + a_2^2 + \cdots + a_n^2)^{1/2} = |c| \| a \| .$$

If $|c| > 1$, **a** is expanded by scalar multiplication, while if $|c| < 1$, **a** is contracted. If $c = 1/ \| a \|$, the resulting vector is defined to be $b = a/ \| a \|$, the n-dimensional unit vector with length 1. A vector has both length and direction. If $c > 0$, scalar multiplication does not change the direction of a vector **a**. However, if $c < 0$, the direction of the vector ca is in opposite direction to the vector **a**. The unit vector $a/ \| a \|$ has the same direction as **a**. The angle θ between two vectors **a** and **b** is defined in terms of their inner product as

$$\cos \theta = a'b/ \| a \| \| b \| = a'b/\sqrt{a'a}\sqrt{b'b}$$

(see Figure 1.2.2.). Since $\cos \theta = 0$ only if $a'b = 0$, **a** and **b** are perpendicular (or orthogonal) when $a'b = 0$.

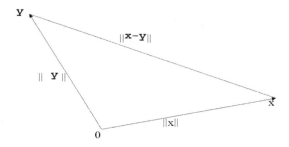

Figure 1.2.2. Inner product of two vectors.

Result 1.2.1. Properties of inner product. Let $a, b,$ and c be n-dimensional vectors and let d be a scalar. Then,

1. $a \bullet b = b \bullet a$

2. $a \bullet (b + c) = a \bullet b + a \bullet c$

3. $d(a \bullet b) = (da) \bullet b = a \bullet (db)$

4. $a \bullet a \geq 0$, with equality if and only if $a = 0$

5. $\| a \pm b \|^2 = \| a \|^2 + \| b \|^2 \pm 2a \bullet b$

6. $|a \bullet b| \leq \| a \| \| b \|$

7. $\| a + b \| \leq \| a \| + \| b \|.$

The last two inequalities in Result 1.2.1 are respectively the Cauchy-Schwarz inequality and the triangle inequality, which we ask the reader to verify in Exercise 1.2. Equality holds in property 6 if and only if $\mathbf{a} = \mathbf{0}$, or $\mathbf{b} = \mathbf{0}$, or $\mathbf{a}$ and $\mathbf{b}$ are scalar multiples of each other. In property 7, equality holds if and only if $\mathbf{a} = \mathbf{0}$, or $\mathbf{b} = \mathbf{0}$, or $\mathbf{b} = c\mathbf{a}$ for some constant $c \geq 0$. Geometrically, the triangle inequality states that the length of one side of a triangle does not exceed the sum of the lengths of the other two sides.

Definition 1.2.2. Outer product of vectors. The outer product of two vectors $\mathbf{a}$ and $\mathbf{b}$ is denoted by $\mathbf{a} \wedge \mathbf{b}$ or $\mathbf{ab}'$ and is obtained by post-multiplying the column vector $\mathbf{a}$ by the row vector $\mathbf{b}'$. There is no restriction on the dimensions of $\mathbf{a}$ and $\mathbf{b}$; if $\mathbf{a}$ is an $m \times 1$ vector and $\mathbf{b}$ is an $n \times 1$ vector, the outer product $\mathbf{ab}'$ is an $m \times n$ matrix.

Example 1.2.1. We illustrate all these vector operations by an example. Let

$$\mathbf{a} = \begin{pmatrix} 2 \\ 3 \\ 4 \end{pmatrix}, \quad \mathbf{b} = \begin{pmatrix} 6 \\ 7 \\ 9 \end{pmatrix} \text{ and } \mathbf{d} = \begin{pmatrix} 10 \\ 20 \end{pmatrix}.$$

Then,

$$\mathbf{a} + \mathbf{b} = \begin{pmatrix} 8 \\ 10 \\ 13 \end{pmatrix}, \quad \mathbf{a} - \mathbf{b} = \begin{pmatrix} -4 \\ -4 \\ -5 \end{pmatrix}, \quad 10\mathbf{b} = \begin{pmatrix} 60 \\ 70 \\ 90 \end{pmatrix},$$

$$\mathbf{a}'\mathbf{b} = 2 \times 6 + 3 \times 7 + 4 \times 9 = 69,$$

$$\mathbf{ab}' = \begin{pmatrix} 2 \\ 3 \\ 4 \end{pmatrix} \begin{pmatrix} 6 & 7 & 9 \end{pmatrix} = \begin{pmatrix} 12 & 14 & 18 \\ 18 & 21 & 27 \\ 24 & 28 & 36 \end{pmatrix}, \text{ and}$$

$$\mathbf{ad}' = \begin{pmatrix} 2 \\ 3 \\ 4 \end{pmatrix} \begin{pmatrix} 10 & 20 \end{pmatrix} = \begin{pmatrix} 20 & 40 \\ 30 & 60 \\ 40 & 80 \end{pmatrix}.$$

However, $\mathbf{a} + \mathbf{d}$, $\mathbf{a}'\mathbf{d}$, and $\mathbf{b}'\mathbf{d}$ are undefined. □

Definition 1.2.3. The set of all linear combinations of the n-dimensional vectors $\{\mathbf{v}_i = (v_{i1}, \cdots, v_{in}), \ v_{ij} \in \mathcal{R}, \ i = 1, 2, \cdots, l\}$ is called their span and is denoted by $\text{Span}\{\mathbf{v}_1, \cdots, \mathbf{v}_l\}$. For example, the vectors $\mathbf{0}$, $\mathbf{v}_1$, $\mathbf{v}_2$, $\mathbf{v}_1 + \mathbf{v}_2$, $10\mathbf{v}_1$, $5\mathbf{v}_1 - 3\mathbf{v}_2$ all belong to $\text{Span}\{\mathbf{v}_1, \mathbf{v}_2\}$. A vector $\mathbf{u}$ is in $\text{Span}\{\mathbf{v}_1, \cdots, \mathbf{v}_l\}$ if and only if there are scalars $c_1, \cdots, c_l$ such that $\mathbf{u} = c_1\mathbf{v}_1 + \cdots + c_l\mathbf{v}_l$.

Definition 1.2.4. Vector space. A vector space is a set

$$\mathcal{V}_n = \{\mathbf{v}_i = (v_{i1}, \cdots, v_{in}), \ v_{ij} \in \mathcal{R}, \ i = 1, 2, \cdots, l\}$$

which is closed under addition and multiplication by a scalar, and contains the vector $\mathbf{0}$. For example, $\mathcal{R}^n$ is a vector space for any positive integer $n = 1, 2, \cdots$. As another example, consider k linear equations in n variables $x_1, \cdots, x_n$:

$$c_{i1}x_1 + \cdots + c_{in}x_n = 0, \quad i = 1, \cdots, k,$$

where c_{ij} are real constants. Then the totality of solutions $(x_1, \cdots, x_n)$ considered as vectors is a subspace of $\mathcal{R}^n$. We discuss solutions of linear equations in Chapter 3.

Definition 1.2.5. Vector subspace. Let $\mathcal{S}_n$ be a space consisting of the vector $\mathbf{0}$ and a subset of vectors in $\mathcal{V}_n$. If $\mathcal{S}_n$ is also a vector space, it is called a subspace of $\mathcal{V}_n$. For example, $\{\mathbf{0}\}$ and $\mathcal{V}_n$ are (trivially) subspaces of $\mathcal{V}_n$. Any plane through the origin is a subspace of $\mathcal{R}^3$.

Definition 1.2.6. Linear dependence and independence of vectors. Let $\{\mathbf{v}_1, \cdots, \mathbf{v}_m\}$ denote n-dimensional vectors in $\mathcal{V}_n$. These m vectors are said to be linearly dependent if and only if there exist scalars $c_1, \cdots, c_m$, not all zero, such that $\sum_{i=1}^m c_i \mathbf{v}_i = \mathbf{0}$. If all the c_i are zero, then $\mathbf{v}_1, \cdots, \mathbf{v}_m$ are said to be linearly independent (LIN) vectors. For example, the null vector $\mathbf{0}$ is a linearly dependent set, as is any set of vectors containing $\mathbf{0}$.

Example 1.2.2. Let $\mathbf{v}_1 = \begin{pmatrix} 1 & -1 & 3 \end{pmatrix}'$ and $\mathbf{v}_2 = \begin{pmatrix} 1 & 1 & 1 \end{pmatrix}'$. Now, $\sum_{i=1}^2 c_i \mathbf{v}_i = \mathbf{0} \Rightarrow c_1 + c_2 = 0, -c_1 + c_2 = 0$, and $3c_1 + c_2 = 0$, for which the only solution is $c_1 = c_2 = 0$. Hence, $\mathbf{v}_1$ and $\mathbf{v}_2$ are LIN vectors. □

Example 1.2.3. The vectors

$$\mathbf{v}_1 = \begin{pmatrix} 1 & -1 \end{pmatrix}', \quad \mathbf{v}_2 = \begin{pmatrix} 1 & 2 \end{pmatrix}', \text{ and } \mathbf{v}_3 = \begin{pmatrix} 2 & 1 \end{pmatrix}'$$

are linearly dependent, which is verified by setting $c_1 = 1$, $c_2 = 1$, and $c_3 = -1$; we see that $\sum_{i=1}^3 c_i \mathbf{v}_i = \mathbf{0}$. □

Result 1.2.2. The following properties hold:

1. If $m > 1$ vectors $\mathbf{v}_1, \cdots, \mathbf{v}_m$ are linearly dependent, we can express at least one of them as a linear combination of the others.

2. If s of the m vectors are linearly dependent, where $s \le m$, then all m vectors are linearly dependent.

3. If $m > n$, then $\mathbf{v}_1, \cdots, \mathbf{v}_m$ are linearly dependent.

4. There can be at most n LIN n-dimensional vectors.

5. The totality of all vectors which are linearly dependent on the n-dimensional vectors $\mathbf{v}_1, \cdots, \mathbf{v}_m$ is a vector space. The dimension of this vector space is the maximum number of LIN vectors in the space. A formal definition follows.

Definition 1.2.7. Basis of a vector space.   Let $\mathbf{v}_1, \cdots, \mathbf{v}_m$ be a set of m LIN vectors in $\mathcal{V}_n$ that span $\mathcal{V}_n$, i.e., each vector in $\mathcal{V}_n$ is obtained as a linear combination of these m vectors. Then, $\{\mathbf{v}_1, \cdots, \mathbf{v}_m\}$ is called a basis (Hamel basis) for $\mathcal{V}_n$ and the dimension of $\mathcal{V}_n$ is $\dim(\mathcal{V}_n) = m$.

Every vector space $\mathcal{V}_n$ has a basis, which is seen as follows. Sequentially choose non null vectors $\mathbf{v}_1, \mathbf{v}_2, \cdots$ in $\mathcal{V}_n$ so that no $\mathbf{v}_i$ is linearly dependent on the preceeding vectors. Suppose that after the choice of m vectors, there is no other LIN vector in $\mathcal{V}_n$, we say that $\mathbf{v}_1, \cdots, \mathbf{v}_m$ is a basis of the m-dimensional vector space $\mathcal{V}_n$. Although a vector space $\mathcal{V}_n$ may be infinite dimensional, we only focus on finite dimensional vector spaces. Every vector in $\mathcal{V}_n$ has a unique representation in terms of a given basis. If we can represent a vector $\mathbf{x}$ in $\mathcal{V}_n$ as $\sum c_i \mathbf{v}_i$ and $\sum d_i \mathbf{v}_i$, then, $\sum (c_i - d_i) \mathbf{v}_i = \mathbf{0}$, which, by Definition 1.2.6 is possible only if $c_i = d_i$ for all i. Note that a basis of a vector space is not unique. However, if $\mathbf{v}_1, \cdots, \mathbf{v}_m$ and $\mathbf{u}_1, \cdots, \mathbf{u}_k$ are two choices for a basis of $\mathcal{V}_n$, then $m = k$. The cardinal number m which is common to all bases of $\mathcal{V}_n$ is the maximum number of LIN vectors in $\mathcal{V}_n$ (or, the minimum number of vectors that span $\mathcal{V}_n$). To verify that $k = m$, let us suppose that on the contrary, $k > m$ and consider the linearly dependent set of vectors $\mathbf{u}_1, \mathbf{v}_1, \cdots, \mathbf{v}_m$. Suppose $\mathbf{v}_i$ depends on the preceeding vectors, then $\mathcal{V}_n$ can be generated by $\mathbf{u}_1, \mathbf{v}_1, \cdots, \mathbf{v}_{i-1}, \mathbf{v}_{i+1}, \cdots, \mathbf{v}_m$. Then, the set of vectors $\mathbf{u}_2, \mathbf{u}_1, \mathbf{v}_1, \cdots, \mathbf{v}_{i-1}, \mathbf{v}_{i+1}, \cdots, \mathbf{v}_m$ are linearly dependent, which in turn implies that we may discard one more $\mathbf{v}$ from this set. We continue this process of discarding a vector $\mathbf{v}$ and including a vector $\mathbf{u}$ until we have the set of vectors $\mathbf{u}_1, \cdots, \mathbf{u}_m$, which spans $\mathcal{V}_n$. Hence, $(k - m)$ of the $\mathbf{u}$ vectors are redundant. The matrix whose columns are the basis of $\mathcal{V}_n$ is called the basis matrix of $\mathcal{V}_n$.

A vector space $\mathcal{V}$ is said to be the **direct sum** of subspaces $\mathcal{V}_1, \cdots, \mathcal{V}_k$, i.e., $\mathcal{V} = \mathcal{V}_1 \oplus \cdots \oplus \mathcal{V}_k$, if a vector $\mathbf{v} \in \mathcal{V}$ can be uniquely written as $\mathbf{v} = \mathbf{v}_1 + \cdots + \mathbf{v}_k$, where $\mathbf{v}_i \in \mathcal{V}_i$. Also, $\mathcal{V}_i \cap \mathcal{V}_j = \{\mathbf{0}\}$, and $\dim(\mathcal{V}) = \dim(\mathcal{V}_1) + \cdots + \dim(\mathcal{V}_k)$.

The m-dimensional vector with 1 for its ith component and zeroes elsewhere is denoted by $\mathbf{e}_i$. The vectors $\mathbf{e}_1, \cdots, \mathbf{e}_m$ are called the standard basis vectors of the vector space $\mathcal{R}^m$, of dimension m. For example, the standard basis vectors in $\mathcal{R}^2$ are $\mathbf{e}_1 = (1, 0)'$ and $\mathbf{e}_2 = (0, 1)'$, while those in $\mathcal{R}^3$ are $\mathbf{e}_1 = (1, 0, 0)'$, $\mathbf{e}_2 = (0, 1, 0)'$, and $\mathbf{e}_3 = (0, 0, 1)'$. Any n-dimensional vector $\mathbf{x}$ can be written as $\mathbf{x} = x_1 \mathbf{e}_1 + \cdots + x_n \mathbf{e}_n$. Any vector space of dimension m is isomorphic to $\mathcal{R}^m$, so the study of m-dimensional vector spaces is equivalent to the study of $\mathcal{R}^m$. Further, there exists an isomorphism between two vector spaces that have the same dimension. Useful notions of distance or angle between vectors in a space $\mathcal{V}_n$ were given in Definitions 1.2.1, Result 1.2.1, and the associated discussion.

Definition 1.2.8. Orthogonal vectors. Two vectors $\mathbf{v}_1$ and $\mathbf{v}_2$ in $\mathcal{V}_n$ are orthogonal if and only if $\mathbf{v}_1 \bullet \mathbf{v}_2 = \mathbf{v}_1' \mathbf{v}_2 = \mathbf{v}_2' \mathbf{v}_1 = 0$; we write $\mathbf{v}_1 \perp \mathbf{v}_2$.

Pythagoras's Theorem states that the n-dimensional vectors $\mathbf{v}_1$ and $\mathbf{v}_2$ are orthogonal if and only if

$$\| \mathbf{v}_1 + \mathbf{v}_2 \|^2 = \| \mathbf{v}_1 \|^2 + \| \mathbf{v}_2 \|^2;$$

this is illustrated in Figure 1.2.3.

Result 1.2.3. If $\mathbf{v}_1, \mathbf{v}_2, \cdots, \mathbf{v}_n$ are nonzero vectors which are mutually orthogonal, i.e., $\mathbf{v}_i'\mathbf{v}_j = 0$, $i \neq j$, $i, j = 1, \cdots, n$, then these vectors are LIN.

Definition 1.2.9. Normal vector. A vector $\mathbf{v}_1$ is said to be a normal vector if $\mathbf{v}_1 \bullet \mathbf{v}_1 = \mathbf{v}_1'\mathbf{v}_1 = 1$.

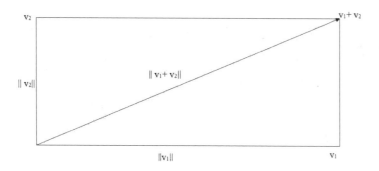

Figure 1.2.3. Pythagoras's theorem.

Definition 1.2.10. Orthonormal basis of $\mathcal{V}_n$. A basis $\{\mathbf{v}_1, \cdots, \mathbf{v}_m\}$ of a vector space $\mathcal{V}_n$ such that $\mathbf{v}_i'\mathbf{v}_j = 0$, for all $i \neq j$, $i, j = 1, \cdots, m$ is called an orthogonal basis. If further, $\mathbf{v}_i'\mathbf{v}_i = 1$ for $i = 1, \cdots, m$, it is called an orthonormal basis of $\mathcal{V}_n$.

Result 1.2.4. Gram-Schmidt orthogonalization. Let $\{\mathbf{v}_1, \cdots, \mathbf{v}_m\}$ denote an arbitrary basis of $\mathcal{V}_n$. To construct an orthonormal basis of $\mathcal{V}_n$ starting from $\{\mathbf{v}_1, \cdots, \mathbf{v}_m\}$, we define

$$\mathbf{y}_1 = \mathbf{v}_1,$$

$$\mathbf{y}_k = \mathbf{v}_k - \sum_{i=1}^{k-1} \frac{\mathbf{y}_i'\mathbf{v}_k}{\|\mathbf{y}_i\|^2}\mathbf{y}_i, \quad k = 2, \cdots, m,$$

$$\mathbf{z}_k = \frac{\mathbf{y}_k}{\|\mathbf{y}_k\|}, \quad k = 1, \cdots, m.$$

It may be easily verified that $\{\mathbf{z}_1, \cdots, \mathbf{z}_m\}$ is an orthonormal basis of $\mathcal{V}_n$. The stages in this process for a basis $\{\mathbf{v}_1, \mathbf{v}_2, \mathbf{v}_3\}$ are shown in Figure 1.2.4.

Example 1.2.4.   We use Result 1.2.4 to find an orthonormal basis starting from the basis vectors $\mathbf{v}_1 = (1, -1, 1)'$, $\mathbf{v}_2 = (-2, 3, -1)'$, and $\mathbf{v}_3 = (1, 2, -4)'$. Let $\mathbf{y}_1 = \mathbf{v}_1$. We compute $\mathbf{y}_1'\mathbf{v}_2 = -6$, and $\mathbf{y}_1'\mathbf{y}_1 = 3$, so that $\mathbf{y}_2 = (0, 1, 1)'$. Next, $\mathbf{y}_1'\mathbf{v}_3 = -5$, $\mathbf{y}_2'\mathbf{v}_3 = -2$, and $\mathbf{y}_2'\mathbf{y}_2 = 2$, so that $\mathbf{y}_3 = (8/3, 4/3, -4/3)'$. It is easily verified that $\{\mathbf{y}_1, \mathbf{y}_2, \mathbf{y}_3\}$ is an orthogonal basis and also that $\mathbf{z}_1 = (1/\sqrt{3}, -1/\sqrt{3}, 1/\sqrt{3})'$, $\mathbf{z}_2 = (0, 1/\sqrt{2}, 1/\sqrt{2})'$, and $\mathbf{z}_3 = (2/\sqrt{6}, 1/\sqrt{6}, -1/\sqrt{6})'$ form a set of orthonormal basis vectors.   □

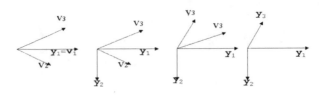

Figure 1.2.4. Gram-Schmidt orthogonalization.

We next describe some elementary properties of matrices and provide illustrations. More detailed properties of special matrices that are relevant to linear model theory are given in Chapter 2.

Definition 1.2.11. Matrix addition and subtraction.   For arbitrary $m \times n$ matrices $\mathbf{A}$ and $\mathbf{B}$, each of the same dimension, $\mathbf{C} = \mathbf{A} \pm \mathbf{B}$ is an $m \times n$ matrix whose (i, j)th element is $c_{ij} = a_{ij} \pm b_{ij}$. For example,

$$\begin{pmatrix} -5 & 4 & 1 \\ -3 & 2 & 6 \end{pmatrix} + \begin{pmatrix} 7 & -9 & 10 \\ 2 & 6 & -1 \end{pmatrix} = \begin{pmatrix} 2 & -5 & 11 \\ -1 & 8 & 5 \end{pmatrix}.$$

Definition 1.2.12. Multiplication of a matrix by a scalar.   For an arbitrary $m \times n$ matrix $\mathbf{A}$, and an arbitrary real scalar c, $\mathbf{B} = c\mathbf{A} = \mathbf{A}c$ is an $m \times n$ matrix whose (i, j)th element is $b_{ij} = ca_{ij}$. For example,

$$5\begin{pmatrix} -5 & 4 & 1 \\ -3 & 2 & 6 \end{pmatrix} = \begin{pmatrix} -25 & 20 & 5 \\ -15 & 10 & 30 \end{pmatrix}.$$

When $c = -1$, we denote $(-1)\mathbf{A}$ as $-\mathbf{A}$, the negative of the matrix $\mathbf{A}$.

Result 1.2.5. Laws of addition and scalar multiplication. Let $\mathbf{A}, \mathbf{B}, \mathbf{C}$ be any $m \times n$ matrices and let a, b, c be any scalars. The following results hold:

1. $(\mathbf{A} + \mathbf{B}) + \mathbf{C} = \mathbf{A} + (\mathbf{B} + \mathbf{C})$ 6. $(a + b)\mathbf{C} = a\mathbf{C} + b\mathbf{C}$
2. $\mathbf{A} + \mathbf{B} = \mathbf{B} + \mathbf{A}$ 7. $(ab)\mathbf{C} = a(b\mathbf{C}) = b(a\mathbf{C})$
3. $\mathbf{A} + (-\mathbf{A}) = (-\mathbf{A}) + \mathbf{A} = 0$ 8. $0\mathbf{A} = 0$
4. $\mathbf{A} + 0 = 0 + \mathbf{A} = \mathbf{A}$ 9. $1\mathbf{A} = \mathbf{A}$.
5. $c(\mathbf{A} + \mathbf{B}) = c\mathbf{A} + c\mathbf{B}$

Definition 1.2.13. Matrix multiplication. For arbitrary matrices $\mathbf{A}$ and $\mathbf{B}$ of respective dimensions $m \times n$ and $n \times p$, $\mathbf{C} = \mathbf{AB}$ is an $m \times p$ matrix whose (i, j)th element is $c_{ij} = \sum_{l=1}^{n} a_{il}b_{lj}$. The product $\mathbf{AB}$ is undefined when the column dimension of $\mathbf{A}$ is not equal to the row dimension of $\mathbf{B}$. For example,

$$\begin{pmatrix} 5 & 4 & 1 \\ -3 & 2 & 6 \end{pmatrix} \begin{pmatrix} 7 \\ -3 \\ 2 \end{pmatrix} = \begin{pmatrix} 25 \\ -15 \end{pmatrix}.$$

In referring to the matrix product $\mathbf{AB}$, we say that $\mathbf{B}$ is pre-multiplied by $\mathbf{A}$, and $\mathbf{A}$ is post-multiplied by $\mathbf{B}$. Provided all the matrices are conformal under multiplication, the following properties hold.

Result 1.2.6. Laws of matrix multiplication. Let a be a scalar, let $\mathbf{A}$ be an $m \times n$ matrix and let matrices $\mathbf{B}$ and $\mathbf{C}$ have appropriate dimensions so that the operations below are defined. Then,

1. $(\mathbf{AB})\mathbf{C} = \mathbf{A}(\mathbf{BC})$ 4. $a(\mathbf{BC}) = (a\mathbf{B})\mathbf{C} = \mathbf{B}(a\mathbf{C})$
2. $\mathbf{A}(\mathbf{B} + \mathbf{C}) = \mathbf{AB} + \mathbf{AC}$ 5. $\mathbf{I}_m\mathbf{A} = \mathbf{A}\mathbf{I}_n = \mathbf{A}$
3. $(\mathbf{A} + \mathbf{B})\mathbf{C} = \mathbf{AC} + \mathbf{BC}$ 6. $0\mathbf{A} = 0$ and $\mathbf{A}0 = 0$.

In general, matrix multiplication is not commutative, i.e., $\mathbf{AB}$ is not necessarily equal to $\mathbf{BA}$. Note that depending on the row and column dimensions of $\mathbf{A}$ and $\mathbf{B}$, it is possible that (i) only $\mathbf{AB}$ is defined and $\mathbf{BA}$ is not, or (ii) both $\mathbf{AB}$ and $\mathbf{BA}$ are defined, but do not have the same dimensions, or (iii) $\mathbf{AB}$ and $\mathbf{BA}$ are defined and have the same dimensions, but $\mathbf{AB} \neq \mathbf{BA}$. Two $n \times n$ matrices $\mathbf{A}$ and $\mathbf{B}$ are said to commute under multiplication if $\mathbf{AB} = \mathbf{BA}$. A collection of $n \times n$ matrices $\mathbf{A}_1, \cdots, \mathbf{A}_k$ is said to be pairwise commutative if $\mathbf{A}_i\mathbf{A}_j = \mathbf{A}_j\mathbf{A}_i$ for $j > i$, $i, j = 1, \cdots, k$. Note that the product $\mathbf{A}^k = \mathbf{A} \cdots \mathbf{A}$ (k times) is defined only if $\mathbf{A}$ is a square matrix. It is easy to verify that $\mathbf{J}_{mn}\mathbf{J}_{np} = n\mathbf{J}_{mp}$.

Example 1.2.5. We show that the product of two upper triangular matrices is upper triangular. Let

$$\mathbf{A} = \begin{pmatrix} a_{11} & a_{12} & a_{13} \\ 0 & a_{22} & a_{23} \\ 0 & 0 & a_{33} \end{pmatrix} \text{ and } \mathbf{B} = \begin{pmatrix} b_{11} & b_{12} & b_{13} \\ 0 & b_{22} & b_{23} \\ 0 & 0 & b_{33} \end{pmatrix}$$

be 3×3 upper triangular matrices. By Definition 1.2.13, their product is

$$\mathbf{AB} = \begin{pmatrix} a_{11}b_{11} & a_{11}b_{12} + a_{12}b_{22} & a_{11}b_{13} + a_{12}b_{23} + a_{13}b_{33} \\ 0 & a_{22}b_{22} & a_{22}b_{23} + a_{23}b_{33} \\ 0 & 0 & a_{33}b_{33} \end{pmatrix},$$

which is upper-triangular.   □

Definition 1.2.14. Matrix transpose. The transpose of an $m \times n$ matrix $\mathbf{A}$ is an $n \times m$ matrix whose columns are the rows of $\mathbf{A}$ in the same order. The transpose of $\mathbf{A}$ is denoted by $\mathbf{A}'$. For example,

$$\mathbf{A} = \begin{pmatrix} 2 & 1 & 6 \\ 4 & 3 & 5 \end{pmatrix}, \quad \mathbf{A}' = \begin{pmatrix} 2 & 4 \\ 1 & 3 \\ 6 & 5 \end{pmatrix}, \quad \mathbf{B} = \begin{pmatrix} 6 & 7 \\ 8 & 9 \end{pmatrix}, \quad \mathbf{B}' = \begin{pmatrix} 6 & 8 \\ 7 & 9 \end{pmatrix}.$$

As we saw earlier, the transpose of an n-dimensional column vector with components $a_1, \cdots, a_n$ is the row vector $(a_1, \cdots, a_n)$. It is often convenient to write a column vector in this transposed form. The transpose of an upper (lower) triangular matrix is a lower (upper) triangular matrix. It may be easily verified that the $n \times n$ unit matrix may be written as $\mathbf{J}_n = \mathbf{1}_n \mathbf{1}_n'$. For any matrix $\mathbf{A}$, each diagonal element of $\mathbf{A}' \mathbf{A}$ is nonnegative.

Result 1.2.7. Laws of transposition. Let $\mathbf{A}$ and $\mathbf{B}$ conform under addition, and let $\mathbf{A}$ and $\mathbf{C}$ conform under multiplication. Let a, b and c denote scalars and let $k \geq 2$ denote a positive integer. Then,

1. $(\mathbf{A}')' = \mathbf{A}$ 4. $\mathbf{A}' = \mathbf{B}'$ if and only if $\mathbf{A} = \mathbf{B}$
2. $(a\mathbf{A} + b\mathbf{B})' = a\mathbf{A}' + b\mathbf{B}'$ 5. $(\mathbf{A}\mathbf{C})' = \mathbf{C}'\mathbf{A}'$
3. $(c\mathbf{A})' = c\mathbf{A}'$ 6. $(\mathbf{A}_1 \cdots \mathbf{A}_k)' = \mathbf{A}_k' \cdots \mathbf{A}_1'.$

Definition 1.2.15. Symmetric matrix. A matrix $\mathbf{A}$ is said to be symmetric if $\mathbf{A}' = \mathbf{A}$. For example,

$$\mathbf{A} = \begin{pmatrix} 1 & 2 & -3 \\ 2 & 4 & 5 \\ -3 & 5 & 9 \end{pmatrix}$$

is a symmetric matrix. Note that a symmetric matrix is always a square matrix. Any diagonal matrix, written as $\mathbf{D} = \text{diag}(d_1, \cdots, d_n)$, is symmetric. Other examples of symmetric matrices include the variance-covariance matrix and the correlation matrix of any random vector, the identity matrix $\mathbf{I}_n$ and the unit matrix $\mathbf{J}_n$. A matrix $\mathbf{A}$ is said to be skew-symmetric if $\mathbf{A}' = -\mathbf{A}$.

Definition 1.2.16. Trace of a matrix. Let $\mathbf{A}$ be an $n \times n$ matrix. The trace of $\mathbf{A}$ is a scalar given by the sum of the diagonal elements of $\mathbf{A}$, i.e., $tr(\mathbf{A}) = \sum_{i=1}^{n} a_{ii}$. For example, if

$$\mathbf{A} = \begin{pmatrix} 2 & -4 & 5 \\ 6 & -7 & 0 \\ 3 & 9 & 7 \end{pmatrix},$$

then $tr(\mathbf{A}) = 2 - 7 + 7 = 2$.

Result 1.2.8. Properties of trace. Provided the matrices are conformable, and given scalars a and b,

1. $tr(\mathbf{I}_n) = n$

2. $tr(a\mathbf{A} \pm b\mathbf{B}) = a tr(\mathbf{A}) \pm b tr(\mathbf{B})$

3. $tr(\mathbf{AB}) = tr(\mathbf{BA})$

4. $tr(\mathbf{ABC}) = tr(\mathbf{CAB}) = tr(\mathbf{BCA})$

5. $tr(\mathbf{A}) = 0$ if $\mathbf{A} = \mathbf{0}$

6. $tr(\mathbf{A}') = tr(\mathbf{A})$

7. $tr(\mathbf{AA}') = tr(\mathbf{A}'\mathbf{A}) = \displaystyle\sum_{i,j=1}^{n} a_{ij}^2$

8. $tr(\mathbf{aa}') = \mathbf{a}'\mathbf{a} = \|\mathbf{a}\|^2 = \displaystyle\sum_{i=1}^{n} a_i^2$.

The trace operation in property 4 is valid under cyclic permutations only.

Definition 1.2.17. Determinant of a matrix. Let $\mathbf{A}$ be an $n \times n$ matrix. The determinant of $\mathbf{A}$ is a scalar given by

$$|\mathbf{A}| = \sum_{j=1}^{n} a_{ij}(-1)^{i+j}|\mathbf{M}_{ij}|, \text{ for any fixed } i, \text{ or}$$

$$|\mathbf{A}| = \sum_{i=1}^{n} a_{ij}(-1)^{i+j}|\mathbf{M}_{ij}|, \text{ for any fixed } j.$$

We call $|\mathbf{M}_{ij}|$ the *minor* corresponding to a_{ij}. The minor $|\mathbf{M}_{ij}|$ is the determinant of the $(n-1) \times (n-1)$ submatrix of $\mathbf{A}$ after deleting the ith row and the jth column from $\mathbf{A}$. The *cofactor* of a_{ij} is the signed minor, i.e., $F_{ij} = (-1)^{i+j}|\mathbf{M}_{ij}|$. We consider two special cases:

1. Suppose $n = 2$. Then $|\mathbf{A}| = a_{11}a_{22} - a_{12}a_{21}$.

2. Suppose $n = 3$. Fix $i = 1$ (row 1). Then

$$F_{11} = (-1)^{1+1}\begin{vmatrix} a_{22} & a_{23} \\ a_{32} & a_{33} \end{vmatrix}; \quad F_{12} = (-1)^{1+2}\begin{vmatrix} a_{21} & a_{23} \\ a_{31} & a_{33} \end{vmatrix};$$

$$F_{13} = (-1)^{1+3}\begin{vmatrix} a_{21} & a_{22} \\ a_{31} & a_{32} \end{vmatrix}$$

and

$$|\mathbf{A}| = a_{11}F_{11} + a_{12}F_{12} + a_{13}F_{13}.$$

For example, if

$$\mathbf{A} = \begin{pmatrix} 2 & -4 & 5 \\ 6 & -7 & 0 \\ 3 & 9 & 7 \end{pmatrix}$$

then,

$$|\mathbf{A}| = 2(-1)^{1+1}\begin{vmatrix} -7 & 0 \\ 9 & 7 \end{vmatrix} - 4(-1)^{1+2}\begin{vmatrix} 6 & 0 \\ 3 & 7 \end{vmatrix} + 5(-1)^{1+3}\begin{vmatrix} 6 & -7 \\ 3 & 9 \end{vmatrix}$$

$$= 2(-49) + 4(42) + 5(75) = 445.$$

Result 1.2.9. Properties of determinants. Let $\mathbf{A}$ be an $n \times n$ matrix and k be any integer. Then

1. $|\mathbf{A}| = |\mathbf{A}'|$.

2. $|c\mathbf{A}| = c^n|\mathbf{A}|$.

3. $|\mathbf{AB}| = |\mathbf{A}||\mathbf{B}|$; $|\mathbf{A}_1 \cdots \mathbf{A}_k| = \prod_{i=1}^{k}|\mathbf{A}_i|$; $|\mathbf{A}^2| = |\mathbf{A}|^2$; and $|\mathbf{A}^k| = |\mathbf{A}|^k$.

4. If $\mathbf{A}$ is a diagonal matrix or an upper (or lower) triangular matrix, the determinant of $\mathbf{A}$ is equal to the product of its diagonal elements, i.e.,

$$|\mathbf{A}| = \prod_{i=1}^{n} a_{ii}.$$

5. If two rows (or columns) of a matrix $\mathbf{A}$ are equal, then $|\mathbf{A}| = 0$.

6. If $\mathbf{A}$ has a row (or column) of zeroes, then $|\mathbf{A}| = 0$.

7. If $\mathbf{A}$ has rows (or columns) that are multiples of each other, then $|\mathbf{A}| = 0$.

8. If a row (or column) of $\mathbf{A}$ is the sum of multiples of two other rows (or columns), then $|\mathbf{A}| = 0$.

9. Let $\mathbf{B}$ be obtained from $\mathbf{A}$ by multiplying one of its rows (or columns) by a nonzero constant c. Then, $|\mathbf{B}| = c|\mathbf{A}|$.

10. Let $\mathbf{B}$ be obtained from $\mathbf{A}$ by interchanging any two rows (or columns). Then, $|\mathbf{B}| = -|\mathbf{A}|$.

11. Let $\mathbf{B}$ be obtained from $\mathbf{A}$ by adding a multiple of one row (or column) to another row (or column). Then, $|\mathbf{B}| = |\mathbf{A}|$.

12. If $\mathbf{A}$ is an $m \times n$ matrix and $\mathbf{B}$ is an $n \times m$ matrix, then $|\mathbf{I}_m + \mathbf{AB}| = |\mathbf{I}_n + \mathbf{BA}|$.

Example 1.2.6. Let $\mathbf{A}$ be a $k \times k$ nonsingular matrix, and let $\mathbf{B}$ and $\mathbf{C}$ be any $k \times n$ and $n \times k$ matrices respectively. Since we can write $\mathbf{A} + \mathbf{BC} = \mathbf{A}(\mathbf{I}_k + \mathbf{A}^{-1}\mathbf{BC})$, we see from property 3 of Result 1.2.9 that $|\mathbf{A} + \mathbf{BC}| = |\mathbf{A}||\mathbf{I}_k + \mathbf{A}^{-1}\mathbf{BC}|$. $\square$

Example 1.2.7. Vandermonde matrix.   An $n \times n$ matrix $\mathbf{A}$ is a Vandermonde matrix if there are scalars $a_1, \cdots, a_n$, such that

$$\mathbf{A} = \begin{pmatrix} 1 & 1 & 1 & \cdots & 1 \\ a_1 & a_2 & a_3 & \cdots & a_n \\ a_1^2 & a_2^2 & a_3^2 & \cdots & a_n^2 \\ \vdots & \vdots & \vdots & \ddots & \vdots \\ a_1^{n-1} & a_2^{n-1} & a_3^{n-1} & \cdots & a_n^{n-1} \end{pmatrix}.$$

The determinant of $\mathbf{A}$ has a simple form:

$$
\begin{aligned}
D \; = \; |\mathbf{A}| &= \prod_{\substack{i,j=1 \\ i<j}}^{n} (a_j - a_i) \\
&= (a_n - a_{n-1})(a_n - a_{n-2}) \cdots (a_n - a_2)(a_n - a_1) \\
&\times \; (a_{n-1} - a_{n-2})(a_{n-1} - a_{n-3}) \cdots (a_{n-1} - a_1) \\
&\times \; \cdots \times (a_2 - a_1).
\end{aligned}
$$

It is easily seen that $|\mathbf{A}| \neq 0$ if and only if $a_i \neq a_j$ for $i < j = 1, \cdots, n$, i.e., $a_1, \cdots, a_n$ are distinct. An example of a Vandermonde matrix is

$$
\mathbf{A} = \begin{pmatrix} 1 & 1 & 1 \\ 1 & -1 & 2 \\ 1 & 1 & 4 \end{pmatrix},
$$

with $a_1 = 1$, $a_2 = -1$, $a_3 = 2$, and $|\mathbf{A}| = -6$. $\quad\square$

Example 1.2.8. Intra-class correlation matrix. We define an $n \times n$ intra-class correlation matrix, which is also called an equicorrelation matrix, by

$$
\mathbf{C} = d \begin{pmatrix} 1 & \rho & \cdots & \rho \\ \rho & 1 & \cdots & \rho \\ \vdots & \vdots & \ddots & \vdots \\ \rho & \rho & \cdots & 1 \end{pmatrix} = d[(1 - \rho)\mathbf{I} + \rho \mathbf{J}],
$$

where $-1 < \rho < 1$ and $d > 0$ is a constant. In an intra-class correlation matrix, all the diagonal elements have the same positive value, and all the off-diagonal elements have the same value which lies between -1 and 1. The determinant of $\mathbf{C}$ is easily computed by seeing that

$$
\begin{aligned}
\begin{vmatrix} 1 & \rho & \cdots & \rho \\ \rho & 1 & \cdots & \rho \\ \vdots & \vdots & \ddots & \vdots \\ \rho & \rho & \cdots & 1 \end{vmatrix}
&= \begin{vmatrix} 1 + (n-1)\rho & \rho & \cdots & \rho \\ 1 + (n-1)\rho & 1 & \cdots & \rho \\ \vdots & & \ddots & \vdots \\ 1 + (n-1)\rho & \rho & \cdots & 1 \end{vmatrix} \\
&= [1 + (n-1)\rho] \begin{vmatrix} 1 & \rho & \cdots & \rho \\ 1 & 1 & \cdots & \rho \\ \vdots & \vdots & \ddots & \vdots \\ 1 & \rho & \cdots & 1 \end{vmatrix} \\
&= [1 + (n-1)\rho] \begin{vmatrix} 1 & \rho & \cdots & \rho \\ 0 & 1 - \rho & \cdots & 0 \\ \vdots & \vdots & \ddots & \vdots \\ 0 & 0 & \cdots & 1 - \rho \end{vmatrix} \\
&= [1 + (n-1)\rho](1 - \rho)^{n-1}
\end{aligned}
$$

and $[1 + (n-1)\rho](1-\rho)^{n-1} \geq 0$ implies that $-\frac{1}{n-1} \leq \rho \leq 1$. So $|\mathbf{C}| = d^n[1 + (n-1)\rho](1-\rho)^{n-1}$. □

Definition 1.2.18. Nonsingular and singular matrices. If $|\mathbf{A}| \neq 0$, then $\mathbf{A}$ is said to be a nonsingular matrix. Otherwise, $\mathbf{A}$ is singular. For example, $\mathbf{A}$ is a nonsingular matrix and $\mathbf{B}$ is a singular matrix, where

$$\mathbf{A} = \begin{pmatrix} 1 & 6 \\ 0 & 3 \end{pmatrix} \text{ and } \mathbf{B} = \begin{pmatrix} 1 & 6 \\ 1/2 & 3 \end{pmatrix}.$$

Definition 1.2.19. Inverse of a matrix. Let $\mathbf{A}$ be an $n \times n$ matrix. If there exists an $n \times n$ matrix $\mathbf{B}$ such that $\mathbf{AB} = \mathbf{I}_n$ (and $\mathbf{BA} = \mathbf{I}_n$), then $\mathbf{B}$ is called the (regular) inverse of $\mathbf{A}$, and is denoted by $\mathbf{A}^{-1}$. A matrix $\mathbf{A}$ is invertible if and only if $|\mathbf{A}| \neq 0$.

Example 1.2.9. We compute the inverse of a matrix $\mathbf{A}$ using the formula

$$\mathbf{A}^{-1} = \tfrac{1}{|\mathbf{A}|}\mathrm{Adj}(\mathbf{A}),$$

where $\mathrm{Adj}(\mathbf{A})$ denotes the adjoint of $\mathbf{A}$, and is defined to be the transpose of the matrix of cofactors of $\mathbf{A}$. Suppose the matrix $\mathbf{A}$, the matrix of cofactors $\mathbf{F}$ and the matrix $\mathrm{Adj}(\mathbf{A})$ are given by

$$\mathbf{A} = \begin{pmatrix} -1 & 2 & 2 \\ 4 & 3 & -2 \\ -5 & 0 & 3 \end{pmatrix}, \quad \mathbf{F} = \begin{pmatrix} 9 & -2 & 15 \\ -6 & 7 & -10 \\ -10 & 6 & -11 \end{pmatrix} \text{ and}$$

$$\mathrm{Adj}(\mathbf{A}) = \begin{pmatrix} 9 & -6 & -10 \\ -2 & 7 & 6 \\ 15 & -10 & -11 \end{pmatrix},$$

then, $|\mathbf{A}| = 17$, and

$$\mathbf{A}^{-1} = \tfrac{1}{|\mathbf{A}|}\mathrm{Adj}(\mathbf{A}) = \begin{pmatrix} 9/17 & -6/17 & -10/17 \\ -2/17 & 7/17 & 6/17 \\ 15/17 & -10/17 & -11/17 \end{pmatrix}$$

is the inverse of $\mathbf{A}$. □

Definition 1.2.20. Reduced row echelon form. An $m \times n$ matrix $\mathbf{A}$ is said to be in **reduced row echelon form** (RREF) if the following conditions are met:

C1. all zero rows are at the bottom of the matrix,

C2. the leading entry of each nonzero row after the first occurs to the right of the leading entry of the previous row,

C3. the leading entry in any nonzero row is 1, and

C4. all entries in the column above and below a leading 1 are zero.

If only C1 and C2 hold, the matrix has *row echelon form*. For example, among the following matrices,

$$\mathbf{A} = \begin{pmatrix} 1 & 0 & 2 & 3 & 0 \\ 0 & 1 & 4 & 5 & 0 \\ 0 & 0 & 0 & 0 & 0 \\ 0 & 0 & 0 & 0 & 0 \end{pmatrix}, \quad \mathbf{B} = \begin{pmatrix} 0 & 1 & 2 & 0 & 3 \\ 0 & 0 & 4 & 0 & 5 \\ 0 & 0 & 0 & 1 & 0 \\ 0 & 0 & 0 & 0 & 0 \end{pmatrix},$$

$$\mathbf{C} = \begin{pmatrix} 0 & 1 & 2 & 3 & 4 \\ 0 & 0 & 0 & 1 & 5 \\ 0 & 0 & 0 & 0 & 0 \end{pmatrix}, \quad \mathbf{D} = \begin{pmatrix} 0 & 0 & 0 & 0 & 0 \\ 0 & 1 & 2 & 0 & 4 \\ 0 & 0 & 0 & 0 & 0 \\ 0 & 0 & 0 & 1 & 5 \\ 0 & 0 & 0 & 0 & 0 \end{pmatrix}, \quad \text{and}$$

$$\mathbf{E} = \begin{pmatrix} 0 & 0 & 0 & 1 & 5 \\ 0 & 1 & 2 & 0 & 4 \end{pmatrix},$$

the matrix $\mathbf{A}$ is in RREF, whereas none of the other matrices is in RREF. In matrix $\mathbf{B}$, row 2 violates C3; matrix $\mathbf{C}$ violates C4, matrix $\mathbf{D}$ violates C1, while matrix $\mathbf{E}$ violates C2.

To verify invertibility and find the inverse (if it exists) of a square matrix $\mathbf{A}$,

(a) Perform elementary row operations on the augmented matrix $(\mathbf{A} \quad \mathbf{I})$ until $\mathbf{A}$ is in RREF.

(b) If $\text{RREF}(\mathbf{A}) \neq \mathbf{I}$, then $\mathbf{A}$ is not invertible.

(c) If $\text{RREF}(\mathbf{A}) = \mathbf{I}$, then the row operations that transformed $\mathbf{A}$ into $\text{RREF}(\mathbf{A})$ will have changed $\mathbf{I}$ into $\mathbf{A}^{-1}$.

Example 1.2.10. We describe an algorithm used to test whether an $n \times n$ matrix $\mathbf{A}$ is invertible, and if it is, to compute its inverse. The first step is to express the matrix $(\mathbf{A} : \mathbf{I})$ in reduced row echelon form, which we denote by $\text{RREF}(\mathbf{A} : \mathbf{I}) = (\mathbf{B} : \mathbf{C})$, say. If $\mathbf{B}$ has a row of zeroes, the matrix $\mathbf{A}$ is singular and is not invertible. Otherwise, the reduced matrix is now in the form $(\mathbf{I} : \mathbf{A}^{-1})$. We use this approach to find the inverse, if it exists, of the matrix

$$\mathbf{A} = \begin{pmatrix} 1 & 0 & -1 \\ 3 & 4 & -2 \\ 3 & 5 & -2 \end{pmatrix}.$$

We row reduce $(\mathbf{A} : \mathbf{I})$:

$$\begin{pmatrix} 1 & 0 & -1 & : & 1 & 0 & 0 \\ 3 & 4 & -2 & : & 0 & 1 & 0 \\ 3 & 5 & -2 & : & 0 & 0 & 1 \end{pmatrix} \sim \begin{pmatrix} 1 & 0 & -1 & : & 1 & 0 & 0 \\ 0 & 4 & 1 & : & -3 & 1 & 0 \\ 0 & 5 & 1 & : & -3 & 0 & 1 \end{pmatrix},$$

$$\begin{pmatrix} 1 & 0 & -1 & : & 1 & 0 & 0 \\ 0 & 4 & 1 & : & -3 & 1 & 0 \\ 0 & 0 & -1/4 & : & 3/4 & -5/4 & 1 \end{pmatrix} \sim \begin{pmatrix} 1 & 0 & -1 & : & 1 & 0 & 0 \\ 0 & 4 & 1 & : & -3 & 1 & 0 \\ 0 & 0 & 1 & : & -3 & 5 & -4 \end{pmatrix},$$

$$\begin{pmatrix} 1 & 0 & 0 & : & -2 & 5 & -4 \\ 0 & 4 & 0 & : & 0 & -4 & 4 \\ 0 & 0 & 1 & : & -3 & 5 & -4 \end{pmatrix} \sim \begin{pmatrix} 1 & 0 & 0 & : & -2 & 5 & -4 \\ 0 & 1 & 0 & : & 0 & -1 & 1 \\ 0 & 0 & 1 & : & -3 & 5 & -4 \end{pmatrix},$$

so that

$$\mathbf{A}^{-1} = \begin{pmatrix} -2 & 5 & -4 \\ 0 & -1 & 1 \\ -3 & 5 & -4 \end{pmatrix}. \quad \square$$

Result 1.2.10. Properties of inverse.   Provided all the inverses exist,

1. $\mathbf{A}^{-1}$ is unique.

2. $(\mathbf{AB})^{-1} = \mathbf{B}^{-1}\mathbf{A}^{-1}$; $(\mathbf{A}_1 \cdots \mathbf{A}_k)^1 = \mathbf{A}_k^{-1} \cdots \mathbf{A}_1^{-1}$.

3. $(c\mathbf{A})^{-1} = (\mathbf{A}c)^{-1} = \frac{1}{c}\mathbf{A}^{-1}$.

4. If $|\mathbf{A}| \neq 0$, then $\mathbf{A}'$ and $\mathbf{A}^{-1}$ are nonsingular matrices and $(\mathbf{A}')^{-1} = (\mathbf{A}^{-1})'$.

5. $(\mathbf{A} + \mathbf{BCD})^{-1} = \mathbf{A}^{-1} - \mathbf{A}^{-1}\mathbf{B}(\mathbf{C}^{-1}+\mathbf{DA}^{-1}\mathbf{B})^{-1}\mathbf{DA}^{-1}$, where $\mathbf{A}, \mathbf{B}, \mathbf{C}$, and $\mathbf{D}$ are respectively $m \times m$, $m \times n$, $n \times n$ and $n \times m$ matrices [Sherman-Morrison-Woodbury theorem].

6. Provided $1 \pm \mathbf{b}'\mathbf{A}^{-1}\mathbf{a} \neq 0$, we have $(\mathbf{A} \pm \mathbf{ab}')^{-1} = \mathbf{A}^{-1} \mp \frac{(\mathbf{A}^{-1}\mathbf{a})(\mathbf{b}'\mathbf{A}^{-1})}{1\pm \mathbf{b}'\mathbf{A}^{-1}\mathbf{a}}$.

7. $|\mathbf{A}^{-1}| = |\mathbf{A}|^{-1}$, i.e., the determinant of the inverse of $\mathbf{A}$ is equal to the reciprocal of $|\mathbf{A}|$.

8. $(\mathbf{I} + a\mathbf{A})^{-1} = \mathbf{I} + \sum_{i=1}^{\infty}(-1)^i a^i \mathbf{A}^i$.

Each of these properties is obtained by verifying that the product of the given matrix and its inverse is the identity matrix (see Exercise 1.21). The inverse in property 5 does not exist in some cases. For example, when we set $\mathbf{A} = \mathbf{I}_n$, $\mathbf{B} = \mathbf{X}$, which is an $n \times k$ matrix of rank k, $\mathbf{D} = \mathbf{X}'$, and $\mathbf{C} = -(\mathbf{X}'\mathbf{X})^{-1}$, we see that $(\mathbf{A} + \mathbf{BCD}) = (\mathbf{I}_n - \mathbf{P})$, where $\mathbf{P} = \mathbf{X}(\mathbf{X}'\mathbf{X})^{-1}\mathbf{X}'$, which is a singular matrix of rank $(n-k)$. Hence, its (regular) inverse does not exist. The matrix $\mathbf{P}$ is the familiar projection matrix, or hat matrix of linear model theory. One may however, interpret this property in terms of a generalized inverse of a matrix, which always exists (see Chapter 3).

Example 1.2.11. Inverse of an intra-class correlation matrix.   We continue with Example 1.2.8. The cofactor of any diagonal element is based on the determinant of an $(n-1) \times (n-1)$ submatrix:

$$d^{n-1}\begin{vmatrix} 1 & \rho & \cdots & \rho \\ \rho & 1 & \cdots & \rho \\ \vdots & \vdots & \ddots & \vdots \\ \rho & \rho & \cdots & 1 \end{vmatrix} = d^{n-1}[1 + (n-2)\rho](1-\rho)^{n-2},$$

while the cofactor of any off-diagonal element is

$$-d^{n-1}\begin{vmatrix} \rho & \rho & \cdots & \rho \\ \rho & 1 & \cdots & \rho \\ \vdots & \vdots & \ddots & \vdots \\ \rho & \rho & \cdots & 1 \end{vmatrix} = -d^{n-1}\rho(1-\rho)^{n-2}.$$

Letting $D = d(1-\rho)[1 + (n-1)\rho]$,

$$\mathbf{A}^{-1} = \frac{1}{D}\begin{pmatrix} 1+(n-2)\rho & -\rho & \cdots & -\rho \\ -\rho & 1+(n-2)\rho & \cdots & -\rho \\ \vdots & \vdots & \ddots & \vdots \\ -\rho & -\rho & \cdots & 1+(n-2)\rho \end{pmatrix}$$

$$= \frac{1}{D}\left([1+(n-1)\rho]\mathbf{I} - \rho\mathbf{J}\right)$$

$$= \frac{1}{d(1-\rho)}\left(\mathbf{I} - \frac{\rho}{1+(n-1)\rho}\mathbf{J}\right).$$

An alternate way to obtain $\mathbf{C}^{-1}$ is using property 6 of Result 1.2.10. Suppose first that $\rho > 0$, and $\mathbf{C} = d[(1-\rho)\mathbf{I} + \rho\mathbf{J}]$, so that $\mathbf{C}^{-1} = d^{-1}[(1-\rho)\mathbf{I} + \rho\mathbf{J}]^{-1}$. In property 6, set $\mathbf{A} = (1-\rho)\mathbf{I}$, and $\mathbf{a} = \mathbf{b} = \sqrt{\rho}\mathbf{1}_n$; then,

$$\mathbf{C}^{-1} = d^{-1}[\frac{1}{1-\rho}\mathbf{I} - \frac{(1-\rho)^{-2}\rho}{1+(1-\rho)^{-1}n\rho}\mathbf{J}]$$

$$= \frac{1}{d(1-\rho)}[\mathbf{I} - \frac{\rho}{1+(n-1)\rho}\mathbf{J}].$$

If $\rho < 0$, it follows that since

$$\mathbf{C} = d[(1-\rho)\mathbf{I} - (\sqrt{-\rho}\mathbf{1}_n)(\sqrt{-\rho}\mathbf{1}_n)'],$$

we have

$$\mathbf{C}^{-1} = \frac{1}{d}[\frac{1}{1-\rho}\mathbf{I} - \frac{(1-\rho)^{-2}\rho}{1+(1-\rho)^{-1}n\rho}\mathbf{J}]$$

$$= \frac{1}{d(1-\rho)}[I - \frac{\rho}{1+(n-1)\rho}\mathbf{J}]. \quad \square$$

Example 1.2.12. Toeplitz matrix.   Consider the $n \times n$ Toeplitz matrix **A** which has the form

$$\mathbf{A} = \begin{pmatrix} 1 & \rho & \rho^2 & \cdots & \rho^{n-1} \\ \rho & 1 & \rho & \cdots & \rho^{n-2} \\ \vdots & \vdots & \vdots & \ddots & \vdots \\ \rho^{n-1} & \rho^{n-2} & \rho^{n-3} & \cdots & 1 \end{pmatrix}.$$

In general, the elements of a Toeplitz matrix satisfy the condition that all the elements on the jth subdiagonal and the jth superdiagonal coincide, for $j \geq 1$. It is easy to verify that, for $|\rho| < 1$, the inverse of **A** is

$$\mathbf{A}^{-1} = \tfrac{1}{1-\rho^2} \begin{pmatrix} 1 & -\rho & 0 & 0 & \cdots & 0 & 0 & 0 \\ -\rho & 1+\rho^2 & -\rho & 0 & \cdots & 0 & 0 & 0 \\ \vdots & \vdots & \vdots & \ddots & \cdots & 0 & 0 & 0 \\ 0 & 0 & 0 & 0 & \cdots & -\rho & 1+\rho^2 & -\rho \\ 0 & 0 & 0 & 0 & \cdots & 0 & -\rho & 1 \end{pmatrix},$$

which has a simple form. □

Definition 1.2.21. Orthogonal matrix.   An $n \times n$ matrix $\mathbf{A}$ is orthogonal if $\mathbf{AA}' = \mathbf{A}'\mathbf{A} = \mathbf{I}_n$. For example,

$$\begin{pmatrix} \cos\theta & -\sin\theta \\ \sin\theta & \cos\theta \end{pmatrix}$$

is a 2×2 orthogonal matrix.

A direct consequence of Definition 1.2.21 is that, for an orthogonal matrix $\mathbf{A}$, $\mathbf{A}' = \mathbf{A}^{-1}$. Suppose $\mathbf{a}_i'$ denotes the ith row of $\mathbf{A}$, then, $\mathbf{AA}' = \mathbf{I}_n$ implies that $\mathbf{a}_i'\mathbf{a}_i = 1$, and $\mathbf{a}_i'\mathbf{a}_j = 0$ for $i \neq j$; so the rows of $\mathbf{A}$ have unit length and are mutually perpendicular (or orthogonal). Since $\mathbf{A}'\mathbf{A} = \mathbf{I}_n$ also, the columns of $\mathbf{A}$ have this property as well. If $\mathbf{A}$ is orthogonal, clearly, $|\mathbf{A}| = \pm 1$. It is also easy to show that the product of two orthogonal matrices $\mathbf{A}$ and $\mathbf{B}$ is itself orthogonal. Usually, orthogonal matrices are used to represent a change of basis, or rotation.

Example 1.2.13. Helmert matrix.   An $n \times n$ Helmert matrix $\mathbf{H}_n$ is an example of an orthogonal matrix and is defined by

$$\mathbf{H}_n = \begin{pmatrix} \frac{1}{\sqrt{n}}\mathbf{1}_n' \\ \mathbf{H}_0 \end{pmatrix},$$

where the ith row of the $(n-1) \times n$ matrix $\mathbf{H}_0$ is defined as follows for $i = 1, \cdots, n-1 : \left(\ \mathbf{1}_i' \ \mid \ -i \mid \ 0 \ \ \mathbf{1}_{n-i-1}' \ \right) / \sqrt{\lambda_i}$, where, $\lambda_i = i(i+1)$. For example, when $n = 4$, we have

$$\mathbf{H}_4 = \begin{pmatrix} 1/\sqrt{4} & 1/\sqrt{4} & 1/\sqrt{4} & 1/\sqrt{4} \\ 1/\sqrt{2} & -1/\sqrt{2} & 0 & 0 \\ 1/\sqrt{6} & 1/\sqrt{6} & -2/\sqrt{6} & 0 \\ 1/\sqrt{12} & 1/\sqrt{12} & 1/\sqrt{12} & -3/\sqrt{12} \end{pmatrix}. \quad □$$

Definition 1.2.22. Linear space of matrices.   A nonempty set of $n \times n$ matrices denoted by $\mathcal{V}$ is called a linear space if

1. for every matrix $\mathbf{A}$ in $\mathcal{V}$, and $\mathbf{B}$ in $\mathcal{V}$, the sum $\mathbf{A} + \mathbf{B}$ is in $\mathcal{V}$, and

2. for every matrix $\mathbf{A}$ in $\mathcal{V}$, and every scalar c, the product $c\mathbf{A}$ is in $\mathcal{V}$.

Note that if $\mathbf{A}_1, \cdots, \mathbf{A}_k$ are in $\mathcal{V}$, and $c_1, \cdots, c_k$ are scalar constants, then $c_1\mathbf{A}_1 + \cdots + c_k\mathbf{A}_k$ is in $\mathcal{V}$. Examples of linear spaces include the set of all $n \times n$ symmetric matrices, and the set $\{\mathbf{0}\}$ containing only the null matrix.

Definition 1.2.23. A subset $\mathcal{V}_1$ of a linear space $\mathcal{V}$ is said to be a subspace of $\mathcal{V}$ if it is itself a linear space. For example, $\{\mathbf{0}\}$ and $\mathcal{V}$ are both subspaces of $\mathcal{V}$, and the set $\mathcal{D}_n$ of all $n \times n$ diagonal matrices is a subspace of the set of all $n \times n$ matrices.

Definition 1.2.24. A basis for a linear space $\mathcal{V}$ is a finite set of linearly independent matrices in $\mathcal{V}$ that span $\mathcal{V}$.

Definition 1.2.25. Let $\mathcal{V}$ be a linear space of matrices and let $\mathcal{V}_1$ be a subspace of $\mathcal{V}$. A matrix $\mathbf{Y}$ in $\mathcal{V}$ which is orthogonal to every matrix in $\mathcal{V}_1$ is said to be orthogonal to $\mathcal{V}_1$ and we write $\mathbf{Y} \perp \mathcal{V}_1$.

If every matrix in a subspace $\mathcal{V}_1$ is orthogonal to every matrix in a subspace $\mathcal{V}_2$, then we say $\mathcal{V}_1$ is orthogonal to $\mathcal{V}_2$ and write $\mathcal{V}_1 \perp \mathcal{V}_2$.

Definition 1.2.26. Let $\mathcal{V}$ be a linear space of matrices, let $\mathcal{V}_1$ and $\mathcal{V}_2$ be subspaces of $\mathcal{V}$, let $\mathbf{Y}$ be a matrix in $\mathcal{V}$, let $\{\mathbf{X}_1, \cdots, \mathbf{X}_s\}$ span $\mathcal{V}_1$, and $\{\mathbf{Z}_1, \cdots, \mathbf{Z}_t\}$ span $\mathcal{V}_2$. We say that $\mathbf{Y} \perp \mathcal{V}_1$ if and only if $\mathbf{Y} \bullet \mathbf{X}_i = \mathbf{0}$, i.e., $\mathbf{Y}$ is orthogonal to $\mathbf{X}_i$ for $i = 1, \cdots, s$. We say that $\mathcal{V}_1 \perp \mathcal{V}_2$ if and only if $\mathbf{X}_i \bullet \mathbf{Z}_j = \mathbf{0}$ for $i = 1, \cdots, s$ and $j = 1, \cdots, t$.

Definition 1.2.27. Orthogonal complement of $\mathcal{V}_1$. The set of all matrices in a linear space $\mathcal{V}$ that is orthogonal to a subspace $\mathcal{V}_1$ of $\mathcal{V}$ is called the orthogonal complement of $\mathcal{V}_1$ relative to $\mathcal{V}$. The orthogonal complement is also a subspace of $\mathcal{V}$, and is denoted by $\mathcal{V}_1^\perp$.

Let $\mathcal{V}_1$ be a subspace of $\mathcal{V}$ and let $\{\mathbf{B}_1, \cdots, \mathbf{B}_k\}$ span $\mathcal{V}_1$. Then, $\mathbf{A}$ is in $\mathcal{V}_1^\perp$ if and only if $\mathbf{A} \bullet \mathbf{B}_j = \mathbf{0}$ for $j = 1, \cdots, k$. We next define three important vector spaces associated with any matrix, viz., the *null space*, the *column space* and the *row space*. These concepts are closely related to properties of systems of linear equations, which are discussed in detail in Chapter 3. A system of homogeneous linear equations is denoted by $\mathbf{Ax} = \mathbf{0}$, while $\mathbf{Ax} = \mathbf{b}$ denotes a system of nonhomogeneous linear equations.

Definition 1.2.28. Null space of a matrix. The null space, $\mathcal{N}(\mathbf{A})$, of an $m \times n$ matrix $\mathbf{A}$ consists of all n-dimensional vectors $\mathbf{x}$ such that $\mathbf{Ax} = \mathbf{0}$, i.e.,

$$\mathcal{N}(\mathbf{A}) = \{\mathbf{x} \in \mathcal{R}^n \text{ such that } \mathbf{Ax} = \mathbf{0}\}.$$

That is, the null space is the set of all solutions to the homogeneous linear system $\mathbf{Ax} = \mathbf{0}$. $\mathcal{N}(\mathbf{A})$ is a subspace of $\mathcal{R}^n$, and its dimension is called the nullity of $\mathbf{A}$. For example, the vector $\mathbf{x} = (1, 2)'$ belongs to the null space of the matrix $\mathbf{A} = \begin{pmatrix} 2 & -1 \\ -4 & 2 \end{pmatrix}$ since $\begin{pmatrix} 2 & -1 \\ -4 & 2 \end{pmatrix} \begin{pmatrix} 1 \\ 2 \end{pmatrix} = \begin{pmatrix} 0 \\ 0 \end{pmatrix}$.

We may use RREF($\mathbf{A}$) to find a basis of the null space of $\mathbf{A}$. We add or delete zero rows until RREF($\mathbf{A}$) is square. We then rearrange the rows to place the leading ones on the main diagonal to obtain $\tilde{\mathbf{H}}$, which is the *Hermite form* of RREF($\mathbf{A}$). The nonzero columns of $\tilde{\mathbf{H}} - \mathbf{I}$ are a basis for $\mathcal{N}(\mathbf{A})$. In general, an $n \times n$ matrix $\tilde{\mathbf{H}}$ is in Hermite form (i) if each diagonal element is either 0 or 1; (ii) if $\tilde{h}_{ii} = 1$, the rest of column i is all zeroes; and (iii) if $\tilde{h}_{ii} = 0$, i.e., the ith row of $\tilde{\mathbf{H}}$ is a vector of zeroes.

Example 1.2.14. We first find a basis for the null space of the matrix

$$\mathbf{A} = \begin{pmatrix} 1 & 0 & -5 & 1 \\ 0 & 1 & 2 & -3 \\ 0 & 0 & 0 & 0 \\ 0 & 0 & 0 & 0 \end{pmatrix}$$

which is in RREF, as we can verify. The augmented matrix of the system $\mathbf{Ax} = \mathbf{0}$ will be

$$\text{RREF}(\mathbf{A}) = \begin{pmatrix} 1 & 0 & -5 & 1 & 0 \\ 0 & 1 & 2 & -3 & 0 \\ 0 & 0 & 0 & 0 & 0 \\ 0 & 0 & 0 & 0 & 0 \end{pmatrix}$$

where $\mathbf{x}' = (x_1, x_2, x_3, x_4)$. We can choose x_3 and x_4 freely; we set $x_3 = s$, and $x_4 = t$. It is clear that the general solution vector is

$$\begin{pmatrix} x_1 \\ x_2 \\ x_3 \\ x_4 \end{pmatrix} = s \begin{pmatrix} 5 \\ -2 \\ 1 \\ 0 \end{pmatrix} + t \begin{pmatrix} -1 \\ 3 \\ 0 \\ 1 \end{pmatrix},$$

so that the vectors $(5, -2, 1, 0)'$ and $(-1, 3, 0, 1)'$ form a basis for $\mathcal{N}(\mathbf{A})$. This basis can also be obtained in an alternate way from RREF($\mathbf{A}$), which in this example coincides with $\mathbf{A}$. Computing

$$\mathbf{I} - \text{RREF}(\mathbf{A}) = \begin{pmatrix} 0 & 0 & 5 & -1 \\ 0 & 0 & -2 & 3 \\ 0 & 0 & 1 & 0 \\ 0 & 0 & 0 & 1 \end{pmatrix},$$

we see that the last two nonzero columns form a basis for $\mathcal{N}(\mathbf{A})$.   □

Definition 1.2.29. Column space of a matrix.   Let $\mathbf{A}$ be an $m \times n$ matrix whose columns are the m-dimensional vectors $\mathbf{a}_1, \mathbf{a}_2, \cdots, \mathbf{a}_n$. The vector space spanned by the n columns of $\mathbf{A}$ is called the column space (or range space) of $\mathbf{A}$, and is denoted by $\mathcal{C}(\mathbf{A})$. The dimension of the column space of $\mathbf{A}$ is the number of LIN columns of $\mathbf{A}$, and is called the column rank of $\mathbf{A}$. For example, given $\mathbf{A} = \begin{pmatrix} 1 & -2 \\ 2 & -4 \end{pmatrix}$, the vector $\mathbf{x}_1 = (-2, 2)'$ is not in $\mathcal{C}(\mathbf{A})$, whereas the vector $\mathbf{x}_2 = (3, 6)'$ is, because

$$\begin{pmatrix} 1 & -2 & -2 \\ 2 & -4 & 2 \end{pmatrix} \sim \begin{pmatrix} 1 & -2 & -2 \\ 0 & 0 & 6 \end{pmatrix} \quad \text{and} \quad \begin{pmatrix} 1 & -2 & 3 \\ 2 & -4 & 6 \end{pmatrix} \sim \begin{pmatrix} 1 & -2 & 3 \\ 0 & 0 & 0 \end{pmatrix}.$$

The row space $\mathcal{R}(\mathbf{A})$ and row rank are defined similarly.

The column space $\mathcal{C}(\mathbf{A})$ and the row space $\mathcal{R}(\mathbf{A})$ of any $m \times n$ matrix $\mathbf{A}$ are subspaces of $\mathcal{R}^m$ and $\mathcal{R}^n$ respectively. The symbol $\mathcal{C}^\perp(\mathbf{A})$ or $\{\mathcal{C}(\mathbf{A})\}^\perp$ represents the orthogonal complement of $\mathcal{C}(\mathbf{A})$.

To find a basis of the column space of $\mathbf{A}$, we first find RREF($\mathbf{A}$). We select the columns of $\mathbf{A}$ which correspond to the columns of RREF($\mathbf{A}$) with leading ones. These are called the leading columns of $\mathbf{A}$ and form a basis for $\mathcal{C}(\mathbf{A})$. The nonzero rows of RREF($\mathbf{A}$) are a basis for $\mathcal{R}(\mathbf{A})$.

Example 1.2.15. We find a basis for $\mathcal{C}(\mathbf{A})$, where the matrix $\mathbf{A}$ and $\mathbf{B} =$ RREF($\mathbf{A}$) are shown below:

$$\mathbf{A} = \begin{pmatrix} 1 & -2 & 2 & 1 & 0 \\ -1 & 2 & -1 & 0 & 0 \\ 2 & -4 & 6 & 4 & 0 \\ 3 & -6 & 8 & 5 & 1 \end{pmatrix} \quad \text{and} \quad \mathbf{B} = \begin{pmatrix} 1 & -2 & 0 & -1 & 0 \\ 0 & 0 & 1 & 1 & 0 \\ 0 & 0 & 0 & 0 & 1 \\ 0 & 0 & 0 & 0 & 0 \end{pmatrix}.$$

We see that columns 1, 3 and 5 are pivot columns and they are linearly independent; they form a basis for $\mathcal{C}(\mathbf{A})$. $\square$

Result 1.2.11. Let $\mathcal{C}(\mathbf{A})$ and $\mathcal{N}(\mathbf{A})$ respectively denote the column and null space of an $m \times n$ matrix $\mathbf{A}$. Then,

1. $\dim[\mathcal{C}(\mathbf{A})] = n - \dim[\mathcal{N}(\mathbf{A})]$.

2. $\mathcal{N}(\mathbf{A}) = \{\mathcal{C}(\mathbf{A})\}^\perp$.

3. $\mathcal{C}(\mathbf{A}'\mathbf{A}) = \mathcal{C}(\mathbf{A}')$, and $\mathcal{R}(\mathbf{A}'\mathbf{A}) = \mathcal{R}(\mathbf{A})$.

4. For any $\mathbf{A}$ and $\mathbf{B}$, $\mathcal{C}(\mathbf{A}\mathbf{B}) \subseteq \mathcal{C}(\mathbf{A})$.

5. $\mathcal{C}(\mathbf{A}\mathbf{C}\mathbf{B}) = \mathcal{C}(\mathbf{A}\mathbf{C})$ if $r(\mathbf{C}\mathbf{B}) = r(\mathbf{C})$.

Definition 1.2.30. Rank of a matrix. Let $\mathbf{A}$ be an $m \times n$ matrix. We say that $\mathbf{A}$ has full row rank if $r(\mathbf{A}) = m$ (which is possible only if $m \leq n$), and has full column rank if $r(\mathbf{A}) = n$ (which is possible only if $n \leq m$). A nonsingular matrix has full row rank and full column rank. We say $\mathbf{A}$ has rank r (denoted by $r(\mathbf{A}) = r$) if its column rank (which is equal to its row rank) is equal to r.

To find the rank of $\mathbf{A}$, we find RREF($\mathbf{A}$). We count the number of leading ones, which is then equal to $r(\mathbf{A})$.

Example 1.2.16. Consider the matrices

$$\mathbf{A} = \begin{pmatrix} 1 & 2 & 2 & -1 \\ 1 & 3 & 1 & -2 \\ 1 & 1 & 3 & 0 \\ 0 & 1 & -1 & -1 \\ 1 & 2 & 2 & -1 \end{pmatrix} \quad \text{and} \quad \mathbf{B} = \begin{pmatrix} 1 & 2 & 2 & -1 \\ 0 & 1 & -1 & -1 \\ 0 & 0 & 0 & 0 \\ 0 & 0 & 0 & 0 \\ 0 & 0 & 0 & 0 \end{pmatrix}$$

where **B**, which is the reduced row echelon form of **A**, has two nonzero rows. Hence, $r(\mathbf{A}) = 2$. $\square$

Result 1.2.12. Properties of rank.

1. An $m \times n$ matrix **A** has rank r if the largest nonsingular square submatrix of **A** has size r.

2. For an $m \times n$ matrix **A**, $r(\mathbf{A}) \leq \min(m, n)$.

3. $r(\mathbf{A} + \mathbf{B}) \leq r(\mathbf{A}) + r(\mathbf{B})$.

4. $r(\mathbf{AB}) \leq \min\{r(\mathbf{A}), r(\mathbf{B})\}$, where **A** and **B** are conformal under multiplication.

5. For nonsingular matrices **A**, **B**, and an arbitrary matrix **C**,

$$r(\mathbf{C}) = r(\mathbf{AC}) = r(\mathbf{CB}) = r(\mathbf{ACB}).$$

6. $r(\mathbf{A}) = r(\mathbf{A}') = r(\mathbf{A}'\mathbf{A}) = r(\mathbf{AA}')$.

7. For any $n \times n$ matrix **A**, $|\mathbf{A}| = 0$ if and only if $r(\mathbf{A}) < n$.

8. $r(\mathbf{A}, \mathbf{b}) \geq r(\mathbf{A})$, i.e., inclusion of a column vector cannot decrease the rank of a matrix.

Definition 1.2.31. Equivalent matrices. Two matrices that have the same dimension and the same rank are said to be equivalent matrices.

Result 1.2.13. Equivalent canonical form of a matrix. An $m \times n$ matrix **A** with $r(\mathbf{A}) = r$ is equivalent to $\mathbf{PAQ} = \begin{pmatrix} \mathbf{I}_r & \mathbf{0} \\ \mathbf{0} & \mathbf{0} \end{pmatrix}$ where **P** and **Q** are respectively $m \times m$ and $n \times n$ matrices, and are obtained as products of elementary matrices, i.e., matrices obtained from the identity matrix using elementary transformations. The matrices **P** and **Q** always exist, but need not be unique. Elementary transformations include

1. interchange of two rows (columns) of **I**, or

2. multiplication of elements of a row (column) of **I** by a nonzero scalar c, or

3. adding to row j (column j) of **I**, c times row i (column i).

Definition 1.2.32. Eigenvalues and eigenvectors of a matrix. The eigenvalues (or characteristic roots) $\lambda_1 \geq \lambda_2 \geq \cdots \geq \lambda_n$ and the corresponding eigenvectors $\mathbf{v}_1, \mathbf{v}_2, \cdots, \mathbf{v}_n$ of an $n \times n$ matrix **A** satisfy the relationship

$$(\mathbf{A} - \lambda_j \mathbf{I})\mathbf{v}_j = \mathbf{0}, \quad j = 1, \cdots, n.$$

The eigenvalues of $\mathbf{A}$ are solutions to the characteristic polynomial equation $P(\lambda) = |(\mathbf{A} - \lambda\mathbf{I})| = 0$, which is a polynomial in λ of degree n. Note that the n eigenvalues of $\mathbf{A}$ are not necessarily all distinct or real-valued. Since $|(\mathbf{A} - \lambda_j\mathbf{I})| = 0$, $\mathbf{A} - \lambda_j\mathbf{I}$ is a singular matrix, for $j = 1, \cdots, n$, and there exists a nonzero n-dimensional vector $\mathbf{v}_j$ which satisfies $(\mathbf{A} - \lambda_j\mathbf{I})\mathbf{v}_j = \mathbf{0}$, i.e., $\mathbf{A}\mathbf{v}_j = \lambda_j\mathbf{v}_j$. The eigenvectors of $\mathbf{A}$ are thus obtained by substituting each λ_j into $\mathbf{A}\mathbf{v}_j = \lambda_j\mathbf{v}_j$, $j = 1, \cdots, n$, and solving the resulting n equations. We say that an eigenvector $\mathbf{v}_j$ is a normalized eigenvector if $\mathbf{v}_j'\mathbf{v}_j = 1$. If λ_j is complex-valued, then $\mathbf{v}_j$ may have complex elements. If some of the eigenvalues of the real matrix $\mathbf{A}$ are complex, then they must clearly be conjugate complex (a conjugate complex pair is defined as $(a + ib), (a - ib)$). Suppose $\mathbf{v}_{j1}$ and $\mathbf{v}_{j2}$ are nonzero eigenvectors of $\mathbf{A}$ corresponding to λ_j, it is easy to see that $\alpha_1\mathbf{v}_{j1} + \alpha_2\mathbf{v}_{j2}$ is also an eigenvector corresponding to λ_j, where α_1 and α_2 are real numbers. That is, we must have $\mathbf{A}(\alpha_1\mathbf{v}_{j1} + \alpha_2\mathbf{v}_{j2}) = \lambda_j(\alpha_1\mathbf{v}_{j1} + \alpha_2\mathbf{v}_{j2})$. The eigenvectors corresponding to any eigenvalue λ_j span a vector space, called the eigenspace of $\mathbf{A}$ for λ_j.

Definition 1.2.33. Eigenspace of a matrix. The eigenspace corresponding to an eigenvalue λ of a matrix $\mathbf{A}$ is the set obtained from $\mathcal{N}(\mathbf{A} - \lambda\mathbf{I}_n)$ by excluding $\mathbf{0}$. The dimension of this eigenspace is $g = n - r(\mathbf{A} - \lambda\mathbf{I}_n)$, and is called the geometric multiplicity of λ.

To find the eigenvectors of $\mathbf{A}$ corresponding to an eigenvalue λ, we find the basis of the null space of $(\mathbf{A} - \lambda\mathbf{I})$. The nonzero columns of $\widetilde{\mathbf{H}} - \mathbf{I}$ are a basis for $\mathcal{N}(\mathbf{A} - \lambda\mathbf{I})$, where $\widetilde{\mathbf{H}}$ denotes the Hermite form of $\mathrm{RREF}(\mathbf{A} - \lambda\mathbf{I})$ (see Example 1.2.19).

Definition 1.2.34. Spectrum of a matrix. The set of distinct (real) eigenvalues $\{\lambda_1, \lambda_2, \cdots, \lambda_k\}$ of $\mathbf{A}$ is called the spectrum of $\mathbf{A}$.

The characteristic polynomial may be written as

$$P(\lambda) = (-1)^n(\lambda - \lambda_1)^{a_1} \cdots (\lambda - \lambda_k)^{a_k}q(\lambda),$$

where $a_1, \cdots, a_k$ are positive integers, a_j is called the algebraic multiplicity of λ_j, $j = 1, \cdots, k$, and $q(\lambda)$ is a polynomial of degree $n - \sum_{j=1}^{k} a_j$ with no real roots. The geometric multiplicity of λ is at most equal to its algebraic multiplicity. This gives a bound on the dimension of the eigenspace of $\mathbf{A}$. In general, if an $n \times n$ matrix $\mathbf{A}$ has k distinct eigenvalues $\lambda_1, \cdots, \lambda_k$ with respective algebraic multiplicities and geometric multiplicities $a_1, \cdots, a_k$ and $g_1, \cdots, g_k$, then, $\sum_{j=1}^{k} g_j \leq \sum_{j=1}^{k} a_j \leq n$. The geometric multiplicity of an eigenvalue λ of a symmetric matrix is equal to its algebraic multiplicity (see Exercise 2.13).

Example 1.2.17. Let $\mathbf{A} = \begin{pmatrix} 1 & 1 \\ 0 & 1 \end{pmatrix}$. Then, $P(\lambda) = (\lambda - 1)^2$, with solutions $\lambda_1 = 1$ (repeated twice), so that $a_1 = 2$. Since $\mathbf{A} - \lambda_1\mathbf{I}_2 = \begin{pmatrix} 0 & 1 \\ 0 & 0 \end{pmatrix}$, with rank 1, the geometric multiplicity of λ_1 is $g_1 = 2 - 1 = 1 < a_1$. □

Example 1.2.18. Let $\mathbf{A} = \begin{pmatrix} 0 & -1 \\ 1 & 0 \end{pmatrix}$. This matrix has no real eigenvalues, since, $P(\lambda) = \lambda^2 + 1$, with solutions $\lambda_1 = i$ and $\lambda_2 = -i$, where $i = \sqrt{-1}$. The corresponding eigenvectors are complex, and are $(i, 1)'$ and $(-i, 1)'$.   □

Example 1.2.19. Let

$$\mathbf{A} = \begin{pmatrix} -1 & 2 & 0 \\ 1 & 2 & 1 \\ 0 & 2 & -1 \end{pmatrix}.$$

Then $|\mathbf{A} - \lambda\mathbf{I}| = -(\lambda + 1)(\lambda - 3)(\lambda + 2) = 0$, yielding solutions $\lambda_1 = -1$, $\lambda_2 = 3$, and $\lambda_3 = -2$, which are the distinct eigenvalues of $\mathbf{A}$. To obtain the eigenvectors corresponding to λ_i, we must solve the homogeneous linear system $(\mathbf{A} - \lambda_i\mathbf{I})\mathbf{v}_i = \mathbf{0}$, or in other words, identify the null space of the matrix $(\mathbf{A} - \lambda_i\mathbf{I})$, by completely reducing the augmented matrix $(\mathbf{A} - \lambda_i\mathbf{I} : \mathbf{0})$. Corresponding to $\lambda_1 = -1$, we see that

$$\mathbf{A} - (-1)\mathbf{I} = \begin{pmatrix} 0 & 2 & 0 \\ 1 & 3 & 1 \\ 0 & 2 & 0 \end{pmatrix}, \quad \text{RREF}(\mathbf{A} + \mathbf{I}) = \begin{pmatrix} 1 & 0 & 1 \\ 0 & 1 & 0 \\ 0 & 0 & 0 \end{pmatrix},$$

which is in Hermite form, i.e., $\text{RREF}(\mathbf{A} + \mathbf{I}) = \tilde{\mathbf{H}}$. The nonzero column of

$$\tilde{\mathbf{H}} - \mathbf{I} = \begin{pmatrix} 0 & 0 & 1 \\ 0 & 0 & 0 \\ 0 & 0 & -1 \end{pmatrix},$$

i.e., $(1, 0, -1)'$ is a basis of $\mathcal{N}(\mathbf{A} - (-1)\mathbf{I})$ and therefore of the eigenspace corresponding to $\lambda_1 = -1$. Using a similar approach, we find that a basis of the eigenspace corresponding to $\lambda_2 = 3$ is $(-1, -2, -1)'$ and corresponding to $\lambda_3 = -2$, it is $(-1, 1/2, -1)'$. These three vectors are the eigenvectors of the matrix $\mathbf{A}$.   □

Result 1.2.14. Let λ be an eigenvalue of $\mathbf{A}$ and let c be a real scalar. Then,

1. λ^k is an eigenvalue of $\mathbf{A}^k$, for any integer k.

2. $c\lambda$ is an eigenvalue of $c\mathbf{A}$.

3. $\lambda + c$ is an eigenvalue of $\mathbf{A} + c\mathbf{I}$, while the eigenvectors of $\mathbf{A} + c\mathbf{I}$ coincide with the eigenvectors of $\mathbf{A}$.

4. $f(\lambda)$ is an eigenvalue of $f(\mathbf{A})$, where $f(.)$ is any polynomial.

To see that property 3 holds, it is easy to verify that $|(\mathbf{A} + c\mathbf{I}) - (\lambda + c)\mathbf{I}| = |\mathbf{A} - \lambda\mathbf{I}| = 0$, so that $\lambda + c$ is an eigenvalue of $\mathbf{A} + c\mathbf{I}$. Also, if $\mathbf{A}\mathbf{v} = \lambda\mathbf{v}$, then $(\mathbf{A} + c\mathbf{I})\mathbf{v} = (\lambda + c)\mathbf{v}$, which shows that $\mathbf{A}$ and $\mathbf{A} + c\mathbf{I}$ have the same eigenvectors.

Result 1.2.15. Sum and product of eigenvalues.   Let $\mathbf{A}$ be an $n \times n$ matrix with eigenvalues $\lambda_1, \lambda_2, \cdots, \lambda_n$. Then,

1. $tr(\mathbf{A}) = \sum\limits_{i=1}^{n} \lambda_i.$

2. $|\mathbf{A}| = \prod\limits_{i=1}^{n} \lambda_i.$

3. $|\mathbf{I}_n \pm \mathbf{A}| = \prod\limits_{i=1}^{n} (1 \pm \lambda_i).$

Let $a_{ij}^{(k)}$ represent the (i,j)th element of an $m \times n$ matrix $\mathbf{A}_k$, $k = 1, 2, \cdots$. For every $i = 1, \cdots, m$ and $j = 1, \cdots, n$, suppose there exists a scalar a_{ij} which is the limit of the sequence of numbers $a_{ij}^{(1)}, a_{ij}^{(2)}, \cdots$, and suppose $\mathbf{A} = \{a_{ij}\}$. We say that the $m \times n$ matrix $\mathbf{A}$ is the limit of the sequence of matrices $\mathbf{A}_k$, $k = 1, 2, \cdots$, or that the sequence $\mathbf{A}_k$, $k = 1, 2, \cdots$ converges to the matrix $\mathbf{A}$, which we denote by $\lim_{k \to \infty} \mathbf{A}_k = \mathbf{A}$. If this limit exists, the sequence of matrices converges, otherwise it diverges. The following infinite series representation of the inverse of the matrix $(\mathbf{I} - \mathbf{A})$ is used in Chapter 5.

Result 1.2.16. For an $n \times n$ matrix $\mathbf{A}$, the infinite series $\sum_{k=0}^{\infty} \mathbf{A}^k$, with $\mathbf{A}^0 = \mathbf{I}$, converges if and only if $\lim_{k \to \infty} \mathbf{A}^k = \mathbf{0}$. Then, $(\mathbf{I} - \mathbf{A})$ is nonsingular and

$$(\mathbf{I} - \mathbf{A})^{-1} = \sum_{k=0}^{\infty} \mathbf{A}^k.$$

Definition 1.2.35. Exponential matrix. For any $n \times n$ matrix $\mathbf{A}$, we define the matrix $e^{\mathbf{A}}$ to be the $n \times n$ matrix given by:

$$e^{\mathbf{A}} = \sum_{i=0}^{\infty} \frac{\mathbf{A}^i}{i!},$$

where the expression on the right is a convergent series, i.e., all the $n \times n$ series $\sum_{i=0}^{\infty} a_{jk}^{(i)}$, $j = 1, \cdots, n$, $k = 1, \cdots, n$ are convergent, $a_{jk}^{(i)}$ being the (j,k)th element of $\mathbf{A}^i$ and $e^{\mathbf{0}} = \mathbf{I}$.

We conclude this section with some definitions of vector and matrix norms.

Definition 1.2.36. Vector norm. A vector norm on $\mathcal{R}^n$ is a function $f : \mathcal{R}^n \to \mathcal{R}$, denoted by $\| \mathbf{v} \|$, such that for every n-dimensional vector $\mathbf{v} \in \mathcal{R}^n$, and every $\alpha \in \mathcal{R}$, we have

1. $f(\mathbf{v}) \geq 0$, with equality if and only if $\mathbf{v} = \mathbf{0}$,

2. $f(\alpha \mathbf{v}) = |\alpha| f(\mathbf{v})$, and

3. $f(\mathbf{u} + \mathbf{v}) \leq f(\mathbf{u}) + f(\mathbf{v})$ for every $\mathbf{u} \in \mathcal{R}^n$.

Specifically, the p-norm of a vector $\mathbf{v} = (v_1, \cdots, v_n)' \in \mathcal{R}^n$, which is also known in the literature as the *Minkowski metric* is defined by

$$\parallel \mathbf{v} \parallel_p = \{|v_1|^p + |v_2|^p + \cdots + |v_n|^p\}^{1/p}, \ p \geq 1.$$

We mention two special cases. The L_1-norm is defined by

$$\parallel \mathbf{v} \parallel_1 = \sum_{i=1}^{n} |v_i|$$

and forms the basis for the definition of LAD regression (see Chapter 8). The L_2-norm, which is also known as the Euclidean norm or the spectral norm is defined by

$$\parallel \mathbf{v} \parallel_2 = \{|v_1|^2 + |v_2|^2 + \cdots + |v_n|^2\}^{1/2} = (\mathbf{v}'\mathbf{v})^{1/2},$$

and is the basis for least squares techniques. In this book, we will denote $\parallel \mathbf{v} \parallel_2$ simply as $\parallel \mathbf{v} \parallel$. An extension is to define the L_2-norm with respect to a nonsingular matrix $\mathbf{A}$ by

$$\parallel \mathbf{v} \parallel_{\mathbf{A}} = (\mathbf{v}'\mathbf{A}\mathbf{v})^{1/2}.$$

Definition 1.2.37. Matrix norm.   A function $f : \mathcal{R}^{m \times n} \to \mathcal{R}$ is called a matrix norm on $\mathcal{R}^{m \times n}$, denoted by $\parallel \mathbf{A} \parallel$, if

1. $f(\mathbf{A}) \geq 0$ for all $m \times n$ real matrices $\mathbf{A}$, with equality if and only if $\mathbf{A} = \mathbf{0}$,

2. $f(\alpha \mathbf{A}) = |\alpha| f(\mathbf{A})$ for all $\alpha \in \mathcal{R}$, and for all $m \times n$ matrices $\mathbf{A}$, and

3. $f(\mathbf{A} + \mathbf{B}) \leq f(\mathbf{A}) + f(\mathbf{B})$ for all $m \times n$ matrices $\mathbf{A}$ and $\mathbf{B}$.

The norm of an $m \times n$ matrix $\mathbf{A} = \{a_{ij}\}$ with respect to the usual inner product is defined by

$$\parallel \mathbf{A} \parallel = [tr(\mathbf{A}'\mathbf{A})]^{1/2} = [\textstyle\sum_{i=1}^{m} \sum_{j=1}^{n} a_{ij}^2]^{1/2}.$$

It is easy to verify that $\parallel \mathbf{A} \parallel \geq 0$, with equality holding only if $\mathbf{A} = \mathbf{0}$. Also, $\parallel c\mathbf{A} \parallel = |c| \parallel \mathbf{A} \parallel$.

Exercises

1.1. Verify the Cauchy-Schwarz inequality for $\mathbf{a} = (-1, 2, 0, -1)$ and $\mathbf{b} = (4, -2, -1, 1)$.

1.2. Verify Properties 6 and 7 in Result 1.2.1.

1.3. Suppose $\mathbf{x}$, $\mathbf{y}$ and $\mathbf{z}$ are orthonormal vectors. Let $\mathbf{u} = a\mathbf{x} + b\mathbf{y}$ and $\mathbf{v} = a\mathbf{x} + b\mathbf{z}$. Find a and b such that the vectors $\mathbf{u}$ and $\mathbf{v}$ are of unit length and the angle between them is 60°.

1.4. Show that $\mathbf{v}_1' = \begin{pmatrix} 1 & 1 & 0 & -1 \end{pmatrix}$, $\mathbf{v}_2' = \begin{pmatrix} 2 & 0 & 1 & -1 \end{pmatrix}$, and $\mathbf{v}_3' = \begin{pmatrix} 0 & -2 & 1 & 1 \end{pmatrix}$ are linearly dependent vectors. Find a set of two linearly independent vectors and express the third as a function of these two.

1.5. Show that the set of vectors $v_1' = (2 \ 3 \ 2)$, $v_2' = (8 \ -6 \ 5)$, and $v_3' = (-4 \ 3 \ 1)$ are linearly independent.

1.6. Verify whether the columns of $\mathbf{A}$ are linearly independent given

$$\mathbf{A} = \begin{pmatrix} -3 & 3 & 3 \\ 2 & 2 & 2 \\ 0 & 1 & 0 \end{pmatrix}.$$

1.7. Verify whether the vector $\mathbf{u} = (2,3)'$ is in the span of the vectors $\mathbf{v}_1 = (1,2)'$ and $\mathbf{v}_2 = (3,5)'$.

1.8. Verify Result 1.2.3.

1.9. Find all matrices that commute with the matrix

$$\mathbf{B} = \begin{pmatrix} b & 1 & 0 \\ 0 & b & 1 \\ 0 & 0 & b \end{pmatrix}.$$

1.10. Given $\mathbf{A} = \begin{pmatrix} a & b \\ 0 & 1 \end{pmatrix}$, find $\mathbf{A}^k$, for all $k \geq 2$.

1.11. If $\mathbf{AB} = \mathbf{BA}$, show that, for any given positive integer k, there exists a matrix $\mathbf{C}$ such that $\mathbf{A}^k - \mathbf{B}^k = (\mathbf{A} - \mathbf{B})\mathbf{C}$.

1.12. For any $n \times n$ matrix $\mathbf{A}$, show that the matrices $\mathbf{A}'\mathbf{A}$ and $\mathbf{AA}'$ are symmetric.

1.13. For any $m \times n$ matrix $\mathbf{A}$, show that $\mathbf{A} = \mathbf{0}$ if and only if $\mathbf{A}'\mathbf{A} = \mathbf{0}$.

1.14. Let $\mathbf{A}$ be an $n \times n$ matrix and let $\mathbf{x}_i$ be an $n \times 1$ vector, $i = 1, \cdots, k$.

(a) Show that $tr(\mathbf{A} \sum_{i=1}^{k} \mathbf{x}_i \mathbf{x}_i') = \sum_{i=1}^{k} \mathbf{x}_i' \mathbf{A} \mathbf{x}_i$.

(b) Show that $tr(\mathbf{B}^{-1}\mathbf{AB}) = tr(\mathbf{A})$.

1.15. Verify Result 1.2.8.

1.16. Find the determinant of the matrix

$$\mathbf{A} = \begin{pmatrix} 1 & 3 & -3 & 1 \\ 5 & 9 & -10 & 3 \\ 1 & 0 & 5 & -2 \\ 2 & 1 & -3 & 1 \end{pmatrix}.$$

1.17. Let

$$\Delta_n = \det \begin{pmatrix} 1+a^2 & a & 0 & \cdots & 0 & 0 \\ a & 1+a^2 & a & \cdots & 0 & 0 \\ 0 & a & 1+a^2 & \cdots & 0 & 0 \\ \vdots & \vdots & \vdots & \ddots & \vdots & \vdots \\ 0 & 0 & 0 & \cdots & 1+a^2 & a \\ 0 & 0 & 0 & \cdots & a & 1+a^2 \end{pmatrix}.$$

Show that $\Delta_n - \Delta_{n-1} = a^2(\Delta_{n-1} - \Delta_{n-2})$, and hence find Δ_n.

1.18. If the row vectors of a square matrix are linearly dependent, show that the determinant of the matrix is zero.

1.19. Evaluate the determinant of

$$\begin{pmatrix} a_1+1 & a_2 & \cdots & a_n \\ a_1 & a_2+1 & \cdots & a_n \\ \vdots & \vdots & \ddots & \vdots \\ a_1 & a_2 & \cdots & a_n+1 \end{pmatrix}.$$

1.20. By reducing the matrix

$$\mathbf{A} = \begin{pmatrix} 1 & 2 & -1 \\ 1 & -2 & -1 \\ 1 & 6 & -1 \end{pmatrix},$$

show that it is singular.

1.21. Verify Result 1.2.10.

1.22. (a) Show that $(\mathbf{I} + \mathbf{AB})^{-1} = \mathbf{I} - \mathbf{A}(\mathbf{I} + \mathbf{BA})^{-1}\mathbf{B}$, provided $\mathbf{AB}$ and $\mathbf{BA}$ exist.

(b) Using (a), show that $(a\mathbf{I}_k + b\mathbf{J}_k)^{-1} = \mathbf{I}_k/a - b\mathbf{J}_k/\{a(a+kb)\}$.

1.23. Let $\mathbf{A}$ be an $n \times n$ orthogonal matrix.

(a) Show that $|\mathbf{A}| = \pm 1$.

(b) Show that $\mathbf{r}_i\mathbf{r}'_j = \delta_{ij}$, and $\mathbf{c}'_i\mathbf{c}_j = \delta_{ij}$, where $\mathbf{r}_i$ is the ith row of $\mathbf{A}$, $\mathbf{c}_i$ is the ith column of $\mathbf{A}$ and δ_{ij} denotes the Kronecker delta, i.e., $\delta_{ij} = 1$ for $i = j$, and $\delta_{ij} = 0$ otherwise.

(c) Show that $\mathbf{AB}$ is orthogonal, where $\mathbf{B}$ is an $n \times n$ orthogonal matrix.

1.24. Let $\mathbf{A}$ be an $n \times n$ symmetric matrix and let $r(\mathbf{A}) = 1$. Show that $|\mathbf{I} + \mathbf{A}| = 1 + tr(\mathbf{A})$.

1.25. Find the dimension of the column space, null space and row space of the matrix

$$\mathbf{A} = \begin{pmatrix} 1 & 1 & 1 \\ 2 & 2 & 2 \\ -1 & 1 & -3 \\ 1 & 2 & 0 \end{pmatrix}.$$

1.26. Prove Result 1.2.11.

1.27. Let $\mathbf{A} = \begin{pmatrix} 1 & 2 & 4 & 3 \\ 3 & -1 & 2 & -2 \\ 5 & -4 & 0 & -7 \end{pmatrix}$. Find the rank of $\mathbf{A}$.

1.28. Verify Result 1.2.16.

1.29. Let $\mathbf{A} = \begin{pmatrix} a+1 & 1 & 1 \\ 1 & a+1 & 1 \\ 1 & 1 & a+1 \end{pmatrix}$. Show that $\mathbf{A} - a\mathbf{I}_3$ has a nonzero eigenvalue of 3. Find the corresponding eigenvector.

1.30. If $\mathbf{A}$ and $\mathbf{B}$ conform under multiplication, show that the nonzero eigenvalues of $\mathbf{AB}$ coincide with the nonzero eigenvalues of $\mathbf{BA}$.

1.31. Let $\mathbf{A}$ be a $k \times k$ matrix and $\mathbf{B}$ be a $k \times k$ nonsingular matrix. Show that $\mathbf{A}$ and $\mathbf{BAB}^{-1}$ have the same eigenvalues. If $\mathbf{Av}_j = \lambda_j \mathbf{v}_j$, i.e., $\mathbf{v}_j$ is an eigenvector corresponding to the eigenvalue λ_j of $\mathbf{A}$, show that $\mathbf{Bv}_j$ is an eigenvector of $\mathbf{BAB}^{-1}$ for λ_j.

1.32. Let $\mathbf{x}$ and $\mathbf{y}$ be real vectors and $\mathbf{A} > \mathbf{0}$. Verify the following results:

(a) $(\mathbf{x}'\mathbf{Ay})^2 \le (\mathbf{x}'\mathbf{Ax})(\mathbf{y}'\mathbf{Ay})$.
(b) $(\mathbf{x}'\mathbf{y})^2 \le (\mathbf{x}'\mathbf{Ax})(\mathbf{y}'\mathbf{A}^{-1}\mathbf{y})$.

Chapter 2

Properties of Special Matrices

In this chapter, we define special matrices that find direct use in the theory of linear models and present some properties of such matrices. We illustrate salient properties of these matrices using several examples. The concepts and results discussed here will be used in subsequent chapters for the development of matrix results and distribution theory.

2.1 Partitioned matrices

Definition 2.1.1. An $m \times n$ partitioned matrix $\mathbf{A}$ is expressed as an array of submatrices (or blocks):

$$\mathbf{A} = \begin{pmatrix} \mathbf{A}_{11} & \mathbf{A}_{12} & \cdots & \mathbf{A}_{1c} \\ \mathbf{A}_{21} & \mathbf{A}_{22} & \cdots & \mathbf{A}_{2c} \\ \vdots & \vdots & \vdots & \vdots \\ \mathbf{A}_{r1} & \mathbf{A}_{r2} & \cdots & \mathbf{A}_{rc} \end{pmatrix}, \tag{2.1.1}$$

where $\mathbf{A}_{ij}$ is an $m_i \times n_j$ submatrix for $i = 1, \cdots, r$, $j = 1, \cdots, c$; $m_1, \cdots, m_r$ and $n_1, \cdots, n_c$ are positive integers such that $\sum_{i=1}^{r} m_i = m$, and $\sum_{j=1}^{c} n_j = n$. Note that each submatrix $\mathbf{A}_{ij}, j = 1, \cdots, c$ has the same number of rows for any i, and similarly that each submatrix $\mathbf{A}_{ij}, i = 1, \cdots, r$ has the same number of columns for any j. For example,

$$\left(\begin{array}{ccc|c} 1 & 3 & 5 & 7 \\ \hline 5 & 4 & 1 & -9 \\ -3 & 2 & 6 & 4 \end{array} \right) \quad \text{and} \quad \left(\begin{array}{cc|cc} 1 & 3 & 5 & 7 \\ \hline 5 & 4 & 1 & -9 \\ -3 & 2 & 6 & 4 \end{array} \right)$$

are two different partitions of the same 3×4 matrix.

Definition 2.1.2. An $m \times n$ matrix $\mathbf{A}$ partitioned as

$$\mathbf{A} = \begin{pmatrix} \mathbf{A}_{11} & \mathbf{A}_{12} & \cdots & \mathbf{A}_{1r} \\ \mathbf{A}_{21} & \mathbf{A}_{22} & \cdots & \mathbf{A}_{2r} \\ \vdots & \vdots & \vdots & \vdots \\ \mathbf{A}_{r1} & \mathbf{A}_{r2} & \cdots & \mathbf{A}_{rr} \end{pmatrix} \qquad (2.1.2)$$

is said to be a block-diagonal matrix if $\mathbf{A}_{ij} = 0$ for $i \neq j$, and is written as

$$\mathbf{A} = \operatorname{diag}(\mathbf{A}_{11}, \mathbf{A}_{22}, \cdots, \mathbf{A}_{rr}).$$

In (2.1.2), if $\mathbf{A}_{ij} = 0$ for $j < i = 1, \cdots, r$, $\mathbf{A}$ is called an upper block-triangular matrix, while if $\mathbf{A}_{ij} = 0$ for $j > i = 1, \cdots, r$, then $\mathbf{A}$ is called a lower block-triangular matrix.

An $m \times n$ matrix $\mathbf{A}$ partitioned only by rows is written as

$$\mathbf{A} = \begin{pmatrix} \mathbf{A}_1 \\ \mathbf{A}_2 \\ \vdots \\ \mathbf{A}_r \end{pmatrix} \qquad (2.1.3)$$

and if it is partitioned only by columns, we write

$$\mathbf{A}' = \begin{pmatrix} \mathbf{A}_1' \\ \mathbf{A}_2' \\ \vdots \\ \mathbf{A}_c' \end{pmatrix} \qquad (2.1.4)$$

or $\mathbf{A} = (\mathbf{A}_1, \mathbf{A}_2, \cdots, \mathbf{A}_c)$. A partitioned n-dimensional column vector is denoted by

$$\mathbf{a} = \begin{pmatrix} \mathbf{a}_1 \\ \mathbf{a}_2 \\ \vdots \\ \mathbf{a}_r \end{pmatrix} \qquad (2.1.5)$$

where $\mathbf{a}_i$ is an n_i-dimensional vector, and $n_i, i = 1, \cdots, r$ are positive integers such that $\sum_{i=1}^{r} n_i = n$. A partitioned n-dimensional row vector is of the form

$$\mathbf{a}' = (\mathbf{a}_1', \cdots, \mathbf{a}_r'). \qquad (2.1.6)$$

Consider a $p \times q$ matrix $\mathbf{B}$ which is partitioned as

$$\mathbf{B} = \begin{pmatrix} \mathbf{B}_{11} & \mathbf{B}_{12} & \cdots & \mathbf{B}_{1h} \\ \mathbf{B}_{21} & \mathbf{B}_{22} & \cdots & \mathbf{B}_{2h} \\ \vdots & \vdots & \vdots & \vdots \\ \mathbf{B}_{l1} & \mathbf{B}_{l2} & \cdots & \mathbf{B}_{lh} \end{pmatrix}, \qquad (2.1.7)$$

where the dimension of $\mathbf{B}_{ij}$ is $p_i \times q_j$, for $i = 1, \cdots, l$, $j = 1, \cdots, h$. We define the following elementary operations on partitioned matrices.

Addition of partitioned matrices. The matrices $\mathbf{A}$ and $\mathbf{B}$ defined in (2.1.1) and (2.1.7) are conformal under addition if $p = m$, $q = n$, $l = r$, $h = c$, $p_i = m_i$, for $i = 1, \cdots, r$, and $q_j = n_j$, for $j = 1, \cdots, c$. Then, the (i, j)th submatrix of $\mathbf{C} = \mathbf{A} \pm \mathbf{B}$ is given by

$$\mathbf{C}_{ij} = \mathbf{A}_{ij} \pm \mathbf{B}_{ij} \quad \text{for} \quad i = 1, \cdots, r \quad \text{and} \quad j = 1, \cdots, c. \tag{2.1.8}$$

For example, when $r = c = l = h = 2$, and the submatrices have conformal dimensions, (2.1.8) becomes

$$\mathbf{A} \pm \mathbf{B} = \begin{pmatrix} \mathbf{A}_{11} \pm \mathbf{B}_{11} & \mathbf{A}_{12} \pm \mathbf{B}_{12} \\ \mathbf{A}_{21} \pm \mathbf{B}_{21} & \mathbf{A}_{22} \pm \mathbf{B}_{22} \end{pmatrix}. \tag{2.1.9}$$

Multiplication of partitioned matrices. The product $\mathbf{AB}$ is defined if $n = p$, $l = c$, and $n_j = p_j$ for $j = 1, \cdots, c$, in which case the submatrix of $\mathbf{C} = \mathbf{AB}$ is given by

$$\mathbf{C}_{ij} = \sum_{k=1}^{c} \mathbf{A}_{ik} \mathbf{B}_{kj}. \tag{2.1.10}$$

When $r = c = l = h = 2$, (2.1.10) simplifies as

$$\mathbf{AB} = \begin{pmatrix} \mathbf{A}_{11}\mathbf{B}_{11} + \mathbf{A}_{12}\mathbf{B}_{21} & \mathbf{A}_{11}\mathbf{B}_{12} + \mathbf{A}_{12}\mathbf{B}_{22} \\ \mathbf{A}_{21}\mathbf{B}_{11} + \mathbf{A}_{22}\mathbf{B}_{21} & \mathbf{A}_{21}\mathbf{B}_{12} + \mathbf{A}_{22}\mathbf{B}_{22} \end{pmatrix}. \tag{2.1.11}$$

Result 2.1.1. Determinant of a lower block-triangular matrix. For nonsingular square matrices $\mathbf{A}$, $\mathbf{A}_{11}$, and $\mathbf{A}_{22}$, where

$$\mathbf{A} = \begin{pmatrix} \mathbf{A}_{11} & \mathbf{0} \\ \mathbf{A}_{21} & \mathbf{A}_{22} \end{pmatrix},$$

we have

$$|\mathbf{A}| = |\mathbf{A}_{11}| |\mathbf{A}_{22}|. \tag{2.1.12}$$

Proof. It is easily verified that $\mathbf{A}$ can be written as

$$\mathbf{A} = \begin{pmatrix} \mathbf{I} & \mathbf{0} \\ \mathbf{0} & \mathbf{A}_{22} \end{pmatrix} \begin{pmatrix} \mathbf{I} & \mathbf{0} \\ \mathbf{A}_{22}^{-1}\mathbf{A}_{21}\mathbf{A}_{11}^{-1} & \mathbf{I} \end{pmatrix} \begin{pmatrix} \mathbf{A}_{11} & \mathbf{0} \\ \mathbf{0} & \mathbf{I} \end{pmatrix}. \tag{2.1.13}$$

Evaluating the determinant of each of the matrices on the right side of (2.1.13) using the cofactor expansion (see Definition 1.2.17), the result follows. ∎

Similarly, we can show that if $\mathbf{A}$ is an upper block-triangular matrix, then $|\mathbf{A}| = |\mathbf{A}_{11}||\mathbf{A}_{22}|$.

Result 2.1.2. Determinant of a partitioned matrix.   Suppose an $n \times n$ matrix $\mathbf{A}$ is partitioned as

$$\mathbf{A} = \begin{pmatrix} \mathbf{A}_{11} & \mathbf{A}_{12} \\ \mathbf{A}_{21} & \mathbf{A}_{22} \end{pmatrix}, \tag{2.1.14}$$

where $\mathbf{A}_{11}$, $\mathbf{A}_{12}$, $\mathbf{A}_{21}$, and $\mathbf{A}_{11}$ are respectively $n_1 \times n_1$, $n_1 \times n_2$, $n_2 \times n_1$, and $n_2 \times n_2$ dimensional submatrices, with $n_1 + n_2 = n$. Suppose $|\mathbf{A}_{22}| \neq 0$. Then,

$$|\mathbf{A}| = |\mathbf{A}_{22}| \, |\mathbf{A}_{11} - \mathbf{A}_{12}\mathbf{A}_{22}^{-1}\mathbf{A}_{21}| . \tag{2.1.15}$$

Proof. From Result 2.1.1, we see that

$$|\mathbf{A}_{22}| \left| \begin{pmatrix} \mathbf{I} & \mathbf{0} \\ -\mathbf{A}_{22}^{-1}\mathbf{A}_{21} & \mathbf{A}_{22}^{-1} \end{pmatrix} \right| = |\mathbf{A}_{22}| \, |\mathbf{A}_{22}^{-1}| = 1.$$

Hence,

$$\begin{aligned} |\mathbf{A}| &= |\mathbf{A}_{22}| \left| \begin{pmatrix} \mathbf{A}_{11} & \mathbf{A}_{12} \\ \mathbf{A}_{21} & \mathbf{A}_{22} \end{pmatrix} \right| \left| \begin{pmatrix} \mathbf{I} & \mathbf{0} \\ -\mathbf{A}_{22}^{-1}\mathbf{A}_{21} & \mathbf{A}_{22}^{-1} \end{pmatrix} \right| \\ &= |\mathbf{A}_{22}| \left| \begin{pmatrix} \mathbf{A}_{11} - \mathbf{A}_{12}\mathbf{A}_{22}^{-1}\mathbf{A}_{21} & \mathbf{A}_{12}\mathbf{A}_{22}^{-1} \\ \mathbf{A}_{21} - \mathbf{A}_{22}\mathbf{A}_{22}^{-1}\mathbf{A}_{21} & \mathbf{I} \end{pmatrix} \right| \\ &= |\mathbf{A}_{22}| \, |\mathbf{A}_{11} - \mathbf{A}_{12}\mathbf{A}_{22}^{-1}\mathbf{A}_{21}| , \end{aligned}$$

using the result on the determinant of an upper block-triangular matrix.   ■

The matrix $\mathbf{A}_{11} - \mathbf{A}_{12}\mathbf{A}_{22}^{-1}\mathbf{A}_{21}$ is called the Schur complement of $\mathbf{A}_{22}$. Note that if $|\mathbf{A}_{11}| \neq 0$, then,

$$|\mathbf{A}| = |\mathbf{A}_{11}| \, |\mathbf{A}_{22} - \mathbf{A}_{21}\mathbf{A}_{11}^{-1}\mathbf{A}_{12}| ; \tag{2.1.16}$$

the matrix $\mathbf{A}_{22} - \mathbf{A}_{21}\mathbf{A}_{11}^{-1}\mathbf{A}_{12}$ is called the Schur complement of $\mathbf{A}_{11}$.

Example 2.1.1. (a)   We will find $|\mathbf{A}|$, where

$$\mathbf{A} = \left(\begin{array}{cc|c} 1 & 2 & 0 \\ 2 & 5 & 0 \\ \hline 4 & 6 & 5 \end{array} \right)$$

has been partitioned into

$$\begin{pmatrix} \mathbf{A}_{11} & \mathbf{A}_{12} \\ \mathbf{A}_{21} & \mathbf{A}_{22} \end{pmatrix}, \quad \text{with } \mathbf{A}_{11} = \begin{pmatrix} 1 & 2 \\ 2 & 5 \end{pmatrix}, \quad \mathbf{A}_{12} = \begin{pmatrix} 0 \\ 0 \end{pmatrix},$$

$$\mathbf{A}_{21} = \begin{pmatrix} 4 & 6 \end{pmatrix} \quad \text{and} \quad \mathbf{A}_{22} = (5).$$

Also, $|\mathbf{A}_{11}| = 1$, and $|\mathbf{A}_{22}| = 5$. From Result 2.1.1, we see that $|\mathbf{A}| = |\mathbf{A}_{11}| \, |\mathbf{A}_{22}| = 5$.

(b) We compute $|\mathbf{A}|$ where

$$\mathbf{A} = \left(\begin{array}{cc|c} 1 & 2 & 1 \\ 2 & 5 & 7 \\ \hline 4 & 6 & 5 \end{array} \right).$$

Here, $\mathbf{A}_{12} = \begin{pmatrix} 1 \\ 7 \end{pmatrix}$, while the other submatrices remain the same as in (a). Using Result 2.1.2, $|\mathbf{A}| = |\mathbf{A}_{22}| \left| \mathbf{A}_{11} - \mathbf{A}_{12}\mathbf{A}_{22}^{-1}\mathbf{A}_{21} \right| = 11.$ $\quad\square$

We next show a result on the inverse of $\mathbf{A}$ partitioned as in (2.1.14). It is straightforward to verify that if $\mathbf{A}_{22}$ is nonsingular, then

$$\begin{aligned}
r\begin{pmatrix} \mathbf{A}_{11} & \mathbf{A}_{12} \\ \mathbf{A}_{21} & \mathbf{A}_{22} \end{pmatrix} &= r\begin{pmatrix} \mathbf{A}_{11} - \mathbf{A}_{12}\mathbf{A}_{22}^{-1}\mathbf{A}_{21} & \mathbf{0} \\ \mathbf{A}_{21} & \mathbf{A}_{22} \end{pmatrix} \\
&= r(\mathbf{A}_{11} - \mathbf{A}_{12}\mathbf{A}_{22}^{-1}\mathbf{A}_{21}) + r(\mathbf{A}_{22}),
\end{aligned}$$

which is used in the proof of the following result.

Result 2.1.3. Inverse of a partitioned matrix. Suppose a nonsingular matrix $\mathbf{A}$ is partitioned as in (2.1.14), and suppose that $\mathbf{B} = \mathbf{A}^{-1}$ is partitioned similar to $\mathbf{A}$.

1. Suppose $|\mathbf{A}_{22}| \neq 0$. Then, the submatrices of the inverse of $\mathbf{A}$ are given by

$$\begin{aligned}
\mathbf{B}_{11} &= (\mathbf{A}_{11} - \mathbf{A}_{12}\mathbf{A}_{22}^{-1}\mathbf{A}_{21})^{-1} \\
\mathbf{B}_{12} &= -\mathbf{B}_{11}\mathbf{A}_{12}\mathbf{A}_{22}^{-1} \\
\mathbf{B}_{21} &= -\mathbf{A}_{22}^{-1}\mathbf{A}_{21}\mathbf{B}_{11} \\
\mathbf{B}_{22} &= \mathbf{A}_{22}^{-1} + \mathbf{A}_{22}^{-1}\mathbf{A}_{21}\mathbf{B}_{11}\mathbf{A}_{12}\mathbf{A}_{22}^{-1}.
\end{aligned} \qquad (2.1.17)$$

2. Suppose $|\mathbf{A}_{11}| \neq 0$. Then, the submatrices of the inverse of $\mathbf{A}$ are

$$\begin{aligned}
\mathbf{B}_{11} &= \mathbf{A}_{11}^{-1} + \mathbf{A}_{11}^{-1}\mathbf{A}_{12}\mathbf{B}_{22}\mathbf{A}_{21}\mathbf{A}_{11}^{-1} \\
\mathbf{B}_{12} &= -\mathbf{A}_{11}^{-1}\mathbf{A}_{12}\mathbf{B}_{22} \\
\mathbf{B}_{21} &= -\mathbf{B}_{22}\mathbf{A}_{21}\mathbf{A}_{11}^{-1} \\
\mathbf{B}_{22} &= (\mathbf{A}_{22} - \mathbf{A}_{21}\mathbf{A}_{11}^{-1}\mathbf{A}_{12})^{-1}.
\end{aligned} \qquad (2.1.18)$$

Proof. We prove property 1. The proof of property 2 is similar and is left to the reader. The matrix $\mathbf{A}$ is nonsingular if and only if the matrix $\mathbf{A}_{11} - \mathbf{A}_{12}\mathbf{A}_{22}^{-1}\mathbf{A}_{21}$ is nonsingular. Since $\mathbf{B}$ is the regular inverse of $\mathbf{A}$, we must have

$$\mathbf{AB} = \begin{pmatrix} \mathbf{A}_{11}\mathbf{B}_{11} + \mathbf{A}_{12}\mathbf{B}_{21} & \mathbf{A}_{11}\mathbf{B}_{12} + \mathbf{A}_{12}\mathbf{B}_{22} \\ \mathbf{A}_{21}\mathbf{B}_{11} + \mathbf{A}_{22}\mathbf{B}_{21} & \mathbf{A}_{21}\mathbf{B}_{12} + \mathbf{A}_{22}\mathbf{B}_{22} \end{pmatrix} = \begin{pmatrix} \mathbf{I} & \mathbf{0} \\ \mathbf{0} & \mathbf{I} \end{pmatrix}.$$

Since $\mathbf{A}_{22}$ is nonsingular, $\mathbf{A}_{21}\mathbf{B}_{11} + \mathbf{A}_{22}\mathbf{B}_{21} = \mathbf{0}$ implies that $\mathbf{B}_{21} = -\mathbf{A}_{22}^{-1}\mathbf{A}_{21}\mathbf{B}_{11}$. Substituting for $\mathbf{B}_{21}$ into $\mathbf{A}_{11}\mathbf{B}_{11} + \mathbf{A}_{12}\mathbf{B}_{21} = \mathbf{I}$, we get

$$\mathbf{A}_{11}\mathbf{B}_{11} + \mathbf{A}_{12}(-\mathbf{A}_{22}^{-1}\mathbf{A}_{21}\mathbf{B}_{11}) = \mathbf{I},$$

so that $\mathbf{B}_{11} = (\mathbf{A}_{11} - \mathbf{A}_{12}\mathbf{A}_{22}^{-1}\mathbf{A}_{21})^{-1}$. Then,

$$\mathbf{B}_{21} = -\mathbf{A}_{22}^{-1}\mathbf{A}_{21}\mathbf{B}_{11} = -\mathbf{A}_{22}^{-1}\mathbf{A}_{21}(\mathbf{A}_{11} - \mathbf{A}_{12}\mathbf{A}_{22}^{-1}\mathbf{A}_{21})^{-1}.$$

Again, since $\mathbf{A}_{21}\mathbf{B}_{12} + \mathbf{A}_{22}\mathbf{B}_{22} = \mathbf{I}$, we see that $\mathbf{B}_{22} = \mathbf{A}_{22}^{-1}(\mathbf{I} - \mathbf{A}_{21}\mathbf{B}_{12})$. Substituting this expression into $\mathbf{A}_{11}\mathbf{B}_{12} + \mathbf{A}_{12}\mathbf{B}_{22} = \mathbf{0}$, and solving for $\mathbf{B}_{12}$, we get $\mathbf{B}_{12} = -\mathbf{B}_{11}\mathbf{A}_{12}\mathbf{A}_{22}^{-1}$, and then

$$\mathbf{B}_{22} = \mathbf{A}_{22}^{-1}(\mathbf{I} - \mathbf{A}_{21}\mathbf{B}_{12}) = \mathbf{A}_{22}^{-1} + \mathbf{A}_{22}^{-1}\mathbf{A}_{21}\mathbf{B}_{11}\mathbf{A}_{12}\mathbf{A}_{22}^{-1},$$

completing the proof. ∎

Example 2.1.1. (continued).   We find the inverse of the matrix in (a). Since $|\mathbf{A}_{22}| = 5 \neq 0$, using (2.1.17) we see that $\mathbf{B}_{11} = \begin{pmatrix} 5 & -2 \\ -2 & 1 \end{pmatrix}$, $\mathbf{B}_{12} = \begin{pmatrix} 0 \\ 0 \end{pmatrix}$, $\mathbf{B}_{21} = \begin{pmatrix} -8/5 & 2/5 \end{pmatrix}$, and $\mathbf{B}_{22} = 1/5$, so that

$$\mathbf{A}^{-1} = \begin{pmatrix} 5 & -2 & 0 \\ -2 & 1 & 0 \\ -8/5 & 2/5 & 1/5 \end{pmatrix}.$$

Since $|\mathbf{A}_{11}| = 1$, we can also use (2.1.18) to get the same result.   □

Example 2.1.2. Suppose an $n \times k$ matrix $\mathbf{A}$ with $r(\mathbf{A}) = k$ is partitioned into $\mathbf{A} = \begin{pmatrix} \mathbf{A}_1 & \mathbf{A}_2 \end{pmatrix}$ where $\mathbf{A}_1$ is an $n \times r$ matrix of rank r and $\mathbf{A}_2$ is an $n \times (k-r)$ matrix of rank $(k-r)$. Let

$$\mathbf{P} = \mathbf{A}(\mathbf{A}'\mathbf{A})^{-1}\mathbf{A}', \quad \mathbf{P}_1 = \mathbf{A}_1(\mathbf{A}_1'\mathbf{A}_1)^{-1}\mathbf{A}_1',$$
$$\mathbf{B} = (\mathbf{I} - \mathbf{P}_1)\mathbf{A}_2, \quad \text{and}$$
$$\mathbf{P}_2 = \mathbf{B}(\mathbf{B}'\mathbf{B})^{-1}\mathbf{B}' = (\mathbf{I} - \mathbf{P}_1)\mathbf{A}_2[\mathbf{A}_2'(\mathbf{I} - \mathbf{P}_1)\mathbf{A}_2]^{-1}\mathbf{A}_2'(\mathbf{I} - \mathbf{P}_1).$$

It is easy to verify that $\mathbf{P} = \mathbf{P}_1 + \mathbf{P}_2$. Using (2.1.11), we first write

$$\mathbf{P} = \begin{pmatrix} \mathbf{A}_1 & \mathbf{A}_2 \end{pmatrix} \begin{pmatrix} \mathbf{A}_1'\mathbf{A}_1 & \mathbf{A}_1'\mathbf{A}_2 \\ \mathbf{A}_2'\mathbf{A}_1 & \mathbf{A}_2'\mathbf{A}_2 \end{pmatrix}^{-1} \begin{pmatrix} \mathbf{A}_1' \\ \mathbf{A}_2' \end{pmatrix}. \tag{2.1.19}$$

We use Result 2.1.3 to evaluate $(\mathbf{A}'\mathbf{A})^{-1}$ in partitioned form as

$$(\mathbf{A}'\mathbf{A})^{-1} = \begin{pmatrix} \mathbf{E} & \mathbf{F} \\ \mathbf{G} & \mathbf{N} \end{pmatrix} \tag{2.1.20}$$

where

$$\mathbf{E} = (\mathbf{A}_1'\mathbf{A}_1)^{-1} + (\mathbf{A}_1'\mathbf{A}_1)^{-1}\mathbf{A}_1'\mathbf{A}_2\mathbf{N}\mathbf{A}_2'\mathbf{A}_1(\mathbf{A}_1'\mathbf{A}_1)^{-1},$$
$$\mathbf{F} = -(\mathbf{A}_1'\mathbf{A}_1)^{-1}\mathbf{A}_1'\mathbf{A}_2\mathbf{N},$$
$$\mathbf{G} = -\mathbf{N}\mathbf{A}_2'\mathbf{A}_1(\mathbf{A}_1'\mathbf{A}_1)^{-1}, \quad \text{and}$$
$$\mathbf{N} = (\mathbf{A}_2'\mathbf{A}_2 - \mathbf{A}_2'\mathbf{A}_1(\mathbf{A}_1'\mathbf{A}_1)^{-1}\mathbf{A}_1'\mathbf{A}_2)^{-1}$$
$$= (\mathbf{A}_2'[\mathbf{I} - \mathbf{A}_1(\mathbf{A}_1'\mathbf{A}_1)^{-1}\mathbf{A}_1']\mathbf{A}_2)^{-1}$$
$$= [\mathbf{A}_2'(\mathbf{I} - \mathbf{P}_1)\mathbf{A}_2]^{-1}. \tag{2.1.21}$$

Substituting (2.1.20) into (2.1.19), we see that

$$
\begin{aligned}
\mathbf{P} &= \mathbf{P}_1 + \mathbf{P}_1\mathbf{A}_2\mathbf{N}\mathbf{A}_2'\mathbf{P}_1 - \mathbf{P}_1\mathbf{A}_2\mathbf{N}\mathbf{A}_2' - \mathbf{A}_2\mathbf{N}\mathbf{A}_2'\mathbf{P}_1 + \mathbf{A}_2\mathbf{N}\mathbf{A}_2' \\
&= \mathbf{P}_1 + (\mathbf{I} - \mathbf{P}_1)\mathbf{A}_2[\mathbf{A}_2'(\mathbf{I} - \mathbf{P}_1)\mathbf{A}_2]^{-1}\mathbf{A}_2'(\mathbf{I} - \mathbf{P}_1) \\
&= \mathbf{P}_1 + \mathbf{P}_2.
\end{aligned}
$$

This example is useful to show that the projection matrix in a linear model can be decomposed into the sum of two (or more) projection matrices. □

Example 2.1.3. Let $\mathbf{X}$ be an $n \times k$ matrix, let $\mathbf{X}_{(i)}$ denote the $(n-1) \times k$ matrix which is obtained by deleting the ith row $\mathbf{x}_i$. We can write the inverse of the symmetric $k \times k$ matrix $\mathbf{X}'\mathbf{X}$ as

$$
\begin{aligned}
(\mathbf{X}'\mathbf{X})^{-1} &= (\mathbf{X}_{(i)}'\mathbf{X}_{(i)} + \mathbf{x}_i\mathbf{x}_i')^{-1} \\
&= (\mathbf{X}_{(i)}'\mathbf{X}_{(i)})^{-1} - \frac{(\mathbf{X}_{(i)}'\mathbf{X}_{(i)})^{-1}\mathbf{x}_i\mathbf{x}_i'(\mathbf{X}_{(i)}'\mathbf{X}_{(i)})^{-1}}{1 + \mathbf{x}_i'(\mathbf{X}_{(i)}'\mathbf{X}_{(i)})^{-1}\mathbf{x}_i}, \quad (2.1.22)
\end{aligned}
$$

which follows directly by using property 5 of Result 1.2.10, setting $\mathbf{A} = \mathbf{X}_{(i)}'\mathbf{X}_{(i)}$, $\mathbf{B} = \mathbf{x}_i$, $\mathbf{C} = 1$, and $\mathbf{D} = \mathbf{x}_i'$. Similarly, if we use the same property and now set $\mathbf{A} = \mathbf{X}'\mathbf{X}$, $\mathbf{B} = -\mathbf{x}_i$, $\mathbf{C} = 1$, and $\mathbf{D} = \mathbf{x}_i'$, we obtain

$$
\begin{aligned}
(\mathbf{X}_{(i)}'\mathbf{X}_{(i)})^{-1} &= (\mathbf{X}'\mathbf{X} - \mathbf{x}_i\mathbf{x}_i')^{-1} \\
&= (\mathbf{X}'\mathbf{X})^{-1} + \frac{(\mathbf{X}'\mathbf{X})^{-1}\mathbf{x}_i\mathbf{x}_i'(\mathbf{X}'\mathbf{X})^{-1}}{1 - \mathbf{x}_i'(\mathbf{X}'\mathbf{X})^{-1}\mathbf{x}_i}. \quad (2.1.23)
\end{aligned}
$$

These results are useful in studying the effect of deleting an observation in a linear regression model (see Chapter 8). □

Example 2.1.4. Let $\mathbf{A}$ be a $k \times k$ nonsingular matrix, while $\mathbf{B}$ and $\mathbf{C}$ are $k \times m$ matrices. We will show that

$$
|\mathbf{A} - \mathbf{B}\mathbf{C}'| = |\mathbf{A}||\mathbf{I} - \mathbf{C}'\mathbf{A}^{-1}\mathbf{B}|. \quad (2.1.24)
$$

From (2.1.16), we see that

$$
\begin{vmatrix} \mathbf{A} & \mathbf{B} \\ \mathbf{C}' & \mathbf{I} \end{vmatrix} = |\mathbf{A}||\mathbf{I} - \mathbf{C}'\mathbf{A}^{-1}\mathbf{B}|, \quad (2.1.25)
$$

while from (2.1.15), we get

$$
\begin{vmatrix} \mathbf{A} & \mathbf{B} \\ \mathbf{C}' & \mathbf{I} \end{vmatrix} = |\mathbf{A} - \mathbf{B}\mathbf{C}'|. \quad (2.1.26)
$$

The required result follows by equating (2.1.26) with (2.1.25). □

2.2   Algorithms for matrix factorization

In this section, we present factorization methods that enable efficient computing in linear model theory and multivariate analysis. Although this is less a
statistical problem than it is a problem in numerical computing, it is useful
for a practicing statistician to have at least a rudimentary knowledge of such
techniques. These methods are especially valuable for an appreciation of the
development and computation of estimates and diagnostic measures in linear
models and are employed by most statistical software in order to produce numerically stable results. The decomposition of a matrix $\mathbf{A}$ into a product of
two or more matrices is useful in computing properties such as the rank, the
determinant or inverse of $\mathbf{A}$. We do not give an exhaustive presentation, and the
reader is referred to Golub and Van Loan (1989) or Stewart (1973) for details.

Result 2.2.1. Full-rank factorization.   Let $\mathbf{A}$ be an $m \times n$ matrix with
$r(\mathbf{A}) = r$. There exists an $m \times r$ matrix $\mathbf{B}$ and an $r \times n$ matrix $\mathbf{C}$ with
$r(\mathbf{B}) = r(\mathbf{C}) = r$ such that

$$\mathbf{A} = \mathbf{BC}. \qquad (2.2.1)$$

Proof.   We show the existence of such matrices $\mathbf{B}$ and $\mathbf{C}$. Since $r(\mathbf{A}) = r$,
the matrix $\mathbf{A}$ has r LIN rows and columns. Assume that the first r rows and
the first r columns are LIN (otherwise, permutation matrices may be used as
described at the end of the proof). The matrix $\mathbf{A}$ can be partitioned as

$$\mathbf{A} = \begin{pmatrix} \mathbf{X} & \mathbf{Y} \\ \mathbf{Z} & \mathbf{W} \end{pmatrix},$$

where $\mathbf{X}$, $\mathbf{Y}$, $\mathbf{Z}$, and $\mathbf{W}$ have respective dimensions $r \times r$, $r \times (n-r)$, $(m-r) \times r$,
and $(m - r) \times (n - r)$, and $\mathbf{X}$ is nonsingular. The first r rows in $\mathbf{A}$ are those of
$\begin{pmatrix} \mathbf{X} & \mathbf{Y} \end{pmatrix}$ and are LIN, so that the rows of $\begin{pmatrix} \mathbf{Z} & \mathbf{W} \end{pmatrix}$ are linear combinations of
those of $\begin{pmatrix} \mathbf{X} & \mathbf{Y} \end{pmatrix}$. Hence, for some matrix $\mathbf{F}$,

$$\begin{pmatrix} \mathbf{Z} & \mathbf{W} \end{pmatrix} = \mathbf{F} \begin{pmatrix} \mathbf{X} & \mathbf{Y} \end{pmatrix}. \qquad (2.2.2)$$

Applying a similar reasoning to the columns of $\mathbf{A}$, we have for a given matrix
$\mathbf{H}$,

$$\begin{pmatrix} \mathbf{Y} \\ \mathbf{W} \end{pmatrix} = \begin{pmatrix} \mathbf{X} \\ \mathbf{Z} \end{pmatrix} \mathbf{H}. \qquad (2.2.3)$$

From (2.2.2), $\mathbf{Z} = \mathbf{FX}$ and $\mathbf{W} = \mathbf{FY}$, while from (2.2.3), $\mathbf{Y} = \mathbf{XH}$. Hence,
$\mathbf{W} = \mathbf{FXH}$, and

$$\mathbf{A} = \begin{pmatrix} \mathbf{X} & \mathbf{Y} \\ \mathbf{Z} & \mathbf{W} \end{pmatrix} = \begin{pmatrix} \mathbf{X} & \mathbf{XH} \\ \mathbf{FX} & \mathbf{FXH} \end{pmatrix} = \begin{pmatrix} \mathbf{I} \\ \mathbf{F} \end{pmatrix} \mathbf{X} \begin{pmatrix} \mathbf{I} & \mathbf{H} \end{pmatrix}. \qquad (2.2.4)$$

Also, since $\mathbf{X}$ is nonsingular, $\mathbf{X}^{-1}$ exists, and hence $\mathbf{Z} = \mathbf{FX}$ implies that
$\mathbf{F} = \mathbf{ZX}^{-1}$, and $\mathbf{Y} = \mathbf{XH}$ implies that $\mathbf{H} = \mathbf{X}^{-1}\mathbf{Y}$. It follows that

$$\mathbf{W} = \mathbf{FY} = \mathbf{ZX}^{-1}\mathbf{Y}.$$

We can write (2.2.4) as

$$\mathbf{A} = \begin{pmatrix} \mathbf{X} & \mathbf{Y} \\ \mathbf{Z} & \mathbf{W} \end{pmatrix} = \begin{pmatrix} \mathbf{X} & \mathbf{Y} \\ \mathbf{Z} & \mathbf{ZX}^{-1}\mathbf{Y} \end{pmatrix} = \begin{pmatrix} \mathbf{I} \\ \mathbf{ZX}^{-1} \end{pmatrix} \mathbf{X} \begin{pmatrix} \mathbf{I} & \mathbf{X}^{-1}\mathbf{Y} \end{pmatrix}. \qquad (2.2.5)$$

Note that (2.2.4) can be further rewritten in two equivalent ways as

$$\mathbf{A} = \begin{pmatrix} \mathbf{X} \\ \mathbf{FX} \end{pmatrix} \begin{pmatrix} \mathbf{I} & \mathbf{H} \end{pmatrix} \quad \text{and} \quad \mathbf{A} = \begin{pmatrix} \mathbf{I} \\ \mathbf{F} \end{pmatrix} \begin{pmatrix} \mathbf{X} & \mathbf{XH} \end{pmatrix}, \qquad (2.2.6)$$

each of which is of the form $\mathbf{A} = \mathbf{BC}$, where $\mathbf{B}$ is an $m \times r$ matrix with full column rank $r = r(\mathbf{A})$, and $\mathbf{C}$ is an $r \times n$ matrix with full row rank $r = r(\mathbf{A})$.

Suppose that the first r rows and columns of $\mathbf{A}$ are not LIN. Let $\mathbf{M} = \mathbf{PAQ}$, where $\mathbf{P}$ and $\mathbf{Q}$ are permutation matrices. We obtain the full-rank factorization $\mathbf{M} = \mathbf{BC}$. By the orthogonality of $\mathbf{P}$ and $\mathbf{Q}$, we have $\mathbf{A} = \mathbf{P}^{-1}\mathbf{MQ}^{-1} = \mathbf{P}'\mathbf{BCQ}' = (\mathbf{P}'\mathbf{B})(\mathbf{CQ}')$, where $\mathbf{P}'\mathbf{B}$ and $\mathbf{CQ}'$ play the same roles as $\mathbf{B}$ and $\mathbf{C}$. This completes the proof. If $\mathbf{A}$ is a symmetric matrix of rank r, it has full-rank factorization $\mathbf{A} = \mathbf{LL}'$ with $r(\mathbf{L}) = r$. ∎

Result 2.2.2. Triangular decomposition. Let $\mathbf{A}$ be an $m \times m$ positive definite symmetric matrix (see Definition 2.4.5). There exists a unique unit lower triangular matrix $\mathbf{L}$ and a unique diagonal matrix $\mathbf{D}$ with positive diagonal elements such that

$$\begin{aligned} \mathbf{A} &= \mathbf{L}^{-1}\mathbf{DL}'^{-1}, \quad &\text{or, equivalently,} \\ \mathbf{LAL}' &= \mathbf{D}, \quad &\text{or, equivalently,} \\ \mathbf{A}^{-1} &= \mathbf{L}'\mathbf{D}^{-1}\mathbf{L}. \end{aligned} \qquad (2.2.7)$$

In the literature, there are three different, but mathematically equivalent versions of the triangular decomposition that go under different names. The first involves $\mathbf{L}^{-1}$ and $\mathbf{D}$, and is known as the Crout decomposition: $\mathbf{A} = (\mathbf{L}^{-1}\mathbf{D})\mathbf{L}'^{-1} = \mathbf{UL}'^{-1}$, say. The second form is called the Doolittle decomposition and combines matrices $\mathbf{D}$ and $\mathbf{L}'^{-1}$: $\mathbf{A} = \mathbf{L}^{-1}(\mathbf{DL}'^{-1}) = \mathbf{L}^{-1}\mathbf{U}'$, say. The third version is the Cholesky decomposition of $\mathbf{A}$, and is obtained by factoring $\mathbf{D}$ into $\mathbf{D} = \mathbf{D}^{1/2}\mathbf{D}^{1/2}$, so that we get $\mathbf{A} = (\mathbf{L}^{-1}\mathbf{D}^{1/2})(\mathbf{D}^{1/2}\mathbf{L}'^{-1}) = \mathbf{VV}'$, say, where $\mathbf{V} = \mathbf{L}^{-1}\mathbf{D}^{1/2}$ is a lower triangular matrix. We show a proof of the Cholesky decomposition here.

Proof. We show a proof by induction on the dimension m. When $m = 1$, $\mathbf{A}$ corresponds to a real scalar, and its Cholesky factorization is $\mathbf{A} = a^2$, where $a = \sqrt{\mathbf{A}}$. Assume the Cholesky decomposition for dimension $m - 1$, where $m > 1$. Suppose we partition $\mathbf{A}$ as

$$\mathbf{A} = \begin{pmatrix} \mathbf{A}_{11} & \mathbf{a}_{12} \\ \mathbf{a}_{21} & a_{22} \end{pmatrix}.$$

By the induction hypothesis, there exists a unique lower triangular $(m-1) \times (m-1)$ matrix $\mathbf{C}_1$ with positive diagonal entries such that $\mathbf{A}_{11} = \mathbf{C}_1\mathbf{C}_1'$. Let

$$\mathbf{C} = \begin{pmatrix} \mathbf{C}_1 & \mathbf{0} \\ \mathbf{c}' & c \end{pmatrix},$$

where $\mathbf{c}$ is an $(m-1)$-dimensional vector, and $c > 0$ is a scalar, both yet unknown. We obtain these from the requirement that $\mathbf{A} = \mathbf{C}\mathbf{C}'$, i.e., $\mathbf{C}_1\mathbf{C}_1' = \mathbf{A}_{11}$, $\mathbf{C}_1\mathbf{c} = \mathbf{a}_{12}$, and $\mathbf{c}'\mathbf{c} + c^2 = a_{22}$. It follows that $\mathbf{c} = \mathbf{C}_1^{-1}\mathbf{a}_{12}$, and $c = (a_{22} - \mathbf{c}'\mathbf{c})^{1/2}$, where $a_{22} - \mathbf{c}'\mathbf{c} > 0$, since $\mathbf{A}$ is positive definite.   ∎

Result 2.2.3. QR decomposition.   Let $\mathbf{A}$ be an $m \times n$ matrix with $r(\mathbf{A}) = n$. Then there exists an $m \times n$ matrix $\mathbf{Q}$ and an $n \times n$ upper triangular matrix $\mathbf{R}$ such that

$$\mathbf{A} = \mathbf{QR}, \qquad\qquad (2.2.8)$$

where $\mathbf{Q}$ is an orthogonal basis for the column space $\mathcal{C}(\mathbf{A})$ of the matrix $\mathbf{A}$.

Proof. Let $\mathbf{a}_1, \cdots, \mathbf{a}_n$ denote the columns of $\mathbf{A}$. The Gram-Schmidt orthogonalization (see Result 1.2.4) can be used to construct an orthogonal set of vectors $\mathbf{b}_1, \cdots, \mathbf{b}_n$ which are defined recursively by

$$\mathbf{b}_1 = \mathbf{a}_1$$

$$\mathbf{b}_i = \mathbf{a}_i - \sum_{j=1}^{i-1} c_{ji}\mathbf{b}_j, \quad i = 2, \cdots, n,$$

where $c_{ij} = \mathbf{a}_j'\mathbf{b}_i/\mathbf{b}_i'\mathbf{b}_i$, $i < j = 1, \cdots, n$. By construction, we define $\mathbf{Q} = (\mathbf{b}_1, \cdots, \mathbf{b}_n)$ to be the required $m \times n$ orthogonal matrix, while $\mathbf{R}$ denotes the $n \times n$ upper-triangular matrix whose (i,j)th element is given by c_{ij}, $i < j = 1, \cdots, n$. Then, the QR decomposition of $\mathbf{A}$ has the form $\mathbf{A} = \mathbf{QR}$.   ∎

The QR decomposition is useful for computing numerically stable estimates of coefficients in a linear model. Various orthogonalization algorithms have been employed in the literature (see Golub and Van Loan, 1989 or Stewart, 1973) which operate directly on the matrix of explanatory variables in a linear model. The QR decomposition also enables us to factor the projection matrix in linear model theory into the product of two orthogonal matrices, which is useful in the study of regression diagnostics (see Chapter 8).

Example 2.2.1.   Let $\mathbf{A} = \mathbf{LL}'$ denote a full-rank factorization of a symmetric matrix $\mathbf{A}$ of rank r, where $\mathbf{L}$ is an $n \times r$ matrix of full column rank. We will show that $\mathbf{L}'\mathbf{L}$ is nonsingular. Let $\mathbf{M}$ be a leading nonsingular submatrix of $\mathbf{L}$, with $r(\mathbf{M}) = r$, so that

$$\mathbf{L} = \begin{pmatrix} \mathbf{M} \\ \mathbf{N} \end{pmatrix}, \mathbf{L}' = \mathbf{M}' \begin{pmatrix} \mathbf{I} & (\mathbf{M}')^{-1}\mathbf{N}' \end{pmatrix} = \mathbf{M}' \begin{pmatrix} \mathbf{I} & \mathbf{S} \end{pmatrix}, \text{say, and}$$

$$\mathbf{L} = \begin{pmatrix} \mathbf{I} \\ \mathbf{S}' \end{pmatrix} \mathbf{M},$$

so that $\mathbf{L'L} = \mathbf{M'(I + SS')M}$. Since $\mathbf{M}$ has full rank, both $\mathbf{M}$ and $\mathbf{M'}$ are non-singular. We show that $\mathbf{I + SS'}$ is also nonsingular. Suppose, on the contrary, it is not. Then, there exists a nonzero vector $\mathbf{u}$ such that $\mathbf{(I + SS')u = 0}$, i.e., $\mathbf{u'(I + SS')u} = 0$, i.e., $\mathbf{u'u + u'S(u'S)'} = 0$, which is possible only if $\mathbf{u = 0}$. This contradicts our assumption, so $\mathbf{I + SS'}$ is nonsingular, and so is $\mathbf{L'L}$. □

In the next three sections, we present results that are crucial for the development of linear model theory and are related to the diagonalization of general matrices, and in particular to symmetric and p.d. matrices. We first give some definitions and basic ideas.

Definition 2.2.1. Diagonability of a matrix.   An $n \times n$ matrix $\mathbf{A}$ is said to be diagonalizable (or diagonable) if there exists an $n \times n$ nonsingular matrix $\mathbf{Q}$ such that

$$\mathbf{Q^{-1}AQ = D}, \tag{2.2.9}$$

where $\mathbf{D}$ is a diagonal matrix. The matrix $\mathbf{Q}$ diagonalizes $\mathbf{A}$ and further, $\mathbf{Q^{-1}AQ = D}$ if and only if $\mathbf{AQ = QD}$, i.e., if and only if $\mathbf{A = QDQ^{-1}}$.

The process of constructing a matrix $\mathbf{Q}$ which diagonalizes $\mathbf{A}$ is referred to as the diagonalization of $\mathbf{A}$; in many cases, we can relate this to the eigensystem of $\mathbf{A}$. In Result 2.2.5, we show how to diagonalize an arbitrary $n \times n$ matrix $\mathbf{A}$. In section 2.3, we show that a symmetric matrix $\mathbf{A}$ is *orthogonally diagonable*.

Definition 2.2.2. Orthogonal diagonability.   An $n \times n$ matrix $\mathbf{A}$ is said to be orthogonally diagonable if and only if there exists an $n \times n$ orthogonal matrix $\mathbf{P}$ such that $\mathbf{P'AP}$ is a diagonal matrix.

Result 2.2.4. Let $\mathbf{A}$ be an $n \times n$ matrix. Suppose there exists an $n \times n$ nonsingular matrix $\mathbf{Q}$ such that $\mathbf{Q^{-1}AQ = D} = \text{diag}(\lambda_1, \cdots, \lambda_n)$. Let $\mathbf{Q} = (\mathbf{q}_1, \cdots, \mathbf{q}_n)$. Then,

1. $r(\mathbf{A})$ is equal to the number of nonzero diagonal elements in $\mathbf{D}$.

2. $|\mathbf{A}| = \prod_{i=1}^{n} \lambda_i = |\mathbf{D}|$.

3. $tr(\mathbf{A}) = \sum_{i=1}^{n} \lambda_i = tr(\mathbf{D})$.

4. The characteristic polynomial of $\mathbf{A}$ is $P(\lambda) = (-1)^n \prod_{i=1}^{n} (\lambda - \lambda_i)$.

5. The eigenvalues of $\mathbf{A}$ are $\lambda_1, \cdots \lambda_n$, which are not necessarily all nonzero, nor are they necessarily distinct.

6. The columns of $\mathbf{Q}$ are the LIN eigenvectors of $\mathbf{A}$, where $\mathbf{q}_i$ corresponds to the eigenvalue λ_i.

Proof. Since $\mathbf{Q}$ is a nonsingular matrix, $r(\mathbf{A}) = r(\mathbf{Q}^{-1}\mathbf{AQ}) = r(\mathbf{D})$, which is clearly equal to the number of nonzero diagonal elements λ_i, $i = 1, \cdots, n$, which proves property 1. The proof of property 2 follows from seeing that

$$|\mathbf{A}| = |\mathbf{Q}^{-1}\mathbf{Q}||\mathbf{A}| = |\mathbf{Q}^{-1}\mathbf{AQ}| = |\mathbf{D}| = \prod_{i=1}^{n} \lambda_i.$$

Similarly, $tr(\mathbf{A}) = tr(\mathbf{QQ}^{-1}\mathbf{A}) = tr(\mathbf{Q}^{-1}\mathbf{AQ}) = tr(\mathbf{D}) = \sum_{i=1}^{n} \lambda_i$, which proves property 3. By property 2, for any scalar λ, $|\mathbf{D} - \lambda\mathbf{I}| = |\mathbf{Q}^{-1}\mathbf{AQ} - \lambda\mathbf{I}| = |\mathbf{Q}^{-1}(\mathbf{A} - \lambda\mathbf{I})\mathbf{Q}| = |\mathbf{A} - \lambda\mathbf{I}|$, so that the characteristic polynomials of $\mathbf{D}$ and $\mathbf{A}$ coincide, which proves property 4, of which property 5 is a direct consequence. Now, $\mathbf{Q}^{-1}\mathbf{AQ} = \mathbf{D}$ implies that $\mathbf{AQ} = \mathbf{QD}$, i.e., $\mathbf{Aq}_i = \lambda_i\mathbf{q}_i$, $i = 1, \cdots, n$. Since λ_i, $i = 1, \cdots, n$ are the eigenvalues of $\mathbf{A}$, property 6 follows. ∎

Result 2.2.5. Diagonability theorem. An $n \times n$ matrix $\mathbf{A}$ having eigenvalues λ_k with algebraic multiplicities a_k, $k = 1, \cdots, s$, with $\sum_{k=1}^{s} a_k = n$, has n LIN eigenvectors if and only if $r(\mathbf{A} - \lambda_k\mathbf{I}) = n - a_k$, $k = 1, \cdots, s$. Then the matrix of eigenvectors $\mathbf{U} = (u_1, \cdots, u_n)$ is nonsingular and $\mathbf{A}$ is diagonable as $\mathbf{U}^{-1}\mathbf{AU} = \mathbf{D} = \text{diag}(\lambda_1, \cdots, \lambda_n)$.

Proof. Sufficiency. Suppose $r(\mathbf{A} - \lambda_k\mathbf{I}) = n - a_k$, $k = 1, \cdots, s$. This implies that $(\mathbf{A} - \lambda_k\mathbf{I})\mathbf{x} = \mathbf{0}$ has exactly $n - (n - a_k) = a_k$ LIN nonzero solutions which are the eigenvectors of $\mathbf{A}$. Corresponding to each λ_k, there exists a set of a_k LIN eigenvectors. We must show that these sets are linearly independent of each other. Suppose that, on the contrary, they are not LIN. Let $(\mathbf{z}_1, \cdots, \mathbf{z}_{a_1})$ and $(\mathbf{y}_1, \cdots, \mathbf{y}_{a_2})$ denote the two sets of vectors and suppose $\mathbf{y}_2$ is a linear combination of $\mathbf{z}_1, \cdots, \mathbf{z}_{a_1}$, i.e., $\mathbf{y}_2 = \sum_{i=1}^{a_1} c_i\mathbf{z}_i$, where not all the c_i's are zero. Now, $\mathbf{Ay}_2 = \sum_{i=1}^{a_1} c_i\mathbf{Az}_i$, which implies that $\lambda_2\mathbf{y}_2 = \sum_{i=1}^{a_1} c_i\lambda_1\mathbf{z}_i = \lambda_1 \sum_{i=1}^{a_1} c_i\mathbf{z}_i = \lambda_1\mathbf{y}_2$, which is impossible, since $\lambda_1 \neq \lambda_2$. Hence, our supposition is incorrect and all the s sets of a_k eigenvectors must be LIN and hence the matrix $\mathbf{U}$ is nonsingular.
Necessity. Suppose $\mathbf{U}^{-1}\mathbf{AU} = \mathbf{D}$ exists. Given $\mathbf{D} = \text{diag}(\lambda_1, \cdots, \lambda_n)$, the matrix $\mathbf{D} - \lambda_k\mathbf{I}$ has exactly a_k zero values on its diagonal since $r(\mathbf{D} - \lambda_k\mathbf{I}) = n - a_k$. Now, $\mathbf{U}^{-1}\mathbf{AU} = \mathbf{D}$, which implies that $\mathbf{A} = \mathbf{UDU}^{-1}$. So, $\mathbf{A} - \lambda_k\mathbf{I} = \mathbf{UDU}^{-1} - \lambda_k\mathbf{I} = \mathbf{U}(\mathbf{D} - \lambda_k\mathbf{I})\mathbf{U}^{-1}$, from which it follows that $r(\mathbf{A} - \lambda_k\mathbf{I}) = r(\mathbf{D} - \lambda_k\mathbf{I}) = n - a_k$. ∎

A general result on the decomposition of an $m \times n$ matrix $\mathbf{A}$ is given by the singular-value decomposition, which is shown in the next result. We leave its proof to the reader.

Result 2.2.6. Let $\mathbf{A}$ be an $m \times n$ matrix of rank r. Let $\mathbf{P}$ be an $m \times m$ orthogonal matrix, let $\mathbf{Q}$ be an $n \times n$ orthogonal matrix, and $\mathbf{D}_1 = \text{diag}(d_1, \cdots, d_r)$ be an $r \times r$ diagonal matrix with $d_i > 0$, $i = 1, \cdots, r$. Suppose we partition $\mathbf{P}$ and

$\mathbf{Q}$ as $\mathbf{P} = \begin{pmatrix} \mathbf{P}_1 & \mathbf{P}_2 \end{pmatrix}$ and $\mathbf{Q} = \begin{pmatrix} \mathbf{Q}_1 & \mathbf{Q}_2 \end{pmatrix}$. The singular-value decomposition of $\mathbf{A}$ is

$$\mathbf{A} = \mathbf{P} \begin{pmatrix} \mathbf{D}_1 & \mathbf{0} \\ \mathbf{0} & \mathbf{0} \end{pmatrix} \mathbf{Q}' = \mathbf{P}_1 \mathbf{D}_1 \mathbf{Q}_1', \text{ or}$$

$$\mathbf{A} = \sum_{i=1}^{r} d_i \mathbf{p}_i \mathbf{q}_i',$$

where $\mathbf{p}_1, \cdots, \mathbf{p}_r$ are the r columns of $\mathbf{P}_1$, and $\mathbf{q}_1, \cdots, \mathbf{q}_r$ are the r columns of $\mathbf{Q}_1$.

The scalars $d_1, \cdots, d_r$, which are called the singular values of $\mathbf{A}$, are the positive square roots of the (not necessarily distinct) nonzero eigenvalues of $\mathbf{A}'\mathbf{A}$, which do not vary with the choice of $\mathbf{P}$ and $\mathbf{Q}$. The m columns of $\mathbf{P}$ are eigenvectors of $\mathbf{A}\mathbf{A}'$, with the first r columns corresponding to the nonzero eigenvalues $d_1^2, \cdots, d_r^2$, while the remaining $m - r$ columns correspond to the zero eigenvalues. Similarly, the n columns of $\mathbf{Q}$ are eigenvectors of $\mathbf{A}'\mathbf{A}$, with the first r columns corresponding to the nonzero eigenvalues $d_1^2, \cdots, d_r^2$, and the remaining $n - r$ columns corresponding to the zero eigenvalues. Once the first r columns of $\mathbf{P}$ are specified, the first r columns of $\mathbf{Q}$ are uniquely determined, and vice versa (see Harville, 1997, section 21.12 for more details).

2.3 Symmetric and idempotent matrices

Recall from Definition 1.2.15 that an $n \times n$ matrix $\mathbf{A}$ is symmetric if $\mathbf{A}' = \mathbf{A}$. We now give several results on symmetric matrices that are useful in the theory of linear models.

Result 2.3.1. Let $\mathbf{A}$ be an $n \times n$ symmetric matrix. There exist vectors $\mathbf{x}_1$ and $\mathbf{x}_2$ such that

$$\frac{\mathbf{x}_1' \mathbf{A} \mathbf{x}_1}{\mathbf{x}_1' \mathbf{x}_1} \leq \frac{\mathbf{x}' \mathbf{A} \mathbf{x}}{\mathbf{x}' \mathbf{x}} \leq \frac{\mathbf{x}_2' \mathbf{A} \mathbf{x}_2}{\mathbf{x}_2' \mathbf{x}_2} \tag{2.3.1}$$

for every nonzero vector $\mathbf{x} \in \mathcal{R}^n$. Here, $\mathbf{x}_1' \mathbf{A} \mathbf{x}_1 / \mathbf{x}_1' \mathbf{x}_1$ and $\mathbf{x}_2' \mathbf{A} \mathbf{x}_2 / \mathbf{x}_2' \mathbf{x}_2$ are respectively the smallest and largest eigenvalues of $\mathbf{A}$, while $\mathbf{x}_1$ and $\mathbf{x}_2$ are the eigenvectors corresponding to these eigenvalues.

Proof. Define $S = \{\mathbf{x} : \mathbf{x}'\mathbf{x} = 1\}$. The quadratic form $\mathbf{x}'\mathbf{A}\mathbf{x}$ is a continuous function of $\mathbf{x}$, and S is a closed and bounded set. Therefore, $\mathbf{x}'\mathbf{A}\mathbf{x}$ attains a maximum and a minimum value over S, i.e., there exist $\mathbf{x}_1$ and $\mathbf{x}_2$ in S such that, for every $\mathbf{x} \in S$,

$$\mathbf{x}_1' \mathbf{A} \mathbf{x}_1 \leq \mathbf{x}' \mathbf{A} \mathbf{x} \leq \mathbf{x}_2' \mathbf{A} \mathbf{x}_2.$$

Clearly, $\mathbf{u} = \mathbf{x}/\sqrt{\mathbf{x}'\mathbf{x}} \in S$, and $\mathbf{u}'\mathbf{A}\mathbf{u} = \mathbf{x}'\mathbf{A}\mathbf{x}/\mathbf{x}'\mathbf{x}$. Therefore, for every $\mathbf{x} \in S$,

$$\mathbf{x}_1' \mathbf{A} \mathbf{x}_1 / \mathbf{x}_1' \mathbf{x}_1 = \mathbf{x}_1' \mathbf{A} \mathbf{x}_1 \leq \mathbf{x}' \mathbf{A} \mathbf{x} / \mathbf{x}' \mathbf{x} \leq \mathbf{x}_2' \mathbf{A} \mathbf{x}_2 = \mathbf{x}_2' \mathbf{A} \mathbf{x}_2 / \mathbf{x}_2' \mathbf{x}_2.$$

By property 3 in Result 2.7.1,

$$\frac{\partial \left(\mathbf{x}' \mathbf{A} \mathbf{x} / \mathbf{x}' \mathbf{x} \right)}{\partial \mathbf{x}} = (\mathbf{x}' \mathbf{x})^{-2} [(\mathbf{x}' \mathbf{x}) 2 \mathbf{A} \mathbf{x} - (\mathbf{x}' \mathbf{A} \mathbf{x}) 2 \mathbf{x}]. \qquad (2.3.2)$$

Since $\mathbf{x}' \mathbf{A} \mathbf{x} / \mathbf{x}' \mathbf{x}$ attains its minimum at $\mathbf{x}_1$ and its maximum at $\mathbf{x}_2$, we set the expression in (2.3.2) to zero, which gives

$$\mathbf{A} \mathbf{x} = \left(\frac{\mathbf{x}' \mathbf{A} \mathbf{x}}{\mathbf{x}' \mathbf{x}} \right) \mathbf{x}, \qquad (2.3.3)$$

so that, by Definition 1.2.32, we conclude that $\mathbf{x}_1' \mathbf{A} \mathbf{x}_1 / \mathbf{x}_1' \mathbf{x}_1$ and $\mathbf{x}_2' \mathbf{A} \mathbf{x}_2 / \mathbf{x}_2' \mathbf{x}_2$ are real eigenvalues of $\mathbf{A}$, with corresponding eigenvectors $\mathbf{x}_1$ and $\mathbf{x}_2$.   ∎

Result 2.3.2. The eigenvalues of every real symmetric matrix are real-valued. That is, if a symmetric matrix has all real-valued elements, its eigenvalues cannot be complex-valued.

Proof.   A proof follows directly from Result 2.3.1. An alternate proof implicitly uses the fundamental theorem of algebra which states that every polynomial equation of the form

$$a_0 + a_1 x + a_2 x^2 + \cdots + a_n x^n = 0$$

where a_0, a_1, a_2, $\cdots$, a_n are arbitrary real numbers, $a_n \neq 0$, has a solution among the complex numbers if $n \geq 1$. This statement is true even if the coefficients a_0, a_1, a_2, $\cdots$, a_n are complex-valued. The idea is that, in order to solve polynomial equations with possibly complex coefficients, it is not necessary to construct numbers more general than complex numbers. The proof follows. Let $\mathbf{A}$ be an $n \times n$ real symmetric matrix. If possible, let $\lambda = \alpha + i \beta$, where $i = \sqrt{-1}$, be a complex eigenvalue of $\mathbf{A}$. Since $\mathbf{A}$ is real, any complex eigenvalues must occur in conjugate pairs. Let $\lambda^* = \alpha - i \beta$ denote the complex conjugate of λ. Let $\mathbf{x} = (x_1, \cdots, x_n)' = \mathbf{a} + i \mathbf{b}$ and $\mathbf{x}^* = \mathbf{a} - i \mathbf{b}$ denote the eigenvectors corresponding to λ and λ^* respectively. By Definition 1.2.32, $\mathbf{A} \mathbf{x} = \lambda \mathbf{x}$, so that

$$\mathbf{x}^{*'} \mathbf{A} \mathbf{x} = \mathbf{x}^{*'} \lambda \mathbf{x} = \lambda \mathbf{x}^{*'} \mathbf{x}. \qquad (2.3.4)$$

We also have $\mathbf{A} \mathbf{x}^* = \lambda^* \mathbf{x}^*$, so that

$$\mathbf{x}^{*'} \mathbf{A} \mathbf{x} = (\mathbf{A} \mathbf{x}^*)' \mathbf{x} = (\lambda^* \mathbf{x}^*)' \mathbf{x} = \lambda^* \mathbf{x}^{*'} \mathbf{x}. \qquad (2.3.5)$$

Equating (2.3.4) and (2.3.5), we get

$$\lambda \mathbf{x}^{*'} \mathbf{x} = \lambda^* \mathbf{x}^{*'} \mathbf{x}.$$

Since $\mathbf{x}^{*'} \mathbf{x}$ is nonzero, being the sum of squares of elements of a nonzero real vector, we must have that $\lambda = \lambda^*$, i.e., $\alpha + i \beta = \alpha - i \beta$, so that λ must be real-valued.   ∎

Result 2.3.3. Let $\mathbf{x}_1$ and $\mathbf{x}_2$ be two eigenvectors corresponding to two distinct eigenvalues λ_1 and λ_2 of an $n \times n$ symmetric matrix $\mathbf{A}$. Then, $\mathbf{x}_1$ and $\mathbf{x}_2$ are orthogonal.

Proof. We are given that $\mathbf{A} = \mathbf{A}'$, and $\mathbf{A}\mathbf{x}_j = \lambda_j \mathbf{x}_j$, $j = 1, 2$. Since $\mathbf{x}_j' \mathbf{A} \mathbf{x}_j$ is a scalar for $j = 1, 2$, we have

$$\lambda_1 \mathbf{x}_2' \mathbf{x}_1 = \mathbf{x}_2' \lambda_1 \mathbf{x}_1 = \mathbf{x}_2' \mathbf{A} \mathbf{x}_1 = \mathbf{x}_1' \mathbf{A} \mathbf{x}_2 = \mathbf{x}_1' \lambda_2 \mathbf{x}_2 = \lambda_2 \mathbf{x}_1' \mathbf{x}_2 = \lambda_2 \mathbf{x}_2' \mathbf{x}_1.$$

Since $\lambda_1 \neq \lambda_2$, we must have $\mathbf{x}_2' \mathbf{x}_1 = 0$. By Definition 1.2.8, $\mathbf{x}_1$ and $\mathbf{x}_2$ are orthogonal. For a more general alternate proof which is applicable when the eigenvalues are not necessarily distinct, see Corollary 21.5.9 in Harville (1997). ∎

Example 2.3.1. Let $\mathbf{A} = \begin{pmatrix} 2 & 2 \\ 2 & -1 \end{pmatrix}$. Then

$$|\mathbf{A} - \lambda \mathbf{I}| = \begin{vmatrix} 2 - \lambda & 2 \\ 2 & -1 - \lambda \end{vmatrix} = -(2 - \lambda)(1 + \lambda) - 4 = 0;$$

the solutions are $\lambda = 3$, and $\lambda = -2$, which are the eigenvalues of $\mathbf{A}$. It is easy to verify that the corresponding eigenvectors are $(2, 1)'$ and $(1, -2)'$, which are clearly orthogonal. □

Result 2.3.4. Spectral decomposition of symmetric matrices. An $n \times n$ matrix $\mathbf{A}$ with eigenvalues λ_k and corresponding eigenvectors $\mathbf{p}_k$, $k = 1, \cdots, n$, is diagonable by an orthogonal matrix $\mathbf{P} = (\mathbf{p}_1, \cdots, \mathbf{p}_n)$ such that

$$\mathbf{P}'\mathbf{A}\mathbf{P} = \mathbf{D} = \operatorname{diag}(\lambda_1, \cdots, \lambda_n), \tag{2.3.6}$$

if and only if $\mathbf{A}$ is symmetric. In other words, every symmetric matrix is orthogonally diagonable. The spectral decomposition of $\mathbf{A}$ is

$$\mathbf{A} = \sum_{k=1}^{n} \lambda_k \mathbf{p}_k \mathbf{p}_k'. \tag{2.3.7}$$

Proof. Necessity. Let $\mathbf{A}$ be any $n \times n$ matrix, and suppose there exists an $n \times n$ orthogonal matrix $\mathbf{P}$ such that $\mathbf{P}'\mathbf{A}\mathbf{P} = \mathbf{D}$, where $\mathbf{D}$ is a diagonal matrix (and hence symmetric). It follows that $\mathbf{A} = \mathbf{P}\mathbf{D}\mathbf{P}'$, so that

$$\mathbf{A}' = (\mathbf{P}\mathbf{D}\mathbf{P}')' = \mathbf{P}\mathbf{D}'\mathbf{P}' = \mathbf{P}\mathbf{D}\mathbf{P}'$$

so that $\mathbf{A}$ is symmetric (see Definition 1.2.15).
Sufficiency. We prove this by induction. Clearly every 1×1 symmetric matrix $\mathbf{A}$ (which corresponds to a scalar) is orthogonally diagonable. Suppose that every $(n - 1) \times (n - 1)$ symmetric matrix $\mathbf{A}$ is orthogonally diagonable, $n \geq 2$. Now consider the symmetric $n \times n$ matrix $\mathbf{A}$ with an eigenvalue equal to λ,

and corresponding normal eigenvector equal to $\mathbf{u}$ (so that $\mathbf{u}'\mathbf{u} = 1$). By Gram-Schmidt orthogonalization (see Result 1.2.4), there exists an $n \times (n-1)$ matrix $\mathbf{V}$ such that the $n \times n$ matrix $(\mathbf{u}, \mathbf{V})$ is orthogonal, and

$$(\mathbf{u}, \mathbf{V})'\mathbf{A}(\mathbf{u}, \mathbf{V}) = \begin{pmatrix} \mathbf{u}'\mathbf{Au} & \mathbf{u}'\mathbf{AV} \\ \mathbf{V}'\mathbf{Au} & \mathbf{V}'\mathbf{AV} \end{pmatrix}. \tag{2.3.8}$$

Since $\mathbf{Au} = \lambda\mathbf{u}$ (by Definition 1.2.32), $\mathbf{u}'\mathbf{Au} = \lambda\mathbf{u}'\mathbf{u} = \lambda$; also

$$\mathbf{V}'\mathbf{Au} = \mathbf{V}'\lambda\mathbf{u} = \lambda\mathbf{V}'\mathbf{u} = \mathbf{0}$$

(by the orthogonal construction), and $\mathbf{u}'\mathbf{AV} = \mathbf{0}$ (transposing $\mathbf{V}'\mathbf{Au}$). Hence (2.3.8) becomes

$$(\mathbf{u}, \mathbf{V})'\mathbf{A}(\mathbf{u}, \mathbf{V}) = \begin{pmatrix} \lambda & \mathbf{0} \\ \mathbf{0} & \mathbf{V}'\mathbf{AV} \end{pmatrix} = \mathrm{diag}(\lambda, \mathbf{V}'\mathbf{AV}).$$

Since $\mathbf{V}'\mathbf{AV}$ is symmetric, it is orthogonally diagonable by the induction hypothesis; i.e., there exists an $(n-1) \times (n-1)$ orthogonal matrix $\mathbf{R}$, and a diagonal matrix $\mathbf{F}$ such that

$$\mathbf{R}'\mathbf{V}'\mathbf{AVR} = \mathbf{F}.$$

Define

$$\mathbf{S} = \mathrm{diag}(1, \mathbf{R}) \quad \text{and} \quad \mathbf{P} = (\mathbf{u}, \mathbf{V})\mathbf{S}.$$

Using the orthogonality of $\mathbf{R}$, it may be verified that

$$\mathbf{S}'\mathbf{S} = \mathrm{diag}(1, \mathbf{R}'\mathbf{R}) = \mathrm{diag}(1, \mathbf{I}_{n-1}) = \mathbf{I}_n,$$

so that $\mathbf{S}$ is orthogonal. The matrix $\mathbf{P}$, being the product of two orthogonal matrices is also orthogonal. Further,

$$\begin{aligned} \mathbf{P}'\mathbf{AP} &= \mathbf{S}'(\mathbf{u}, \mathbf{V})'\mathbf{A}(\mathbf{u}, \mathbf{V})\mathbf{S} \\ &= \mathbf{S}'\mathrm{diag}(\lambda, \mathbf{V}'\mathbf{AV})\mathbf{S} \\ &= \mathrm{diag}(\lambda, \mathbf{R}'\mathbf{V}'\mathbf{AVR}) \\ &= \mathrm{diag}(\lambda, \mathbf{F}), \end{aligned}$$

so that $\mathbf{P}'\mathbf{AP}$ is a diagonal matrix. To summarize, using the eigenvectors of $\mathbf{A}$, we have constructed an orthogonal matrix $\mathbf{P}$ such that $\mathbf{P}'\mathbf{AP}$ is a diagonal matrix. $\blacksquare$

Result 2.3.5. Let $\mathbf{A}$ be an $n \times n$ nonsingular symmetric matrix. Then $\mathbf{A}$ and $\mathbf{A}^{-1}$ have the same eigenvectors, while the eigenvalues of $\mathbf{A}^{-1}$ are the reciprocals of the eigenvalues of $\mathbf{A}$.

Proof. By Result 2.3.4, we have $\mathbf{P}'\mathbf{AP} = \mathbf{D}$. Since $\mathbf{P}$ is an orthogonal matrix, this implies $\mathbf{A} = \mathbf{PDP}'$. Let $\mathbf{B} = \mathbf{PD}^{-1}\mathbf{P}'$, where $\mathbf{D}^{-1}$ denotes the regular inverse of the diagonal matrix $\mathbf{D}$, which is itself diagonal with elements that are the reciprocals of the diagonal elements of $\mathbf{D}$, which in turn are the eigenvalues of $\mathbf{A}$. The matrix $\mathbf{B}$ is clearly symmetric and its eigenvalues are the reciprocals of the eigenvalues of $\mathbf{A}$, while its eigenvector matrix is $\mathbf{P}$. Now,

$$\mathbf{AB} = \mathbf{PDP'PD^{-1}P'} = \mathbf{PDD^{-1}P'} = \mathbf{PP'} = \mathbf{I}_n$$

and similarly, $\mathbf{BA} = \mathbf{I}_n$. Hence, $\mathbf{B} = \mathbf{A}^{-1}$. ∎

Result 2.3.6. Let $\mathbf{A}$ be a symmetric $n \times n$ matrix with eigenvalues $\lambda_1, \cdots, \lambda_n$. Then

1. $tr(\mathbf{A}) = \sum_{i=1}^{n} \lambda_i$.

2. $tr(\mathbf{A}^s) = \sum_{i=1}^{n} \lambda_i^s$.

3. $tr(\mathbf{A}^{-1}) = \sum_{i=1}^{n} 1/\lambda_i$, provided $\mathbf{A}$ is nonsingular.

Proof. By Result 2.3.4, there exists an orthogonal matrix $\mathbf{P}$ such that $\mathbf{P'AP} = \mathbf{D}$, where $\mathbf{D} = \mathrm{diag}(\lambda_1, \cdots, \lambda_n)$. Since $\mathbf{P}$ is orthogonal, $\mathbf{P'P} = \mathbf{PP'} = \mathbf{I}_n$ and

$$\textstyle\sum_{i=1}^{n} \lambda_i = tr(\mathbf{D}) = tr(\mathbf{P'AP}) = tr(\mathbf{PP'A}) = tr(\mathbf{A}),$$

proving property 1. Note that property 1 holds for all square matrices. To prove property 2, once again, from the orthogonality of $\mathbf{P}$, it follows that

$$\mathbf{D}^s = (\mathbf{P'AP})(\mathbf{P'AP}) \cdots (\mathbf{P'AP}) = (\mathbf{P'A^sP})$$

and so $\sum_{i=1}^{n} \lambda_i^s = tr(\mathbf{D}^s) = tr(\mathbf{P'A^sP}) = tr(\mathbf{A}^s)$. To show property 3, note that

$$\mathbf{D}^{-1} = (\mathbf{P'AP})^{-1} = \mathbf{P'A^{-1}P},$$

from which the result follows directly. ∎

Result 2.3.7. Let $\mathbf{A}$ and $\mathbf{B}$ be $m \times n$ matrices. Let $\mathbf{C}$ be a $p \times m$ matrix with $r(\mathbf{C}) = m$, and let $\mathbf{D}$ be an $n \times p$ matrix with $r(\mathbf{D}) = n$.

1. If $\mathbf{CA} = \mathbf{CB}$, then $\mathbf{A} = \mathbf{B}$.

2. If $\mathbf{AD} = \mathbf{BD}$, then $\mathbf{A} = \mathbf{B}$.

3. If $\mathbf{CAD} = \mathbf{CBD}$, then $\mathbf{A} = \mathbf{B}$.

Proof. We prove only property 3 here; the proofs of the first two properties follow as special cases. Since $\mathbf{C}$ and $\mathbf{D}$ have respectively full row and column ranks, let $\mathbf{L}$ and $\mathbf{R}$ denote their respective left and right inverses (which exist). Then, $\mathbf{CAD} = \mathbf{CBD}$ implies

$$\mathbf{A} = \mathbf{IAI} = \mathbf{LCADR} = \mathbf{LCBDR} = \mathbf{IBI} = \mathbf{B}$$

which proves the result. ∎

Result 2.3.8. Let $\mathbf{A}$ be an $m \times n$ matrix.

1. For $n \times p$ matrices $\mathbf{B}$ and $\mathbf{C}$, $\mathbf{AB} = \mathbf{AC}$ if and only if $\mathbf{A}'\mathbf{AB} = \mathbf{A}'\mathbf{AC}$.

2. For $p \times n$ matrices $\mathbf{E}$ and $\mathbf{F}$, $\mathbf{EA}' = \mathbf{FA}'$ if and only if $\mathbf{EA}'\mathbf{A} = \mathbf{FA}'\mathbf{A}$.

Proof. To prove property 1, note that if $\mathbf{AB} = \mathbf{AC}$, then $\mathbf{A}'\mathbf{AB} = \mathbf{A}'\mathbf{AC}$ holds. Now suppose that $\mathbf{A}'\mathbf{AB} = \mathbf{A}'\mathbf{AC}$ holds. We must show that this implies $\mathbf{AB} = \mathbf{AC}$. We have $\mathbf{0} = (\mathbf{A}'\mathbf{AB} - \mathbf{A}'\mathbf{AC}) = (\mathbf{B}' - \mathbf{C}')(\mathbf{A}'\mathbf{AB} - \mathbf{A}'\mathbf{AC}) = (\mathbf{AB} - \mathbf{AC})'(\mathbf{AB} - \mathbf{AC})$, which implies that $\mathbf{AB} - \mathbf{AC} = \mathbf{0}$ (see Exercise 2.11). The proof of property 2 follows directly by transposing relevant matrices in property 1.   ∎

Definition 2.3.1. An $n \times n$ matrix $\mathbf{A}$ is said to be idempotent if $\mathbf{A}^2 = \mathbf{A}$. We say that $\mathbf{A}$ is symmetric and idempotent if $\mathbf{A}' = \mathbf{A}$ and $\mathbf{A}^2 = \mathbf{A}$.

Examples of symmetric and idempotent matrices include the identity matrix $\mathbf{I}_n$, the matrix $\bar{\mathbf{J}}_n = \frac{1}{n}\mathbf{J}_n$ and the centering matrix $\mathbf{C}_n = \mathbf{I}_n - \bar{\mathbf{J}}_n$. We complete this section with some properties of idempotent matrices.

Result 2.3.9. Properties of idempotent matrices.

1. $\mathbf{A}'$ is idempotent if and only if $\mathbf{A}$ is idempotent.

2. $\mathbf{I} - \mathbf{A}$ is idempotent if and only if $\mathbf{A}$ is idempotent.

3. If $\mathbf{A}$ is an $n \times n$ idempotent matrix, then $r(\mathbf{A}) = tr(\mathbf{A})$ and $r(\mathbf{I}_n - \mathbf{A}) = n - tr(\mathbf{A})$.

4. If $r(\mathbf{A}) = n$ for an $n \times n$ idempotent matrix $\mathbf{A}$, then we must have $\mathbf{A} = \mathbf{I}_n$.

Proof. To prove property 1, assume first that $\mathbf{A}'\mathbf{A}' = \mathbf{A}'$. That $\mathbf{A}$ is idempotent follows by transposing both sides. The proof that $\mathbf{A}'$ is idempotent if $\mathbf{A}$ is idempotent is similar. To prove property 2, assume first that $\mathbf{I} - \mathbf{A}$ is idempotent, which implies that $(\mathbf{I} - \mathbf{A}) = (\mathbf{I} - \mathbf{A})(\mathbf{I} - \mathbf{A})$, from which idempotency of $\mathbf{A}$ follows immediately. The converse is similarly proved. To show property 3, let $r = r(\mathbf{A})$. By the full-rank factorization in Result 2.2.1, there exists an $n \times r$ matrix $\mathbf{P}$ and an $r \times n$ matrix $\mathbf{Q}$, each of rank r, such that $\mathbf{A} = \mathbf{PQ}$. Now,

$$\mathbf{PQPQ} = \mathbf{A}^2 = \mathbf{A} = \mathbf{PQ},$$

so that, by property 3 of Result 2.3.7, $\mathbf{QP} = \mathbf{I}_r$. Using properties of trace (see Result 1.2.8), $tr(\mathbf{A}) = tr(\mathbf{PQ}) = tr(\mathbf{QP}) = tr(\mathbf{I}_r) = r$. A simple extension of this idea proves the second part, i.e., $r(\mathbf{I}_n - \mathbf{A}) = n - tr(\mathbf{A}) = n - r$. To prove property 4, suppose that the $n \times n$ idempotent matrix $\mathbf{A}$ has rank n, so that $\mathbf{A}^{-1}$ exists. Then,

$$\mathbf{A} = \mathbf{I}_n\mathbf{A} = \mathbf{A}^{-1}\mathbf{AA} = \mathbf{A}^{-1}\mathbf{A}^2 = \mathbf{A}^{-1}\mathbf{A} = \mathbf{I}_n$$

which proves the result. The only nonsingular idempotent matrix is the identity matrix. ∎

Result 2.3.10. Let $\mathbf{A}$ be an $n \times n$ symmetric matrix. $\mathbf{A}$ is idempotent of rank m if and only if m of its eigenvalues are equal to 1 and the remaining $(n - m)$ eigenvalues are equal to 0.

Proof. Let $\mathbf{A}' = \mathbf{A}$, and let $\lambda_1, \cdots, \lambda_n$ denote the eigenvalues of $\mathbf{A}$, which are not necessarily all distinct. By Result 2.3.4, there exists an orthogonal matrix $\mathbf{P}$ such that $\mathbf{A} = \mathbf{PDP}'$, where $\mathbf{D} = \text{diag}(\lambda_1, \cdots, \lambda_n)$. Also,

$$\mathbf{A}^2 = \mathbf{PDP}'\mathbf{PDP}' = \mathbf{PD}^2\mathbf{P}',$$

where $\mathbf{D}^2 = \text{diag}(\lambda_1^2, \cdots, \lambda_n^2)$. Suppose $\mathbf{A}^2 = \mathbf{A}$, i.e., $\mathbf{A}$ is idempotent. This must imply that $\mathbf{D}^2 = \mathbf{D}$, or $\lambda_j^2 - \lambda_j = 0$, which in turn implies that each eigenvalue is either 0 or 1. Conversely, let us suppose that each eigenvalue of $\mathbf{A}$ is either 0 or 1. This implies that $\lambda_j^2 = \lambda_j$ for all j, i.e., $\mathbf{A}^2 = \mathbf{A}$, so that $\mathbf{A}$ is idempotent. Clearly, $r(\mathbf{D})$ is equal to the number of nonzero eigenvalues in $\mathbf{A}$, which is also equal to $r(\mathbf{A})$ (since $\mathbf{P}$ is a nonsingular matrix). ∎

2.4 Nonnegative definite quadratic forms and matrices

We introduce quadratic forms and matrices of quadratic forms, and describe their properties. First, we define a linear form in a vector $\mathbf{x}$, as well as a bilinear form in $\mathbf{x}$ and $\mathbf{y}$.

Definition 2.4.1. Linear form in x. Given an arbitrary vector $\mathbf{a} = (a_1, \cdots, a_n)'$, a linear form in $\mathbf{x} = (x_1, \cdots, x_n)'$ is a function that assigns to each vector $\mathbf{x} \in \mathcal{R}^n$ the value

$$\mathbf{a}'\mathbf{x} = \sum_{i=1}^{n} a_i x_i = a_1 x_1 + \cdots + a_n x_n. \tag{2.4.1}$$

Note that the linear form $\mathbf{a}'\mathbf{x}$ can also be written as $\mathbf{x}'\mathbf{a}$ and is a homogeneous polynomial of degree 1 with coefficient vector $\mathbf{a}$. For example, $4x_1 + 5x_2 - 3x_3$ is a linear form in $\mathbf{x} = (x_1, x_2, x_3)'$ with coefficient vector $\mathbf{a} = (4, 5, -3)'$. Two linear forms $\mathbf{a}'\mathbf{x}$ and $\mathbf{b}'\mathbf{x}$ are identically equal for all $\mathbf{x}$ if and only if $\mathbf{a} = \mathbf{b}$.

Definition 2.4.2. Bilinear form in x and y. Given an arbitrary $m \times n$ matrix $\mathbf{A} = \{a_{ij}\}$, a bilinear form is a function that assigns to each pair of vectors $\mathbf{x} = (x_1, \cdots, x_m)' \in \mathcal{R}^m$ and $\mathbf{y} = (y_1, \cdots, y_n)' \in \mathcal{R}^n$, the value

$$\mathbf{x}'\mathbf{A}\mathbf{y} = \sum_{i=1}^{m} \sum_{j=1}^{n} a_{ij} x_i y_j, \tag{2.4.2}$$

and $\mathbf{A}$ is the matrix of the bilinear form. The form in (2.4.2) can also be written as $\mathbf{y}'\mathbf{A}'\mathbf{x}$.

Two bilinear forms $\mathbf{x}'\mathbf{Ay}$ and $\mathbf{x}'\mathbf{By}$ are identically equal if and only if $\mathbf{A} = \mathbf{B}$. A bilinear form $\mathbf{x}'\mathbf{Ay}$ is symmetric if $\mathbf{x}'\mathbf{Ay} = \mathbf{y}'\mathbf{A}'\mathbf{x}$ for all $\mathbf{x}$ and $\mathbf{y}$, i.e., if and only if the matrix of the bilinear form is (square) symmetric, i.e., $\mathbf{A} = \mathbf{A}'$.

Example 2.4.1.   The expression $x_1y_1+2x_1y_2+4x_2y_1+7x_2y_2+2x_3y_1-2x_3y_2$ is a bilinear form in $\mathbf{x} = (x_1, x_2, x_3)'$ and $\mathbf{y} = (y_1, y_2)'$, with the matrix of the bilinear form given by

$$\mathbf{A} = \begin{pmatrix} 1 & 2 \\ 4 & 7 \\ 2 & -2 \end{pmatrix}.$$

An example of a symmetric bilinear form in $\mathbf{x} = (x_1, x_2, x_3)'$ and $\mathbf{y} = (y_1, y_2, y_3)'$ is $x_1y_1 + 2x_1y_2 - 3x_1y_3 + 2x_2y_1 + 7x_2y_2 + 6x_2y_3 - 3x_3y_1 + 6x_3y_2 + 5x_3y_3$, the matrix of the bilinear form being

$$\mathbf{A} = \begin{pmatrix} 1 & 2 & -3 \\ 2 & 7 & 6 \\ -3 & 6 & 5 \end{pmatrix}. \quad \square$$

Definition 2.4.3. Quadratic form in x.   Given an arbitrary $n \times n$ matrix $\mathbf{A} = \{a_{ij}\}$, a quadratic form is a function that assigns to each vector $\mathbf{x} = (x_1, \cdots, x_n)' \in \mathcal{R}^n$, the value

$$\mathbf{x}'\mathbf{Ax} = \sum_{i=1}^{n}\sum_{j=1}^{n} a_{ij}x_ix_j, \qquad (2.4.3)$$

which is a homogeneous polynomial of degree two.

Example 2.4.2.   The expression $x_1^2 + 7x_2^2 + 4x_3^2 + 4x_1x_2 + 10x_1x_3 - 4x_2x_3$ is a quadratic form in $\mathbf{x} = (x_1, x_2, x_3)'$, the matrix of the quadratic form being $\mathbf{A} = \begin{pmatrix} 1 & 2 & 5 \\ 2 & 7 & -2 \\ 5 & -2 & 4 \end{pmatrix}$. When $\mathbf{x} = \mathbf{0}$, then $\mathbf{x}'\mathbf{Ax} = 0$ for all $\mathbf{A}$. $\square$

Let $\mathbf{A} = \{a_{ij}\}$ and $\mathbf{B} = \{b_{ij}\}$ be two arbitrary $n \times n$ matrices. We say $\mathbf{x}'\mathbf{Ax}$ and $\mathbf{x}'\mathbf{Bx}$ are identically equal if and only if $\mathbf{A} + \mathbf{A}' = \mathbf{B} + \mathbf{B}'$. If $\mathbf{A}$ and $\mathbf{B}$ are symmetric matrices, then $\mathbf{x}'\mathbf{Ax}$ and $\mathbf{x}'\mathbf{Bx}$ are identically equal if and only if $\mathbf{A} = \mathbf{B}$. For any matrix $\mathbf{A}$, note that $\mathbf{C} = (\mathbf{A} + \mathbf{A}')/2$ is always symmetric and $\mathbf{x}'\mathbf{Ax} = \mathbf{x}'\mathbf{Cx}$. Hence, we may assume without loss of generality that corresponding to a given quadratic form, there exists a unique symmetric matrix $\mathbf{A}$ which is the matrix of that quadratic form. Let $\mathbf{x}'\mathbf{Ax}$ be a quadratic form in $\mathbf{x}$ and let $\mathbf{y} = \mathbf{C}^{-1}\mathbf{x}$, where $\mathbf{C}$ is an $n \times n$ nonsingular matrix. Then, $\mathbf{x}'\mathbf{Ax} = \mathbf{y}'\mathbf{C}'\mathbf{ACy} = \mathbf{y}'\mathbf{By}$, say. We refer to $\mathbf{A}$ and $\mathbf{B}$ as congruent matrices.

Definition 2.4.4. Nonnegative definite (n.n.d.) quadratic form. An arbitrary quadratic form $\mathbf{x}'\mathbf{Ax}$ is said to be nonnegative definite if $\mathbf{x}'\mathbf{Ax} \geq 0$ for every vector $\mathbf{x} \in \mathcal{R}^n$. The matrix $\mathbf{A}$ is called a nonnegative definite matrix.

Definition 2.4.5. Positive definite (p.d.) quadratic form. A nonnegative definite quadratic form $\mathbf{x}'\mathbf{Ax}$ is said to be positive definite if $\mathbf{x}'\mathbf{Ax} > 0$ for all nonnull vectors $\mathbf{x} \in \mathcal{R}^n$ and $\mathbf{x}'\mathbf{Ax} = 0$ only when $\mathbf{x}$ is the null vector, i.e., when $\mathbf{x} = \mathbf{0}$. The matrix $\mathbf{A}$ is called a positive definite matrix.

Definition 2.4.6. Positive semidefinite (p.s.d.) quadratic form. A nonnegative definite quadratic form $\mathbf{x}'\mathbf{Ax}$ is said to be positive semidefinite if $\mathbf{x}'\mathbf{Ax} \geq 0$ for every $\mathbf{x} \in \mathcal{R}^n$ and $\mathbf{x}'\mathbf{Ax} = 0$ for some nonnull $\mathbf{x}$. The matrix $\mathbf{A}$ is called a positive semidefinite matrix.

Example 2.4.3. The quadratic form $x_1^2 + \cdots + x_n^2 = \mathbf{x}'\mathbf{I}_n\mathbf{x} > 0$ for every nonnull $\mathbf{x} \in \mathcal{R}^n$ and is p.d. The quadratic form $(x_1 + \cdots + x_n)^2 = \mathbf{x}'\mathbf{11}'\mathbf{x} = \mathbf{x}'\mathbf{J}_n\mathbf{x} \geq 0$ for every $\mathbf{x} \in \mathcal{R}^n$ and is equal to 0 when $\mathbf{x} = (1 - n, 1, \cdots, 1)'$; it is a p.s.d. quadratic form. $\square$

A quadratic form $\mathbf{x}'\mathbf{Ax}$ is respectively nonpositive definite, or negative definite or negative semidefinite if $-\mathbf{x}'\mathbf{Ax}$ is nonnegative definite, or positive definite or positive semidefinite. The only symmetric $n \times n$ matrix which is both nonnegative definite and nonpositive definite is the null matrix. A quadratic form is said to be indefinite if $\mathbf{x}'\mathbf{Ax} > 0$ for some vectors $\mathbf{x}$ in $\mathcal{R}^n$ and $\mathbf{x}'\mathbf{Ax} \leq 0$ for some other vectors $\mathbf{x}$ in $\mathcal{R}^n$. The matrices of such quadratic forms have the corresponding names as well. In general, we will assume p.d. matrices to be symmetric.

Result 2.4.1. Let $\mathbf{P}$ be an $n \times m$ matrix and let $\mathbf{A}$ be an $n \times n$ n.n.d. matrix. Then the matrix $\mathbf{P}'\mathbf{AP}$ is n.n.d. If $r(\mathbf{P}) < m$, then $\mathbf{P}'\mathbf{AP}$ is p.s.d. If $\mathbf{A}$ is p.d. and $r(\mathbf{P}) = m$, then $\mathbf{P}'\mathbf{AP}$ is p.d.

Proof. Since $\mathbf{A}$ is n.n.d., by Definition 2.4.4, $\mathbf{x}'\mathbf{Ax} \geq 0$ for every $\mathbf{x} \in \mathcal{R}^n$. Suppose $\mathbf{x} = \mathbf{Py}$, $\mathbf{y} \in \mathcal{R}^m$. Then,

$$\mathbf{y}'(\mathbf{P}'\mathbf{AP})\mathbf{y} = (\mathbf{Py})'\mathbf{A}(\mathbf{Py}) = \mathbf{x}'\mathbf{Ax} \geq 0 \qquad (2.4.4)$$

which implies, by Definition 2.4.4 that $\mathbf{P}'\mathbf{AP}$ is n.n.d. If $r(\mathbf{P}) < m$, then by property 4 of Result 1.2.12, we see that $r(\mathbf{P}'\mathbf{AP}) \leq r(\mathbf{P}) < m$, so that $\mathbf{P}'\mathbf{AP}$ is p.s.d. Further, if $\mathbf{A}$ is p.d., the quadratic form $(\mathbf{Py})'\mathbf{A}(\mathbf{Py}) = 0$ only when $\mathbf{Py} = \mathbf{0}$, which implies that $\mathbf{y} = \mathbf{0}$ (since $r(\mathbf{P}) = m$). Thus, in (2.4.4), $\mathbf{y}'(\mathbf{P}'\mathbf{AP})\mathbf{y} = 0$ only when $\mathbf{y} = \mathbf{0}$, i.e., $\mathbf{P}'\mathbf{AP}$ is p.d. ∎

Result 2.4.2. Properties of nonnegative definite matrices.

1. If an $n \times n$ matrix $\mathbf{A}$ is p.d. (or p.s.d.), and $c > 0$ is a positive scalar, then $c\mathbf{A}$ is also p.d. (or p.s.d.).

2. If two $n \times n$ matrices $\mathbf{A}$ and $\mathbf{B}$ are both n.n.d., then $\mathbf{A} + \mathbf{B}$ is n.n.d. If, in addition, either $\mathbf{A}$ or $\mathbf{B}$ is p.d., then $\mathbf{A} + \mathbf{B}$ is also p.d.

3. Any principal submatrix of a n.n.d. matrix is n.n.d. Any principal submatrix of a p.d. (or p.s.d.) matrix is p.d. (or p.s.d).

Proof. To prove property 1, we see that by Definitions 2.4.5 and 2.4.6, the matrix $\mathbf{A}$ is p.d. (or p.s.d.) if the quadratic form $\mathbf{x}'\mathbf{A}\mathbf{x}$ is p.d. (or p.s.d.), or since $c > 0$, if $c\mathbf{x}'\mathbf{A}\mathbf{x} = \mathbf{x}'c\mathbf{A}\mathbf{x}$ is p.d. (or p.s.d.). This implies that $c\mathbf{A}$ is p.d. (or p.s.d.). Property 2 follows since $\mathbf{A}$ and $\mathbf{B}$ are both n.n.d., so that we have by Definition 2.4.4 that for every nonnull vector $\mathbf{x} \in \mathcal{R}^n$, $\mathbf{x}'\mathbf{A}\mathbf{x} \geq 0$ and $\mathbf{x}'\mathbf{B}\mathbf{x} \geq 0$. Hence, $\mathbf{x}'\mathbf{A}\mathbf{x} + \mathbf{x}'\mathbf{B}\mathbf{x} = \mathbf{x}'(\mathbf{A} + \mathbf{B})\mathbf{x} \geq 0$, which implies that the matrix $\mathbf{A} + \mathbf{B}$ is n.n.d. In addition, suppose that $\mathbf{A}$ is p.d. Then, we must have by Definition 2.4.6 that $\mathbf{x}'\mathbf{A}\mathbf{x} > 0$, while $\mathbf{x}'\mathbf{B}\mathbf{x} \geq 0$ for every nonnull $\mathbf{x} \in \mathcal{R}^n$. Hence, $\mathbf{x}'(\mathbf{A}+\mathbf{B})\mathbf{x} = \mathbf{x}'\mathbf{A}\mathbf{x} + \mathbf{x}'\mathbf{B}\mathbf{x} > 0$, so that $\mathbf{A}+\mathbf{B}$ is p.d. To prove property 3, consider the principal submatrix of an $n \times n$ matrix $\mathbf{A}$ obtained by deleting all its rows and columns except its $i_1, i_2, \cdots, i_m$th, where $i_1 < i_2 < \cdots < i_m$. We can write the resulting submatrix as $\mathbf{P}'\mathbf{A}\mathbf{P}$, where $\mathbf{P}$ is the $n \times m$ matrix of rank m, whose columns are the $i_1, i_2, \cdots, i_m$th columns of $\mathbf{I}_n$. If $\mathbf{A}$ is n.n.d., it follows from Result 2.4.1 that $\mathbf{P}'\mathbf{A}\mathbf{P}$ is too. In particular, the principal minors of a p.d. matrix are all positive. ∎

Result 2.4.3.

1. An $n \times n$ p.d. matrix $\mathbf{A}$ is nonsingular and its inverse is also a p.d. matrix.

2. If a p.s.d. matrix $\mathbf{A}$ is nonsingular, then it is invertible, and its inverse is p.s.d.

Proof. To prove property 1, suppose that, on the contrary, the p.d. matrix $\mathbf{A}$ is singular, with $r(\mathbf{A}) < n$. The columns of $\mathbf{A}$ are linearly dependent and hence there exists a vector $\mathbf{v} \neq \mathbf{0}$ such that $\mathbf{A}\mathbf{v} = \mathbf{0}$, which implies that $\mathbf{v}'\mathbf{A}\mathbf{v} = 0$, which is a contradiction to our assumption that $\mathbf{A}$ is p.d. Hence $\mathbf{A}$ must be nonsingular, and let $\mathbf{A}^{-1}$ denote the regular inverse of $\mathbf{A}$. Since $\mathbf{A}$ is p.d., by Result 2.4.1, $(\mathbf{A}^{-1})'\mathbf{A}\mathbf{A}^{-1}$ is p.d. But $(\mathbf{A}^{-1})' = (\mathbf{A}^{-1})'\mathbf{A}\mathbf{A}^{-1}$, implying that $(\mathbf{A}^{-1})'$ is p.d. and so is $\mathbf{A}^{-1}$. The proof of property 2 is similar, and follows from Result 2.4.1. ∎

Result 2.4.4. Let $\mathbf{A}$ be an $n \times n$ symmetric matrix and let $\mathbf{D} = \text{diag}(\lambda_1, \cdots, \lambda_n)$ be an $n \times n$ diagonal matrix such that $\mathbf{P}'\mathbf{A}\mathbf{P} = \mathbf{D}$. Then,

1. $\mathbf{A}$ is p.s.d. if and only if $\lambda_j \geq 0$, $j = 1, \cdots, n$, with equality holding for at least one j, and

2. $\mathbf{A}$ is p.d. if and only if $\lambda_j > 0$, $j = 1, \cdots, n$.

Proof. From Result 2.3.4, we know that there exists an orthogonal matrix $\mathbf{P}$ which diagonalizes $\mathbf{A}$. Since $\mathbf{P}$ is orthogonal, $\mathbf{P}' = \mathbf{P}^{-1}$, and hence

$$\mathbf{A} = (\mathbf{P}^{-1})'\mathbf{D}\mathbf{P}^{-1} = \mathbf{P}\mathbf{D}\mathbf{P}'.$$

We can also show that $\mathbf{A}$ is p.d. (or p.s.d.) if and only if $\mathbf{A}'$ is p.d. (or p.s.d.). Together with Result 2.4.1, this completes the proof. ∎

Result 2.4.5. Diagonability of p.d. (p.s.d.) matrices. An $n \times n$ symmetric matrix $\mathbf{A}$ is diagonable by an $n \times n$ matrix $\mathbf{P}$ with $r(\mathbf{P}) = n$ (or $r(\mathbf{P}) < n$) such that $\mathbf{A} = \mathbf{P}\mathbf{P}'$ if and only if $\mathbf{A}$ is p.d. (or p.s.d.).

Proof. Let $\mathbf{A} = \mathbf{P}\mathbf{P}'$. Then

$$\mathbf{x}'\mathbf{A}\mathbf{x} = \mathbf{x}'\mathbf{P}\mathbf{P}'\mathbf{x} = (\mathbf{P}'\mathbf{x})'(\mathbf{P}'\mathbf{x}) \geq 0 \qquad (2.4.5)$$

for every nonnull $\mathbf{x} \in \mathcal{R}^n$. If $r(\mathbf{P}) = n$, then the columns of $\mathbf{P}$ form a basis for $\mathcal{R}^n$, so that $\mathbf{P}'\mathbf{x} = \mathbf{0}$ only if $\mathbf{x} = \mathbf{0}$. Hence, $\mathbf{A}$ is p.d. If $r(\mathbf{P}) < n$, there exists some nonnull $\mathbf{x} \in \mathcal{R}^n$, such that $\mathbf{P}'\mathbf{x} = \mathbf{0}$, so that (2.4.5) holds with equality for some nonnull $\mathbf{x}$, so that $\mathbf{A}$ is p.s.d. To prove the converse, since $\mathbf{A}$ is symmetric, by Result 2.3.4, we have $\mathbf{A} = \mathbf{Q}\mathbf{D}\mathbf{Q}'$, where $\mathbf{D} = \mathrm{diag}(\lambda_1, \cdots, \lambda_n)$, $\lambda_j > 0$, $j = 1, \cdots, n$ if $\mathbf{A}$ is p.d. (or $\lambda_j \geq 0$, $j = 1, \cdots, n$ if $\mathbf{A}$ is p.s.d). Define

$$\mathbf{D}^{1/2} = \mathrm{diag}(d_1, \cdots, d_n) \quad \text{where} \quad d_j = \begin{cases} \sqrt{\lambda_j} & \text{if } \lambda_j > 0 \\ 0 & \text{if } \lambda_j = 0. \end{cases}$$

Then, $\mathbf{A} = \mathbf{Q}\mathbf{D}^{1/2}\mathbf{D}^{1/2}\mathbf{Q}' = \mathbf{P}\mathbf{P}'$, where $\mathbf{P} = \mathbf{Q}\mathbf{D}^{1/2}$. ∎

Result 2.4.5 can be used to define the square root of a positive definite (or positive semidefinite) symmetric matrix $\mathbf{A}$. We may write

$$\mathbf{A} = \mathbf{Q}\mathbf{D}^{1/2}\mathbf{D}^{1/2}\mathbf{Q}' = \mathbf{Q}\mathbf{D}^{1/2}\mathbf{Q}'\mathbf{Q}\mathbf{D}^{1/2}\mathbf{Q}',$$

where $\mathbf{Q}$ is orthogonal. Suppose we set $\mathbf{B} = \mathbf{Q}\mathbf{D}^{1/2}\mathbf{Q}'$, we see that $\mathbf{A} = \mathbf{B}\mathbf{B} = \mathbf{B}^2$, i.e., the matrix $\mathbf{B}$ is the square root of the matrix $\mathbf{A}$, and we can write $\mathbf{B} = \mathbf{A}^{1/2}$.

Example 2.4.4. For all p.d. $k \times k$ matrices $\mathbf{A}$, we show that

$$\exp\{-\tfrac{1}{2}tr(\mathbf{A}^{-1}\mathbf{B})\}/|\mathbf{A}|^b \leq (2b)^{kb}\exp(-kb)/|\mathbf{B}|^b,$$

with equality holding only when $\mathbf{A} = \mathbf{B}/2b$, where $\mathbf{B}$ is a $k \times k$ symmetric p.d. matrix, and $b > 0$ is a scalar. If $\mathbf{B}^{1/2}$ denotes the symmetric square root of $\mathbf{B}$, then $\mathbf{B}^{1/2}\mathbf{B}^{1/2} = \mathbf{B}$, and $tr(\mathbf{A}^{-1}\mathbf{B}) = tr\{(\mathbf{A}^{-1}\mathbf{B}^{1/2})\mathbf{B}^{1/2}\} = tr(\mathbf{B}^{1/2}\mathbf{A}^{-1}\mathbf{B}^{1/2})$. Since

$$\mathbf{x}'\mathbf{B}^{1/2}\mathbf{A}^{-1}\mathbf{B}^{1/2}\mathbf{x} = (\mathbf{B}^{1/2}\mathbf{x})'\mathbf{A}^{-1}(\mathbf{B}^{1/2}\mathbf{x}) > 0$$

if $\mathbf{x} \neq \mathbf{0}$, the matrix $\mathbf{B}^{1/2}\mathbf{A}^{-1}\mathbf{B}^{1/2}$ is p.d. Let $\lambda_j > 0$, $j = 1, \cdots, k$ denote the eigenvalues of this matrix. Then

$$tr(\mathbf{A}^{-1}\mathbf{B}) = tr(\mathbf{B}^{1/2}\mathbf{A}^{-1}\mathbf{B}^{1/2}) = \sum_{j=1}^{k}\lambda_j, \quad \text{and}$$

$$|\mathbf{B}^{1/2}\mathbf{A}^{-1}\mathbf{B}^{1/2}| = |\mathbf{A}^{-1}||\mathbf{B}^{1/2}||\mathbf{B}^{1/2}| = |\mathbf{B}|/|\mathbf{A}| = \prod_{j=1}^{k}\lambda_j,$$

so that $|\mathbf{A}| = |\mathbf{B}| / \prod_{j=1}^{k} \lambda_j$. From these results, we see that

$$\frac{\exp\{-\frac{1}{2}tr(\mathbf{A}^{-1}\mathbf{B})\}}{|\mathbf{A}|^b} = \frac{\left(\prod_{j=1}^{k} \lambda_j\right)^b \exp(-\frac{1}{2}\sum_{j=1}^{k} \lambda_j)}{|\mathbf{B}|^b}$$

$$= \frac{\prod_{j=1}^{k} \lambda_j^b \exp(-\frac{1}{2}\lambda_j)}{|\mathbf{B}|^b}.$$

It can be verified that the function $\lambda_j^b \exp(-\frac{1}{2}\lambda_j)$ attains a maximum value of $(2b)^b \exp(-b)$ at $\lambda_j = 2b$, $j = 1, \cdots, k$, from which the result follows.   □

Result 2.4.6.   Let $\mathbf{P}$ be a p.d. matrix. For any vector $\mathbf{b}$,

$$\sup_{\mathbf{h} \neq \mathbf{0}} \frac{(\mathbf{h}'\mathbf{b})^2}{\mathbf{h}'\mathbf{P}\mathbf{h}} = \mathbf{b}'\mathbf{P}^{-1}\mathbf{b}. \tag{2.4.6}$$

Proof.   For every constant $a \in \mathcal{R}$,

$$\begin{aligned} 0 \ &\leq \ \| (\mathbf{v} - a\mathbf{u}) \|^2 \\ &= \ a^2 \| \mathbf{u} \|^2 - 2a\mathbf{u}'\mathbf{v} + \| \mathbf{v} \|^2 \\ &= \ \{a \| \mathbf{u} \| - \frac{\mathbf{u}'\mathbf{v}}{\| \mathbf{u} \|}\}^2 + \| \mathbf{v} \|^2 - \frac{(\mathbf{u}'\mathbf{v})^2}{\| \mathbf{u} \|^2}. \end{aligned}$$

For nonzero $\mathbf{u}$, the Cauchy-Schwarz inequality implies that

$$\sup_{\mathbf{v} \neq \mathbf{0}} \left\{ \frac{(\mathbf{u}'\mathbf{v})^2}{\mathbf{v}'\mathbf{v}} \right\} = \mathbf{u}'\mathbf{u}. \tag{2.4.7}$$

Since $\mathbf{P}$ is p.d., there exists a nonsingular matrix $\mathbf{R}$ such that $\mathbf{P} = \mathbf{R}\mathbf{R}'$. Set $\mathbf{v} = \mathbf{R}'\mathbf{h}$, and $\mathbf{u} = \mathbf{R}^{-1}\mathbf{b}$. Then, (2.4.7) yields (2.4.6) after simplification.   ■

The next example shows a useful matrix inequality called the extended Cauchy-Schwarz inequality.

Example 2.4.5.   Let $\mathbf{b}$ and $\mathbf{d}$ be two n-dimensional vectors, and let $\mathbf{B}$ be an $n \times n$ p.d. matrix. We will show that

$$(\mathbf{b}'\mathbf{d})^2 \leq (\mathbf{b}'\mathbf{B}\mathbf{b})(\mathbf{d}'\mathbf{B}^{-1}\mathbf{d}), \tag{2.4.8}$$

with equality if and only if $\mathbf{b} = a\mathbf{B}^{-1}\mathbf{d}$, or if $\mathbf{d} = a\mathbf{B}\mathbf{b}$, for some constant a. Since (2.4.8) holds trivially when $\mathbf{b} = \mathbf{0}$ or $\mathbf{d} = \mathbf{0}$, let us consider nonzero vectors. Let $\lambda_1, \cdots, \lambda_n$ denote the eigenvalues of $\mathbf{B}$, and let $\mathbf{v}_1, \cdots, \mathbf{v}_n$ denote the corresponding normalized eigenvectors. Since $\mathbf{B}^{1/2} = \sum_{i=1}^{n} \sqrt{\lambda_i}\mathbf{v}_i\mathbf{v}_i'$, and $\mathbf{B}^{-1/2} = \sum_{i=1}^{n} \mathbf{v}_i\mathbf{v}_i'/\sqrt{\lambda_i}$, we see that

$$\mathbf{b}'\mathbf{d} = \mathbf{b}'\mathbf{Id} = \mathbf{b}'\mathbf{B}^{1/2}\mathbf{B}^{-1/2}\mathbf{d} = (\mathbf{B}^{1/2}\mathbf{b})'(\mathbf{B}^{-1/2}\mathbf{d}).$$

Apply the Cauchy-Schwarz inequality (see Result 1.2.1) to the vectors $\mathbf{B}^{1/2}\mathbf{b}$ and $\mathbf{B}^{-1/2}\mathbf{d}$ to obtain the inequality in (2.4.8). $\square$

We end this section with a result on the spectral decomposition of a symmetric, n.n.d. matrix.

Result 2.4.7. Let $\mathbf{A}$ be an $n \times n$ symmetric n.n.d. matrix. We can write $\mathbf{A}$ in the form

$$\mathbf{A} = \mathbf{Q}\begin{pmatrix} \mathbf{D}_1 & \mathbf{0} \\ \mathbf{0} & \mathbf{0} \end{pmatrix}\mathbf{Q}', \tag{2.4.9}$$

where $\mathbf{Q}$ is an $n \times n$ orthogonal matrix and $\mathbf{D}_1$ is a diagonal matrix with positive diagonal elements.

Proof. The proof follows directly from Result 2.3.4 and the nonnegativity of eigenvalues of a n.n.d. matrix. ∎

2.5 Simultaneous diagonalization of matrices

We present results that deal with finding a matrix $\mathbf{P}$ that will simultaneously diagonalize two $n \times n$ matrices with different properties in terms of symmetry and nonnegative definiteness.

Result 2.5.1. Let $\mathbf{A}$ and $\mathbf{B}$ be two $n \times n$ symmetric matrices. There exists an orthogonal matrix $\mathbf{P}$ such that $\mathbf{P}'\mathbf{AP}$ and $\mathbf{P}'\mathbf{BP}$ are both diagonal if and only if $\mathbf{AB} = \mathbf{BA}$.

Proof. Sufficiency. Suppose that $\mathbf{AB} = \mathbf{BA}$. Since $\mathbf{A}$ is symmetric, there exists an orthogonal matrix $\mathbf{R}$ such that $\mathbf{R}'\mathbf{AR} = \mathbf{D} = \mathrm{diag}(\lambda_i \mathbf{I}_{m_i})$, where λ_i is a distinct eigenvalue of $\mathbf{A}$ with multiplicity m_i, $i = 1, \cdots, s$, say. Suppose further that $\mathbf{R}'\mathbf{BR} = \mathbf{C} = \{\mathbf{C}_{ij}\}$, where the matrix $\mathbf{C}$ has been partitioned conformably with $\mathbf{D}$. Then,

$$\mathbf{CD} = \mathbf{R}'\mathbf{BRR}'\mathbf{AR} = \mathbf{R}'\mathbf{BAR} = \mathbf{R}'\mathbf{ABR} = \mathbf{R}'\mathbf{ARR}'\mathbf{BR} = \mathbf{DC},$$

or $\mathbf{C}_{ij}\lambda_j = \lambda_i\mathbf{C}_{ij}$, $i \neq j$. For $i \neq j$, since $\lambda_i \neq \lambda_j$, we must have $\mathbf{C}_{ij} = \mathbf{0}$. That is, the matrix $\mathbf{C}$ must be block-diagonal with $\mathbf{C} = \mathrm{diag}\{\mathbf{C}_{ii}\}$. Since $\mathbf{C}$ is symmetric, $\mathbf{C}_{ii}$ must be symmetric. Hence, for $i = 1, \cdots, s$, there exist orthogonal matrices $\mathbf{Q}_i$ such that $\mathbf{Q}_i'\mathbf{C}_{ii}\mathbf{Q}_i = \Delta_i$, which is diagonal. Let $\mathbf{Q} = \mathrm{diag}\{\mathbf{Q}_i\}$; then $\mathbf{Q}'\mathbf{Q} = \mathbf{I}$. Define $\mathbf{P} = \mathbf{RQ}$; we have $\mathbf{P}'\mathbf{P} = \mathbf{I}$ and

$$\begin{aligned}
\mathbf{P}'\mathbf{AP} &= \mathbf{Q}'\mathbf{R}'\mathbf{ARQ} = \mathbf{Q}'\mathbf{DQ} = \mathrm{diag}\{\lambda_i\mathbf{Q}_i'\mathbf{Q}_i\} = \mathrm{diag}\{\lambda_i\mathbf{I}_{m_i}\}, \text{ and} \\
\mathbf{P}'\mathbf{BP} &= \mathbf{Q}'\mathbf{R}'\mathbf{BRQ} = \mathbf{Q}'\mathbf{CQ} = \mathrm{diag}\{\Delta_i\} = \Delta.
\end{aligned}$$

Necessity. Let $\mathbf{P}'\mathbf{AP} = \mathbf{D}$, $\mathbf{P}'\mathbf{BP} = \Delta$, where $\mathbf{D}$ and Δ are diagonal matrices. Now, $\mathbf{D}\Delta = \Delta\mathbf{D}$, which implies that

$$\mathbf{AB} = \mathbf{PP'APP'BPP'} = \mathbf{PD\Delta P'} = \mathbf{P\Delta DP'} = \mathbf{PP'BPP'APP'} = \mathbf{BA},$$

and completes the proof. ∎

This result extends to $n \times n$ symmetric matrices $\mathbf{A}_1, \cdots, \mathbf{A}_k$, $k > 2$; these matrices are simultaneously diagonable by an orthogonal matrix $\mathbf{P}$ if and only if they commute under multiplication in pairs.

Result 2.5.2.   Let $\mathbf{A}$ be an $n \times n$ p.d. matrix and let $\mathbf{B}$ be an $n \times n$ symmetric matrix. There exists a nonsingular matrix $\mathbf{P}$ such that $\mathbf{P'AP} = \mathbf{I}$ and $\mathbf{P'BP} = \Lambda = \text{diag}(\lambda_1, \cdots, \lambda_n)$, where λ_i are solutions to $|\mathbf{B} - \lambda\mathbf{A}| = 0$.

Proof. Since $\mathbf{A}$ is p.d., there exists a nonsingular matrix $\mathbf{R}$ such that $\mathbf{R'AR} = \mathbf{I}$, so that $\mathbf{A} = (\mathbf{R'})^{-1}\mathbf{R}^{-1}$. Also, since $\mathbf{B}$ is symmetric, $\mathbf{R'BR}$ is symmetric. By Result 2.3.4, there exists an orthogonal matrix $\mathbf{Q}$ such that

$$\mathbf{Q'R'BRQ} = \mathbf{D} = \text{diag}(\lambda_1, \cdots, \lambda_n),$$

where λ_i's are solutions to the characteristic equation $|\mathbf{R'BR} - \lambda\mathbf{I}| = 0$. Note that $|\mathbf{R'BR} - \lambda\mathbf{I}| = |\mathbf{R'BR} - \lambda\mathbf{R'AR}| = |\mathbf{R'BR} - \mathbf{R'}\lambda\mathbf{AR}| = |\mathbf{R'}||\mathbf{B} - \lambda\mathbf{A}||\mathbf{R}| = 0$. Hence, the λ_i's are also solutions of $|\mathbf{B} - \lambda\mathbf{A}| = 0$. Let $\mathbf{P} = \mathbf{RQ}$. Then,

$$\mathbf{P'BP} = \mathbf{Q'R'BRQ} = \mathbf{D} \quad \text{and} \quad \mathbf{P'AP} = \mathbf{Q'R'ARQ} = \mathbf{Q'Q} = \mathbf{I},$$

which proves the result. ∎

The problem of finding the solutions for λ to the equation $|\mathbf{B} - \lambda\mathbf{A}| = 0$ is called the *generalized eigenvalue problem*, and reduces to the problem of finding the eigenvalues of $\mathbf{B}$ when $\mathbf{A} = \mathbf{I}$. Since $|\mathbf{B} - \lambda\mathbf{A}| = |\mathbf{R}|^2|\mathbf{R'BR} - \lambda\mathbf{I}| = |\mathbf{A}^{-1}\mathbf{B} - \lambda\mathbf{I}| = |\mathbf{BA}^{-1} - \lambda\mathbf{I}|$, the generalized eigenvalue problem is equivalent to that of finding the eigenvalues of $\mathbf{R'BR}$ or $\mathbf{A}^{-1}\mathbf{B}$ or $\mathbf{BA}^{-1}$.

2.6   Geometrical perspectives

We discuss orthogonal projections and projection matrices and their relevance to linear model theory. Recall that if $\mathbf{u}, \mathbf{v} \in \mathcal{R}^n$, we say that $\mathbf{u} \perp \mathbf{v}$ if $\mathbf{u'v} = 0$. If $\mathbf{u} \in \mathcal{R}^n$ and $\mathcal{V}$ is a subspace of $\mathcal{R}^n$, $\mathbf{u} \perp \mathcal{V}$ if $\mathbf{u'v} = 0$ for every $\mathbf{v} \in \mathcal{V}$. Likewise, if $\mathcal{U}$ and $\mathcal{V}$ are two subspaces of $\mathcal{R}^n$, then $\mathcal{U} \perp \mathcal{V}$ if $\mathbf{u'v} = 0$ for every $\mathbf{u} \in \mathcal{U}$ and for every $\mathbf{v} \in \mathcal{V}$. The vector space $\mathcal{R}^n$ is said to be the direct sum of subspaces $\mathcal{U}$ and $\mathcal{V}$ if any vector $\mathbf{y} \in \mathcal{R}^n$ can be uniquely expressed as $\mathbf{y} = \mathbf{y}_1 + \mathbf{y}_2$, where $\mathbf{y}_1 \in \mathcal{U}$ and $\mathbf{y}_2 \in \mathcal{V}$. We denote this by

$$\mathcal{R}^n = \mathcal{U} \oplus \mathcal{V}.$$

We now build upon the basic ideas that we introduced in Chapter 1. We begin with the definition of the projection of an n-dimensional vector.

Definition 2.6.1.   The orthogonal projection of a vector $\mathbf{v}_1$ onto another vector $\mathbf{v}_2$ is given by

$$(\mathbf{v}_1'\mathbf{v}_2/\mathbf{v}_2'\mathbf{v}_2)\mathbf{v}_2 = (\mathbf{v}_1'\mathbf{v}_2/\parallel \mathbf{v}_2 \parallel)(1/\parallel \mathbf{v}_2 \parallel)\mathbf{v}_2.$$

Since the length of $\mathbf{v}_2/\parallel \mathbf{v}_2 \parallel$ is unity, the length of the projection is

$$|\mathbf{v}_1'\mathbf{v}_2|/\parallel \mathbf{v}_2 \parallel = \parallel \mathbf{v}_1 \parallel |\mathbf{v}_1'\mathbf{v}_2|/(\parallel \mathbf{v}_1 \parallel \parallel \mathbf{v}_2 \parallel) = \parallel \mathbf{v}_1 \parallel |\cos(\theta)|,$$

where θ is the angle between $\mathbf{v}_1$ and $\mathbf{v}_2$.

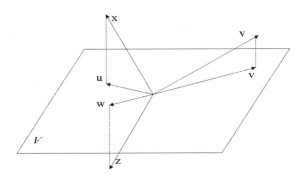

Figure 2.6.1. Projection of three vectors onto a two-dimensional subspace $\mathcal{V}$ of a three-dimensional space.

Figure 2.6.1 illustrates the projection of three vectors $\mathbf{x}, \mathbf{y}$, and $\mathbf{z}$ onto vectors $\mathbf{u}, \mathbf{v}$, and $\mathbf{w}$ in a two-dimensional subspace $\mathcal{V}$ of a three-dimensional space. We next discuss the notion of a projection of a vector onto a subspace of the n-dimensional Euclidean space. This concept is basic to an understanding of the geometry of the least squares approach which is a classical estimation tool in linear model theory. We show that such a projection exists, it is unique and the corresponding matrices of the projection are unique as well. This is graphically represented in Figure 2.6.2, which illustrates the projection of a 2-dimensional vector $\mathbf{y}$ onto a vector $\mathbf{u}$ which belongs to a subspace $\mathcal{V}$, and a vector $\mathbf{v}$ which belongs to $\mathcal{V}^\perp$, the orthogonal complement of $\mathcal{V}$. The orthogonal complement of any subspace $\mathcal{V}$ of $\mathcal{R}^n$ is defined below.

Definition 2.6.2. Orthogonal complement.   For any subspace $\mathcal{V} \subset \mathcal{R}^n$, the orthogonal complement of $\mathcal{V}$, written as $\mathcal{V}^\perp$ is the subspace of $\mathcal{R}^n$ which consists of vectors in $\mathcal{R}^n$ that are orthogonal to every vector in $\mathcal{V}$. Then, $\mathcal{V} \cap \mathcal{V}^\perp$ is empty.

The null space of any $n \times k$ matrix $\mathbf{X}$ is the orthogonal complement of the column space of $\mathbf{X}'$, i.e., $\mathcal{N}(\mathbf{X}) = \mathcal{C}(\mathbf{X}')^\perp$. The next result discusses the orthogonal decomposition of an n-dimensional vector.

Result 2.6.1. Every vector $\mathbf{y} \in \mathcal{R}^n$ can be expressed uniquely as

$$\mathbf{y} = \mathbf{u} + \mathbf{v}, \quad \mathbf{u} \in \mathcal{V}, \mathbf{v} \in \mathcal{V}^{\perp}, \qquad (2.6.1)$$

where $\mathcal{V}$ is a subspace of $\mathcal{R}^n$. Further, if $\mathbf{X}$ is an $n \times k$ basis matrix for $\mathcal{V}$, i.e., $\mathcal{V} = \mathcal{C}(\mathbf{X})$, and the columns of $\mathbf{X}$ are LIN, then the projection of $\mathbf{y}$ onto $\mathcal{V}$ is given by $\mathbf{X}(\mathbf{X}'\mathbf{X})^{-1}\mathbf{X}'\mathbf{y}$. We can write $\mathcal{R}^n = \mathcal{V} \oplus \mathcal{V}^{\perp}$.

Proof.   If possible, let there be two such decompositions of $\mathbf{y}$, i.e., suppose $\mathbf{y} = \mathbf{u}_1 + \mathbf{v}_1$ and $\mathbf{y} = \mathbf{u}_2 + \mathbf{v}_2$, where $\mathbf{u}_1, \mathbf{u}_2 \in \mathcal{V}$, and $\mathbf{v}_1, \mathbf{v}_2 \in \mathcal{V}^{\perp}$. It follows that $\mathbf{u}_1 - \mathbf{u}_2 + \mathbf{v}_1 - \mathbf{v}_2 = \mathbf{0}$. However, $\mathbf{u}_1 - \mathbf{u}_2 \in \mathcal{V}$, while $\mathbf{v}_1 - \mathbf{v}_2 \in \mathcal{V}^{\perp}$. Therefore, we must have $\mathbf{u}_1 = \mathbf{u}_2$, and $\mathbf{v}_1 = \mathbf{v}_2$, i.e., the decomposition of $\mathbf{y}$ is unique. To prove the second part of the result, suppose that $\mathbf{v} = \mathbf{X}(\mathbf{X}'\mathbf{X})^{-1}\mathbf{X}'\mathbf{y}$. Clearly, $\mathbf{v} \in \mathcal{V}$. We must now show that $\mathbf{y} - \mathbf{v} \in \mathcal{V}^{\perp}$. Let $\mathbf{u} \in \mathcal{V}$. We can write $\mathbf{u} = \mathbf{Xc}$, for some vector $\mathbf{c}$. Hence,

$$(\mathbf{y} - \mathbf{v})'\mathbf{u} = (\mathbf{y} - \mathbf{X}(\mathbf{X}'\mathbf{X})^{-1}\mathbf{X}'\mathbf{y})'\mathbf{Xc} = \mathbf{y}'\mathbf{Xc} - \mathbf{y}'\mathbf{X}(\mathbf{X}'\mathbf{X})^{-1}\mathbf{X}'\mathbf{Xc} = 0,$$

so that $\mathbf{y} - \mathbf{v} \in \mathcal{V}^{\perp}$. That is, the projection of $\mathbf{y}$ onto $\mathcal{V}$ is $\mathbf{X}(\mathbf{X}'\mathbf{X})^{-1}\mathbf{X}'\mathbf{y}$, which is a linear function of $\mathbf{y}$. That $\mathcal{R}^n = \mathcal{V} \oplus \mathcal{V}^{\perp}$ follows directly from the definition of the direct sum of a vector space (see the discussion following Definition 1.2.7). ∎

Definition 2.6.3. Projection matrix. The matrix $\mathbf{P}_{\mathcal{V}} = \mathbf{X}(\mathbf{X}'\mathbf{X})^{-1}\mathbf{X}'$ is called the projection matrix, since premultiplying $\mathbf{y} \in \mathcal{R}^n$ by this matrix gives the projection of the vector $\mathbf{y}$ onto $\mathcal{V}$. The matrix $\mathbf{P}_{\mathcal{V}}$ (which is simply denoted by $\mathbf{P}$ when it is clear which subspace we are projecting onto) is the unique linear function which assigns to each $\mathbf{y}$ its projection onto the subspace $\mathcal{V}$, which is itself a vector.

Result 2.6.2. The projection matrix $\mathbf{P}$ and the matrix is $\mathbf{I}_n - \mathbf{P}$ are symmetric and idempotent, and further $\mathbf{PX} = \mathbf{X}$.

Proof. We see that

$$\mathbf{P}' = [\mathbf{X}(\mathbf{X}'\mathbf{X})^{-1}\mathbf{X}']' = \mathbf{X}(\mathbf{X}'\mathbf{X})^{-1}\mathbf{X}', \text{ and}$$
$$\mathbf{P}^2 = \mathbf{PP} = \mathbf{X}(\mathbf{X}'\mathbf{X})^{-1}\mathbf{X}'\mathbf{X}(\mathbf{X}'\mathbf{X})^{-1}\mathbf{X}' = \mathbf{X}(\mathbf{X}'\mathbf{X})^{-1}\mathbf{X}',$$

so that symmetry and idempotency of $\mathbf{P}$ follow directly from Definition 1.2.15 and Definition 2.3.1. To show this in another way, observe that $\mathbf{Pc} \in \mathcal{V}$, and $(\mathbf{I}_n - \mathbf{P})\mathbf{d} \in \mathcal{V}^{\perp}$ for some vectors $\mathbf{c}$ and $\mathbf{d}$, so that by Definition 1.2.8, $\mathbf{c}'\mathbf{P}'(\mathbf{I}_n - \mathbf{P})\mathbf{d} = 0$, which in turn implies that $\mathbf{P}'(\mathbf{I}_n - \mathbf{P}) = \mathbf{0}$, that is, $\mathbf{P}' = \mathbf{P}'\mathbf{P}$. Then,

$$\mathbf{P} = (\mathbf{P}')' = (\mathbf{P}'\mathbf{P})' = \mathbf{P}'\mathbf{P} = \mathbf{P}',$$

which implies that $\mathbf{P}$ is symmetric. Since $\mathbf{P}^2 = \mathbf{P}$, it is also idempotent. That $r(\mathbf{P}) = k$ follows directly from property 3 of Result 2.3.9. It is easy to verify that

$\mathbf{PX} = \mathbf{X}$. The proof of the symmetry and idempotency of $\mathbf{I}_n - \mathbf{P}$ is obtained in a similar manner. ∎

Result 2.6.3. The column space $\mathcal{C}(\mathbf{P})$ of $\mathbf{P}$ is $\mathcal{V}$, and the column space $\mathcal{C}(\mathbf{I}_n - \mathbf{P})$ is $\mathcal{V}^\perp$. If $\dim(\mathcal{V}) = k$, then $tr(\mathbf{P}) = r(\mathbf{P}) = k$ and $tr(\mathbf{I}_n - \mathbf{P}) = r(\mathbf{I}_n - \mathbf{P}) = n - k$.

Proof. Since $\mathbf{Py} = \mathbf{u} \in \mathcal{V}$, it follows that $\mathcal{C}(\mathbf{P}) \subset \mathcal{V}$. Also, if $\mathbf{x} \in \mathcal{V}$, then by Result 2.6.1, the unique orthogonal decomposition of $\mathbf{x}$ is $\mathbf{x} = \mathbf{x} + \mathbf{0}$, which implies that $\mathbf{x} = \mathbf{Px} \in \mathcal{C}(\mathbf{P})$. The two spaces therefore coincide, and $\dim(\mathcal{V}) = r(\mathbf{P})$. Since the projection matrix $\mathbf{P}$ is symmetric and idempotent, it follows from Result 2.3.9 that

$$r(\mathbf{P}) = tr(\mathbf{P}) = tr[\mathbf{X}(\mathbf{X}'\mathbf{X})^{-1}\mathbf{X}'] = tr[\mathbf{X}'\mathbf{X}(\mathbf{X}'\mathbf{X})^{-1}] = tr(\mathbf{I}_k) = k.$$

That $r(\mathbf{I}_n - \mathbf{P}) = n - k$ follows immediately. ∎

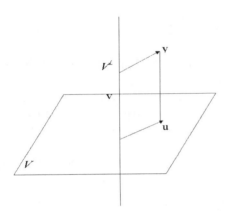

Figure 2.6.2. Projection of a 2-dimensional vector $\mathbf{y}$ onto a subspace $\mathcal{V}$ and its orthogonal complement $\mathcal{V}^\perp$.

Result 2.6.4. The matrix $\mathbf{I}_n - \mathbf{P}$ represents the orthogonal projection onto $\mathcal{V}^\perp$.

Proof. From Result 2.6.2, recall that $\mathbf{P}$ is the $n \times n$ symmetric, idempotent projection matrix of $\mathbf{y}$. Using the identity $\mathbf{y} = \mathbf{Py} + (\mathbf{I}_n - \mathbf{P})\mathbf{y}$, it follows from Result 2.6.1 that $\mathbf{v} = (\mathbf{I}_n - \mathbf{P})\mathbf{y}$, so that $\mathbf{I}_n - \mathbf{P}$ represents the matrix of the orthogonal projection onto $\mathcal{V}^\perp$. Then,

$$(\mathbf{Py})'(\mathbf{I}_n - \mathbf{P})\mathbf{y} = \mathbf{y}'(\mathbf{P} - \mathbf{P}^2)\mathbf{y} = 0,$$

which implies orthogonality of the components of $\mathbf{y}$ that belong respectively to $\mathcal{V}$ and $\mathcal{V}^\perp$. But, $\mathbf{P}$ and $\mathbf{I}_n - \mathbf{P}$ respectively span the orthogonal subspaces $\mathcal{V}$ and $\mathcal{V}^\perp$ (see Result 2.6.3), from which the result follows. ∎

Result 2.6.5. If $\mathbf{v} \in \mathcal{V}$, then,

1. $\| \mathbf{y} - \mathbf{v} \|^2 = \| \mathbf{y} - \mathbf{Py} \|^2 + \| \mathbf{Py} - \mathbf{v} \|^2$.

2. $\| \mathbf{y} - \mathbf{Py} \|^2 \leq \| \mathbf{y} - \mathbf{v} \|^2$ for all $\mathbf{v} \in \mathcal{V}$ with equality holding if and only if $\mathbf{v} = \mathbf{Py}$.

Proof. To prove property 1, we note that since $\mathbf{Py}$ is the projection of $\mathbf{y}$ onto $\mathcal{V}$, $\mathbf{y} - \mathbf{Py} \in \mathcal{V}^\perp$ and $\mathbf{Py} - \mathbf{v} \in \mathcal{V}$. Hence, $\mathbf{y} - \mathbf{Py} \perp \mathbf{Py} - \mathbf{v}$, so that the cross term is zero in

$$\| \mathbf{y} - \mathbf{v} \|^2 = \| (\mathbf{y} - \mathbf{Py}) + (\mathbf{Py} - \mathbf{v}) \|^2.$$

We therefore get $\| \mathbf{y} - \mathbf{v} \|^2 = \| \mathbf{y} - \mathbf{Py} \|^2 + \| \mathbf{Py} - \mathbf{v} \|^2$. To prove property 2, first note that since $\| \mathbf{y} - \mathbf{v} \|^2 = \| \mathbf{y} - \mathbf{Py} \|^2 + \| \mathbf{Py} - \mathbf{v} \|^2$, and $\| \mathbf{Py} - \mathbf{v} \|^2 \geq 0$, we must have $\| \mathbf{y} - \mathbf{Py} \|^2 \leq \| \mathbf{y} - \mathbf{v} \|^2$ for all $\mathbf{v} \in \mathcal{V}$. It is also obvious that $\| \mathbf{Py} - \mathbf{v} \|^2 = 0$, and we get equality if and only if $\mathbf{v} = \mathbf{Py}$, i.e., $\mathbf{v} \in \mathcal{V}$ is the vector closest to $\mathbf{y}$. ∎

Result 2.6.6. Let $\mathbf{X}$ be an $n \times k$ matrix of rank k and with column space $\mathcal{C}(\mathbf{X})$. There exists an $(n - k) \times n$ matrix $\mathbf{Z}$ such that $\mathbf{ZX} = \mathbf{0}$, and $\mathcal{C}(\mathbf{X}) = \mathcal{N}(\mathbf{Z})$.

Proof. Let $\Omega = \mathcal{C}(\mathbf{X})$. By Definition 2.6.3 and Result 2.6.3, we see that $\mathbf{P}_\Omega = \mathbf{X}(\mathbf{X}'\mathbf{X})^{-1}\mathbf{X}'$ has rank k, while the $n \times n$ matrix $\mathbf{I}_n - \mathbf{P}_\Omega = \mathbf{I}_n - \mathbf{X}(\mathbf{X}'\mathbf{X})^{-1}\mathbf{X}'$ has rank $n - k$. Let $\mathbf{Z}$ consist of any $n - k$ LIN rows of $\mathbf{I}_n - \mathbf{P}_\Omega$. Since $(\mathbf{I}_n - \mathbf{P}_\Omega)\mathbf{P}_\Omega = \mathbf{0}$ by Result 2.6.4, we have $\mathbf{ZX} = \mathbf{0}$. Further, by Definition 2.6.2, $\mathcal{N}(\mathbf{Z}) = \mathcal{C}(\mathbf{Z}')^\perp = \mathcal{C}(\mathbf{I}_n - \mathbf{P}_\Omega)^\perp = \Omega$. ∎

Result 2.6.7. Let $\Omega \subset \mathcal{R}^n$, $\Omega_1 \subset \Omega$, $\Omega_1^\perp \subset \Omega$, and let $\mathbf{P}_\Omega$, $\mathbf{P}_{\Omega_1}$ and $\mathbf{P}_{\Omega_1^\perp}$ denote the corresponding projection operators. Then,

1. $\mathbf{P}_\Omega \mathbf{P}_{\Omega_1} = \mathbf{P}_{\Omega_1} \mathbf{P}_\Omega = \mathbf{P}_{\Omega_1}$.

2. $\mathbf{P}_\Omega \mathbf{P}_{\Omega_1^\perp} = \mathbf{P}_{\Omega_1^\perp} \mathbf{P}_\Omega = \mathbf{P}_{\Omega_1^\perp}$.

3. $\mathbf{P}_{\Omega_1} \mathbf{P}_{\Omega_1^\perp} = \mathbf{P}_{\Omega_1^\perp} \mathbf{P}_{\Omega_1} = \mathbf{0}$.

4. $\mathbf{P}_\Omega = \mathbf{P}_{\Omega_1} + \mathbf{P}_{\Omega_1^\perp \cap \Omega}$.

Proof. Since by Result 2.6.3, $\Omega_1 = \mathcal{C}(\mathbf{P}_{\Omega_1})$, we see that $\mathbf{P}_\Omega \mathbf{P}_{\Omega_1} = \mathbf{P}_{\Omega_1}$. By symmetry of these projection matrices, property 1 follows. This implies that a vector $\mathbf{v}$ projected first onto Ω and then onto Ω_1 stays in Ω_1. The proof of property 2 is similar. To prove property 3, write $\mathbf{P}_{\Omega_1^\perp} \mathbf{P}_{\Omega_1} = \mathbf{P}_{\Omega_1^\perp}(\mathbf{P}_\Omega - \mathbf{P}_{\Omega_1^\perp}) = \mathbf{P}_{\Omega_1^\perp} \mathbf{P}_\Omega - \mathbf{P}_{\Omega_1^\perp}^2 = \mathbf{P}_{\Omega_1^\perp} - \mathbf{P}_{\Omega_1^\perp} = \mathbf{0}$. To prove property 4, which states property 3 in an alternate way, consider $\mathbf{P}_\Omega \mathbf{y} = \mathbf{P}_{\Omega_1} \mathbf{y} + (\mathbf{P}_\Omega - \mathbf{P}_{\Omega_1})\mathbf{y}$, where $\mathbf{P}_\Omega \mathbf{y} \in \Omega$, and $\mathbf{P}_{\Omega_1} \mathbf{y} \in \Omega$. We also see that $(\mathbf{P}_\Omega - \mathbf{P}_{\Omega_1})\mathbf{y} \in \Omega$. Thus, $\mathbf{P}_\Omega \mathbf{y} = \mathbf{P}_{\Omega_1} \mathbf{y} + (\mathbf{P}_\Omega - \mathbf{P}_{\Omega_1})\mathbf{y}$ corresponds to the unique orthogonal decomposition described in Result 2.6.1, so that $\mathbf{P}_\Omega = \mathbf{P}_{\Omega_1} + \mathbf{P}_{\Omega_1^\perp \cap \Omega}$. ∎

2.7 Vector and matrix differentiation

We first define derivatives of vectors, matrices, products of vectors and matrices, as well as scalar functions of vectors and matrices, results which commonly appear in linear model theory (see Magnus and Neudecker, 1988 for more details). We assume throughout that all the derivatives exist and are continuous.

Definition 2.7.1. Let $\beta = (\beta_1, \cdots, \beta_k)'$ be a k-dimensional vector and let $f(\beta)$ denote a scalar function of β. The first partial differential of f with respect to β is defined to be the k-dimensional vector of partial differentials $\partial f/\partial \beta_i$:

$$\partial f(\beta)/\partial \beta = \partial f/\partial \beta = \begin{pmatrix} \partial f/\partial \beta_1 \\ \partial f/\partial \beta_2 \\ \vdots \\ \partial f/\partial \beta_k \end{pmatrix}. \tag{2.7.1}$$

Also,

$$\partial f/\partial \beta' = \begin{pmatrix} \partial f/\partial \beta_1, & \partial f/\partial \beta_2, & \cdots, & \partial f/\partial \beta_k \end{pmatrix}. \tag{2.7.2}$$

Definition 2.7.2. The second partial differential of f with respect to β is defined to be the $k \times k$ matrix of partial differentials $\partial^2 f/\partial \beta_i \partial \beta_j$:

$$\partial^2 f/\partial \beta \partial \beta' = \begin{pmatrix} \partial^2 f/\partial \beta_1^2 & \partial^2 f/\partial \beta_1 \partial \beta_2 & \cdots & \partial^2 f/\partial \beta_1 \partial \beta_k \\ \partial^2 f/\partial \beta_1 \partial \beta_2 & \partial^2 f/\partial \beta_2^2 & \cdots & \partial^2 f/\partial \beta_2 \partial \beta_k \\ \vdots & \vdots & \cdots & \vdots \\ \partial^2 f/\partial \beta_1 \partial \beta_k & \partial^2 f/\partial \beta_2 \partial \beta_k & \cdots & \partial^2 f/\partial \beta_k^2 \end{pmatrix}. \tag{2.7.3}$$

Example 2.7.1. Let $\beta = (\beta_1, \beta_2)'$ and let $f(\beta) = (\beta_1^2 - 2\beta_1 \beta_2)$. Then,

$$\partial f/\partial \beta' = \begin{pmatrix} 2\beta_1 - 2\beta_2, & -2\beta_1 \end{pmatrix}$$

and

$$\partial^2 f/\partial \beta \partial \beta' = \begin{pmatrix} 2 & -2 \\ -2 & 0 \end{pmatrix}.$$

Result 2.7.1. Let f and g represent scalar functions of a k-dimensional vector β, and let a and b be real constants. Then

$$
\begin{aligned}
\partial(af + bg)/\partial \beta_j &= a\partial f/\partial \beta_j + b\partial g/\partial \beta_j \\
\partial(fg)/\partial \beta_j &= f\partial g/\partial \beta_j + g\partial f/\partial \beta_j \\
\partial(f/g)/\partial \beta_j &= (1/g^2)\{g\partial f/\partial \beta_j - f\partial g/\partial \beta_j\}.
\end{aligned} \tag{2.7.4}
$$

Definition 2.7.3. Let $\mathbf{A} = \{a_{ij}\}$ be an $m \times n$ matrix and let $f(\mathbf{A})$ be a real function of $\mathbf{A}$. The first partial differential of f with respect to $\mathbf{A}$ is defined as the $m \times n$ matrix of partial differentials $\partial f/\partial a_{ij}$:

$$
\begin{aligned}
\partial f(\mathbf{A})/\partial \mathbf{A} &= \{\partial f/\partial a_{ij}\}, i = 1, \cdots, m, j = 1, \cdots, n \\
&= \begin{pmatrix} \partial f/\partial a_{11} & \partial f/\partial a_{12} & \cdots & \partial f/\partial a_{1n} \\ \vdots & \vdots & & \vdots \\ \partial f/\partial a_{m1} & \partial f/\partial a_{m2} & \cdots & \partial f/\partial a_{mn} \end{pmatrix}.
\end{aligned} \quad (2.7.5)
$$

The results that follow give rules for finding partial derivatives of vector or matrix functions of matrices and vectors and are useful in the first step in linear model theory, viz., obtaining a solution to the least squares minimization problem.

Result 2.7.2. Let β denote an n-dimensional vector and let $\mathbf{A}$ be an $m \times n$ matrix. Then

$$\partial \mathbf{A}\beta/\partial \beta' = \mathbf{A}, \text{ and } \partial \beta' \mathbf{A}'/\partial \beta = \mathbf{A}'. \quad (2.7.6)$$

Proof. We may write

$$
\mathbf{A}\beta = \begin{pmatrix} a_{11}\beta_1 + \cdots + a_{1n}\beta_n \\ a_{21}\beta_1 + \cdots + a_{2n}\beta_n \\ \vdots \\ a_{m1}\beta_1 + \cdots + a_{mn}\beta_n \end{pmatrix},
$$

so that by Definition 2.7.2, $\partial \mathbf{A}\beta/\partial \beta'$ is given by

$$
\begin{aligned}
&\begin{pmatrix} \partial(a_{11}\beta_1 + \cdots + a_{1n}\beta_n)/\partial \beta_1 & \cdots & \partial(a_{11}\beta_1 + \cdots + a_{1n}\beta_n)/\partial \beta_n \\ \partial(a_{21}\beta_1 + \cdots + a_{2n}\beta_n)/\partial \beta_1 & \cdots & \partial(a_{21}\beta_1 + \cdots + a_{2n}\beta_n)/\partial \beta_n \\ \vdots & & \vdots \\ \partial(a_{m1}\beta_1 + \cdots + a_{mn}\beta_n)/\partial \beta_1 & \cdots & \partial(a_{m1}\beta_1 + \cdots + a_{mn}\beta_n)/\partial \beta_n \end{pmatrix} \\
&= \begin{pmatrix} a_{11} & \cdots & a_{1n} \\ \vdots & \vdots & \vdots \\ a_{m1} & & a_{mn} \end{pmatrix} = \mathbf{A}.
\end{aligned} \quad (2.7.7)
$$

That $\partial \beta' \mathbf{A}'/\partial \beta = \mathbf{A}'$ follows by transposing both sides of (2.7.7). ∎

Result 2.7.3. Let β be an n-dimensional vector and let $\mathbf{A}$ be an $n \times n$ matrix. Then

$$
\begin{aligned}
\partial \beta' \mathbf{A}\beta/\partial \beta &= (\mathbf{A} + \mathbf{A}')\beta \\
\partial \beta' \mathbf{A}\beta/\partial \beta' &= \beta'(\mathbf{A} + \mathbf{A}') \\
\partial^2 \beta' \mathbf{A}\beta/\partial \beta \, \partial \beta' &= \mathbf{A} + \mathbf{A}'.
\end{aligned} \quad (2.7.8)
$$

Further, if $\mathbf{A}$ is a symmetric matrix,

$$
\begin{aligned}
\partial \beta' \mathbf{A}\beta/\partial \beta &= 2\mathbf{A}\beta \\
\partial \beta' \mathbf{A}\beta/\partial \beta' &= 2\beta' \mathbf{A} \\
\partial^2 \beta' \mathbf{A}\beta/\partial \beta \, \partial \beta' &= 2\mathbf{A}.
\end{aligned} \quad (2.7.9)
$$

Proof. We will prove the result for a symmetric matrix $\mathbf{A}$. Clearly,

$$\beta'\mathbf{A}\beta = \sum_{i,j=1}^{n} a_{ij}\beta_i\beta_j$$

so that

$$
\begin{aligned}
\partial\beta'\mathbf{A}\beta/\partial\beta_r &= \sum_{\substack{j=1 \\ r\neq j}}^{n} a_{rj}\beta_j + \sum_{\substack{i=1 \\ r\neq i}}^{n} a_{ir}\beta_i + 2a_{rr}\beta_r \\
&= 2\sum_{j=1}^{n} a_{rj}\beta_j \quad \text{(by symmetry of } \mathbf{A}) \\
&= 2\mathbf{a}_r'\beta
\end{aligned}
$$

where $\mathbf{a}_r'$ denotes the rth row vector of $\mathbf{A}$. By Definition 2.7.3, we get

$$\frac{\partial\beta'\mathbf{A}\beta}{\partial\beta} = \begin{pmatrix} \partial\beta'\mathbf{A}\beta/\partial\beta_1 \\ \partial\beta'\mathbf{A}\beta/\partial\beta_2 \\ \vdots \\ \partial\beta'\mathbf{A}\beta/\partial\beta_n \end{pmatrix} = 2\begin{pmatrix} \mathbf{a}_1' \\ \mathbf{a}_2' \\ \vdots \\ \mathbf{a}_n'. \end{pmatrix}\beta = 2\mathbf{A}\beta \qquad (2.7.10)$$

The second result follows by transposing both sides of (2.7.10). To show the last result, we again take the first partial derivative of $\partial\beta'\mathbf{A}\beta/\partial\beta' = 2\beta'\mathbf{A}$, and use Result 2.7.2. ∎

Result 2.7.4. Let $\mathbf{C}$ be an $m \times n$ matrix, α be an m-dimensional vector and β be an n-dimensional vector. Then

$$\frac{\partial\alpha'\mathbf{C}\beta}{\partial\mathbf{C}} = \alpha\beta'. \qquad (2.7.11)$$

Proof. Since

$$\alpha'\mathbf{C}\beta = \sum_{i=1}^{m}\sum_{j=1}^{n} c_{ij}\alpha_i\beta_j,$$

we have

$$\partial(\alpha'\mathbf{C}\beta)/\partial c_{kl} = \alpha_k\beta_l$$

which is the (k,l)th element of $\alpha\beta'$, from which the result follows. ∎

We next give a few useful results without proof.

Result 2.7.5. Let $\mathbf{A}$ be an $n \times n$ matrix. Then,

$$\frac{\partial tr(\mathbf{A})}{\partial\mathbf{A}} = \mathbf{I}_n, \text{ and} \qquad (2.7.12)$$

$$\frac{\partial|\mathbf{A}|}{\partial\mathbf{A}} = [\text{Adj}(\mathbf{A})]'$$

where $\text{Adj}(\mathbf{A})$ denotes the adjoint of $\mathbf{A}$.

Result 2.7.6.   Suppose $\mathbf{A}$ is an $n \times n$ matrix with $|\mathbf{A}| > 0$. Then

$$\frac{\partial \ln |\mathbf{A}|}{\partial \mathbf{A}} = (\mathbf{A}')^{-1}. \qquad (2.7.13)$$

Result 2.7.7   Let $\mathbf{A}$ be an $m \times n$ matrix and let $\mathbf{B}$ be an $n \times m$ matrix. Then

$$\frac{\partial tr(\mathbf{AB})}{\partial \mathbf{A}} = \mathbf{B}'. \qquad (2.7.14)$$

Result 2.7.8.   Let Ω be a symmetric matrix, let $\mathbf{y}$ be an n-dimensional vector, let β a k-dimensional vector, and let $\mathbf{X}$ be an $n \times k$ matrix. Then

$$\begin{aligned}
\partial(\mathbf{y} - \mathbf{X}\beta)'\Omega(\mathbf{y} - \mathbf{X}\beta)/\partial\beta &= -2\mathbf{X}'\Omega(\mathbf{y} - \mathbf{X}\beta), \text{ and} \\
\partial^2(\mathbf{y} - \mathbf{X}\beta)'\Omega(\mathbf{y} - \mathbf{X}\beta)/\partial\beta\partial\beta' &= 2\mathbf{X}'\Omega\mathbf{X}. \qquad (2.7.15)
\end{aligned}$$

The next definition deals with partial derivatives of a matrix (or a vector) with respect to some scalar θ. We see that in this case, the partial differential is itself a matrix or vector of the same dimension whose elements are the partial derivatives with respect to θ of each element of that matrix or vector.

Definition 2.7.4.   Let $\mathbf{A}$ be an $m \times n$ matrix which is a function of a scalar θ, then

$$\begin{aligned}
\partial\mathbf{A}/\partial\theta &= \{\partial a_{ij}/\partial\theta\}, i = 1, \cdots, m, j = 1, \cdots, n \\
&= \begin{pmatrix} \partial a_{11}/\partial\theta & \partial a_{12}/\partial\theta & \cdots & \partial a_{1n}/\partial\theta \\ \vdots & \vdots & & \vdots \\ \partial a_{m1}/\partial\theta & \partial a_{m2}/\partial\theta & \cdots & \partial a_{mn}/\partial\theta \end{pmatrix}. \qquad (2.7.16)
\end{aligned}$$

2.8   Special operations on matrices

Definition 2.8.1. Kronecker product of matrices.   Let $\mathbf{A} = \{a_{ij}\}$ be an $m \times n$ matrix and $\mathbf{B} = \{b_{ij}\}$ be a $p \times q$ matrix. The Kronecker product of $\mathbf{A}$ and $\mathbf{B}$ is denoted by $\mathbf{A} \otimes \mathbf{B}$ and is defined to be the $mp \times nq$ matrix

$$\mathbf{A} \otimes \mathbf{B} = \begin{pmatrix} a_{11}\mathbf{B} & a_{12}\mathbf{B} & \cdots & a_{1n}\mathbf{B} \\ a_{21}\mathbf{B} & a_{22}\mathbf{B} & \cdots & a_{2n}\mathbf{B} \\ \vdots & \vdots & \vdots & \vdots \\ a_{m1}\mathbf{B} & a_{m2}\mathbf{B} & \cdots & a_{mn}\mathbf{B} \end{pmatrix}. \qquad (2.8.1)$$

The matrix in (2.8.1) is a partitioned matrix whose (i, j)th entry is a $p \times q$ submatrix $a_{ij}\mathbf{B}$. The Kronecker product $\mathbf{A} \otimes \mathbf{B}$ can be defined regardless of the dimensions of $\mathbf{A}$ and $\mathbf{B}$. The Kronecker product is also referred to in the literature as the *direct product* or the *tensor product*.

Example 2.8.1.   Consider two matrices $\mathbf{A}$ and $\mathbf{B}$ where

$$\mathbf{A} = \begin{pmatrix} 3 & 4 & -1 \\ 2 & 0 & 0 \end{pmatrix}, \text{ and } \mathbf{B} = \begin{pmatrix} 5 & -1 \\ 3 & 3 \end{pmatrix}.$$

Then,

$$\mathbf{A} \otimes \mathbf{B} = \begin{pmatrix} 15 & -3 & 20 & -4 & -5 & 1 \\ 9 & 9 & 12 & 12 & -3 & -3 \\ 10 & -2 & 0 & 0 & 0 & 0 \\ 6 & 6 & 0 & 0 & 0 & 0 \end{pmatrix},$$

and

$$\mathbf{B} \otimes \mathbf{A} = \begin{pmatrix} 15 & 20 & -5 & -3 & -4 & 1 \\ 10 & 0 & 0 & -2 & 0 & 0 \\ 9 & 12 & -3 & 9 & 12 & -3 \\ 6 & 0 & 0 & 6 & 0 & 0 \end{pmatrix}. \qquad \square$$

In general, $\mathbf{A} \otimes \mathbf{B}$ is not equal to $\mathbf{B} \otimes \mathbf{A}$. The elements in these two products are the same, except that they are in different positions. The definition $\mathbf{A} \otimes \mathbf{B}$ extends naturally to more than two matrices:

$$\mathbf{A} \otimes \mathbf{B} \otimes \mathbf{C} = A \otimes (\mathbf{B} \otimes \mathbf{C}) \quad \text{and} \quad \overset{k}{\underset{i=1}{\otimes}} \mathbf{A}_i = \mathbf{A}_1 \otimes \mathbf{A}_2 \otimes \cdots \otimes \mathbf{A}_k. \qquad (2.8.2)$$

Result 2.8.1. Properties of Kronecker product. Let $\mathbf{A}$ be an $m \times n$ matrix. Then

1. For a positive scalar c, we have $c \otimes \mathbf{A} = \mathbf{A} \otimes c = c\mathbf{A}$.

2. For any diagonal matrix $D = \text{diag}(d_1, \cdots, d_k)$, we have

$$\mathbf{A} \otimes \mathbf{D} = \text{diag}(d_1 \mathbf{A}, \cdots, d_k \mathbf{A}).$$

3. $\mathbf{I} \otimes \mathbf{A} = \text{diag}(\mathbf{A}, \mathbf{A}, \cdots, \mathbf{A})$.

4. $\mathbf{I}_m \otimes \mathbf{I}_p = \mathbf{I}_{mp}$.

5. For a $p \times q$ matrix $\mathbf{B}$, we have $(\mathbf{A} \otimes \mathbf{B})' = \mathbf{A}' \otimes \mathbf{B}'$.

6. $(\mathbf{A} \otimes \mathbf{B})(\mathbf{C} \otimes \mathbf{D}) = (\mathbf{AC}) \otimes (\mathbf{BD})$, where we assume that relevant matrices are conformal for multiplication.

7. $r(\mathbf{A} \otimes \mathbf{B}) = r(\mathbf{A})r(\mathbf{B})$.

8. $(\mathbf{A} + \mathbf{B}) \otimes (\mathbf{C} + \mathbf{D}) = (\mathbf{A} \otimes \mathbf{C}) + (\mathbf{A} \otimes \mathbf{D}) + (\mathbf{B} \otimes \mathbf{C}) + (\mathbf{B} \otimes \mathbf{D})$.

9. Suppose $\mathbf{A}$ is an $n \times n$ matrix, and $\mathbf{B}$ is an $m \times m$ matrix. The nm eigenvalues of $\mathbf{A} \otimes \mathbf{B}$ are products of the n eigenvalues $\lambda_i, i = 1, \cdots, n$ of $\mathbf{A}$ and the m eigenvalues $\gamma_j, j = 1, \cdots, m$ of $\mathbf{B}$.

10. $|\mathbf{A} \otimes \mathbf{B}| = |\mathbf{A}|^m |\mathbf{B}|^n = \left[\prod_{i=1}^{n} \lambda_i \right]^m \left[\prod_{j=1}^{m} \gamma_j \right]^n$.

11. Provided all the inverses exist, $(\mathbf{A} \otimes \mathbf{B})^{-1} = \mathbf{A}^{-1} \otimes \mathbf{B}^{-1}$.

Moser and Sawyer (1998) present algorithms for sums of squares and covariance matrices using Kronecker products.

Definition 2.8.2. Vectorization of matrices.   Given an $m \times n$ matrix $\mathbf{A}$ with columns $\mathbf{a}_1, \mathbf{a}_2, \cdots, \mathbf{a}_n$, we define $vec(\mathbf{A}) = (\mathbf{a}'_1, \mathbf{a}'_2, \cdots, \mathbf{a}'_n)'$ to be an mn-dimensional column vector.

Result 2.8.2. Properties of the vec operator.

1. Given $m \times n$ matrices $\mathbf{A}$ and $\mathbf{B}$, $vec(\mathbf{A} + \mathbf{B}) = vec(\mathbf{A}) + vec(\mathbf{B})$.

2. If $\mathbf{A}$, $\mathbf{B}$ and $\mathbf{C}$ are respectively $m \times n$, $n \times p$ and $p \times q$ matrices, then

   (i) $vec(\mathbf{AB}) = (\mathbf{I}_p \otimes \mathbf{A})vec(\mathbf{B}) = (\mathbf{B}' \otimes \mathbf{I}_m)vec(\mathbf{A})$.

   (ii) $vec(\mathbf{ABC}) = (\mathbf{C}' \otimes \mathbf{A})vec(\mathbf{B})$.

   (iii) $vec(\mathbf{ABC}) = (\mathbf{I}_q \otimes \mathbf{AB})vec(\mathbf{C}) = (\mathbf{C}'\mathbf{B}' \otimes \mathbf{I}_n)vec(\mathbf{A})$.

3. If $\mathbf{A}$ is $m \times n$ and $\mathbf{B}$ is $n \times m$,

$$vec(\mathbf{B}')'vec(\mathbf{A}) = vec(\mathbf{A}')'vec(\mathbf{B}) = tr(\mathbf{AB}).$$

4. If $\mathbf{A}$, $\mathbf{B}$ and $\mathbf{C}$ are respectively $m \times n$, $n \times p$ and $p \times m$ matrices,

$$
\begin{aligned}
tr(\mathbf{ABC}) &= vec(\mathbf{A}')'(\mathbf{C}' \otimes \mathbf{I}_n)vec(\mathbf{B}) \\
&= vec(\mathbf{A}')'(\mathbf{I}_m \otimes \mathbf{B})vec(\mathbf{C}) \\
&= vec(\mathbf{B}')'(\mathbf{A} \otimes \mathbf{I}_p)vec(\mathbf{C}) \\
&= vec(\mathbf{B}')'(\mathbf{I}_n \otimes \mathbf{C})vec(\mathbf{A}) \\
&= vec(\mathbf{C}')'(\mathbf{B}' \otimes \mathbf{I}_m)vec(\mathbf{A}) \\
&= vec(\mathbf{C}')'(\mathbf{I}_p \otimes \mathbf{A})vec(\mathbf{B})
\end{aligned}
$$

Definition 2.8.3. Direct sum of matrices.   The direct sum of two matrices $\mathbf{A}$ and $\mathbf{B}$ (which can be of any dimension) is defined as

$$\mathbf{A} \oplus \mathbf{B} = \begin{pmatrix} \mathbf{A} & \mathbf{0} \\ \mathbf{0} & \mathbf{B} \end{pmatrix}. \tag{2.8.3}$$

This operation extends naturally to more than two matrices:

$$\overset{k}{\underset{i=1}{\oplus}} \mathbf{A}_i = \sum_{i=1}^{k}{}^{+} \mathbf{A}_i = \mathbf{A}_1 \oplus \mathbf{A}_2 \oplus \cdots \oplus \mathbf{A}_k = \begin{pmatrix} \mathbf{A}_1 & \mathbf{0} & \cdots & \mathbf{0} \\ \mathbf{0} & \mathbf{A}_2 & \cdots & \mathbf{0} \\ \vdots & \vdots & \vdots & \vdots \\ \mathbf{0} & \mathbf{0} & \mathbf{0} & \mathbf{A}_k \end{pmatrix}. \tag{2.8.4}$$

This definition applies to vectors as well.

2.9 Linear optimization

The technique of Lagrange multipliers (sometimes called undetermined multipliers) is used to find the stationary points of a function of several variables subject to one or more constraints. Consider the problem of finding the minimum of a function $f(x_1, x_2)$ subject to a constraint relating x_1 and x_2 which is written as

$$g(x_1, x_2) = 0. \qquad (2.9.1)$$

One approach to the minimization is, of course, (a) to express x_2 as a function $h(x_1)$ of x_1 by solving (2.9.1), (b) to substitute $x_2 = h(x_1)$ into $f(x_1, x_2)$ to obtain $f(x_1, h(x_1))$, and (c) to minimize this function of a single variable x_1 in the "usual" way using differential calculus. A difficulty with this approach is that explicitly obtaining $h(x_1)$ may be difficult in some cases. A simpler, and more elegant method is the Lagrange multiplier approach, which incorporates a parameter λ into the minimization problem. Suppose $\mathbf{x} = (x_1, \cdots, x_d)' \in \mathcal{D} \subset \mathcal{R}^d$; the constraint equation $g(\mathbf{x}) = 0$ geometrically represents a surface $\mathcal{S}$ in $\mathcal{D}$. We denote the gradient of the function $f(\mathbf{x})$ at any point P on $\mathcal{S}$ by ∇f and wish to find the stationary point of $f(\mathbf{x})$ within the surface. To do this, we compute the component $\nabla^{\mathcal{S}} f$ of ∇f which lies in $\mathcal{S}$ and set $\nabla^{\mathcal{S}} f = 0$. Consider the Taylor expansion of $g(\mathbf{x})$

$$g(\mathbf{x} + \varepsilon) = g(\mathbf{x}) + \varepsilon' \nabla g(\mathbf{x})$$

for some small ε. If the point $\mathbf{x} + \varepsilon$ lies within the surface $\mathcal{S}$, then we have $g(\mathbf{x} + \varepsilon) = g(\mathbf{x})$, and $\varepsilon' \nabla g(\mathbf{x}) = 0$, i.e., the vector ∇g is orthogonal to the surface $g(\mathbf{x}) = 0$. We obtain $\nabla^{\mathcal{S}} f$ by adding to ∇f some multiple of ∇g:

$$\nabla^{\mathcal{S}} f = \nabla f + \lambda \nabla g. \qquad (2.9.2)$$

Let

$$L(\mathbf{x}, \lambda) = f(\mathbf{x}) + \lambda g(\mathbf{x}) \qquad (2.9.3)$$

denote the Lagrangian function. Note that $\partial L / \partial \lambda = 0$ leads to the constraint condition $g(\mathbf{x}) = 0$. The stationarity condition for minimizing L is $\nabla L = 0$, where ∇L is given by the right side of (2.9.2). We find the stationary point of $L(\mathbf{x}, \lambda)$ with respect to both $\mathbf{x}$ and λ, using $d+1$ equations, leading to stationary solutions $\widetilde{\mathbf{x}}$ and $\widetilde{\lambda}$. If we are not interested in λ, we can eliminate it from the stationarity equations without the necessity of finding its value (hence λ is called the "undetermined multiplier"). This technique can be extended to the situation where there are K constraints, $g_j(\mathbf{x}) = 0$, $j = 1, \cdots, K$. In this case, the Lagrangian function becomes

$$L(\mathbf{x}, \lambda) = f(\mathbf{x}) + \sum_{j=1}^{K} \lambda_j g_j(\mathbf{x}), \qquad (2.9.4)$$

where $\lambda = (\lambda_1, \cdots, \lambda_K)'$ denotes the vector of Lagrangian multipliers. We minimize (2.9.4) with respect to $\mathbf{x}$ and λ (see Dixon, 1972).

Exercises

2.1. Let $\mathbf{P} = (\mathbf{A} \quad \mathbf{B})$, where $\mathbf{P}$ is an $n \times n$ orthogonal matrix. Show that $\mathbf{A}'\mathbf{A}$ is an idempotent matrix.

2.2. Suppose an $m \times n$ matrix $\mathbf{A}$ is partitioned as $\mathbf{A} = \begin{pmatrix} \mathbf{A}_{11} & \mathbf{A}_{12} \\ \mathbf{A}_{21} & \mathbf{A}_{22} \end{pmatrix}$, where $\mathbf{A}_{11}, \mathbf{A}_{12}, \mathbf{A}_{21}$, and $\mathbf{A}_{22}$ are respectively $r \times r$, $r \times (n-r)$, $(n-r) \times r$, and $(n-r) \times (n-r)$ submatrices, such that $r(\mathbf{A}_{11}) = r(\mathbf{A}) = r > 0$. Show that $\mathbf{A}_{22} = \mathbf{A}_{21}\mathbf{A}_{11}^{-1}\mathbf{A}_{12}$.

2.3. Suppose an $n \times n$ matrix $\mathbf{A}$ is partitioned as $\begin{pmatrix} \mathbf{P} & \mathbf{x} \\ \mathbf{x}' & 1 \end{pmatrix}$, where $\mathbf{P}$ is an $(n-1) \times (n-1)$ dimensional nonsingular matrix, and $\mathbf{x}$ is an $(n-1)$-dimensional vector. Show that $\mathbf{x}'\mathbf{P}^{-1}\mathbf{x} = 1 - |\mathbf{P} - \mathbf{xx}'|/|\mathbf{P}|$.

2.4. Let $\mathbf{A}, \mathbf{B}, \mathbf{C}$, and $\mathbf{D}$ be $m \times p$, $p \times q$, $n \times m$, and $n \times q$ matrices respectively, and let $\mathbf{E} = \mathbf{D} - \mathbf{CAB}$.

   (a) Show that $r \begin{pmatrix} \mathbf{0} & \mathbf{B} \\ \mathbf{A} & \mathbf{0} \end{pmatrix} = r \begin{pmatrix} \mathbf{B} & \mathbf{0} \\ \mathbf{0} & \mathbf{A} \end{pmatrix} = r(\mathbf{A}) + r(\mathbf{B})$.

   (b) Show that $r \begin{pmatrix} \mathbf{A} & \mathbf{AB} \\ \mathbf{CA} & \mathbf{D} \end{pmatrix} = r \begin{pmatrix} \mathbf{D} & \mathbf{CA} \\ \mathbf{AB} & \mathbf{A} \end{pmatrix} = r(\mathbf{A}) + r(\mathbf{E})$.

2.5. Consider the partition in Example 2.1.2, and suppose that $\mathbf{A}_2$ contains only one column, i.e., $r = k - 1$. Show that

$$\mathbf{P} = \mathbf{P}_1 + \frac{(\mathbf{I}-\mathbf{P}_1)\mathbf{A}_2\mathbf{A}_2'(\mathbf{I}-\mathbf{P}_1)}{\mathbf{A}_2'(\mathbf{I}-\mathbf{P}_1)\mathbf{A}_2}.$$

2.6. [Rao and Toutenberg, 1995, p. 295]. Let $\mathbf{A}$ be an $n \times k$ matrix and $\mathbf{B}$ be a $k \times n$ matrix with $n \geq k$.

   (a) Show that $\begin{vmatrix} -\lambda\mathbf{I}_n & -\mathbf{A} \\ \mathbf{B} & \mathbf{I}_k \end{vmatrix} = (-\lambda)^{n-k}|\mathbf{BA}-\lambda\mathbf{I}_k| = |\mathbf{AB} - \lambda\mathbf{I}_n|$.

   (b) Hence, show that the n eigenvalues of $\mathbf{AB}$ are equal to the k eigenvalues of $\mathbf{BA}$, together with the eigenvalue 0, which has a multiplicity of $(n-k)$.

   (c) Let $\mathbf{v}$ denote a nonzero eigenvector corresponding to a nonzero eigenvalue λ of $\mathbf{AB}$. Show that $\mathbf{u} = \mathbf{Bv}$ is a nonzero eigenvector of $\mathbf{BA}$ corresponding to this λ.

2.7. Let $\mathbf{A} = \mathbf{aa}'$, where $\mathbf{a}$ is a nonzero n-dimensional vector. Show that the only nonzero eigenvalue of $\mathbf{A}$ is $\lambda = \mathbf{a}'\mathbf{a}$ with corresponding eigenvector $\mathbf{a}$.

2.8. Let $\mathbf{A}$ be a $k \times k$ nonsingular matrix, and let $\mathbf{B}$ and $\mathbf{C}$ be respectively $k \times n$ and $n \times k$ matrices. Show that $|\mathbf{A} + \mathbf{BC}| = |\mathbf{A}||\mathbf{I}_n + \mathbf{CA}^{-1}\mathbf{B}|$.

2.9. Let $\mathbf{B}$ and $\mathbf{C}$ be $k \times n$ and $n \times k$ matrices respectively. Show that $|\mathbf{I}_k + \mathbf{BC}| = |\mathbf{I}_n + \mathbf{CB}|$.

2.10. Show that $|\mathbf{A} + \mathbf{aa}'| = (1 + \mathbf{a}'\mathbf{A}^{-1}\mathbf{a})|\mathbf{A}|$, where $\mathbf{A}$ is a $k \times k$ nonsingular matrix and $\mathbf{a}$ is a k-dimensional vector.

2.11. If $(\mathbf{AB} - \mathbf{AC})'(\mathbf{AB} - \mathbf{AC}) = \mathbf{0}$, show that we must have $\mathbf{AB} - \mathbf{AC} = \mathbf{0}$.

2.12. Let $\mathbf{A}$ be an $n \times n$ symmetric matrix with eigenvalues $\lambda_1, \cdots, \lambda_n$.

    (a) Show that $r(\mathbf{A})$ is equal to the number of nonzero eigenvalues of $\mathbf{A}$.

    (b) Show that $\| \mathbf{A} \| = (\sum_{i=1}^{n} \lambda_i^2)^{1/2}$.

2.13. Let $\mathbf{A}$ be an $n \times n$ symmetric matrix which has k distinct eigenvalues $\lambda_1, \cdots, \lambda_k$ with geometric multiplicities $g_1, \cdots, g_k$ and algebraic multiplicities $a_1, \cdots, a_k$. Show that $\sum_{j=1}^{k} g_j = \sum_{j=1}^{k} a_j = n$, and that $g_j = a_j$ $(= m_j)$, for $j = 1, \cdots, k$.

2.14. Let $\mathbf{x}$ be an n-dimensional nonzero vector. Is

    ((a) $\frac{\mathbf{xx}'}{\mathbf{x}'\mathbf{x}}$ symmetric and idempotent ?

    (b) $\mathbf{xx}'$ symmetric and idempotent ?

2.15. Let $\mathbf{A}$ be an $n \times n$ symmetric matrix, let $\mathbf{B}$ and $\mathbf{U}$ be $k \times k$ and $n \times k$ matrices such that $\mathbf{U}'\mathbf{U} = \mathbf{I}_k$, and $\mathbf{AU} = \mathbf{UB}$. Show that there exists an $n \times (n-k)$ matrix $\mathbf{V}$ such that the $n \times n$ matrix $\begin{pmatrix} \mathbf{U} & \mathbf{V} \end{pmatrix}$ is orthogonal and $\begin{pmatrix} \mathbf{U} & \mathbf{V} \end{pmatrix}' \mathbf{A} \begin{pmatrix} \mathbf{U} & \mathbf{V} \end{pmatrix} = \begin{pmatrix} \mathbf{B} & \mathbf{0} \\ \mathbf{0} & \mathbf{V}'\mathbf{AV} \end{pmatrix}$.

2.16. Show that every symmetric idempotent matrix is nonnegative definite.

2.17. Let $\mathbf{A}$ be an $n \times n$ matrix. Show that the nonzero eigenvalues of $\mathbf{AA}'$ coincide with the nonzero eigenvalues of $\mathbf{A}'\mathbf{A}$.

2.18. Let $\mathbf{A}$ and $\mathbf{B}$ be $n \times k$ and $k \times n$ matrices respectively, with $n \geq k$.

    (a) Show that the n eigenvalues of $\mathbf{AB}$ are equal to the p eigenvalues of $\mathbf{BA}$, together with the eigenvalue 0 with multiplicity $(n - k)$.

    (b) If $\mathbf{x}$ is a nonzero eigenvector of $\mathbf{AB}$ corresponding to a nonzero eigenvalue λ, show that $\mathbf{y} = \mathbf{Bx}$ is a nonzero eigenvector of $\mathbf{BA}$ corresponding to λ.

2.19. Let $\mathbf{Q}$ be an $n \times n$ nonsingular matrix which diagonalizes a nonsingular matrix $\mathbf{A}$. Show that $\mathbf{A}^{-1}$ is also diagonalized by $\mathbf{Q}$.

2.20. Let $\mathbf{A}$ be an $n \times n$ symmetric matrix of rank r. Suppose $tr(\mathbf{A}) = tr(\mathbf{A}^2) = p$.

    (a) Show that $0 \leq p \leq r$.

    (b) If $tr(\mathbf{A}) = r$, show that $\mathbf{A}$ must be idempotent of rank r.

2.21. Suppose $\mathbf{A}_1$ and $\mathbf{A}_2$ are respectively $n \times p$ and $n \times q$ matrices of ranks p and q, and suppose the columns of $\mathbf{A}_1$ are LIN of the columns of $\mathbf{A}_2$. Let $\mathbf{B} = \mathbf{I} - \mathbf{A}_1(\mathbf{A}_1'\mathbf{A}_1)^{-1}\mathbf{A}_1'$. Show that $\mathbf{C} = \mathbf{A}_2'\mathbf{B}\mathbf{A}_2$ is nonsingular.

2.22. Let $\mathbf{P}$ be an $n \times n$ orthogonal matrix and let $\mathbf{A}$ be an $n \times n$ symmetric and idempotent matrix. Show that the matrix $\mathbf{P}'\mathbf{A}\mathbf{P}$ is symmetric and idempotent.

2.23. Let $\mathbf{A} = \begin{pmatrix} 2 & -1 & -1 \\ -1 & 1 & 1 \\ -1 & 1 & 4 \end{pmatrix}$. Verify that $\mathbf{A}$ is a p.d. matrix. Find a matrix $\mathbf{B}$ such that $\mathbf{A} = \mathbf{B}\mathbf{B}'$.

2.24. Let $\mathbf{A} = (1 - a)\mathbf{I}_n + a\mathbf{J}_n$. For what values of a is the matrix $\mathbf{A}$ p.d. ?

2.25. Let $\mathbf{B}$ be an $n \times n$ p.d. matrix and let $\mathbf{A}$ be an $n \times n$ symmetric matrix. Show that there exists a positive real number λ such that $\mathbf{B} - \lambda\mathbf{A}$ is p.d.

2.26. Let $\mathbf{A}$ be an $n \times n$ symmetric matrix and $\mathbf{x}$ be an n-dimensional vector.

  (a) If $\mathbf{x}'\mathbf{A}\mathbf{x} = 0$ for all $\mathbf{x}$, show that $\mathbf{A} = \mathbf{0}$.

  (b) Let $\mathbf{A}$ be p.s.d. Show that if $\mathbf{x}'\mathbf{A}\mathbf{x} = 0$, then $\mathbf{A}\mathbf{x} = \mathbf{0}$.

2.27. Let $\mathbf{A}$ and $\mathbf{B}$ be $n \times n$ symmetric matrices such that $\mathbf{A} + \mathbf{B}$ is nonsingular. Let $\mathbf{x}$, $\mathbf{a}$ and $\mathbf{b}$ be n-dimensional vectors. If $\mathbf{c} = (\mathbf{A} + \mathbf{B})^{-1}(\mathbf{A}\mathbf{a} + \mathbf{B}\mathbf{b})$, show that $(\mathbf{x} - \mathbf{a})'\mathbf{A}(\mathbf{x} - \mathbf{a}) + (\mathbf{x} - \mathbf{b})'\mathbf{B}(\mathbf{x} - \mathbf{b}) = (\mathbf{x} - \mathbf{c})'(\mathbf{A} + \mathbf{B})(\mathbf{x} - \mathbf{c}) + (\mathbf{a} - \mathbf{b})'\mathbf{A}(\mathbf{A} + \mathbf{B})^{-1}\mathbf{B}(\mathbf{a} - \mathbf{b})$.

2.28. Let $\mathbf{A}$, $\mathbf{B}$, and $\mathbf{C}$ be $m \times m$, $n \times n$ and $n \times m$ matrices respectively, and suppose $\mathbf{A}$ and $\mathbf{B}$ are p.d. Show that

  (a) $(\mathbf{A}^{-1} + \mathbf{C}'\mathbf{B}^{-1}\mathbf{C})^{-1} = \mathbf{A} - \mathbf{A}\mathbf{C}'(\mathbf{C}\mathbf{A}\mathbf{C}' + \mathbf{B})^{-1}\mathbf{C}\mathbf{A}$,

  (b) $(\mathbf{A}^{-1} + \mathbf{C}'\mathbf{B}^{-1}\mathbf{C})^{-1}\mathbf{C}'\mathbf{B}^{-1} = \mathbf{A}\mathbf{C}'(\mathbf{C}\mathbf{A}\mathbf{C}' + \mathbf{B})^{-1}$.

2.29. Let $\mathbf{A}_1, \cdots, \mathbf{A}_k$ be $n \times n$ matrices.

  (a) Show that a necessary condition for $\mathbf{A}_1, \cdots, \mathbf{A}_k$ to be simultaneously diagonalizable (by an $n \times n$ nonsingular matrix $\mathbf{P}$) is that $\mathbf{A}_j\mathbf{A}_i = \mathbf{A}_i\mathbf{A}_j$, $j > i = 1, \cdots, k$, i.e., $\mathbf{A}_1, \cdots, \mathbf{A}_k$ commute in pairs.

  (b) If $\mathbf{A}_1, \cdots, \mathbf{A}_k$ are symmetric, show that the condition in (a) is necessary and sufficient.

2.30. Let $\mathbf{A}$ and $\mathbf{B}$ be $n \times n$ symmetric n.n.d. matrices. Show that there exists a nonsingular matrix $\mathbf{P}$ such that $\mathbf{P}'\mathbf{A}\mathbf{P}$ and $\mathbf{P}'\mathbf{B}\mathbf{P}$ are both diagonal.

2.31. For square matrices $\mathbf{A}$ and $\mathbf{B}$, show that $tr(\mathbf{A} \otimes \mathbf{B}) = tr(\mathbf{A})tr(\mathbf{B})$.

2.32. If $\mathbf{u} = \mathbf{P}_\mathcal{V}\mathbf{y}$, $\mathbf{y} \in \mathcal{R}^n$, show that $\mathbf{P}_\mathcal{V}$ must be unique.

Chapter 3

Generalized Inverses and Solutions to Linear Systems

The notion of a generalized inverse of a matrix has its origin in the theory of simultaneous linear equations. A generalized inverse of a matrix $\mathbf{A}$ is some matrix $\mathbf{G}$ such that $\mathbf{Gb}$ is a solution to a set of consistent linear equations $\mathbf{Ax} = \mathbf{b}$ (Rao and Mitra, 1971). We give the definition and properties of generalized inverses of matrices in section 3.1, while in section 3.2, we discuss solutions to systems of linear equations. Both topics play a fundamental role in the development of linear model theory.

3.1 Generalized inverses

Definition 3.1.1. A generalized inverse (g-inverse) of an $m \times n$ matrix $\mathbf{A}$ is any $n \times m$ matrix $\mathbf{G}$ which satisfies the relation

$$\mathbf{AGA} = \mathbf{A}. \qquad (3.1.1)$$

The matrix $\mathbf{G}$ is also referred to in the literature as "conditional inverse" or "pseudo-inverse". We will refer to $\mathbf{G}$ as g-inverse and denote it by $\mathbf{A}^-$ (pronounced $\mathbf{A}$ minus).

Result 3.1.1. A g-inverse $\mathbf{G}$ of a real matrix $\mathbf{A}$ always exists. In general, $\mathbf{G}$ is not unique except in the special case where $\mathbf{A}$ is a square nonsingular matrix.

Proof. To show the existence of $\mathbf{G}$, we recall the full-rank factorization of an $m \times n$ matrix $\mathbf{A}$, with $r(\mathbf{A}) = r$ given by $\mathbf{A} = \mathbf{BC}$ where $\mathbf{B}$ and $\mathbf{C}$ are $m \times r$ and $r \times n$ matrices respectively, each with rank r, and $\mathbf{B}'\mathbf{B}$ and $\mathbf{CC}'$ are nonsingular (see Result 2.2.1). It is easy to verify that the $n \times m$ matrix defined by

$$\mathbf{A}_1^- = \mathbf{C}'(\mathbf{CC}')^{-1}(\mathbf{B}'\mathbf{B})^{-1}\mathbf{B}' \qquad (3.1.2)$$

satisfies (3.1.1) and is a g-inverse of $\mathbf{A}$. For arbitrary $n \times m$ matrices $\mathbf{E}$ and $\mathbf{F}$, let

$$\mathbf{A}_2^- = \mathbf{A}_1^- \mathbf{A} \mathbf{A}_1^- + (\mathbf{I}_n - \mathbf{A}_1^- \mathbf{A})\mathbf{E} + \mathbf{F}(\mathbf{I}_m - \mathbf{A}\mathbf{A}_1^-). \tag{3.1.3}$$

By direct multiplication, it is easy to verify that $\mathbf{A}_2^-$ satisfies (3.1.1). Inserting different matrices $\mathbf{E}$ and $\mathbf{F}$ into (3.1.3) generates an infinite number of g-inverses of $\mathbf{A}$, starting from $\mathbf{A}_1^-$. The only matrix $\mathbf{A}$ which has a unique g-inverse is a square matrix with $|\mathbf{A}| \neq 0$. Use the notation $\mathbf{A}^-$ for $\mathbf{G}$ in (3.1.1), and pre-multiply and post-multiply both sides by $\mathbf{A}^{-1}$ to get

$$\mathbf{A}^{-1}\mathbf{A}\mathbf{A}^-\mathbf{A}\mathbf{A}^{-1} = \mathbf{A}^{-1}\mathbf{A}\mathbf{A}^{-1}, \quad \text{i.e.,} \quad \mathbf{A}^- = \mathbf{A}^{-1},$$

and completes the proof. ∎

Result 3.1.2. Algorithm to compute $\mathbf{A}^-$. Let $\mathbf{B}_{11}$ denote a submatrix of $\mathbf{A}$ with $r(\mathbf{B}_{11}) = r(\mathbf{A}) = r$. Let $\mathbf{R}$ and $\mathbf{S}$ denote elementary permutation matrices that bring $\mathbf{B}_{11}$ to the leading position, i.e.,

$$\mathbf{RAS} = \begin{pmatrix} \mathbf{B}_{11} & \mathbf{B}_{12} \\ \mathbf{B}_{21} & \mathbf{B}_{22} \end{pmatrix} = \mathbf{B}, \text{ say.}$$

Then,

$$\mathbf{A}^- = \mathbf{SB}^-\mathbf{R} = \{\mathbf{R}'(\mathbf{B}^-)'\mathbf{S}'\}' \tag{3.1.4}$$

is a g-inverse of $\mathbf{A}$, where

$$\mathbf{B}^- = \begin{pmatrix} \mathbf{B}_{11}^{-1} & \mathbf{0} \\ \mathbf{0} & \mathbf{0} \end{pmatrix}. \tag{3.1.5}$$

Proof. Since $\mathbf{R}$ and $\mathbf{S}$ are orthogonal, $\mathbf{R}' = \mathbf{R}^{-1}$ and $\mathbf{S}' = \mathbf{S}^{-1}$, so that $\mathbf{A} = \mathbf{R}'\mathbf{BS}'$. It is easy to verify that $\mathbf{B}^-$ satisfies (3.1.1), so that it is a g-inverse of $\mathbf{B}$ (see Exercise 2.2). Now,

$$\mathbf{AA}^-\mathbf{A} = \mathbf{R}'\mathbf{BS}'\mathbf{SB}^-\mathbf{RR}'\mathbf{BS}' = \mathbf{R}'\mathbf{BB}^-\mathbf{BS}' = \mathbf{R}'\mathbf{BS}' = \mathbf{A}$$

since $\mathbf{RR}' = \mathbf{I}_m$ and $\mathbf{S}'\mathbf{S} = \mathbf{I}_n$. ∎

To summarize the algorithm, we find a submatrix $\mathbf{B}_{11}$ of order r of $\mathbf{A}$, and compute $(\mathbf{B}_{11}^{-1})'$. In $\mathbf{A}$, we replace each element of $\mathbf{B}_{11}$ by the corresponding element of $(\mathbf{B}_{11}^{-1})'$, and replace all other elements of $\mathbf{A}$ by 0. We transpose the resulting matrix to obtain $\mathbf{A}^-$.

Example 3.1.1. We will find a g-inverse of the rectangular matrix

$$\mathbf{A} = \begin{pmatrix} 4 & 1 & 2 & 0 \\ 1 & 1 & 5 & 15 \\ 3 & 1 & 3 & 5 \end{pmatrix}$$

using Result 3.1.2. We first verify that $r(\mathbf{A}) = 2$. Next, suppose $\mathbf{B}_{11} = \begin{pmatrix} 4 & 1 \\ 1 & 1 \end{pmatrix}$; then $|\mathbf{B}_{11}| = 3$. Application of Result 3.1.2 gives the corresponding g-inverse as

$$\mathbf{A}^- = \begin{pmatrix} 1/3 & -1/3 & 0 \\ -1/3 & 4/3 & 0 \\ 0 & 0 & 0 \\ 0 & 0 & 0 \end{pmatrix}.$$

Suppose, we now choose another nonsingular submatrix of $\mathbf{A}$ of rank 2, i.e., we let $\mathbf{B}_{11} = \begin{pmatrix} 1 & 15 \\ 1 & 5 \end{pmatrix}$, with $|\mathbf{B}_{11}| = -10$. Using the algorithm, we find the corresponding g-inverse to be

$$\mathbf{A}^- = \begin{pmatrix} 0 & 0 & 0 \\ 0 & -1/2 & 3/2 \\ 0 & 0 & 0 \\ 0 & 1/10 & -1/10 \end{pmatrix}. \qquad \square$$

In this example, we see that a unique g-inverse of $\mathbf{A}$ does not exist. Result 3.1.3 shows this formally.

Example 3.1.2. Let $\mathbf{A}$ be an $m \times n$ matrix with a g-inverse $\mathbf{G}$. The following results can be verified using (3.1.1).

1. For nonsingular matrices $\mathbf{P}$ and $\mathbf{Q}$, a g-inverse of $\mathbf{PAQ}$ is the matrix $\mathbf{Q}^{-1}\mathbf{GP}^{-1}$. This is clear from $\mathbf{PAQQ}^{-1}\mathbf{GP}^{-1}\mathbf{PAQ} = \mathbf{PAQ}$, since $\mathbf{PP}^{-1} = \mathbf{I}_m$, $\mathbf{QQ}^{-1} = \mathbf{I}_n$, and $\mathbf{AGA} = \mathbf{A}$.

2. A g-inverse of $\mathbf{GA}$ is $\mathbf{GA}$ since $\mathbf{GAGAGA} = \mathbf{GAGA} = \mathbf{GA}$.

3. Let c be a scalar. A g-inverse of $c\mathbf{A}$ is $\mathbf{G}/c$, which is verified by seeing that $c\mathbf{A}(\mathbf{G}/c)c\mathbf{A} = c\mathbf{AGA} = c\mathbf{A}$.

4. A g-inverse of the unit matrix $\mathbf{J}_n$ is $\mathbf{I}_n/n$, which is verified by $\mathbf{J}_n(\mathbf{I}_n/n)\mathbf{J}_n = n\mathbf{J}_n/n = \mathbf{J}_n$. $\quad \square$

Example 3.1.3. Let

$$\mathbf{A} = \begin{pmatrix} 2 & 2 & 6 \\ 2 & 3 & 8 \\ 6 & 8 & 22 \end{pmatrix},$$

with $|\mathbf{A}| = 0$. Let $\mathbf{B}_{11} = \begin{pmatrix} 2 & 6 \\ 2 & 8 \end{pmatrix}$, with $|\mathbf{B}_{11}| = 4$. Using the algorithm in Result 3.1.2, we find the g-inverse corresponding to $\mathbf{B}_{11}$ to be

$$\mathbf{A}^- = \begin{pmatrix} 2 & -3/2 & 0 \\ 0 & 0 & 0 \\ -1/2 & 1/2 & 0 \end{pmatrix}.$$

Again, let $\mathbf{B}_{11} = \begin{pmatrix} 2 & 2 \\ 2 & 3 \end{pmatrix}$, with $|\mathbf{B}_{11}| = 2$. Using the algorithm, we find the corresponding g-inverse

$$\mathbf{A}^- = \begin{pmatrix} 3/2 & -1 & 0 \\ -1 & 1 & 0 \\ 0 & 0 & 0 \end{pmatrix},$$

which is symmetric. □

The previous example demonstrates that even if $\mathbf{A}$ is an $n \times n$ symmetric matrix, its g-inverse $\mathbf{A}^-$ is not necessarily symmetric. However, we can always construct a symmetric g-inverse of a symmetric matrix. To see this, note that if $\mathbf{A}^-$ is any g-inverse of a symmetric matrix $\mathbf{A}$, so is $\mathbf{A}^{-\prime}$ (see Result 3.1.3), and therefore, the symmetric matrix $\frac{1}{2}(\mathbf{A}^- + \mathbf{A}^{-\prime})$ is a g-inverse of $\mathbf{A}$. In general, we may also obtain a symmetric g-inverse by applying the same permutation in the algorithm of Result 3.1.2 to the rows and to the columns. This would result in a symmetric $\mathbf{B}_{11}$ and therefore a symmetric g-inverse.

Result 3.1.3. Let $\mathbf{A}^-$ be a g-inverse of a symmetric matrix $\mathbf{A}$. Then $(\mathbf{A}^-)'$ is also a g-inverse of $\mathbf{A}$.

Proof. By (3.1.1), we have $\mathbf{AA}^-\mathbf{A} = \mathbf{A}$. Transposing both sides, and using $\mathbf{A}' = \mathbf{A}$, we get the result. ∎

Result 3.1.4. If $\mathbf{A}^-$ is a g-inverse of $\mathbf{A}$, then

$$r(\mathbf{A}) \leq r(\mathbf{A}^-) \leq \min(n, m). \tag{3.1.6}$$

Proof. The proof follows directly from property 4 of Result 1.2.12. ∎

Result 3.1.5. Let $\mathbf{A}$ be an $m \times n$ matrix of rank r. Then

1. $\mathbf{A}^-\mathbf{A}$ and $\mathbf{AA}^-$ are idempotent.

2. $(\mathbf{I} - \mathbf{A}^-\mathbf{A})$ and $(\mathbf{I} - \mathbf{AA}^-)$ are idempotent.

3. $r(\mathbf{A}^-\mathbf{A}) = r(\mathbf{A}) = r$ and $r(\mathbf{I} - \mathbf{A}^-\mathbf{A}) = n - r(\mathbf{A}) = n - r$.

4. $tr(\mathbf{A}^-\mathbf{A}) = tr(\mathbf{AA}^-) = r$.

Proof. Using (3.1.1), we see that $(\mathbf{A}^-\mathbf{A})(\mathbf{A}^-\mathbf{A}) = \mathbf{A}^-\mathbf{A}$ and $(\mathbf{AA}^-)(\mathbf{AA}^-) = \mathbf{AA}^-$, proving property 1. We can prove property 2 by a similar application of (3.1.1). To prove property 3, we see that since $(\mathbf{I} - \mathbf{A}^-\mathbf{A})$ is idempotent, it follows from property 3 of Result 2.3.9 that $r(\mathbf{I} - \mathbf{A}^-\mathbf{A}) = tr(\mathbf{I} - \mathbf{A}^-\mathbf{A}) = n - r(\mathbf{A}) = n - r$. The result for $\mathbf{A}^-\mathbf{A}$ follows immediately. Property 4 follows from property 3 and the idempotency of $\mathbf{AA}^-$ and $\mathbf{A}^-\mathbf{A}$. ∎

Definition 3.1.2. If $\mathbf{A}^-\mathbf{A} = \mathbf{A}\mathbf{A}^-$, then $\mathbf{A}^-$ is called a commuting g-inverse of $\mathbf{A}$, where $\mathbf{A}$ is a square matrix (Englefield, 1966).

Result 3.1.6. Let $\mathbf{D} = \mathrm{diag}(d_1, \cdots, d_n)$. Then, $\mathbf{D}^-$ is a diagonal matrix with the ith diagonal element given by $1/d_i$ if $d_i \neq 0$ and by 0 if $d_i = 0$.

Proof. It is easy to verify that $\mathbf{D}^-$ satisfies (3.1.1). ■

Result 3.1.7. Let $\mathbf{A}$ be a symmetric matrix of rank r. Let $\lambda_1, \cdots, \lambda_n$ denote the eigenvalues of $\mathbf{A}$ and let $\mathbf{x}_1, \cdots, \mathbf{x}_n$ denote the corresponding eigenvectors of $\mathbf{A}$. A g-inverse of $\mathbf{A}$ is given by $\mathbf{A}^- = \mathbf{X}\mathbf{D}^-\mathbf{X}'$, where $\mathbf{X} = (\mathbf{x}_1, \cdots, \mathbf{x}_n)'$ and $\mathbf{D}^- = \mathrm{diag}(d_1, \cdots, d_n)$, where $d_i = 1/\lambda_i$ if $\lambda_i \neq 0$ and $d_i = 0$ if $\lambda_i = 0$.

Proof. Note that there are exactly r nonzero eigenvalues, and without loss of generality, we can label them as the first r values, viz., $\lambda_1, \cdots, \lambda_r$. Since $\mathbf{A}$ is symmetric, we have by Result 2.3.4 that

$$\mathbf{A} = \mathbf{X}\mathbf{D}\mathbf{X}' \text{ with } \mathbf{X}\mathbf{X}' = \mathbf{X}'\mathbf{X} = \mathbf{I}_n.$$

Since $\mathbf{D}^-$ is a g-inverse of $\mathbf{D}$,

$$\mathbf{A}\mathbf{A}^-\mathbf{A} = \mathbf{X}\mathbf{D}\mathbf{X}'\mathbf{X}\mathbf{D}^-\mathbf{X}'\mathbf{X}\mathbf{D}\mathbf{X}' = \mathbf{X}\mathbf{D}\mathbf{D}^-\mathbf{D}\mathbf{X}' = \mathbf{X}\mathbf{D}\mathbf{X}' = \mathbf{A},$$

so that $\mathbf{X}\mathbf{D}^-\mathbf{X}'$ is a g-inverse of $\mathbf{A}$. ■

Result 3.1.8. Let $\mathbf{G}$ be a g-inverse of the symmetric matrix $\mathbf{A}'\mathbf{A}$, where $\mathbf{A}$ is any $m \times n$ matrix. Then,

1. $\mathbf{G}'$ is also a g-inverse of $\mathbf{A}'\mathbf{A}$.

2. $\mathbf{G}\mathbf{A}'$ is a g-inverse of $\mathbf{A}$, so that

$$\mathbf{A}\mathbf{G}\mathbf{A}'\mathbf{A} = \mathbf{A}. \tag{3.1.7}$$

3. $\mathbf{A}\mathbf{G}\mathbf{A}'$ is invariant to $\mathbf{G}$, i.e.,

$$\mathbf{A}\mathbf{G}_1\mathbf{A}' = \mathbf{A}\mathbf{G}_2\mathbf{A}', \tag{3.1.8}$$

   for any two g-inverses $\mathbf{G}_1$ and $\mathbf{G}_2$ of $\mathbf{A}'\mathbf{A}$.

4. Whether or not $\mathbf{G}$ is symmetric, $\mathbf{A}\mathbf{G}\mathbf{A}'$ is.

Proof. To prove property 1, we see that since $\mathbf{G}$ is a g-inverse of $\mathbf{A}'\mathbf{A}$, we have from (3.1.1) that $\mathbf{A}'\mathbf{A}\mathbf{G}\mathbf{A}'\mathbf{A} = \mathbf{A}'\mathbf{A}$. Transposing both sides,

$$\mathbf{A}'\mathbf{A}\mathbf{G}'\mathbf{A}'\mathbf{A} = \mathbf{A}'\mathbf{A}, \tag{3.1.9}$$

so $\mathbf{G}'$ satisfies (3.1.1) and is a g-inverse of $\mathbf{A}'\mathbf{A}$. Using property 1 of Result 2.3.8, we see that the result $\mathbf{A}'\mathbf{A}\mathbf{G}\mathbf{A}'\mathbf{A} = \mathbf{A}'\mathbf{A}$ implies (3.1.7), proving property 2. To prove property 3, let $\mathbf{G}_1$ and $\mathbf{G}_2$ be two distinct g-inverses of $\mathbf{A}'\mathbf{A}$. From (3.1.7),

$$\mathbf{AG_1A'A = A} \quad \text{and} \quad \mathbf{AG_2A'A = A},$$

i.e., $\mathbf{A'AG_1'A' = A'AG_2'A'}$. By property 1 of Result 2.3.8, this implies $\mathbf{AG_1'A' = AG_2'A'}$; transposing both sides, $\mathbf{AG_1A' = AG_2A'}$, i.e., $\mathbf{AGA'}$ is invariant to the choice of a g-inverse. This is an important result. It was mentioned earlier that every symmetric matrix must have a symmetric g-inverse. Let $\mathbf{G_1}$ denote a symmetric g-inverse and let $\mathbf{G}$ denote any other g-inverse of $\mathbf{A'A}$. Since

$$(\mathbf{AG_1A'})' = \mathbf{AG_1'A' = AG_1A'}$$

(since $\mathbf{G_1 = G_1'}$), $\mathbf{AG_1A'}$ is symmetric when $\mathbf{G_1}$ is symmetric. Consider $(\mathbf{AGA'})' = \mathbf{AG'A'}$. By property 1 and property 3, we have

$$\mathbf{AG'A' = AGA'},$$

so that $\mathbf{AGA'}$ is symmetric for any $\mathbf{G}$, proving property 4. ∎

We will see later that Result 3.1.8, especially property 3, is very important for the discussion of inference for the less than full-rank linear model.

Example 3.1.4.   Suppose

$$\mathbf{X} = \begin{pmatrix} 1 & 1 & 0 & 0 \\ 1 & 1 & 0 & 0 \\ 1 & 1 & 0 & 0 \\ 1 & 0 & 1 & 0 \\ 1 & 0 & 1 & 0 \\ 1 & 0 & 0 & 1 \end{pmatrix}.$$

It is easy to verify that

$$\mathbf{A = X'X} = \begin{pmatrix} 6 & 3 & 2 & 1 \\ 3 & 3 & 0 & 0 \\ 2 & 0 & 2 & 0 \\ 1 & 0 & 0 & 1 \end{pmatrix},$$

with rank 3. Two distinct g-inverses of $\mathbf{X'X}$ are

$$\mathbf{G_1} = \begin{pmatrix} 0 & 0 & 0 & 0 \\ 0 & 1/3 & 0 & 0 \\ 0 & 0 & 1/2 & 0 \\ 0 & 0 & 0 & 1 \end{pmatrix}$$

and

$$\mathbf{G_2} = \begin{pmatrix} 0 & 1/3 & 0 & 0 \\ 0 & 0 & 0 & 0 \\ 0 & -1/3 & 1/2 & 0 \\ 0 & -1/3 & 0 & 1 \end{pmatrix}$$

which correspond to the full rank submatrices

$$\mathbf{A}_{11} = \begin{pmatrix} 3 & 0 & 0 \\ 0 & 2 & 0 \\ 0 & 0 & 1 \end{pmatrix}$$

and

$$\mathbf{A}_{11} = \begin{pmatrix} 3 & 0 & 0 \\ 2 & 2 & 0 \\ 1 & 0 & 1 \end{pmatrix}$$

respectively. It is easy to verify that

$$\mathbf{X}\mathbf{G}_1\mathbf{X}' = \mathbf{X}\mathbf{G}_2\mathbf{X}' = \begin{pmatrix} 1/3 & 1/3 & 1/3 & 0 & 0 & 0 \\ 1/3 & 1/3 & 1/3 & 0 & 0 & 0 \\ 1/3 & 1/3 & 1/3 & 0 & 0 & 0 \\ 0 & 0 & 0 & 1/2 & 1/2 & 0 \\ 0 & 0 & 0 & 1/2 & 1/2 & 0 \\ 0 & 0 & 0 & 0 & 0 & 1 \end{pmatrix}. \quad \square$$

Example 3.1.5. Let $\lambda_1, \cdots, \lambda_k$ and $\mathbf{x}_1, \cdots, \mathbf{x}_k$ denote the eigenvalues and corresponding eigenvectors of a symmetric matrix $\mathbf{B} = \mathbf{A}'\mathbf{A}$, where $\mathbf{A}$ is an $n \times k$ matrix. Suppose the first r eigenvalues are nonzero, while the last $(k - r)$ are zero. We first write down the spectral decomposition of $\mathbf{B}$. Let $\Lambda = \mathrm{diag}(\lambda_1, \cdots, \lambda_r, 0, \cdots, 0)$ and let $\mathbf{X} = (\mathbf{x}_1, \cdots, \mathbf{x}_r, \mathbf{x}_{r+1}, \cdots, \mathbf{x}_k)$. By Result 2.3.4,

$$\mathbf{B} = \mathbf{X}\Lambda\mathbf{X}' = \sum_{i=1}^{r} \lambda_i \mathbf{x}_i \mathbf{x}_i'.$$

Let $\mathbf{C} = \sum_{i=1}^{r} \mathbf{x}_i \mathbf{x}_i'/\lambda_i$, and let $\Lambda^- = \mathrm{diag}(1/\lambda_1, \cdots, 1/\lambda_r, 0, \cdots, 0)$. We can verify that $\Lambda\Lambda^-\Lambda = \Lambda$, so that Λ^- is a g-inverse of Λ, and that $\mathbf{C} = \mathbf{X}\Lambda^-\mathbf{X}'$. Since $\mathbf{X}\mathbf{X}' = \mathbf{X}'\mathbf{X} = \mathbf{I}$,

$$\mathbf{BCB} = (\mathbf{X}\Lambda\mathbf{X}')(\mathbf{X}\Lambda^-\mathbf{X}')(\mathbf{X}\Lambda\mathbf{X}') = \mathbf{X}\Lambda\Lambda^-\Lambda\mathbf{X}' = \mathbf{X}\Lambda\mathbf{X}' = \mathbf{B},$$

so that $\mathbf{C}$ is a g-inverse of $\mathbf{B}$. This result is useful in the discussion of estimable functions in the less than full rank linear model. $\square$

Example 3.1.6. Let $\mathbf{B}$ be an $m \times n$ matrix and let $\mathbf{A}$ and $\mathbf{C}$ respectively denote nonsingular $m \times m$ and $n \times n$ matrices. We will show that $\mathbf{G}$ is a g-inverse of $\mathbf{ABC}$ if and only if $\mathbf{G} = \mathbf{C}^{-1}\mathbf{H}\mathbf{A}^{-1}$, $\mathbf{H}$ being any g-inverse of $\mathbf{B}$. By Definition 3.1.1, $\mathbf{G}$ is a g-inverse of $\mathbf{ABC}$ if and only if $\mathbf{ABCGABC} = \mathbf{ABC}$, i.e., if and only if $\mathbf{BCGAB} = \mathbf{B}$, i.e., if and only if $\mathbf{G} = \mathbf{C}^{-1}\mathbf{H}\mathbf{A}^{-1}$. Two special cases of this condition are given in Exercise 3.13. $\square$

Result 3.1.9. An $m \times p$ matrix $\mathbf{B}$ is in the column space of an $m \times n$ matrix $\mathbf{A}$, i.e., $\mathcal{C}(\mathbf{B}) \subset \mathcal{C}(\mathbf{A})$ if and only if $\mathbf{AA}^-\mathbf{B} = \mathbf{B}$, or equivalently, if and only if $(\mathbf{I} - \mathbf{AA}^-)\mathbf{B} = \mathbf{0}$. Similarly, any $q \times n$ matrix $\mathbf{C}$ is in the row space of $\mathbf{A}$, i.e., $\mathcal{R}(\mathbf{C}) \subset \mathcal{R}(\mathbf{A})$ if and only if $\mathbf{C} = \mathbf{CA}^-\mathbf{A}$, or equivalently, if and only if $\mathbf{C}(\mathbf{I} - \mathbf{A}^-\mathbf{A}) = \mathbf{0}$.

Proof.   The proof of the sufficiency is obvious. To prove necessity, $\mathcal{C}(\mathbf{B}) \subset \mathcal{C}(\mathbf{A})$ implies that there exists a matrix $\mathbf{M}$ such that $\mathbf{B} = \mathbf{AM}$. Then,

$$\mathbf{AA}^-\mathbf{B} = \mathbf{AA}^-\mathbf{AM} = \mathbf{AM} = \mathbf{B}.$$

The proof of the other result is similar.   ∎

Result 3.1.10. G-inverse of a partitioned matrix.   Let $\mathbf{A} = \begin{pmatrix} \mathbf{A}_{11} & \mathbf{A}_{12} \\ \mathbf{A}_{21} & \mathbf{A}_{22} \end{pmatrix}$ be an $m \times n$ partitioned matrix, $\mathbf{A}_{ij}$ having dimension $m_i \times n_j$, $i, j = 1, 2$, and with $r(\mathbf{A}) < m$. Let $\mathbf{E} = \mathbf{A}_{22} - \mathbf{A}_{21}\mathbf{A}_{11}^-\mathbf{A}_{12}$, $\mathcal{C}(\mathbf{A}_{12}) \subset \mathcal{C}(\mathbf{A}_{11})$, and $\mathcal{R}(\mathbf{A}_{21}) \subset \mathcal{R}(\mathbf{A}_{11})$. A g-inverse of $\mathbf{A}$ is

$$\begin{pmatrix} \mathbf{A}_{11}^- + \mathbf{A}_{11}^-\mathbf{A}_{12}\mathbf{E}^-\mathbf{A}_{21}\mathbf{A}_{11}^- & -\mathbf{A}_{11}^-\mathbf{A}_{12}\mathbf{E}^- \\ -\mathbf{E}^-\mathbf{A}_{21}\mathbf{A}_{11}^- & \mathbf{E}^- \end{pmatrix}$$

$$= \begin{pmatrix} \mathbf{A}_{11}^- & \mathbf{0} \\ \mathbf{0} & \mathbf{0} \end{pmatrix} + \begin{pmatrix} -\mathbf{A}_{11}^-\mathbf{A}_{12} \\ \mathbf{I}_{n_2} \end{pmatrix} \mathbf{E}^- \left(-\mathbf{A}_{21}\mathbf{A}_{11}^-, \quad \mathbf{I}_{m_2} \right).$$

Proof.   By Result 3.1.9, $\mathbf{A}_{12} = \mathbf{A}_{11}\mathbf{A}_{11}^-\mathbf{A}_{12}$ and $\mathbf{A}_{21} = \mathbf{A}_{21}\mathbf{A}_{11}^-\mathbf{A}_{11}$. Hence,

$$\begin{pmatrix} \mathbf{A}_{11} & \mathbf{A}_{12} \\ \mathbf{A}_{21} & \mathbf{A}_{22} \end{pmatrix} = \begin{pmatrix} \mathbf{A}_{11} & \mathbf{A}_{11}\mathbf{A}_{11}^-\mathbf{A}_{12} \\ \mathbf{A}_{21}\mathbf{A}_{11}^-\mathbf{A}_{11} & \mathbf{A}_{22} \end{pmatrix}.$$

The result follows by using Exercise 3.14, setting $\mathbf{A} = \mathbf{A}_{11}$, $\mathbf{D} = \mathbf{A}_{22}$, $\mathbf{B} = \mathbf{A}_{11}^-\mathbf{A}_{12}$, and $\mathbf{C} = \mathbf{A}_{21}\mathbf{A}_{11}^-$, so that $\mathbf{CA}_{11}\mathbf{B} = \mathbf{A}_{21}\mathbf{A}_{11}^-\mathbf{A}_{11}\mathbf{A}_{11}^-\mathbf{A}_{12} = \mathbf{A}_{21}\mathbf{A}_{11}^-\mathbf{A}_{12}$.   ∎

Example 3.1.7.   Let

$$\mathbf{A} = \left(\begin{array}{cc|cc} 4 & 4 & 0 & 0 \\ 1 & 1 & 0 & 0 \\ \hline 0 & 0 & 3 & 5 \end{array} \right) = \left(\begin{array}{c|c} \mathbf{A}_{11} & \mathbf{0} \\ \hline \mathbf{0} & \mathbf{A}_{22} \end{array} \right).$$

Let

$$\mathbf{A}_{11}^- = \begin{pmatrix} 1/4 & 0 \\ 0 & 0 \end{pmatrix}, \quad \text{and} \quad \mathbf{A}_{22}^- = \begin{pmatrix} 0 \\ 1/5 \end{pmatrix}.$$

Using Result 3.1.10,

$$\mathbf{A}^- = \begin{pmatrix} 1/4 & 0 & 0 \\ 0 & 0 & 0 \\ 0 & 0 & 0 \\ 0 & 0 & 1/5 \end{pmatrix} = \begin{pmatrix} \mathbf{A}_{11}^- & \mathbf{0} \\ \mathbf{0} & \mathbf{A}_{22}^- \end{pmatrix}.$$

is a g-inverse of $\mathbf{A}$ $\quad\square$.

Result 3.1.11. Let $\Omega = \mathcal{C}(\mathbf{A})$, where $\mathbf{A}$ is an $m \times n$ matrix of rank r, and let $(\mathbf{A}'\mathbf{A})^-$ denote any g-inverse of the $n \times n$ symmetric matrix $\mathbf{A}'\mathbf{A}$. Then, $\mathbf{P} = \mathbf{A}(\mathbf{A}'\mathbf{A})^-\mathbf{A}'$ represents the matrix of the orthogonal projection of the n-dimensional vector $\mathbf{y}$ onto Ω .

Proof. Let $\mathbf{c} = \mathbf{A}'\mathbf{y}$. Then $(\mathbf{A}'\mathbf{A})^-\mathbf{c}$ is a solution of $\mathbf{A}'\mathbf{Ab} = \mathbf{c}$. Since by Definition 3.1.1,

$$\mathbf{A}'\mathbf{A}[(\mathbf{A}'\mathbf{A})^-\mathbf{c}] = \mathbf{A}'\mathbf{A}(\mathbf{A}'\mathbf{A})^-\mathbf{A}'\mathbf{Ab} = \mathbf{A}'\mathbf{Ab} ,$$

we see that $(\mathbf{A}'\mathbf{A})^-\mathbf{c}$ must be a solution of $\mathbf{A}'\mathbf{Ab} = \mathbf{A}'\mathbf{y}$. Let $\mathbf{t} = \mathbf{A}(\mathbf{A}'\mathbf{A})^-\mathbf{c}$. Then, we can write $\mathbf{y} = \mathbf{t} + (\mathbf{y} - \mathbf{t})$ where

$$\mathbf{A}'(\mathbf{y} - \mathbf{t}) = \mathbf{A}'\mathbf{y} - \mathbf{A}'\mathbf{A}(\mathbf{A}'\mathbf{A})^-\mathbf{A}'\mathbf{Ab} = \mathbf{A}'\mathbf{y} - \mathbf{A}'\mathbf{Ab} = \mathbf{0}.$$

Hence, we have an orthogonal decomposition of the vector $\mathbf{y}$, with $\mathbf{t} \in \mathcal{C}(\mathbf{A})$, and $\mathbf{y} - \mathbf{t} \in \mathcal{C}(\mathbf{A})^\perp$, the orthogonal complement of $\mathcal{C}(\mathbf{A})$. The matrix $\mathbf{P} = \mathbf{A}(\mathbf{A}'\mathbf{A})^-\mathbf{A}'$ is therefore the matrix of this unique orthogonal projection (see Definition 2.6.3), and the proof is complete. ∎

Note that if the columns of $\mathbf{A}$ are LIN, then $\mathbf{P} = \mathbf{A}(\mathbf{A}'\mathbf{A})^{-1}\mathbf{A}'$, since the unique g-inverse of $\mathbf{A}'\mathbf{A}$ is $(\mathbf{A}'\mathbf{A})^{-1}$ (see Result 3.1.1).

Result 3.1.12. The matrix of the orthogonal projection of $\mathbf{y}$ onto $\mathcal{N}(\mathbf{A})$ is $\mathbf{I}_n - \mathbf{P} = \mathbf{I}_n - \mathbf{A}(\mathbf{A}'\mathbf{A})^-\mathbf{A}'$.

Proof. Let us denote $\Omega = \mathcal{N}(\mathbf{A})$, so that by Definition 2.6.2, $\Omega^\perp = \mathcal{C}(\mathbf{A}')$. By Definition 2.6.3, $\mathbf{P}_{\Omega^\perp} = \mathbf{A}(\mathbf{A}'\mathbf{A})^-\mathbf{A}'$, from which it follows that $\mathbf{P}_\Omega = \mathbf{I}_n - \mathbf{P}_{\Omega^\perp} = \mathbf{I}_n - \mathbf{A}(\mathbf{A}'\mathbf{A})^-\mathbf{A}'$. If the columns of $\mathbf{A}'$ are LIN, then the unique g-inverse of $\mathbf{A}'\mathbf{A}$ is $(\mathbf{A}'\mathbf{A})^{-1}$ and hence the matrix of the orthogonal projection in this case is $\mathbf{I}_n - \mathbf{A}(\mathbf{A}'\mathbf{A})^{-1}\mathbf{A}'$. ∎

Example 3.1.8. For an $m \times n$ matrix $\mathbf{A}$, and an $m \times p$ matrix $\mathbf{B}$, we show that $\begin{pmatrix} \mathbf{A}^- \\ \mathbf{B}^- \end{pmatrix}$ is a g-inverse of $(\mathbf{A} \quad \mathbf{B})$ if and only if, by Definition 3.1.1,

$$\begin{aligned}
(\mathbf{A} \quad \mathbf{B}) &= (\mathbf{A} \quad \mathbf{B}) \begin{pmatrix} \mathbf{A}^- \\ \mathbf{B}^- \end{pmatrix} (\mathbf{A} \quad \mathbf{B}) \\
&= (\mathbf{A} \quad \mathbf{B}) \begin{pmatrix} \mathbf{A}^-\mathbf{A} & \mathbf{A}^-\mathbf{B} \\ \mathbf{B}^-\mathbf{A} & \mathbf{B}^-\mathbf{B} \end{pmatrix} \\
&= (\mathbf{A}\mathbf{A}^-\mathbf{A} + \mathbf{B}\mathbf{B}^-\mathbf{A}, \quad \mathbf{A}\mathbf{A}^-\mathbf{B} + \mathbf{B}\mathbf{B}^-\mathbf{B})
\end{aligned}$$

i.e., if and only if $\mathbf{A}\mathbf{A}^-\mathbf{B} = \mathbf{0}$, and $\mathbf{B}\mathbf{B}^-\mathbf{A} = \mathbf{0}$. $\quad\square$

Definition 3.1.3. Moore-Penrose inverse. The Moore-Penrose inverse $\mathbf{A}^+$ of an $m \times n$ matrix $\mathbf{A}$ satisfies the following conditions:

1. $\mathbf{A}\mathbf{A}^{+}\mathbf{A} = \mathbf{A}$, i.e., $\mathbf{A}^{+}$ is a g-inverse of $\mathbf{A}$,

2. $\mathbf{A}^{+}\mathbf{A}\mathbf{A}^{+} = \mathbf{A}^{+}$, i.e., $\mathbf{A}$ is a g-inverse of $\mathbf{A}^{+}$,

3. $(\mathbf{A}\mathbf{A}^{+})' = \mathbf{A}\mathbf{A}^{+}$, and

4. $(\mathbf{A}^{+}\mathbf{A})' = \mathbf{A}^{+}\mathbf{A}$.

If a g-inverse $\mathbf{G}$ of $\mathbf{A}$ satisfies only conditions 1 and 3, it is called a reflexive g-inverse of $\mathbf{A}$. We will not discuss these alternative inverses, except to mention that $\mathbf{A}^{+}$ is unique. The reader may refer to Rao and Mitra (1971) or to Pringle and Rayner (1971) for details.

3.2   Solutions to linear systems

Least squares estimation of the parameters in a linear statistical model starts with the mathematical problem of solving a system of linear equations involving those parameters and the data. These equations are called normal equations. In this chapter, we discuss systems of linear equations and some properties of solutions to such systems. A linear system of m equations in n unknown variables $\mathbf{x} = (x_1, \cdots, x_n)$ is written as

$$
\begin{array}{ccccc}
a_{11}x_1+ & a_{12}x_2+ & \cdots & +a_{1n}x_n & = & b_1 \\
a_{21}x_1+ & a_{22}x_2+ & \cdots & +a_{2n}x_n & = & b_2 \\
\vdots & \vdots & \vdots\ \vdots & & \vdots \\
a_{m1}x_1+ & a_{m2}x_2+ & \cdots & +a_{mn}x_n & = & b_m
\end{array}
$$

or in matrix form as

$$\mathbf{A}\mathbf{x} = \mathbf{b} \tag{3.2.1}$$

where $\mathbf{A} = \{a_{ij}\}$ is an $m \times n$ coefficient matrix, $\mathbf{b} = (b_1, \cdots, b_m)'$ is called the right side and a_{ij}'s and b_i's are fixed scalars. Solving (3.2.1) is the process of finding a solution, provided it exists, i.e., a value of $\mathbf{x}$ which satisfies (3.2.1). The matrix $\mathbf{B_A} = (\ \mathbf{A}\quad \mathbf{b}\ )$ is called the augmented matrix. In multivariate problems, we will find it necessary to solve each of L linear systems

$$\mathbf{A}\mathbf{x}_l = \mathbf{b}_l, \quad l = 1, \cdots, L. \tag{3.2.2}$$

Let $\mathbf{X}$ be an $n \times L$ matrix with columns $\mathbf{x}_l$, $l = 1, \cdots, L$, and let $\mathbf{B}$ be an $m \times L$ matrix with columns $\mathbf{b}_l$, $l = 1, \cdots, L$; then (3.2.2) can be written collectively as a linear system in $\mathbf{X}$ as

$$\mathbf{A}\mathbf{X} = \mathbf{B}. \tag{3.2.3}$$

A solution is any $n \times L$ matrix $\mathbf{X}$ that satisfies (3.2.3). Note that (3.2.1) is a special case of (3.2.3) when $L = 1$. We present definitions and results for the system (3.2.3). They will be directly valid for (3.2.1) with $L = 1$. The linear system $\mathbf{AX} = \mathbf{B}$ is said to be homogeneous if $\mathbf{B} = \mathbf{0}$, i.e., the system is

$$\mathbf{AX} = \mathbf{0}, \tag{3.2.4}$$

and is said to be nonhomogeneous if $\mathbf{B} \neq \mathbf{0}$. The collection of solutions to (3.2.3) is the set of all $n \times L$ matrices $\mathbf{X}$ that satisfy $\mathbf{AX} = \mathbf{B}$ and is called the solution set of the system.

Definition 3.2.1. Consistent linear system. A linear system $\mathbf{AX} = \mathbf{B}$ is said to be consistent if it has at least one solution; otherwise, if no solution exists, the system is inconsistent.

Example 3.2.1. When $L = 1$, the system

$$\begin{pmatrix} 1 & 3 \\ 2 & 6 \end{pmatrix} \begin{pmatrix} x_1 \\ x_2 \end{pmatrix} = \begin{pmatrix} 5 \\ 10 \end{pmatrix},$$

which may be written out as

$$\begin{array}{rcrcl} x_1 & + & 3x_2 & = & 5 \\ 2x_1 & + & 6x_2 & = & 10 \end{array}$$

has a solution given by $x_1 = 2, x_2 = 1$, and is consistent. Note that row 2 in the coefficient matrix is twice row 1 and the same relationship exists between the corresponding elements of the right side. This linear system is said to be compatible. It is easy to see that the system

$$\begin{pmatrix} 1 & 3 \\ 2 & 6 \end{pmatrix} \begin{pmatrix} x_1 \\ x_2 \end{pmatrix} = \begin{pmatrix} 5 \\ 19 \end{pmatrix}$$

is not consistent. Note that in this example, $|\mathbf{A}| = 0$. $\square$

Definition 3.2.2. A linear system $\mathbf{AX} = \mathbf{B}$ is said to be compatible if every linear relationship that exists among the rows of $\mathbf{A}$ also exists among the corresponding rows of $\mathbf{B}$.

We state two results without proof.

Result 3.2.1. A linear system $\mathbf{AX} = \mathbf{B}$ is consistent if and only if it is compatible.

For consistency of the system $\mathbf{AX} = \mathbf{B}$, we do not require existence of linear relationships among the rows of $\mathbf{A}$. For instance, when the rows of $\mathbf{A}$ are LIN, so that $\mathbf{A}^{-1}$ exists, (3.2.3) is consistent. However, Result 3.2.1 shows that should there exist linear relationships among the rows of $\mathbf{A}$, the same relationships should exist among the rows of $\mathbf{B}$. Solutions to linear equations exist if and only if the equations are consistent; hereafter, we assume consistency.

Result 3.2.2. The linear system $\mathbf{AX} = \mathbf{B}$ is consistent

1. if and only if $\mathcal{C}(\mathbf{A}, \mathbf{B}) = \mathcal{C}(\mathbf{A})$; or

2. if and only if $r(\mathbf{A}, \mathbf{B}) = r(\mathbf{A})$; or

3. if $\mathbf{A}$ has full row rank m.

A homogeneous linear system $\mathbf{AX} = \mathbf{0}$ is always consistent; its (nonempty) solution set is a linear space called the solution space. For $L = 1$ and for an $n \times n$ matrix $\mathbf{A}$, the solution space corresponding to $\mathbf{Ax} = \mathbf{0}$ is

$$\mathcal{N}(\mathbf{A}) = \{\mathbf{x} : (\mathbf{I} - \mathbf{A})\mathbf{x} = \mathbf{x}\} \subset \mathcal{C}(\mathbf{I} - \mathbf{A}). \tag{3.2.5}$$

Also, $\mathcal{N}(\mathbf{I} - \mathbf{A}) = \{\mathbf{x} : \mathbf{Ax} = \mathbf{x}\} \subset \mathcal{C}(\mathbf{A})$. The solution set of a nonhomogeneous system (3.2.1) is *not* a linear space. This is seen directly by noting that the null matrix $\mathbf{0}$ is not a solution to the system.

Result 3.2.3.   For every $m \times L$ matrix $\mathbf{B}$ for which $\mathbf{AX} = \mathbf{B}$ is consistent, $\mathbf{GB}$ is a solution to the system if and only if the $n \times m$ matrix $\mathbf{G}$ is a g-inverse of $\mathbf{A}$.

Proof.   Let $\mathbf{G}$ be a g-inverse of $\mathbf{A}$ and suppose $\mathbf{X}^0$ is any solution to $\mathbf{AX} = \mathbf{B}$. Then, by (3.1.1)

$$\mathbf{A}(\mathbf{GB}) = (\mathbf{AG})\mathbf{B} = \mathbf{AGAX}^0 = \mathbf{AX}^0 = \mathbf{B},$$

so $\mathbf{GB}$ is a solution. Conversely, suppose that $\mathbf{GB}$ is a solution to $\mathbf{AX} = \mathbf{B}$. Suppose that $\mathbf{B} = (\mathbf{a}_j, \mathbf{0}, \cdots, \mathbf{0})$, where $\mathbf{a}_j$ denotes the jth column of $\mathbf{A}$. Then, one solution to $\mathbf{AX} = \mathbf{B}$ is the matrix $(\mathbf{1}_j, \mathbf{0}, \cdots, \mathbf{0})$, where $\mathbf{1}_j$ is the n-dimensional unit vector. Hence,

$$\mathbf{AG}(\mathbf{a}_j, \mathbf{0}, \cdots, \mathbf{0}) = (\mathbf{a}_j, \mathbf{0}, \cdots, \mathbf{0})$$

or $\mathbf{AGa}_j = \mathbf{a}_j, j = 1, \cdots, n$, i.e., $\mathbf{AGA} = \mathbf{A}$. By (3.1.1), $\mathbf{G}$ is a g-inverse of $\mathbf{A}$. ∎

Let $\mathbf{A}$ be any $n \times n$ nonsingular matrix, and $\mathbf{G}$ be any $n \times n$ matrix. $\mathbf{GB}$ is a solution to $\mathbf{AX} = \mathbf{B}$ for every $n \times L$ matrix $\mathbf{B}$ if and only if $\mathbf{G} = \mathbf{A}^{-1}$.

Example 3.2.2.   A g-inverse of the coefficient matrix $\mathbf{A} = \begin{pmatrix} 1 & 3 \\ 2 & 6 \end{pmatrix}$ for the consistent linear system in Example 3.2.1 is $\mathbf{A}^- = \begin{pmatrix} 0 & 0 \\ 1/3 & 0 \end{pmatrix}$ and $\mathbf{A}^- \mathbf{b} = (0 \quad 5/3)'$ is a solution.   □

For convenience of notation, we use $\mathbf{Z}^0$ to denote a solution to the homogeneous system $\mathbf{AZ} = \mathbf{0}$ (in $\mathbf{Z}$) and $\mathbf{X}^0$ to denote a solution to the nonhomogeneous system $\mathbf{AX} = \mathbf{B}$ (in $\mathbf{X}$).

Result 3.2.4. An $n \times L$ matrix $\mathbf{Z}^0$ is a solution to the homogeneous system $\mathbf{AZ} = \mathbf{0}$ (in $\mathbf{Z}$) if and only if, for some matrix $\mathbf{Y}$,

$$\mathbf{Z}^0 = (\mathbf{I} - \mathbf{A}^- \mathbf{A})\mathbf{Y}. \tag{3.2.6}$$

When $L = 1$, we see that for some column vector $\mathbf{y}$

$$\mathbf{z}^0 = (\mathbf{I} - \mathbf{A}^- \mathbf{A})\mathbf{y} \tag{3.2.7}$$

is a solution to $\mathbf{Az} = \mathbf{0}$ (in $\mathbf{z}$), $\mathcal{N}(\mathbf{A}) = \mathcal{C}(\mathbf{I} - \mathbf{A}^- \mathbf{A})$ and

$$\dim[\mathcal{N}(\mathbf{A})] = n - r(\mathbf{A}). \tag{3.2.8}$$

Proof. Let $\mathbf{Z}^0 = (\mathbf{I} - \mathbf{A}^- \mathbf{A})\mathbf{Y}$ for some $n \times L$ matrix $\mathbf{Y}$; using (3.1.1),

$$\mathbf{AZ}^0 = (\mathbf{A} - \mathbf{AA}^- \mathbf{A})\mathbf{Y} = (\mathbf{A} - \mathbf{A})\mathbf{Y} = \mathbf{0},$$

so that $\mathbf{Z}^0$ solves $\mathbf{AZ} = \mathbf{0}$. Conversely, if $\mathbf{Z}^0$ is a solution to $\mathbf{AZ} = \mathbf{0}$, then

$$\mathbf{Z}^0 = \mathbf{Z}^0 - \mathbf{A}^-(\mathbf{AZ}^0) = (\mathbf{I} - \mathbf{A}^- \mathbf{A})\mathbf{Z}^0,$$

i.e., there exists a matrix $\mathbf{Y} = \mathbf{Z}^0$ satisfying (3.2.6). As a special case, when $L = 1$, we have (3.2.7), from which it directly follows that $\mathcal{N}(\mathbf{A}) = \mathcal{C}(\mathbf{I} - \mathbf{A}^- \mathbf{A})$. From property 1 and property 2 of Result 1.2.11, we have

$$\dim[\mathcal{N}(\mathbf{A})] = \dim[\mathcal{C}(\mathbf{I} - \mathbf{A}^- \mathbf{A})] = r(\mathbf{I} - \mathbf{A}^- \mathbf{A}) = n - r(\mathbf{A}) . \quad \blacksquare$$

If $r(\mathbf{A}) = n$, i.e., if $\mathbf{A}$ has full column rank, then $\dim[\mathcal{N}(\mathbf{A})] = 0$, and the system $\mathbf{Az} = \mathbf{0}$ has a unique solution, viz., $\mathbf{0}$. If $r(\mathbf{A}) < n$, then the homogeneous system $\mathbf{Az} = \mathbf{0}$ has an infinite number of solutions.

Result 3.2.5. Let $\mathbf{AZ} = \mathbf{0}$ denote a system of homogeneous linear equations. The dimension of its solution space is $L\{n - r(\mathbf{A})\}$.

Proof. Clearly, a matrix $\mathbf{Z}^0$ is a solution to $\mathbf{AZ} = \mathbf{0}$ if and only if each column of $\mathbf{Z}^0$ is a solution to $\mathbf{AZ} = \mathbf{0}$. We consider two cases. First, suppose that $r(\mathbf{A}) = n$. From the discussion below Result 3.2.4, the only solution to $\mathbf{AZ} = \mathbf{0}$ is the $n \times L$ null matrix. Next, suppose that $r(\mathbf{A}) < n$, let $s = n - r(\mathbf{A})$, and let $\mathbf{Z}_1, \mathbf{Z}_2, \cdots, \mathbf{Z}_s$ be any s LIN solutions to $\mathbf{AZ} = \mathbf{0}$. Clearly, the Ls matrices $(\mathbf{Z}_1, \mathbf{0}, \cdots, \mathbf{0}), \cdots (\mathbf{Z}_s, \mathbf{0}, \cdots, \mathbf{0}), \cdots, (\mathbf{0}, \cdots, \mathbf{0}, \mathbf{Z}_1), \cdots, (\mathbf{0}, \cdots, \mathbf{0}, \mathbf{Z}_s)$, each of which has dimension $n \times L$, form a basis of the solution space of $\mathbf{AZ} = \mathbf{0}$. The dimension of this solution space is $Ls = L\{n - r(\mathbf{A})\}$. $\quad \blacksquare$

Result 3.2.6. Let $\mathbf{X}^*$ be any particular solution to a consistent linear system $\mathbf{AX} = \mathbf{B}$. A matrix $\mathbf{X}^0$ is a solution to this system if and only if

$$\mathbf{X}^0 = \mathbf{X}^* + \mathbf{Z}^0, \tag{3.2.9}$$

for some $\mathbf{Z}^0$ which is a solution to the homogeneous system $\mathbf{AZ} = \mathbf{0}$.

Proof. If $\mathbf{X}^0 = \mathbf{X}^* + \mathbf{Z}^0$, then $\mathbf{AX}^0 = \mathbf{AX}^* + \mathbf{AZ}^0 = \mathbf{B} + \mathbf{0} = \mathbf{B}$, so that $\mathbf{X}^0$ is a solution to (3.2.3). To prove the converse, if $\mathbf{X}^0$ solves the system $\mathbf{AX} = \mathbf{B}$, defining $\mathbf{Z}^0 = \mathbf{X}^0 - \mathbf{X}^*$, we see that $\mathbf{X}^0 = \mathbf{X}^* + \mathbf{Z}^0$. Since

$$\mathbf{AZ}^0 = \mathbf{AX}^0 - \mathbf{AX}^* = \mathbf{B} - \mathbf{B} = \mathbf{0},$$

we see that $\mathbf{Z}^0$ solves $\mathbf{AZ} = \mathbf{0}$. ■

Hence, all matrices in the solution set $\mathbf{AX} = \mathbf{B}$ can be generated from

$$\mathbf{X} = \mathbf{X}^* + \mathbf{Z}$$

where $\mathbf{X}^*$ is any particular solution of (3.2.3) and $\mathbf{Z}$ ranges over all matrices in the solution space of $\mathbf{AZ} = \mathbf{0}$. When $L = 1$, we replace matrices $\mathbf{X}, \mathbf{X}^0, \mathbf{X}^*, \mathbf{Z}$, and $\mathbf{Z}^0$ respectively by vectors $\mathbf{x}, \mathbf{x}^0, \mathbf{x}^*, \mathbf{z}$, and $\mathbf{z}^0$.

Result 3.2.7.   A matrix $\mathbf{X}^0$ is a solution to the system $\mathbf{AX} = \mathbf{B}$ if and only if, for some matrix $\mathbf{Y}$,

$$\mathbf{X}^0 = \mathbf{A}^-\mathbf{B} + (\mathbf{I} - \mathbf{A}^-\mathbf{A})\mathbf{Y}. \tag{3.2.10}$$

Proof.   The proof follows directly from Result 3.2.3, Result 3.2.4 and Result 3.2.6. ■

A special case of Result 3.2.7 for $L = 1$ states that $\mathbf{x}^0$ is a solution to $\mathbf{Ax} = \mathbf{b}$ if and only if, for some column vector $\mathbf{y}$,

$$\mathbf{x}^0 = \mathbf{A}^-\mathbf{b} + (\mathbf{I} - \mathbf{A}^-\mathbf{A})\mathbf{y}. \tag{3.2.11}$$

Example 3.2.2 (continued).   Let $\mathbf{y} = (y_1, y_2)'$. We see that

$$\mathbf{A}^-\mathbf{b} + (\mathbf{I} - \mathbf{A}^-\mathbf{A})\mathbf{y} = \begin{pmatrix} y_1 \\ 5/3 - 1/3y_1 \end{pmatrix}. \tag{3.2.12}$$

The solution set then consists of all vectors of the general form (3.2.12).   □

Example 3.2.3.   Consider the system of equations $\mathbf{Ax} = \mathbf{b}$ where

$$\mathbf{A} = \begin{pmatrix} 1 & -2 & 3 & 2 \\ 1 & 0 & 1 & -3 \\ 1 & 2 & -3 & 0 \end{pmatrix}, \quad \mathbf{x} = \begin{pmatrix} x_1 \\ x_2 \\ x_3 \\ x_4 \end{pmatrix}, \quad \text{and } \mathbf{b} = \begin{pmatrix} 2 \\ -4 \\ -4 \end{pmatrix}.$$

This system is consistent (see Exercise 3.15). A g-inverse of $\mathbf{A}$ is

$$\mathbf{A}^- = \begin{pmatrix} 1/2 & 0 & 1/2 \\ -1 & 3/2 & -1/2 \\ -1/2 & 1 & -1/2 \\ 0 & 0 & 0 \end{pmatrix},$$

and a solution to the system of equations is $\mathbf{x} = \mathbf{A}^-\mathbf{b} = (-1, -6, -3, 0)'$. Another solution is $\mathbf{x}_1 = \mathbf{A}^-\mathbf{b} + (\mathbf{I} - \mathbf{A}^-\mathbf{A})\mathbf{y}$, for an arbitrary 4-dimensional vector $\mathbf{y}$.   □

Result 3.2.8. If $\mathbf{A}$ is nonsingular, then $\mathbf{AX} = \mathbf{B}$ has a unique solution given by $\mathbf{A}^{-1}\mathbf{B}$.

Proof. By property 3 of Result 3.2.2, the system $\mathbf{AX} = \mathbf{B}$ is consistent and a solution is given by (3.2.10).   ■

Result 3.2.9. Let $\mathbf{AX} = \mathbf{B}$ denote a consistent linear system. For any $n \times q$ matrix $\mathbf{C}$, the value of $\mathbf{C}'\mathbf{X}$ is the same for every solution to the system $\mathbf{AX} = \mathbf{B}$ if and only if $\mathcal{R}(\mathbf{C}') \subset \mathcal{R}(\mathbf{A})$, i.e., if and only if every row of $\mathbf{C}'$ belongs to $\mathcal{R}(\mathbf{A})$.

Proof.   If $\mathcal{R}(\mathbf{C}') \subset \mathcal{R}(\mathbf{A})$, there exists a matrix $\mathbf{F}$ such that $\mathbf{C}' = \mathbf{FA}$. Let $\mathbf{X}^*$ and $\mathbf{X}^0$ respectively denote any solution and a particular solution to $\mathbf{AX} = \mathbf{B}$. Then, $\mathbf{C}'\mathbf{X}^* = \mathbf{FAX}^* = \mathbf{FB} = \mathbf{FAX}^0 = \mathbf{C}'\mathbf{X}^0$, i.e., $\mathbf{C}'\mathbf{X}$ is the same for each solution to $\mathbf{AX} = \mathbf{B}$. To prove the converse, it follows by Result 3.2.7 that for every $\mathbf{Y}$, the value of $\mathbf{C}'[\mathbf{A}^-\mathbf{B} + (\mathbf{I} - \mathbf{A}^-\mathbf{A})\mathbf{Y}]$ remains the same. Let $\mathbf{Y} = (\mathbf{y}, \mathbf{0}, \cdots, \mathbf{0})$. It follows that $\mathbf{C}'(\mathbf{I} - \mathbf{A}^-\mathbf{A})\mathbf{y} = \mathbf{0}$ for every n-dimensional vector $\mathbf{y}$, i.e., $\mathbf{C}'\mathbf{A}^-\mathbf{A} = \mathbf{C}'$, i.e., $\mathcal{R}(\mathbf{C}') \subset \mathcal{R}(\mathbf{A})$.   ■

When $L = 1$, and $\mathbf{c}$ is an n-dimensional vector, the value of $\mathbf{c}'\mathbf{x}$ is the same for every solution to $\mathbf{Ax} = \mathbf{b}$ if and only if $\mathbf{c}' \in \mathcal{R}(\mathbf{A})$ (see Exercise 3.18). We will recall this result in the discussion of estimability in the less than full rank linear model theory in Chapter 4.

We next state without proof (see Harville, 1997, p. 155) a result on *absorption*, which enables us to solve a linear system with an arbitrary number of equations in an arbitrary number of unknown variables. Consider the linear system $\mathbf{AX} = \mathbf{B}$, where $\mathbf{A}$, $\mathbf{B}$ and $\mathbf{X}$ are respectively $m \times n$, $m \times L$ and $n \times L$ matrices partitioned as

$$\mathbf{A} = \begin{pmatrix} \mathbf{A}_{11} & \mathbf{A}_{12} \\ \mathbf{A}_{21} & \mathbf{A}_{22} \end{pmatrix}, \quad \mathbf{B} = \begin{pmatrix} \mathbf{B}_1 \\ \mathbf{B}_2 \end{pmatrix}, \text{ and } \mathbf{X} = \begin{pmatrix} \mathbf{X}_1 \\ \mathbf{X}_2 \end{pmatrix},$$

where $\mathbf{A}_{11}$ is $m_1 \times n_1$, $\mathbf{A}_{12}$ is $m_1 \times n_2$, $\mathbf{A}_{21}$ is $m_2 \times n_1$, $\mathbf{A}_{22}$ is $m_2 \times n_2$, $\mathbf{X}_1$ is $n_1 \times L$, $\mathbf{X}_2$ is $n_2 \times L$, $\mathbf{B}_1$ is $m_1 \times L$, and $\mathbf{B}_2$ is $m_2 \times L$. We can express $\mathbf{AX} = \mathbf{B}$ as

$$\mathbf{A}_{11}\mathbf{X}_1 + \mathbf{A}_{12}\mathbf{X}_2 = \mathbf{B}_1,$$
$$\mathbf{A}_{21}\mathbf{X}_1 + \mathbf{A}_{22}\mathbf{X}_2 = \mathbf{B}_2.$$

The following result implicitly requires solving the first m_1 equations in $\mathbf{AX} = \mathbf{B}$ for $\mathbf{X}_1$ in terms of $\mathbf{X}_2$, substituting this solution for $\mathbf{X}_1$ into the last m_2 equations, thereby absorbing the first m_1 equations into the last m_2 equations, solving the resulting *reduced* linear system, and finally back-solving for $\mathbf{X}_1$. This procedure is called *absorption*, and is useful, for example, in the context of solving the system of normal equations in a two-way fixed-effects ANOVA model without interaction (see Example 4.2.6).

Result 3.2.10. Absorption.   Consider the linear system $\mathbf{AX} = \mathbf{B}$, where $\mathbf{A}$, $\mathbf{B}$ and $\mathbf{X}$ are partitioned as above. Suppose $\mathcal{C}(\mathbf{A}_{12}) \subset \mathcal{C}(\mathbf{A}_{11})$, $\mathcal{C}(\mathbf{B}_1) \subset \mathcal{C}(\mathbf{A}_{11})$, and $\mathcal{R}(\mathbf{A}_{21}) \subset \mathcal{R}(\mathbf{A}_{11})$. The matrix $\mathbf{X}^* = \begin{pmatrix} \mathbf{X}_1^* \\ \mathbf{X}_2^* \end{pmatrix}$ is a solution to $\mathbf{AX} = \mathbf{B}$ if and only if

(i) $\mathbf{X}_2^*$ is a solution to the linear system (in $\mathbf{X}_2$)

$$(\mathbf{A}_{22} - \mathbf{A}_{21}\mathbf{D})\mathbf{X}_2 = \mathbf{B}_2 - \mathbf{A}_{21}\mathbf{C}, \text{ and}$$

(ii) $\mathbf{X}_1^*$ and $\mathbf{X}_2^*$ form a solution to the system (in $\mathbf{X}_1$ and $\mathbf{X}_2$)

$$\mathbf{A}_{11}\mathbf{X}_1 + \mathbf{A}_{12}\mathbf{X}_2 = \mathbf{B}_1,$$

where $\mathbf{C} = \mathbf{A}_{11}^{-}\mathbf{B}_1$ and $\mathbf{D} = \mathbf{A}_{11}^{-}\mathbf{A}_{12}$.   ∎

Exercises

3.1. Find a g-inverse of

(a) $\mathbf{A} = \begin{pmatrix} 1 & 2 \\ 1 & 1 \\ -1 & 0 \end{pmatrix}$, and (b) $\mathbf{A} = \begin{pmatrix} 1 & 2 & 4 & 3 \\ 3 & -1 & 2 & -2 \\ 5 & -4 & 0 & -7 \end{pmatrix}$.

3.2. Suppose an $m \times n$ matrix $\mathbf{B}$ is partitioned as $\mathbf{B} = \begin{pmatrix} \mathbf{A}_1'\mathbf{A}_1 & \mathbf{A}_1'\mathbf{A}_2 \\ \mathbf{A}_2'\mathbf{A}_1 & \mathbf{A}_2'\mathbf{A}_2 \end{pmatrix}$. Show that a g-inverse of $\mathbf{B}$ is given by

$$\mathbf{B}^- = \begin{pmatrix} (\mathbf{A}_1'\mathbf{A}_1)^- & 0 \\ 0 & 0 \end{pmatrix} + \begin{pmatrix} -(\mathbf{A}_1'\mathbf{A}_1)^-\mathbf{A}_1'\mathbf{A}_2 \\ \mathbf{I} \end{pmatrix} \mathbf{S}^- \begin{pmatrix} -\mathbf{A}_2'\mathbf{A}_1(\mathbf{A}_1'\mathbf{A}_1)^- & \mathbf{I} \end{pmatrix},$$

where $\mathbf{S} = \mathbf{A}_2'\mathbf{A}_2 - \mathbf{A}_2'\mathbf{A}_1(\mathbf{A}_1'\mathbf{A}_1)^-\mathbf{A}_1'\mathbf{A}_2$.

3.3. Let $\mathbf{K}$ be an idempotent matrix, let $\mathbf{B} = \mathbf{KAK}$, and let $\mathbf{B}^-$ denote a g-inverse of $\mathbf{B}$. Show that $\mathbf{KB}^-\mathbf{K}$ is also a g-inverse of $\mathbf{B}$.

3.4. Let $\mathbf{G}$ be a g-inverse of a matrix $\mathbf{A}'\mathbf{A}$. Show that

(a) $\mathbf{AG}'\mathbf{A}'\mathbf{A} = \mathbf{A}$.

(b) $\mathbf{A}'\mathbf{AGA}' = \mathbf{A}'$.

(c) $\mathbf{A}'\mathbf{AG}'\mathbf{A}' = \mathbf{A}'$.

(d) $\mathbf{AG}'\mathbf{A}' = \mathbf{AGA}'$

(e) $\mathbf{AG}'\mathbf{A}'$ is symmetric.

3.5. Show that $\mathbf{B}^-\mathbf{A}^-$ is a g-inverse of $\mathbf{AB}$ if and only if $\mathbf{A}^-\mathbf{ABB}^-$ is idempotent.

3.6. Let $\mathbf{A}$ be an $n \times n$ symmetric matrix of rank $r < n$, and let $\mathbf{A} = \mathbf{CC}'$, where $r(\mathbf{C}) = r$. If $\mathbf{A}^-$ denotes a symmetric g-inverse of $\mathbf{A}$, show that $(\mathbf{A}^-\mathbf{C})(\mathbf{A}^-\mathbf{C})'$ is also a g-inverse of $\mathbf{A}$.

3.7. Let $\mathbf{A}$ have rank r, and let $\mathbf{P}_1$ and $\mathbf{P}_2$ be nonsingular matrices such that

$$\mathbf{P}_1\mathbf{A}\mathbf{P}_2 = \mathbf{Q} = \begin{pmatrix} \mathbf{I}_r & \mathbf{0} \\ \mathbf{0} & \mathbf{0} \end{pmatrix}.$$

Show that $\mathbf{G}$ is a g-inverse of $\mathbf{A}$ if and only if it can be written as $G = \mathbf{P}_2\mathbf{Q}^-\mathbf{P}_1$, where

$$\mathbf{Q}^- = \begin{pmatrix} \mathbf{I}_r & \mathbf{U} \\ \mathbf{V} & \mathbf{W} \end{pmatrix}$$

for arbitrary matrices $\mathbf{U}, \mathbf{V}$, and $\mathbf{W}$.

3.8. [Englefield, 1966]. Let $\mathbf{A}$ be an $n \times n$ matrix. If $r(\mathbf{A}) = r \leq n$, show that any one of the following conditions is necessary and sufficient for the existence of a commuting g-inverse of $\mathbf{A}$:

(a) $r(\mathbf{A}) = r(\mathbf{A}^2)$,

(b) there exists a nonsingular matrix $\mathbf{B}$ such that $\mathbf{B}\mathbf{A}\mathbf{B}^{-1} = \begin{pmatrix} \mathbf{A}_1 & \mathbf{0} \\ \mathbf{0} & \mathbf{0} \end{pmatrix}$,

where $\mathbf{A}_1$ is an $r \times r$ nonsingular matrix.

3.9. Show that a symmetric matrix $\mathbf{A}$ always has a commuting g-inverse and that it is also possible to construct a symmetric commuting g-inverse of $\mathbf{A}$.

3.10. Let $\mathbf{G}_1$ and $\mathbf{G}_2$ be two g-inverses of an $m \times n$ matrix $\mathbf{A}$. Let $\mathbf{x}$ be any vector such that $\mathbf{A}\mathbf{G}_1\mathbf{x} = \mathbf{x}$. Show that $\mathbf{A}\mathbf{G}_2\mathbf{x} = \mathbf{x}$.

3.11. In Example 3.1.5, let $\mathbf{D} = \mathbf{CB}$. Show that $\mathbf{x}'_i\mathbf{D} = \mathbf{x}'_i$, $i = 1, \cdots, r$, while $\mathbf{x}'_i\mathbf{D} = \mathbf{0}$, $i = r+1, \cdots, k$.

3.12. Show that $\mathbf{PX} = \mathbf{X}$, where $\mathbf{P} = \mathbf{X}(\mathbf{X}'\mathbf{X})^-\mathbf{X}'$ denotes the projection matrix onto $\mathcal{C}(\mathbf{X})$.

3.13. Let $\mathbf{H}$ be any g-inverse of an $m \times n$ matrix $\mathbf{B}$ and let $\mathbf{A}$ and $\mathbf{C}$ respectively denote nonsingular $m \times m$ and $n \times n$ matrices. Show that

(a) $\mathbf{G}$ is a g-inverse of $\mathbf{AB}$ if and only if $\mathbf{G} = \mathbf{HA}^{-1}$; and

(b) $\mathbf{G}$ is a g-inverse of $\mathbf{BC}$ if and only if $\mathbf{G} = \mathbf{C}^{-1}\mathbf{H}$.

3.14. Given the matrices defined in Exercise 2.4, show that a g-inverse of the matrix $\begin{pmatrix} \mathbf{A} & \mathbf{AB} \\ \mathbf{CA} & \mathbf{D} \end{pmatrix}$ is

$$\begin{pmatrix} \mathbf{A}^- + \mathbf{BE}^-\mathbf{C} & -\mathbf{BE}^- \\ -\mathbf{E}^-\mathbf{C} & \mathbf{E}^- \end{pmatrix} = \begin{pmatrix} \mathbf{A}^- & \mathbf{0} \\ \mathbf{0} & \mathbf{0} \end{pmatrix} + \begin{pmatrix} -\mathbf{B} \\ \mathbf{I}_q \end{pmatrix} \mathbf{E}^- \begin{pmatrix} -\mathbf{C}, & \mathbf{I}_n \end{pmatrix}.$$

3.15. Show that the system of equations $\mathbf{Ax} = \mathbf{b}$ in Example 3.2.3 is consistent.

3.16. Solve the system of linear equations $\mathbf{Ax} = \mathbf{b}$ where

$$
\mathbf{A} = \begin{pmatrix} 2 & -2 & 0 & 4 \\ -1 & 0 & 3 & 1 \\ 6 & -6 & 1 & 8 \\ 1 & 2 & -7 & -16 \end{pmatrix}, \text{ and } \mathbf{b} = \begin{pmatrix} 2 \\ 6 \\ 12 \\ -7 \end{pmatrix}.
$$

3.17. Show that $\mathbf{c}'\mathbf{x}$ has a unique value for each solution to $\mathbf{Ax} = \mathbf{b}$ if and only if $\mathbf{c}'\mathbf{A}^{-}\mathbf{A} = \mathbf{c}'$, where $\mathbf{A}^{-}$ is any g-inverse of the matrix $\mathbf{A}$.

3.18. Consider the matrix $\begin{pmatrix} \mathbf{A} & \mathbf{b} \\ \mathbf{c}' & 0 \end{pmatrix}$ where $\mathbf{A}$ is an $m \times n$ matrix, $\mathbf{b}$ is an m-dimensional vector which belongs to the row space of $\mathbf{A}$, and $\mathbf{c}$ is an n-dimensional vector which belongs to the column space of $\mathbf{A}$. Show that the value of $\mathbf{c}'\mathbf{x}$ is the same at all solutions of $\mathbf{Ax} = \mathbf{b}$ and is given by $\mathbf{c}'\mathbf{A}^{-}\mathbf{b}$ where $\mathbf{A}^{-}$ is a g-inverse of $\mathbf{A}$.

Chapter 4

The General Linear Model

The theory of linear statistical models underlies several important and widely used procedures such as univariate and multivariate regression analysis, analysis of variance, analysis of covariance, random-effects modeling, time series analysis, spatial analysis, etc. In this chapter, we introduce the general linear model to explain an unknown response vector as a linear function of known predictors and an unknown vector of model parameters. We discuss general results for the situation where the matrix of predictors need not have full rank. We define the notion of estimability of linear functions of the vector of model parameters, and derive the least squares estimates of such functions. The Gauss-Markov theorem guarantees an important optimality property for these estimates. The results in this chapter are distribution free, so that we do not need to specify a probability distribution for the model errors.

4.1 Model definition and examples

Given data $(Y_i, X_{i1}, X_{i2}, \cdots, X_{ik})$, $i = 1, \cdots, N$, the general linear model has the form

$$\mathbf{y} = \mathbf{X}\beta + \varepsilon \qquad (4.1.1)$$

where $\mathbf{y} = (Y_1, \cdots, Y_N)'$ is an N-dimensional vector of observed responses, $\beta = (\beta_0, \beta_1, \cdots, \beta_k)'$ is a $(k+1)$-dimensional vector of unknown parameters, $\mathbf{X}$ is an $N \times (k+1)$ matrix of rank r of known predictors, and $\varepsilon = (\varepsilon_1, \cdots, \varepsilon_N)'$ is an N-dimensional random vector of unobserved errors. The matrix $\mathbf{X}$ is written as

$$\mathbf{X} = \begin{pmatrix} 1 & X_{11} & \cdots & X_{1k} \\ 1 & X_{21} & \cdots & X_{2k} \\ \vdots & \vdots & \vdots & \vdots \\ 1 & X_{N1} & \cdots & X_{Nk} \end{pmatrix}.$$

For convenience of notation, we let $p = k + 1$. Unless specified otherwise, we assume that the first column of $\mathbf{X}$ is the vector $\mathbf{1}_N = (1, \cdots, 1)'$, so that the first coefficient β_0 is the intercept. We can write $\mathbf{X} = (\mathbf{1}_N, \widetilde{\mathbf{X}})$, where $\widetilde{\mathbf{X}}$ is an $N \times k$ matrix. There are k coefficients $\beta_1, \cdots, \beta_k$ which correspond to the explanatory variables $X_1, \cdots, X_k$. Note that we may also write the model (4.1.1) as

$$Y_i = \beta_0 + \beta_1 X_{i1} + \cdots + \beta_k X_{ik} + \varepsilon_i, \quad i = 1, \cdots, N, \qquad (4.1.2)$$

or as

$$Y_i = \mathbf{x}_i'\beta + \varepsilon_i, \quad i = 1, \cdots, N, \qquad (4.1.3)$$

where $\mathbf{x}_i = (1, X_{i1}, \cdots, X_{ik})'$ denotes a $p \times 1$ vector corresponding to the explanatory variables on the ith subject. Suppose

$$E(\varepsilon) = \mathbf{0}, \quad \text{and} \quad Cov(\varepsilon) = \sigma^2 \mathbf{I}_N, \qquad (4.1.4)$$

i.e., the errors are uncorrelated, each with zero mean and the same variance σ^2. In Chapter 7, where we discuss detailed inference for the linear model, we will assume some probability distribution for the error vector, usually the normal distribution. Here, we see that it follows from (4.1.4) and the properties of the expectation and covariance operators that

$$\begin{aligned} E(\mathbf{y}) &= E(\mathbf{X}\beta + \varepsilon) = \mathbf{X}\beta + \mathbf{E}(\varepsilon) = \mathbf{X}\beta, \quad \text{and} \\ Cov(\mathbf{y}) &= Cov(\mathbf{X}\beta + \varepsilon) = Cov(\varepsilon) = \sigma^2 \mathbf{I}_N. \end{aligned} \qquad (4.1.5)$$

Multiple regression models, fixed-effects and random-effects analysis of variance (ANOVA) models, and analysis of covariance (ANACOVA) models that are frequently encountered in applied statistics all fall under this umbrella. In regression models, the X_j's may be continuous or categorical observed variables, whereas in the family of ANOVA models, the explanatory variables generally correspond to levels of different factors of interest in designed experiments. The symmetric matrix $\mathbf{X}'\mathbf{X}$, and the symmetric, idempotent matrices $\mathbf{P} = \mathbf{X}(\mathbf{X}'\mathbf{X})^-\mathbf{X}'$ (the projection matrix, or hat matrix, or prediction matrix), and $\mathbf{I} - \mathbf{P}$ play a central role in the development of statistical theory for linear models. If $r(\mathbf{X}'\mathbf{X}) = p$, we have the full rank model, while $r(\mathbf{X}'\mathbf{X}) = r < p$ corresponds to the non-full rank model, or the design model. The multiple regression model is a "full rank linear model", whereas the ANOVA models are examples of "less than full rank linear models". In this chapter, we describe the form of the general linear model, derive the least squares estimates of relevant parameters and prove an important theorem called the Gauss-Markov Theorem. This theorem states a useful optimality result for the least squares estimator of linear parametric functions of the parameter vector β. We begin with some examples of the linear model.

Example 4.1.1. Simple linear regression.   Suppose there is a single continuous-valued response (dependent variable) Y, and a single continuous-valued predictor (independent variable) X, and we wish to explain the variability in Y due to X. The simple regression model has the form (4.1.2) with $k = 1$:

$$Y_i = \beta_0 + \beta_1 X_i + \varepsilon_i, \quad i = 1, \cdots, N. \qquad (4.1.6)$$

We have postulated a straight line relationship between X and Y, with intercept β_0 and slope β_1. Both β_0 and β_1 are unknown model parameters, which must be estimated together with the error variance σ^2, based on data pairs (X_i, Y_i), $i = 1, \cdots, N$. The usual interpretation for β_0 is that it is the value assumed by Y when $X = 0$. When $\beta_0 = 0$, (4.1.6) reduces to a simple regression model without intercept, represented by a straight line through the origin. The coefficient β_1 is the change in Y for a unit increase in X. When $\beta_1 > 0$, there is a positive association between X and Y, so that Y is expected to increase as X increases. When $\beta_1 < 0$, there is an inverse or negative relationship between the two variables, while if $\beta_1 = 0$, Y is unaffected by changes in X. When β_1 is very close to zero, we interpret it as a weak, or virtually nonexistent regression relationship. A scatterplot of Y versus X is one of the first exploratory data analysis (EDA) steps that enables a quick assessment of the validity of a linear model fit to the data.

Suppose we transform both the response and predictor variables as follows: $Y^* = c_1 + c_2 Y$, and $X^* = d_1 + d_2 X$. We will investigate the effect of this data transformation on the regression coefficients. Suppose the regression model on the transformed variables is

$$Y^* = \beta_0^* + \beta_1^* X^*.$$

After some algebra, we can see that

$$\beta_1^* = c_2 \beta_1 / d_2, \text{ and } \beta_0^* = c_1 - \{c_2 d_1 \beta_1 / d_2\} + c_2 \beta_0.$$

The slope is unaffected by a shift in the location but is affected by a scale change, while the intercept is affected by both a location shift and a scale change. □

Example 4.1.2. Multiple linear regression. We relate a single continuous-valued response Y to multiple predictors $X_1, \cdots, X_k$, $k > 1$, using a linear model of the form (4.1.2), which represents a hyperplane in $\mathcal{R}^p$. The response surface has a linear functional form whose parameters are the coefficients β_j, $j = 1, \cdots, k$, which are called partial regression coefficients. We interpret β_j as the amount by which Y changes when X_j is increased by one unit, while all other predictor variables are held at fixed values. The coefficient β_0 corresponds to the constant term. If a particular β_j is zero, the interpretation is that the corresponding predictor X_j is unrelated to Y (in a linear model), and may be dropped from the regression. A multivariate scatterplot is recommended as a preliminary step which enables us to assess the usefulness of a linear model fit to such data. Let $\overline{Y} = \sum_{i=1}^{N} Y_i / N$ and $\overline{X}_j = \sum_{i=1}^{N} X_{ij} / N$, $j = 1, \cdots, k$. By expressing each observation on the response and the predictors in terms of deviations from their respective means, we may write (4.1.2) in *deviations form* as

$$y_i = \beta_1 x_{i1} + \cdots + \beta_k x_{ik} + \varepsilon_i,$$

where $y_i = Y_i - \overline{Y}$, and $x_{ij} = X_{ij} - \overline{X}_j$, $j = 1, \cdots, k$.

The *centered and scaled form* of the multiple regression model is

$$Y_i^* = \beta_1^* X_{i1}^* + \beta_2^* X_{i2}^* + \cdots + \beta_k^* X_{ik}^* + \varepsilon_i$$

where $\beta_j^* = \beta_j (S_{jj}/S_{yy})^{1/2}$, $j = 1, \cdots, k$ and

$$X_{ij}^* = (X_{ij} - \overline{X}_j)/\sqrt{S_{jj}}, \text{ and } Y_i^* = (Y_i - \overline{Y})/\sqrt{S_{yy}},$$

for $i = 1, \cdots, N$, $j = 1, \cdots, k$. Let $\mathbf{X}^*$ denote the regression matrix of centered and scaled variables, i.e.,

$$\mathbf{X}^* = \begin{pmatrix} X_{11}^* & X_{12}^* & \cdots & X_{1k}^* \\ X_{21}^* & X_{22}^* & \cdots & X_{2k}^* \\ \vdots & \vdots & \vdots & \vdots \\ X_{N1}^* & X_{N2}^* & \cdots & X_{Nk}^* \end{pmatrix}$$

so that $\mathbf{X}^{*\prime}\mathbf{X}^*$ denotes the $k \times k$ correlation matrix of the explanatory variables, excluding the intercept column, which becomes zero by the centering.

Standardized coefficients describe the relative importance of the explanatory variables in the model. They are the partial regression coefficients in the model where each variable is normalized by subtracting its sample mean and dividing by its sample standard deviation. A comparison of the different forms yields the following relationship between the partial regression coefficients and the corresponding standardized coefficients:

$$\beta_j^* = \beta_j s_{X_j}/s_Y, \quad j = 1, \cdots, k.$$

We see that the standardized coefficients have the same sign as the β_j's. A standardized coefficient of 0.6 means that an increase of one standard deviation in the independent variable is expected to cause a change of 0.6 standard deviations in the response variable. An elasticity measures the percent change in the response variable Y corresponding to an increase of 1% in the explanatory variable. We end this example with the notion of column-equilibrating the matrix $\mathbf{X}$. This consists of dividing each column of $\mathbf{X}$ by the sum of squares of its elements. The sum of squares of the elements in each column of the resulting matrix $\mathbf{X}_E$, say, should be 1. □

Example 4.1.3. One-way fixed-effects ANOVA model.   Consider the model

$$Y_{ij} = \mu + \tau_i + \varepsilon_{ij}, \quad j = 1, \cdots, n_i, \ i = 1, \cdots, a, \qquad (4.1.7)$$

which can be written in the form (4.1.1) with

$$
\begin{aligned}
\mathbf{y} &= (Y_{11}, \cdots, Y_{1,n_1}, \cdots, Y_{a1}, \cdots, Y_{a,n_a})', \\
\varepsilon &= (\varepsilon_{11}, \cdots, \varepsilon_{1,n_1}, \cdots, \varepsilon_{a1}, \cdots, \varepsilon_{a,n_a})', \\
\beta &= (\mu, \tau_1, \cdots, \tau_a)', \\
\mathbf{X} &= [\ \mathbf{1}_N \ \ \overset{a}{\underset{i=1}{\overset{+}{\sum}}} \ \mathbf{1}_{n_i}\ ],
\end{aligned}
$$

where $N = \sum_{i=1}^{a} n_i$, $E(\varepsilon) = \mathbf{0}$, $Cov(\varepsilon) = \sigma^2 \mathbf{I}_N$, and the direct sum of vectors was introduced in Definition 2.8.3. In general, Y_{ij} represents the observed response from the jth subject in the ith group, where $j = 1, \cdots, n_i$, and $i = 1, \cdots, a$. The design or incidence matrix $\mathbf{X}$ consists of 1's and 0's and $p = a + 1$. The ith column of $\mathbf{X}$ has 1's in its $\sum_{k=1}^{i-1}(n_k + 1)$th row to its $\sum_{k=1}^{i} n_k$th row, and zeroes elsewhere. It is easy to verify that $r(\mathbf{X}) = r = a$, since the last a columns of the design matrix add up to the first column, imposing one dependence. For example, when $a = 3$, $n_1 = 3$, $n_2 = 2$, and $n_3 = 1$, we write

$$
\begin{aligned}
Y_{1j} &= \mu + \tau_1 + \varepsilon_{1j}, \quad j = 1, 2, 3 \\
Y_{2h} &= \mu + \tau_2 + \varepsilon_{2h}, \quad h = 1, 2 \\
Y_{31} &= \mu + \tau_3 + \varepsilon_{31},
\end{aligned}
$$

so that $E(Y_{1j}) = \mu + \tau_1$, $j = 1, 2, 3$, $E(Y_{2h}) = \mu + \tau_2$, $h = 1, 2$, and $E(Y_{31}) = \mu + \tau_3$. In this case, the response vector is $\mathbf{y} = (Y_1, Y_2, \cdots, Y_6)'$, the parameter vector is $\beta = (\mu, \tau_1, \tau_2, \tau_3)'$, the error vector is $\varepsilon = (\varepsilon_1, \varepsilon_2, \cdots, \varepsilon_6)'$, and the design matrix is

$$
\mathbf{X} = \begin{pmatrix}
1 & 1 & 0 & 0 \\
1 & 1 & 0 & 0 \\
1 & 1 & 0 & 0 \\
1 & 0 & 1 & 0 \\
1 & 0 & 1 & 0 \\
1 & 0 & 0 & 1
\end{pmatrix},
$$

with $r(\mathbf{X}) = 3$. When $n_i = n$ for $i = 1, \cdots, a$, we say the model is *balanced*, otherwise it is an *unbalanced* model. Using Kronecker product notation (see Definition 2.8.1), it is easy to verify that the design matrix in a balanced model can be written as

$$
\mathbf{X} = [(\mathbf{1}_a, \mathbf{I}_a) \otimes \mathbf{1}_n]. \quad \square
$$

Example 4.1.4. One-way random-effects ANOVA model. Consider the balanced version of the model in (4.1.7):

$$
Y_{ij} = \mu + \tau_i + \varepsilon_{ij}, \quad j = 1, \cdots, n, \ i = 1, \cdots, a,
$$

where the errors are independently distributed with $E(\varepsilon_{ij}) = 0$, and $Var(\varepsilon_{ij}) = \sigma_\varepsilon^2$. Unlike the fixed-effects model, the τ_i's are no longer fixed unknown constants, but are themselves assumed to be independent random variables, with $E(\tau_i) = 0$, and $Var(\tau_i) = \sigma_\tau^2$. We also assume that the τ_i's and ε_{ij}'s are independently distributed. In this case, it is straightforward to verify that

$$
Cov(Y_{ij}, Y_{i',j'}) = \begin{cases}
\sigma_\tau^2 + \sigma_\varepsilon^2, & i = i', j = j', \\
\sigma_\tau^2, & i = i', j \neq j', \\
0, & i \neq i'.
\end{cases} \tag{4.1.8}
$$

Concisely, we can write

$$
\begin{aligned}
\mathbf{y} &= (\mathbf{1}_a \otimes \mathbf{1}_n)\mu + (\mathbf{I}_a \otimes \mathbf{1}_n)\tau + \varepsilon, \text{ and} \\
Cov(\mathbf{y}) &= \mathbf{I}_a \otimes (\sigma_\tau^2 \mathbf{J}_n + \sigma_\varepsilon^2 \mathbf{I}_n).
\end{aligned}
\tag{4.1.9}
$$

The quantity

$$
\rho = \frac{\sigma_\tau^2}{\sigma_\tau^2 + \sigma_\varepsilon^2}
\tag{4.1.10}
$$

is called the intra-class correlation. We will discuss inference for random-effects models in Chapter 10. We will also study mixed-effects models which are useful, for instance, in designed experiments where some factors are fixed, while others are random.   □

In the general linear model (4.1.1), the parameter vector β and the error variance σ^2 are usually unknown. The least squares approach, which is described in the next section, is a simple and elegant procedure that enables estimation of functions of the parameters in a linear model.

4.2   The least squares approach

Given data on the response variable and predictors, either from an observational study or from a designed experiment, the objective is inference on the model parameters, or functions of the model parameters, as well as predictions for the response variable based on the general linear model (4.1.1). The method of least squares, which was introduced in the early 19th century, enables such inference using minimal assumptions. In particular, we need not specify any parametric form for the probability distribution of the errors ε_i. In the full rank linear model, i.e., when $r(\mathbf{X}) = p$, the least squares approach enables us to construct the best linear unbiased estimator of the parameter vector β, "best" in the sense of having minimum variance in the class of all linear unbiased estimators. When $r(\mathbf{X}) = r < p$, we will obtain least squares estimates of certain linear functions of β, although, as we shall see, there does not exist a unique estimator for β itself. In order to proceed with inference beyond point estimation and prediction for the linear model, i.e., in order to construct confidence interval estimates or to do hypothesis tests, it is usual to assume some parametric form for the error distribution. The simplest and most popular distributional assumption is the assumption of normality of the linear model errors. In Chapter 5, we introduce suitable families of multivariate probability distributions, including the multivariate normal distribution, and return to classical inference for linear models in Chapter 7. We now describe the least squares principle.

Geometrically, the response $\mathbf{y} = (Y_1, \cdots, Y_N)$ represents a point (or a vector from the origin $\mathbf{0}$) in the N-dimensional Euclidean space $\mathcal{R}^N$. Let $\tilde{\mathbf{x}}_j = (X_{1,j}, \cdots, X_{N,j})'$, $j = 1, \cdots, k$, so that $\mathbf{X} = (\mathbf{1}_N, \tilde{\mathbf{X}}) = (\mathbf{1}_N, \tilde{\mathbf{x}}_1, \cdots, \tilde{\mathbf{x}}_k)$, and let $\mathcal{C}(\mathbf{X})$ denote the vector subspace of $\mathcal{R}^N$ defined by these columns of $\mathbf{X}$ (see

Definition 1.2.29). The vector $\mathbf{X}\beta = \beta_0 \mathbf{1}_N + \beta_1 \tilde{\mathbf{x}}_1 + \cdots + \beta_k \tilde{\mathbf{x}}_k$ is in $\mathcal{C}(\mathbf{X})$. When $r(\mathbf{X}) = p$, the p LIN columns of $\mathbf{X}$ span the p-dimensional *estimation space* $\Omega = \mathcal{C}(\mathbf{X})$. In Figure 4.2.1 (a), the points $\mathbf{0}, \mathbf{y}$, and $\mathbf{X}\beta$ form a triangle in $\mathcal{R}^N$, whose sides are the vectors $\mathbf{y}, \mathbf{X}\beta$, and $\varepsilon = \mathbf{y} - \mathbf{X}\beta$. The method of least squares consists of minimizing $\varepsilon'\varepsilon = \| \mathbf{y} - \mathbf{X}\beta \|^2$ with respect to β, or equivalently minimizing $\| \mathbf{y} - \theta \|^2$ where $\theta = \mathbf{X}\beta \in \mathcal{C}(\mathbf{X})$. As θ varies in $\mathcal{C}(\mathbf{X})$, the square of the length of the vector $\mathbf{y} - \theta$ will be minimum when $\theta = \widehat{\theta}$, for $\widehat{\theta}$ in $\mathcal{C}(\mathbf{X})$. Then, $\mathbf{X}'(\mathbf{y} - \widehat{\theta}) = \mathbf{0}$ or $\mathbf{X}'\widehat{\theta} = \mathbf{X}'\mathbf{y}$. The vector $\widehat{\theta}$ denotes the unique orthogonal projection of $\mathbf{y}$ onto $\mathcal{C}(\mathbf{X})$, so $\mathbf{X}\widehat{\beta}$ (which is equal to $\widehat{\theta}$) is unique. In other words, when $\mathbf{X}$ has full rank p, the least squares estimate of β is the vector $\widehat{\beta}$ which uniquely minimizes the quadratic form $(\mathbf{y} - \mathbf{X}\beta)'(\mathbf{y} - \mathbf{X}\beta)$, which denotes the squared length of the vector joining $\mathbf{y}$ and $\mathbf{X}\beta$ in Figure 4.2.1 (a). From Figure 4.2.1 (b), we see that this quadratic form is minimum when $\mathbf{X}\widehat{\beta}$ joins the origin $\mathbf{0}$ to the foot of the perpendicular (denoted by $\widehat{\mathbf{y}}$) from $\mathbf{y}$ onto the estimation space Ω. The fitted vector $\widehat{\mathbf{y}} = \mathbf{X}\widehat{\beta}$ is orthogonal to $\widehat{\varepsilon} = \mathbf{y} - \mathbf{X}\widehat{\beta}$. The residual vector $\widehat{\varepsilon}$ lies in the subspace $\Omega^\perp = \mathcal{C}^\perp(\mathbf{X})$ of $\mathcal{R}^N$, called the *error space*. Any vector in the estimation space is orthogonal to any vector in the error space, i.e., the estimation space is orthogonal to the estimation space. The dimensions of the estimation and error spaces are respectively r and $N - r$.

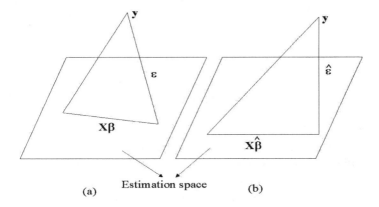

Figure 4.2.1. Geometry of least squares.

Starting from the general linear model (4.1.1), consider the function of β

$$S(\beta) = \varepsilon'\varepsilon = \sum_{i=1}^{N}(Y_i - \mathbf{x}_i'\beta)^2 = (\mathbf{y} - \mathbf{X}\beta)'(\mathbf{y} - \mathbf{X}\beta)$$

$$= \mathbf{y}'\mathbf{y} - 2\beta'\mathbf{X}'\mathbf{y} + \beta'\mathbf{X}'\mathbf{X}\beta. \qquad (4.2.1)$$

The least squares solution of β is chosen to minimize (4.2.1). Differentiating (4.2.1) with respect to the vector β (see Result 2.7.8) yields the set of p *normal equations*

$$\mathbf{X}'\mathbf{X}\beta^0 = \mathbf{X}'\mathbf{y}, \tag{4.2.2}$$

which admits a solution if $r(\mathbf{X}'\mathbf{X}, \mathbf{X}'\mathbf{y}) = r(\mathbf{X}'\mathbf{X})$ (see Result 3.2.2). We ask the reader to verify this (Exercise 4.1). The set of normal equations has a unique solution if and only if the matrix $\mathbf{X}'\mathbf{X}$ has full rank p, i.e., $(\mathbf{X}'\mathbf{X})^{-1}$ exists. Otherwise, when $r(\mathbf{X}'\mathbf{X}) = r < p$, there are infinitely many solutions to (4.2.2), one of which is

$$\beta^0 = \mathbf{G}\mathbf{X}'\mathbf{y}, \tag{4.2.3}$$

$\mathbf{G} = (\mathbf{X}'\mathbf{X})^-$ being a generalized inverse of the symmetric $p \times p$ matrix $\mathbf{X}'\mathbf{X}$. We saw in Result 3.1.1 that $\mathbf{G}$ is not unique. What a solution β^0 "estimates" depends on which g-inverse of $\mathbf{X}'\mathbf{X}$ we use! It is clear that β^0 cannot be regarded as an estimator of β, but merely as one possible solution to the set of normal equations (4.2.2). On the other hand, when $r(\mathbf{X}'\mathbf{X}) = p$, the solution to (4.2.2) is the unique ordinary least squares (OLS) estimator of β denoted by

$$\widehat{\beta} = (\mathbf{X}'\mathbf{X})^{-1}\mathbf{X}'\mathbf{y}. \tag{4.2.4}$$

The solution β^0 indeed minimizes the sum of squares function $S(\beta)$ since

$$
\begin{aligned}
S(\beta) &= (\mathbf{y} - \mathbf{X}\beta^0 + \mathbf{X}\beta^0 - \mathbf{X}\beta)'(\mathbf{y}-\mathbf{X}\beta^0+\mathbf{X}\beta^0-\mathbf{X}\beta) \\
&= (\mathbf{y} - \mathbf{X}\beta^0)'(\mathbf{y}-\mathbf{X}\beta^0) + (\mathbf{y} - \mathbf{X}\beta^0)'\mathbf{X}(\beta^0 - \beta) \\
&\quad + (\beta^0-\beta)'\mathbf{X}'(\mathbf{y} - \mathbf{X}\beta^0)+(\beta^0 - \beta)'\mathbf{X}'\mathbf{X}(\beta^0 - \beta) \\
&= S(\beta^0) + (\beta^0 - \beta)'\mathbf{X}'\mathbf{X}(\beta^0 - \beta), \tag{4.2.5}
\end{aligned}
$$

since $(\beta^0-\beta)'\mathbf{X}'(\mathbf{y} - \mathbf{X}\beta^0) = (\mathbf{y} - \mathbf{X}\beta^0)'\mathbf{X}(\beta^0 - \beta) = \mathbf{0}$ by (4.2.2). The last term on the right side of (4.2.5) is non-negative, so that $S(\beta)-S(\beta^0) \geq 0$ for all $\beta \in \mathcal{R}^p$. The minimum value $S(\beta^0)$ is denoted by SSE, and provides the basis for an estimate of the error variance σ^2.

Letting $\widehat{\mathbf{y}} = \mathbf{X}\beta^0$, the least squares estimate of the error variance is

$$\widehat{\sigma}^2 = \frac{1}{N-r}(\mathbf{y} - \widehat{\mathbf{y}})'(\mathbf{y} - \widehat{\mathbf{y}}), \tag{4.2.6}$$

for which a computationally simple form is obtained after some algebraic simplification as

$$\widehat{\sigma}^2 = \frac{1}{N-r}(\mathbf{y}'\mathbf{y} - \beta^{0'}\mathbf{X}'\mathbf{y}). \tag{4.2.7}$$

Example 4.2.1.   Let $Y_1, \cdots, Y_N$ be a random sample from a normal population with mean θ and variance σ^2. In the framework of (4.1.1),

$$Y_i = \theta + \varepsilon_i, \quad i = 1, \cdots, N,$$

where ε_i are independently distributed with $E(\varepsilon_i) = 0$, and $Var(\varepsilon_i) = \sigma^2$. In matrix notation, let $\mathbf{y} = (Y_1, \cdots, Y_N)'$, $\varepsilon = (\varepsilon_1, \cdots, \varepsilon_N)'$, $\mathbf{X} = (1, \cdots, 1)' = \mathbf{1}_N$, and $\beta = \theta$. Since $\mathbf{X}'\mathbf{X} = N$, and $\mathbf{X}'\mathbf{y} = \sum_{i=1}^{N} Y_i$, the least squares estimate of the scalar parameter θ and its variance are

$$\widehat{\theta} = \sum_{i=1}^{N} Y_i/N = \overline{Y}, \text{ and } Var(\widehat{\theta}) = \sigma^2(\mathbf{1}'_N \mathbf{1}_N)^{-1} = \sigma^2/N. \quad \square$$

Definition 4.2.1. Fitted vector. The vector of fitted values $\widehat{\mathbf{y}}$ is uniquely defined as a function of the solution vector β^0:

$$\widehat{\mathbf{y}} = \mathbf{X}\beta^0 = \mathbf{X}\mathbf{G}\mathbf{X}'\mathbf{y}. \tag{4.2.8}$$

For the full rank model, the fitted vector has the form $\mathbf{X}(\mathbf{X}'\mathbf{X})^{-1}\mathbf{X}'\mathbf{y}$.

Definition 4.2.2. Residual vector. The vector of least squares residuals $\widehat{\varepsilon}$ is also uniquely defined as a function of the solution vector β^0:

$$\widehat{\varepsilon} = \mathbf{y} - \widehat{\mathbf{y}} = (\mathbf{I}_N - \mathbf{X}\mathbf{G}\mathbf{X}')\mathbf{y}. \tag{4.2.9}$$

For the full rank model, the residual vector has the form $[\mathbf{I}_N - \mathbf{X}(\mathbf{X}'\mathbf{X})^{-1}\mathbf{X}']\mathbf{y}$.

By property 3 of Result 3.1.8, $\mathbf{X}\mathbf{G}\mathbf{X}'$ is invariant to the choice of $\mathbf{G}$, so that the fitted vector $\widehat{\mathbf{y}}$ and the residual vector $\widehat{\varepsilon}$ are unique. In other words, each of the infinite solution vectors to the normal equations yields the same predictions and the same residual summaries. We denote by $\mathbf{P}$ the matrix $\mathbf{X}\mathbf{G}\mathbf{X}'$ in the situation when $r(\mathbf{X}) < p$, and the matrix $\mathbf{X}(\mathbf{X}'\mathbf{X})^{-1}\mathbf{X}'$ in the full rank case. $\mathbf{P} = \mathbf{X}\mathbf{G}\mathbf{X}'$ is the linear transformation matrix representing the orthogonal projection from the N-dimensional space $\mathcal{R}^N$ onto the estimation space $\mathcal{C}(\mathbf{X})$, while $\mathbf{I} - \mathbf{P} = (\mathbf{I} - \mathbf{X}\mathbf{G}\mathbf{X}')$ represents the orthogonal projection of $\mathcal{R}^N$ onto the error space $\mathcal{C}^\perp(\mathbf{X})$. The N-dimensional vector $\mathbf{y}$ can be uniquely decomposed as

$$\mathbf{y} = \mathbf{P}\mathbf{y} + (\mathbf{I} - \mathbf{P})\mathbf{y}, \tag{4.2.10}$$

where $\mathbf{P}\mathbf{y} \in \mathcal{C}(\mathbf{X})$ and $(\mathbf{I} - \mathbf{P})\mathbf{y} \in \mathcal{C}^\perp(\mathbf{X})$ (see section 2.6). Result 4.2.1 gives some properties of the matrices $\mathbf{P}$, $\mathbf{I} - \mathbf{P}$, and $\mathbf{H} = \mathbf{G}\mathbf{X}'\mathbf{X}$, while Result 4.2.2 follows as an immediate consequence.

Result 4.2.1. Properties of the matrices $\mathbf{P}$, $\mathbf{I} - \mathbf{P}$ and $\mathbf{H}$. Suppose $r(\mathbf{X}) = r$. Then,

1. $\mathbf{P}$ and $\mathbf{I} - \mathbf{P}$ are symmetric and idempotent matrices.

2. $r(\mathbf{P}) = r$, and $r(\mathbf{I} - \mathbf{P}) = N - r$.

3. $\mathbf{P}(\mathbf{I} - \mathbf{P}) = \mathbf{0}$.

4. $\mathbf{H}$ is idempotent, with $r(\mathbf{H}) = r$. Further, $\mathbf{X'XH} = \mathbf{X'X}$.

Proof. Using Definitions 1.2.15 and 2.3.1, it is straightforward to verify that $\mathbf{P'} = \mathbf{P}$, $\mathbf{P}^2 = \mathbf{P}$, $(\mathbf{I} - \mathbf{P})' = \mathbf{I} - \mathbf{P}$, and $(\mathbf{I} - \mathbf{P})^2 = \mathbf{I} - \mathbf{P}$, proving property 1. Together with property 3 of Result 2.3.9, this gives the results in property 2. An algebraic verification of property 3 again follows from the symmetry and idempotency of $\mathbf{P}$:

$$\mathbf{P}(\mathbf{I} - \mathbf{P}) = \mathbf{P} - \mathbf{P}^2 = \mathbf{P} - \mathbf{P} = \mathbf{0}.$$

Geometrically, we see that $\mathbf{P}(\mathbf{I} - \mathbf{P})$ must be $\mathbf{0}$ by Definition 1.2.8, since $\mathbf{P} \in \mathcal{C}(\mathbf{X})$ and $\mathbf{I} - \mathbf{P} \in \mathcal{C}^{\perp}(\mathbf{X})$, and these are orthogonal subspaces of $\mathcal{R}^N$. Idempotency of $\mathbf{H}$ is a direct consequence of the fact that $\mathbf{X'XGX'} = \mathbf{X'}$ (see Exercise 3.4), so that $\mathbf{H}^2 = \mathbf{GX'XGX'X} = \mathbf{GX'X} = \mathbf{H}$. Hence, $r(\mathbf{H}) = r(\mathbf{X'X}) = r(\mathbf{X}) = r$. Now, $\mathbf{X'XH} = \mathbf{X'XGX'X} = \mathbf{X'X}$, which also follows immediately. Note that the matrix $\mathbf{H}$ need not be symmetric, since $\mathbf{G}$ is not necessarily symmetric. ■

Corollary 4.2.1. When $r(\mathbf{X}) = p$, $\mathbf{P}$ and $\mathbf{I} - \mathbf{P}$ are symmetric and idempotent matrices, such that $\mathbf{P}(\mathbf{I} - \mathbf{P}) = \mathbf{0}$, with $r(\mathbf{P}) = p$, and $r(\mathbf{I} - \mathbf{P}) = N - p$.

Proof.   Symmetry and idempotency have been verified in Result 4.2.1. From property 3 of Result 2.3.9,

$$r(\mathbf{P}) = tr(\mathbf{P}) = tr[\mathbf{X}(\mathbf{X'X})^{-1}\mathbf{X'}] = tr[\mathbf{X'X}(\mathbf{X'X})^{-1}] = tr(\mathbf{I}_p) = p,$$

(also see property 4 in Result 1.2.8). That $r(\mathbf{I} - \mathbf{P}) = N - p$ can be shown in the same way. ■

Result 4.2.2.   For the general linear model (4.1.1),

$$\widehat{\mathbf{y}}'(\mathbf{y} - \widehat{\mathbf{y}}) = \sum_{i=1}^{N} \widehat{Y}_i(Y_i - \widehat{Y}_i) = 0.$$

Proof.   Clearly, $\widehat{\mathbf{y}} \in \mathcal{C}(\mathbf{X})$, while $\widehat{\varepsilon} = (\mathbf{y} - \widehat{\mathbf{y}}) \in \mathcal{C}^{\perp}(\mathbf{X})$, so that their inner product must be zero (see Definition 1.2.8). Since $\mathbf{P}$ is symmetric, and $\mathbf{P}(\mathbf{I} - \mathbf{P}) = \mathbf{0}$, it follows that

$$
\begin{aligned}
\sum_{i=1}^{N} \widehat{Y}_i(Y_i - \widehat{Y}_i) &= \widehat{\mathbf{y}}'(\mathbf{y} - \widehat{\mathbf{y}}) = (\mathbf{Py})'(\mathbf{y} - \mathbf{Py}) \\
&= \mathbf{y'P'}(\mathbf{I} - \mathbf{P})\mathbf{y} = 0. \blacksquare
\end{aligned}
$$

In Figure 4.2.1 (a), $\mathbf{y}$, $\widehat{\mathbf{y}}$ and $\widehat{\varepsilon}$ are the sides of a right triangle. An application of Pythagoras's Theorem gives

$$\mathbf{y'y} = \widehat{\mathbf{y}}'\widehat{\mathbf{y}} + \widehat{\varepsilon}'\widehat{\varepsilon}.$$

We next characterize these squared distances in terms of quadratic forms in $\mathbf{y}$.

Definition 4.2.3. Sums of squares. Let SST, SSR and SSE respectively denote the total variation in Y, the variation explained by the fitted model, and the unexplained (residual) variation. We define these sums of squares by

$$
\begin{aligned}
SST &= \mathbf{y}'\mathbf{y} = \sum_{i=1}^{N} Y_i^2, \\
SSR &= \hat{\mathbf{y}}'\hat{\mathbf{y}} = \mathbf{y}'\mathbf{P}\mathbf{y} = \beta^{0\prime}\mathbf{X}'\mathbf{X}\beta^0, \text{ and} \\
SSE &= \hat{\varepsilon}'\hat{\varepsilon} = \mathbf{y}'(\mathbf{I}_N - \mathbf{P})\mathbf{y} = \mathbf{y}'\mathbf{y} - \beta^{0\prime}\mathbf{X}'\mathbf{X}\beta^0.
\end{aligned}
\tag{4.2.11}
$$

SST refers to the total sum of squares, and the ANOVA decomposition represents a partition of SST as

$$
SST = SSR + SSE, \tag{4.2.12}
$$

where SSR is the model sum of squares and SSE is the error sum of squares. The ANOVA decomposition in (4.2.12) can also be written as

$$
\mathbf{y}'\mathbf{y} = \mathbf{y}'\mathbf{X}\mathbf{G}\mathbf{X}'\mathbf{y} + \mathbf{y}'(\mathbf{I}_N - \mathbf{X}\mathbf{G}\mathbf{X}')\mathbf{y}.
$$

Orthogonality of the fitted vector $\hat{\mathbf{y}}$ and the residual vector $\hat{\varepsilon}$ is necessary for an unambiguous partition of SST as the sum of SSR and SSE. The dimensions of the linear spaces $\mathcal{R}^N$, $\mathcal{C}(\mathbf{X})$ and $\mathcal{C}^{\perp}(\mathbf{X})$ also split as $N = r + (N - r)$. In some cases, it is useful to express the ANOVA decomposition in terms of mean corrected sums of squares:

$$
SST_c = SSR_c + SSE \tag{4.2.13}
$$

where

$$
\begin{aligned}
SST_c &= \sum_{i=1}^{N}(Y_i - \overline{Y})^2 = \mathbf{y}'\mathbf{y} - N\overline{Y}^2, \text{ and} \\
SSR_c &= \beta^{0\prime}\mathbf{X}'\mathbf{y} - N\overline{Y}^2.
\end{aligned}
\tag{4.2.14}
$$

We can also express the ANOVA decomposition in terms of the sum of squares due to the mean

$$
SSM = N\overline{Y}^2 \tag{4.2.15}
$$

as

$$
SST = SSM + SSR_c + SSE. \tag{4.2.16}
$$

Note that the error sum of squares can also be written as

$$
SSE = \hat{\varepsilon}'\hat{\varepsilon} = (\mathbf{y} - \hat{\mathbf{y}})'(\mathbf{y} - \hat{\mathbf{y}}), \tag{4.2.17}
$$

so that the least squares estimate of the error variance is

$$\widehat{\sigma}^2 = \frac{SSE}{N-r}. \tag{4.2.18}$$

Example 4.2.2.   We continue with Example 4.1.1. In the simple linear regression model, $\mathbf{y} = (Y_1, \cdots, Y_N)'$ and $\mathbf{x} = (X_1, \cdots, X_N)'$ are vectors in $\mathcal{R}^N$. Let

$$S(\beta_0, \beta_1) = \varepsilon'\varepsilon = \sum_{i=1}^{N} \varepsilon_i^2 = \sum_{i=1}^{N}(Y_i - \beta_0 - \beta_1 X_i)^2.$$

Minimizing $S(\beta_0, \beta_1)$ with respect to β_0 and β_1, and setting the normal equations equal to zero,

$$\frac{\partial}{\partial \beta_0} S(\beta_0, \beta_1) = -2\sum_{i=1}^{N}(Y_i - \beta_0 - \beta_1 X_i) = 0$$

$$\Rightarrow \quad N\widehat{\beta}_0 + \widehat{\beta}_1 \sum_{i=1}^{N} X_i = \sum_{i=1}^{N} Y_i$$

$$\frac{\partial}{\partial \beta_1} S(\beta_0, \beta_1) = -2\sum_{i=1}^{N} X_i(Y_i - \beta_0 - \beta_1 X_i) = 0$$

$$\Rightarrow \quad \widehat{\beta}_0 \sum_{i=1}^{N} X_i + \widehat{\beta}_1 \sum_{i=1}^{N} X_i^2 = \sum_{i=1}^{N} X_i Y_i.$$

Solving these equations simultaneously for the parameters, we obtain

$$\widehat{\beta}_1 = \frac{\displaystyle\sum_{i=1}^{N}(X_i - \overline{X})(Y_i - \overline{Y})}{\displaystyle\sum_{i=1}^{N}(X_i - \overline{X})^2} = \frac{\displaystyle\sum_{i=1}^{N} X_i Y_i - N\overline{X}\overline{Y}}{\displaystyle\sum_{i=1}^{N} X_i^2 - N\overline{X}^2},$$

$$\widehat{\beta}_0 = \overline{Y} - \widehat{\beta}_1 \overline{X}, \tag{4.2.19}$$

and

$$\widehat{\sigma}^2 = \sum_{i=1}^{N}(Y_i - \widehat{\beta}_0 - \widehat{\beta}_1 X_i)^2/(N-2).$$

We give a geometric interpretation. Consider the vector $\varepsilon = (Y_1 - \beta_0 - \beta_1 X_1, \cdots, Y_N - \beta_0 - \beta_1 X_N)'$ for arbitrary coefficients β_0 and β_1. The least squares criterion chooses β_0 and β_1 such that the squared length

$$\| \varepsilon \|^2 = \| \mathbf{y} - \beta_0 \mathbf{1}_N - \beta_1 \mathbf{x} \|^2 = \sum_{i=1}^{N}(Y_i - \beta_0 - \beta_1 X_i)^2$$

is a minimum (see Figure 4.2.2). Varying (β_0, β_1) varies $\beta_0 \mathbf{1}_N + \beta_1 \mathbf{x}$ through all the vectors in the space spanned by $\mathbf{1}_N$ and $\mathbf{x}$ (point A). The choice of (β_0, β_1)

minimizing $\| \varepsilon \|$ corresponds to the projection of the response vector $\mathbf{y}$ onto this plane, such that the vector $\widehat{\varepsilon}$ is orthogonal to the plane (point B). The least squares estimates $\widehat{\beta}_0$ and $\widehat{\beta}_1$ are these minimizing values. The vector of "fitted" or "predicted" values is $\widehat{\mathbf{y}} = \widehat{\beta}_0 \mathbf{1}_N + \widehat{\beta}_1 \mathbf{x}$, i.e., the ith predicted value is $\widehat{Y}_i = \widehat{\beta}_0 + X_i \widehat{\beta}_1$, $i = 1, \cdots, N$.

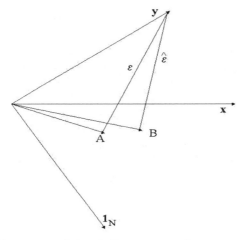

Figure 4.2.2. Geometry of simple linear regression.

The least squares residual vector is $\widehat{\varepsilon} = \mathbf{y} - \widehat{\beta}_0 \mathbf{1}_N - \widehat{\beta}_1 \mathbf{x}$, i.e., the ith residual is $\widehat{\varepsilon}_i = Y_i - \widehat{Y}_i$, $i = 1, \cdots, N$. The least squares predictor $\widehat{\mathbf{y}}$ is the vector with the smallest error, i.e., the vector corresponding to the shortest error vector, $\widehat{\varepsilon}$. This happens when $\widehat{\mathbf{y}} \perp \widehat{\varepsilon}$. $\square$

Example 4.2.3. Consider the linear model

$$\begin{pmatrix} Y_1 \\ Y_2 \\ Y_3 \end{pmatrix} = \begin{pmatrix} 1 & -1 & 1 \\ 1 & 0 & -2 \\ 1 & 1 & 1 \end{pmatrix} \begin{pmatrix} \beta_0 \\ \beta_1 \\ \beta_2 \end{pmatrix} + \begin{pmatrix} \varepsilon_1 \\ \varepsilon_2 \\ \varepsilon_3 \end{pmatrix}.$$

We can verify that the columns of $\mathbf{X}$ are mutually orthogonal. The least squares estimate of $\beta = (\beta_0, \beta_1, \beta_2)'$ is

$$\widehat{\beta} = \begin{pmatrix} \frac{1}{3}(Y_1 + Y_2 + Y_3) \\ -\frac{1}{2}(Y_1 - Y_3) \\ \frac{1}{6}(Y_1 - 2Y_2 + Y_3) \end{pmatrix}.$$

Suppose we set $\beta_2 = 0$ in the above model. The resulting model is

$$\begin{pmatrix} Y_1 \\ Y_2 \\ Y_3 \end{pmatrix} = \begin{pmatrix} 1 & -1 \\ 1 & 0 \\ 1 & 1 \end{pmatrix} \begin{pmatrix} \beta_0 \\ \beta_1 \end{pmatrix} + \begin{pmatrix} \varepsilon_1 \\ \varepsilon_2 \\ \varepsilon_3 \end{pmatrix},$$

and the least squares estimate of β_0 and β_1 are $\widehat{\beta}_0 = \frac{1}{3}(Y_1 + Y_2 + Y_3)$, and $\widehat{\beta}_1 = -\frac{1}{2}(Y_1 - Y_3)$, which are unchanged by omitting the parameter β_2. It is not difficult to see that this is a consequence of the orthogonality of $\mathbf{X}$, which leads to a diagonal $\mathbf{X'X}$ matrix.   □

Measuring the adequacy of the least squares fit is an important practical problem. Recall that the vectors $\mathbf{y}$, $\widehat{\mathbf{y}}$ and $\widehat{\varepsilon}$ form a right triangle, with the latter two vectors containing the right angle. Either the angle between the vectors $\mathbf{y}$ and $\widehat{\mathbf{y}}$ (which lies between zero and 90°) or their relative lengths can be used to assess adequacy of fit (see Figure 4.2.3). When the model provides a good fit (as in (a)), the angle between $\mathbf{y}$ and $\widehat{\mathbf{y}}$ is small, and the two vectors have nearly the same length. On the contrary, the angle is large and $\widehat{\mathbf{y}}$ is much shorter than $\mathbf{y}$ if there is a poor fit (as in (b)). If $\mathbf{y} \perp \mathcal{C}(\mathbf{X})$, the projection of $\mathbf{y}$ onto $\mathcal{C}(\mathbf{X})$ is the null vector, i.e., $\widehat{\mathbf{y}} = \mathbf{0}$. The square of the cosine of the angle between $\mathbf{y}$ and $\widehat{\mathbf{y}}$, which is also equal to the square of the relative lengths of $\widehat{\mathbf{y}}$ and $\mathbf{y}$ is called the coefficient of determination, i.e., $R^2 = \| \widehat{\mathbf{y}} \|^2 / \| \mathbf{y} \|^2$. In other words, we can interpret R^2 as the proportion by which the fitted vector $\widehat{\mathbf{y}}$ is shorter than the observed response vector $\mathbf{y}$. We give a formal definition.

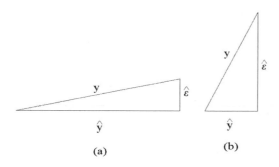

Figure 4.2.3.   Adequacy of least squares.

Definition 4.2.4. R-square.   We define the coefficient of determination of the linear model as the proportion of the total variation in Y explained by the explanatory variables, i.e.,

$$R^2 = \frac{SSR}{SST} = 1 - \frac{SSE}{SST}. \qquad (4.2.20)$$

Clearly, $0 \leq R^2 \leq 1$.

This measure, which is also the multiple correlation coefficient between Y and the set of predictors $(X_1, \cdots, X_k)$ (see Definition 5.2.8), is widely used to assess goodness of fit of the linear regression. A value of R^2 close to 0 indicates a poor linear regression fit, while a value close to 1 indicates a good fit. An R^2 of 0 says that the linear model does not explain any variation in the response Y. In a simple regression model, it is possible that (a) the values of Y lie randomly around the horizontal line $Y = \overline{Y}$, or (b) the observations lie on a circle. An R^2 of 1 can occur only when all the Y values lie on the estimated regression line. In this case, it is easily verified that R^2 is the square of the simple product-moment correlation between X and Y. One disadvantage with using R^2 as a measure of goodness of fit is that it does not account for the number of degrees of freedom associated with SSR. We define a measure that makes this degree of freedom correction in the context of a full rank model.

Definition 4.2.5. Adjusted R-square. The adjusted R^2, or the corrected R^2 is defined as

$$
\begin{aligned}
R^2_{adj.} &= 1 - \frac{\widehat{Var}(\hat{\varepsilon})}{\widehat{Var}(\mathbf{y})} = 1 - \frac{\sum_{i=1}^N \hat{\varepsilon}_i^2/(N-p)}{\sum_{i=1}^N (Y_i - \overline{Y})^2/(N-1)} \\
&= 1 - \frac{SSE}{SST_c} = 1 - \frac{N-1}{N-p}(1 - R^2)
\end{aligned}
\tag{4.2.21}
$$

where p is the total number of parameters in the fitted model including the intercept, SST_c is the total mean corrected sum of squares and SSE denotes the error sum of squares with $(N-p)$ degrees of freedom.

Since an "adjustment" has been made for the corresponding degrees of freedom in the relevant sums of squares, $R^2_{adj.}$ is useful for comparing different regression fits to the same data as well as for comparing different data sets, although in the latter situation, its usefulness is rather limited. It is a gross initial indicator, and one is better off using other model comparison criteria. The adjusted R^2 is closely related to Mallows' C_p statistic, which we describe in Chapter 8. We next derive a general formula for the mean of a quadratic form which is useful for obtaining the covariance matrix of β^0.

Result 4.2.3. Suppose $E(\mathbf{x}) = \mu$, and $Var(\mathbf{x}) = \Sigma$, then,

$$
E(\mathbf{x}'\mathbf{A}\mathbf{x}) = tr(\mathbf{A}\Sigma) + \mu'\mathbf{A}\mu.
\tag{4.2.22}
$$

Proof. Similar to the well known univariate expression $E(X^2) = Var(X) + \{E(X)\}^2$, we can write in the vector case

$$
\begin{aligned}
E(\mathbf{x}\mathbf{x}') &= \Sigma + \mu\mu', \text{i.e.,} \\
E(\mathbf{x} - \mu)(\mathbf{x} - \mu)' &= \Sigma.
\end{aligned}
$$

Since $tr(\mathbf{x}'\mathbf{A}\mathbf{x}) = tr(\mathbf{A}\mathbf{x}\mathbf{x}')$ from property 4 of Result 1.2.8,

$$
\begin{aligned}
E(\mathbf{x}'\mathbf{A}\mathbf{x}) &= E[tr(\mathbf{A}\mathbf{x}\mathbf{x}')] = tr[\mathbf{A}E(\mathbf{x}\mathbf{x}')] = tr[\mathbf{A}\Sigma + \mathbf{A}\mu\mu'] \\
&= tr(\mathbf{A}\Sigma) + tr(\mu'\mathbf{A}\mu) = tr(\mathbf{A}\Sigma) + \mu'\mathbf{A}\mu,
\end{aligned}
$$

which completes the proof. ■

Result 4.2.4.   The following properties hold.

1. We have

$$E(\beta^0) = \mathbf{H}\beta \quad \text{and} \quad Cov(\beta^0) = \sigma^2 \mathbf{GX'XG'}, \tag{4.2.23}$$

where $\mathbf{H} = \mathbf{GX'X}$.

2. The expectation and covariance of the vector of fitted values and the residual vector are

$$E(\widehat{\mathbf{y}}) = \mathbf{X}\beta, \quad \text{and} \quad Cov(\widehat{\mathbf{y}}) = \sigma^2 \mathbf{P},$$
$$E(\widehat{\varepsilon}) = \mathbf{0}, \quad \text{and} \quad Cov(\widehat{\varepsilon}) = \sigma^2(\mathbf{I} - \mathbf{P}). \tag{4.2.24}$$

3. The expectation of the mean square error is

$$E(\widehat{\sigma}^2) = \sigma^2. \tag{4.2.25}$$

Proof. The expected value of the solution vector β^0 is

$$E(\beta^0) = \mathbf{GX'}E(\mathbf{y}) = \mathbf{GX'X}\beta = \mathbf{H}\beta,$$

so that β^0 is an unbiased estimate of $\mathbf{H}\beta$. Note that $\mathbf{H}$ is a function of the design matrix $\mathbf{X}$ and of $\mathbf{G}$, a g-inverse of $\mathbf{X'X}$. The variance-covariance matrix of β^0 is

$$Cov(\beta^0) = \mathbf{GX'}Cov(\mathbf{y})\mathbf{XG'} = \mathbf{GX'}(\sigma^2\mathbf{I}_N)\mathbf{XG'} = \sigma^2\mathbf{GX'XG'}.$$

By a suitable choice of g-inverse, we would obtain $Cov(\beta^0) = \sigma^2\mathbf{G}$. To see this, recall from Result 2.3.4 that there exists a $p \times p$ orthogonal matrix $\mathbf{P}$ such that $\mathbf{P'X'XP}$ is a diagonal matrix whose r nonzero elements are the eigenvalues of $\mathbf{X'X}$. Let $\mathbf{A}_{11}$ denote the leading $r \times r$ principal submatrix of $\mathbf{P'X'XP}$. Then,

$$\mathbf{G}^* = \mathbf{P} \begin{pmatrix} \mathbf{A}_{11}^{-1} & \mathbf{0} \\ \mathbf{0} & \mathbf{0} \end{pmatrix} \mathbf{P'}$$

is a symmetric g-inverse of $\mathbf{X'X}$ and we can verify that $\mathbf{G}^*\mathbf{X'XG}^{*\prime} = \mathbf{G}^*$. If $\beta^0 = \mathbf{G}^*\mathbf{X'y}$, then $Cov(\beta^0) = \sigma^2\mathbf{G}^*$. To prove property 2, we see that $E(\widehat{\mathbf{y}}) = \mathbf{XGX'}E(\mathbf{y}) = \mathbf{XGX'X}\beta = \mathbf{X}\beta$, and $E(\widehat{\varepsilon}) = E(\mathbf{y}-\widehat{\mathbf{y}}) = \mathbf{0}$. Now,

$$\begin{aligned} SSE &= (\mathbf{y} - \mathbf{X}\beta^0)'(\mathbf{y} - \mathbf{X}\beta^0) \\ &= \mathbf{y}'(\mathbf{I}_N - \mathbf{XGX'})'(\mathbf{I}_N - \mathbf{XGX'})\mathbf{y} \\ &= \mathbf{y}'(\mathbf{I}_N - \mathbf{XGX'})\mathbf{y} \end{aligned} \tag{4.2.26}$$

since $\mathbf{I}_N - \mathbf{XGX'}$ is a symmetric and idempotent matrix (see Exercise 4.2). Since $\mathbf{XGX'}$ is unique, so is SSE. Using Result 4.2.3,

$$\begin{aligned} E(SSE) &= E[\mathbf{y}'(\mathbf{I}_N - \mathbf{XGX'})\mathbf{y}] \\ &= tr[\sigma^2(\mathbf{I}_N - \mathbf{XGX'})] + \beta'\mathbf{X'}(\mathbf{I}_N - \mathbf{XGX'})\mathbf{X}\beta \\ &= \sigma^2(N - r). \end{aligned} \tag{4.2.27}$$

Therefore, the least squares estimator $\widehat{\sigma}^2$ is an unbiased estimate of σ^2, and is again invariant to the choice of $\mathbf{G}$. ∎

Corollary 4.2.2. In the full rank model, the properties of the least squares estimator of β follow as a special case of Result 4.2.4 and are given below:

$$E(\widehat{\beta}) = \beta \quad \text{and} \quad Cov(\widehat{\beta}) = \sigma^2(\mathbf{X'X})^{-1}. \tag{4.2.28}$$

Example 4.2.4. Let Y_1, Y_2, and Y_3 be independently distributed with $E(Y_i) = i\theta$, and $Var(Y_i) = \sigma^2$, for $i = 1, 2, 3$. We first set this up as a full rank linear model of the form (4.1.1), with

$$\mathbf{y} = \begin{pmatrix} Y_1 \\ Y_2 \\ Y_3 \end{pmatrix}, \quad \varepsilon = \begin{pmatrix} \varepsilon_1 \\ \varepsilon_2 \\ \varepsilon_3 \end{pmatrix}, \quad \mathbf{X} = \begin{pmatrix} 1 \\ 2 \\ 3 \end{pmatrix}, \quad \beta = \theta.$$

The least squares estimator of θ is $\widehat{\theta} = (\mathbf{X'X})^{-1}\mathbf{X'y} = \frac{1}{14}(Y_1 + 2Y_2 + 3Y_3)$, with variance $Var(\widehat{\theta}) = \sigma^2/14$. The estimator is unbiased for θ since $E(\widehat{\theta}) = \frac{1}{14}\{\theta + 2(2\theta) + 3(3\theta)\} = \theta$. The fitted vector $\widehat{\mathbf{y}}$ and the residual vector $\widehat{\varepsilon}$ are respectively given by

$$\widehat{\mathbf{y}} = \begin{pmatrix} \widehat{\theta} \\ 2\widehat{\theta} \\ 3\widehat{\theta} \end{pmatrix} = \begin{pmatrix} \frac{1}{14}(Y_1 + 2Y_2 + 3Y_3) \\ \frac{1}{7}(Y_1 + 2Y_2 + 3Y_3) \\ \frac{3}{14}(Y_1 + 2Y_2 + 3Y_3) \end{pmatrix}, \quad \widehat{\varepsilon} = \mathbf{y} - \widehat{\mathbf{y}} = \begin{pmatrix} Y_1 - \widehat{\theta} \\ Y_2 - 2\widehat{\theta} \\ Y_3 - 3\widehat{\theta} \end{pmatrix}.$$

The error sum of squares is

$$\begin{aligned} SSE &= \widehat{\varepsilon}'\widehat{\varepsilon} = (Y_1^2 + Y_2^2 + Y_3^2) - \widehat{\theta}(Y_1 + 2Y_2 + 3Y_3) \\ &= (Y_1^2 + Y_2^2 + Y_3^2) - \frac{1}{14}(Y_1 + 2Y_2 + 3Y_3)^2, \end{aligned}$$

and the mean square error (MSE) is $\widehat{\sigma}^2 = SSE/(N - p) = SSE/2$. □

Numerical Example 4.1. Simple linear regression. A company which markets and repairs small computers needs to forecast the number of service engineers required over the next few years. This requires consideration of the length of service calls, which in turn depends on the number of components that need to be repaired or replaced. The data set consists of the number of components repaired, X, and the length of the service call in minutes, Y, for a random sample of 20 calls (Chatterjee and Price, 1991). We illustrate fitting a simple linear regression model to explain the relationship between Y and X.

The estimated simple correlation between Y and X is $\widehat{\rho} = 0.965$, indicating a high, positive linear relationship between the two variables. The fitted simple linear regression model is

$$\widehat{Y} = 37.21 + 9.97X,$$

with $\hat{\sigma} = \sqrt{MSE} = 18.75$. The estimated standard errors of the least squares estimates are $s.e.(\hat{\beta}_0) = 7.99$, and $s.e.(\hat{\beta}_1) = 0.72$. Both coefficients are significantly different from zero at the 5% level of significance. The coefficient of determination, $R^2 = 0.90$, which is the square of the simple correlation coefficient, while $R^2_{adj.} = 0.89$.   ▲

Numerical Example 4.2. Multiple linear regression.   The data consists of health records of 30 employees who were regular members of a company's health club. The variables are Y, the time in a one-mile run (in seconds), X_1, the weight (in pounds), X_2, the resting pulse rate per minute, X_3, the arm and leg strength (no. of pounds a subject was able to lift), and X_4, the time in a 1/4-mile run (in seconds) (see Chatterjee and Hadi, 1988). The following matrix shows the pairwise correlations between the variables (Y, X_1, X_2, X_3, X_4):

$$\begin{pmatrix} 1.000 & 0.798 & 0.501 & 0.452 & 0.848 \\ 0.798 & 1.000 & 0.420 & 0.734 & 0.643 \\ 0.501 & 0.420 & 1.000 & 0.063 & 0.539 \\ 0.452 & 0.734 & 0.063 & 1.000 & 0.410 \\ 0.848 & 0.643 & 0.539 & 0.410 & 1.000 \end{pmatrix}.$$

The fitted multiple regression model is

$$\widehat{Y} = -8.863 + 1.243X_1 - 0.502X_2 - 0.476X_3 + 3.938X_4.$$

Least squares estimates of the parameters are shown below, and $R^2 = 0.85$.

Least squares estimates for Numerical Example 4.2.

Parameter	d.f.	Estimate	s.e.	t-value	Pr> t
Intercept	1	−8.863	55.520	−0.16	0.875
X_1	1	1.243	0.284	4.37	0.0002
X_2	1	−0.502	0.867	−0.58	0.568
X_3	1	−0.476	0.241	−1.98	0.059
X_4	1	3.938	0.752	5.23	< .0001

Entries in the last two columns pertain to inference based on normality of errors, which will be discussed in Chapter 7. ▲

Although the normal equations in (4.2.2) presumably consist of p equations in p unknowns, there are only r LIN equations, since the remaining $(p - r)$ equations are linear combinations of these. To obtain a solution of β, $(p - r)$ additional *consistent* equations, say, $\mathbf{a}'_j\beta = b_j$, $j = 1, \cdots, (p - r)$, are required, satisfying the condition that $\mathbf{a}_j$ is not a linear combination of the rows of $\mathbf{X}'\mathbf{X}$. Suppose that, on the contrary, $\mathbf{a}'_j$ is such a linear combination. Then, we can either obtain the corresponding additional equation from (4.2.2), or we will face inconsistency, i.e., we will obtain two different values for $\mathbf{a}'_j\beta^0$. In other words, this condition requires that $\mathbf{a}'_j\beta$ is a *non-estimable* function (see section 4.3). Suppose we represent the $(p - r)$ additional equations in the form $\mathbf{A}\beta = \mathbf{b}$;

each equation (row) must correspond to a non-estimable function. We will refer to these additional equations as *constraints*; they are generally chosen by inspection, and are included for the purpose of solving the normal equations. In section 4.6, we will talk about linear restrictions on the parameter vector β which arise as an integral part of the model specification.

Example 4.2.5. We continue with Example 4.1.3. In the one-way fixed-effects ANOVA model, we have seen that $r(\mathbf{X}) = a < p$, so that the least squares solution β^0 is not unique. Let $Y_{i\cdot}$ and $\overline{Y}_{i\cdot}$ respectively denote the total and average of the sample observations under the ith treatment. Let $Y_{\cdot\cdot}$ and $\overline{Y}_{\cdot\cdot}$ respectively denote the grand total and average of all the sample observations. We have used the "dot" subscript notation which implies summation over the subscript that it replaces. Symbolically, $Y_{i\cdot} = \sum_{j=1}^{n_i} Y_{ij}$, $\overline{Y}_{i\cdot} = Y_{i\cdot}/n_i$, $i = 1, \cdots, a$, $Y_{\cdot\cdot} = \sum_{i=1}^{a} \sum_{j=1}^{n_i} Y_{ij}$, and $\overline{Y}_{\cdot\cdot} = Y_{\cdot\cdot}/N$, where $N = \sum_{i=1}^{a} n_i$ is the total number of observations. The method of least squares consists of minimizing the sum of squares

$$S(\mu, \tau_1, \cdots, \tau_a) = \sum_{i=1}^{a} \sum_{j=1}^{n_i} \varepsilon_{ij}^2 = \sum_{i=1}^{a} \sum_{j=1}^{n_i} (Y_{ij} - \mu - \tau_i)^2 ;$$

the $(a+1)$ normal equations are

$$\left.\frac{\partial S}{\partial \mu}\right|_{\mu^0, \tau_i^0} = 0, \text{ and } \left.\frac{\partial S}{\partial \tau_i}\right|_{\mu^0, \tau_i^0} = 0, \quad i = 1, \cdots, a,$$

which have the form

$$N\mu^0 + \sum_{i=1}^{a} n_i \tau_i^0 = Y_{\cdot\cdot} \text{ and}$$
$$n_i(\mu^0 + \tau_i^0) = Y_{i\cdot}, \quad i = 1, \cdots, a.$$

Note that the sum of the last a normal equations is equal to the first; the $a+1$ normal equations are linearly dependent and hence no unique solution exists. In other words, there are $p = a+1$ parameters, and $r(\mathbf{X}) = a$, so we can set one element of β^0 equal to zero, and solve for the remaining a parameters uniquely. In general, we may obtain a solution to the normal equations subject to a constraint such as $\mu^0 = 0$, or $\tau_a^0 = 0$.

If we set $\mu^0 = 0$, we obtain the solution $\beta^0 = (0, \overline{Y}_{1\cdot}, \cdots, \overline{Y}_{a\cdot})'$. The g-inverse that corresponds to this solution is obtained by deleting the first row and column from $\mathbf{X'X}$ in the algorithm in Result 3.1.2 as

$$\mathbf{G} = \begin{pmatrix} 0 & \mathbf{0} \\ \mathbf{0} & \mathbf{D} \end{pmatrix}.$$

where $\mathbf{D} = \text{diag}(1/n_1, \cdots, 1/n_a)$ is an $a \times a$ diagonal matrix. The projection matrix $\mathbf{P}$ has the block diagonal form

$$\mathbf{P} = \text{diag}\left(\tfrac{1}{n_1}\mathbf{J}_{n_1}, \cdots, \tfrac{1}{n_a}\mathbf{J}_{n_a}\right)$$

and the fitted vector $\widehat{\mathbf{y}}$ is

$$\widehat{\mathbf{y}} = \mathbf{P}\mathbf{y} = (\overline{Y}_1.\mathbf{1}'_{n_1}, \cdots, \overline{Y}_a.\mathbf{1}'_{n_a})'.$$

The ANOVA decomposition can be written as

$$\sum_{i=1}^{a}\sum_{j=1}^{n_i} Y_{ij}^2 = \sum_{i=1}^{a} n_i \overline{Y}_i^2. + \sum_{i=1}^{a}\sum_{j=1}^{n_i} (Y_{ij} - \overline{Y}_i.)^2.$$

Suppose we impose an alternate constraint $\sum_{i=1}^{a} n_i \tau_i^0 = 0$ on the normal equations, we obtain the solution vector

$$\beta^0 = (\overline{Y}.., \overline{Y}_1. - \overline{Y}.., \cdots, \overline{Y}_a. - \overline{Y}..).$$

Subject to this constraint, the estimate of the overall mean μ is the grand sample average of all the N observations, while the estimate of the ith treatment effect τ_i is the difference between the average of the sample observations under the ith treatment and the grand average. The estimate of the error variance in both cases is

$$\widehat{\sigma}^2 = \frac{SSE}{(N-a)}, \tag{4.2.29}$$

where

$$SSE = \sum_{i=1}^{a}\sum_{j=1}^{n_i} Y_{ij}^2 - \sum_{i=1}^{a} n_i \overline{Y}_i^2.. \tag{4.2.30}$$

Neither of these solutions for β is unique; a solution depends on the constraint under which we choose to solve the normal equations.   □

Although this might seem like an unfortunate event, since we would be afraid that it might lead two different data analysts to draw two completely different inferences, we show that estimation and inference is indeed unique for certain functions of the parameters called "estimable functions" which are described in the next section. We conclude this section with an example of another fixed-effects linear model.

Example 4.2.6. Two-way cross-classified model.   Suppose an experiment has two factors, Factor A at a levels, and Factor B at b levels. In a cross-classified model, every level of Factor A can be studied with every level of Factor B. We introduce two relevant models.

Additive model.   This model involves only main effects due to each factor and has the form

$$Y_{ijk} = \mu + \tau_i + \beta_j + \varepsilon_{ijk}, \quad k = 1, \cdots, n, \ i = 1, \cdots, a, \ j = 1, \cdots, b, \quad (4.2.31)$$

where Y_{ijk} denotes the kth replicate in the (i,j)th cell, μ is the overall mean, τ_i denotes the effect due to the ith level of Factor A, β_j is the effect due to the jth level of Factor B, and the errors ε_{ijk} are iid with zero means and variance σ^2. If $n = 1$, we can write (4.2.31) in the form (4.1.1) with $N = ab$, $p = a + b + 1$, and

$$\mathbf{X} = \begin{pmatrix} \mathbf{1}_b & \mathbf{1}_b & \mathbf{0} & \cdots & \mathbf{0} & \mathbf{I}_b \\ \mathbf{1}_b & \mathbf{0} & \mathbf{1}_b & \cdots & \mathbf{0} & \mathbf{I}_b \\ \vdots & \vdots & \vdots & \ddots & \vdots & \mathbf{I}_b \\ \mathbf{1}_b & \mathbf{0} & \mathbf{0} & \cdots & \mathbf{1}_b & \mathbf{I}_b \end{pmatrix},$$

$$\mathbf{y} = \begin{pmatrix} Y_{11} & \cdots & Y_{1b} & \cdots & Y_{a1} & \cdots & Y_{ab} \end{pmatrix}',$$

with $r(\mathbf{X}) = a + b - 1$. Let $N = nab$. In the balanced case, $\mathbf{X}$ is an $N \times p$ design matrix, with $p = (a + b + 1)$, while $r(\mathbf{X}) = (a + b - 1)$, since there are two linear dependencies. The normal equations $\mathbf{X}'\mathbf{X}\beta^0 = \mathbf{X}'\mathbf{y}$ have the form

$$nab\mu^0 + nb\sum_{i=1}^{a}\tau_i^0 + na\sum_{j=1}^{b}\beta_j^0 = Y_{...}$$

$$nb\mu^0 + nb\tau_i^0 + n\sum_{j=1}^{b}\beta_j^0 = Y_{i..}, \quad i = 1, \cdots, a$$

$$na\mu^0 + n\sum_{i=1}^{a}\tau_i^0 + na\beta_j^0 = Y_{.j.}, \quad j = 1, \cdots, b.$$

We impose two constraints $\sum_{i=1}^{a}\tau_i^0 = 0$, and $\sum_{j=1}^{b}\beta_j^0 = 0$, i.e., $\mathbf{A}'\beta = \mathbf{0}$, with

$$\mathbf{A}' = \begin{pmatrix} 0 & 1 & \cdots & 1 & 0 & \cdots & 0 \\ 0 & 0 & \cdots & 0 & 1 & \cdots & 1 \end{pmatrix}, \quad \beta = (\mu, \tau_1, \cdots, \tau_a, \beta_1 \cdots, \beta_b)', \text{ and solve}$$

the resulting system of normal equations to obtain

$$\mu^0 = \overline{Y}_{...}$$

$$\tau_i^0 = \overline{Y}_{i..} - \overline{Y}_{...}, \quad i = 1, \cdots, a$$

$$\beta_j^0 = \overline{Y}_{.j.} - \overline{Y}_{...}, \quad j = 1, \cdots, b.$$

Searle (1971, p. 266) has described the use of *absorbing equations* for solution of the normal equations (see Result 3.2.10). The fitted values are

$$\widehat{Y}_{ijk} = \mu^0 + \tau_i^0 + \beta_j^0 = \overline{Y}_{i..} + \overline{Y}_{.j.} - \overline{Y}_{...}.$$

Model with interaction. In some experiments, we find that the difference in response between the levels of Factor A is not the same at all levels of Factor B. In this case, there is *interaction* between the two factors. A general model which involves main effects due to each factor as well as interaction between them is

$$Y_{ijk} = \mu + \tau_i + \beta_j + (\tau\beta)_{ij} + \varepsilon_{ijk}, \quad k = 1, \cdots, n, \; i = 1, \cdots, a, \; j = 1, \cdots, b, \tag{4.2.32}$$

where $(\tau\beta)_{ij}$ denotes the interaction effect between the ith level of Factor A and jth level of Factor B, and the other terms have been defined earlier. The interaction term is sometimes denoted in the literature by γ_{ij}. We can write $\mu_{ij} = \mu + \tau_i + \beta_j + \gamma_{ij}$, so that $\gamma_{ij} = \mu_{ij} - \mu - \tau_i - \beta_j$ is what is left over from additivity. If $n = 1$, i.e., there is no replication, we can show that we cannot separate interaction from the error (see Exercise 4.10). Let $N = nab$, and let $Y_{...} = \sum_{k=1}^{n}\sum_{j=1}^{b}\sum_{i=1}^{a}Y_{ijk}$, $Y_{i..} = \sum_{k=1}^{n}\sum_{j=1}^{b}Y_{ijk}$, $Y_{.j.} = \sum_{k=1}^{n}\sum_{i=1}^{a}Y_{ijk}$, and $Y_{ij.} = \sum_{k=1}^{n}Y_{ijk}$. The normal equations obtained by minimizing

$$\sum_{k=1}^{n}\sum_{j=1}^{b}\sum_{i=1}^{a}(Y_{ijk} - \mu - \tau_i - \beta_j - \gamma_{ij})^2$$

are given by

$$Y_{\cdots} = abn\mu^0 + bn\sum_{i=1}^{a}\tau_i^0 + an\sum_{j=1}^{b}\beta_j^0 + n\sum_{i=1}^{a}\sum_{j=1}^{b}\gamma_{ij}^0$$

$$Y_{i\cdot\cdot} = bn\mu^0 + bn\tau_i^0 + n\sum_{j=1}^{b}\beta_j^0 + n\sum_{j=1}^{b}\gamma_{ij}^0, \quad i = 1,\cdots,a$$

$$Y_{\cdot j\cdot} = an\mu^0 + n\sum_{i=1}^{a}\tau_i^0 + an\beta_j^0 + n\sum_{i=1}^{a}\gamma_{ij}^0, \quad j = 1,\cdots,b$$

$$Y_{ij\cdot} = n\mu^0 + n\tau_i^0 + n\beta_j^0 + n\gamma_{ij}^0, \quad i = 1,\cdots,a, j = 1,\cdots,b.$$

Only the last set of ab equations is LIN, and the remaining equations can be derived from these, by adding over i, or over j, or both. In matrix form, the design matrix $\mathbf{X}$ has dimension $nab \times (1 + a + b + ab)$, but its rank is only ab, since there are $(a + b + 1)$ linearly independent constraints. Of the constraints $\sum_{i=1}^{a}\tau_i^0 = 0$, $\sum_{i=1}^{a}\beta_j^0 = 0$, $\sum_{i=1}^{a}\gamma_{ij}^0 = 0$, $j = 1,\cdots,b$, and $\sum_{j=1}^{b}\gamma_{ij}^0 = 0$, $i = 1,\cdots,a$, only $(a+b+1)$ are LIN, since $\sum_{i=1}^{a}\sum_{j=1}^{b}\gamma_{ij}^0 = 0$, so that $r(\mathbf{X'X}) = ab$. Imposing these constraints, the normal equations yield the following solutions:

$$\mu^0 = \overline{Y}_{\cdots}$$
$$\tau_i^0 = \overline{Y}_{i\cdot\cdot} - \overline{Y}_{\cdots}, \quad i = 1,\cdots,a$$
$$\beta_j^0 = \overline{Y}_{\cdot j\cdot} - \overline{Y}_{\cdots}, \quad j = 1,\cdots,b, \text{ and}$$
$$(\tau\beta)_{ij}^0 = \overline{Y}_{ij\cdot} - \overline{Y}_{i\cdot\cdot} - \overline{Y}_{\cdot j\cdot} + \overline{Y}_{\cdots}, \quad i = 1,\cdots,a, j = 1,\cdots,b.$$

$$(4.2.33)$$

A numerical example illustrating these and further inference is described in Chapter 7.   □

Example 4.2.7. Two-factor nested model.   In some multi-factor experiments, the levels of one factor, say Factor B, are similar, but not identical for different levels of another factor, Factor A. Then, the levels of Factor B may be considered to be nested within (under) the levels of Factor A, and we have a nested or hierarchical model. The two-way nested model has the form

$$Y_{ijk} = \mu + \tau_i + \beta_{j(i)} + \varepsilon_{(ij)k}, \quad\quad (4.2.34)$$

for $k = 1,\cdots,n_{ij}$, $j = 1,\cdots,b_i$, and $i = 1,\cdots,a$. There are a levels of Factor A, and b_i levels of Factor B nested within each of the levels of Factor A in this unbalanced model. For example, suppose that a clinical trial involves a counties, and there are b_i hospitals in the ith county, and that data is collected on a sample of n_{ij} patients from the jth hospital in the ith county. The analysis of such data requires a nested or hierarchical model. Notice that we cannot include an interaction term between Factor A and Factor B since every level of Factor B does not appear with every level of Factor A. If $n_{ij} = n$, and $b_i = b$ for all i, j, we have a balanced model with $N = nab$ observations. The total number of model parameters in this case is $p = 1 + a + ab$ corresponding to μ, τ_i, and $\beta_{j(i)}$, $j = 1, \cdots, b$, $i = 1, \cdots, a$.

In the unbalanced case, the normal equations are obtained by minimizing the function

$$\sum_{i=1}^{a} \sum_{j=1}^{b_i} \sum_{k=1}^{n_{ij}} (Y_{ijk} - \mu^0 - \tau_i^0 - \beta_{j(i)}^0)^2,$$

and have the form

$$Y_{...} = N\mu^0 + \sum_{i=1}^{a} n_{i.}\tau_i^0 + \sum_{i=1}^{a}\sum_{j=1}^{b_i} n_{ij}\beta_{j(i)}^0,$$

$$Y_{i..} = n_{i.}\mu^0 + n_{i.}\tau_i^0 + \sum_{j=1}^{b_i} n_{ij}\beta_{j(i)}^0, \quad i = 1, \cdots, a,$$

$$Y_{ij.} = n_{ij}(\mu^0 + \tau_i^0 + \beta_{j(i)}^0), \quad j = 1, \cdots, b_i; \ i = 1, \cdots, a,$$

where $n_{i.} = \sum_{j=1}^{b_i} n_{ij}$, and $N = \sum_{i=1}^{a} \sum_{j=1}^{b_i} n_{ij}$. We may verify that the first equation is obtained by summing the last set of equations over both i and j, while the next set of a equations are obtained by summing the last set over j. Although the total number of parameters in the unbalanced model is $p = 1 + a + \sum_{i=1}^{a} b_i$, the number of LIN normal equations is only $\sum_{i=1}^{a} b_i$. We impose the following $(a + 1)$ constraints. We assume that $\sum_{i=1}^{a} n_{i.}\tau_i^0 = 0$, and $\sum_{j=1}^{b_i} n_{ij}\beta_{j(i)}^0 = 0$, $i = 1, \cdots, a$. The least squares solutions of the parameters under these constraints are

$$\mu^0 = \overline{Y}_{...},$$
$$\tau_i^0 = \overline{Y}_{i..} - \overline{Y}_{...}, \ i = 1, \cdots, a, \text{ and}$$
$$\beta_{j(i)}^0 = \overline{Y}_{ij.} - \overline{Y}_{i..}, \ j = 1, \cdots, b_i, \ i = 1, \cdots, a.$$

The fitted values are $\widehat{Y}_{ijk} = \overline{Y}_{ij.}$, and the residuals are $\widehat{\varepsilon}_{ijk} = Y_{ijk} - \overline{Y}_{ij.}$. For the balanced model, the least squares solutions are obtained by setting $n_{ij} = n$, and $b_i = b$ in the above formulas. In Example 7.4.6, we generalize the two-stage nested model to an m-stage nested model. $\square$

Numerical examples for these ANOVA models will be described in Chapter 7, where we discuss inference for the balanced models. In Chapter 9, we discuss unbalanced ANOVA models.

4.3 Estimable functions

In the previous section, we saw that unless $r(\mathbf{X}) = p$, β^0 is not unique. Although in the full rank model, we can estimate any function of β, we must restrict ourselves to estimating only certain linear functions of β when $r(\mathbf{X}) < p$. Such a linear function of β is called an *estimable function*. In other words, a linear function of β for which a (unique) estimator based on β^0 exists, which is invariant to the solution β^0, is called an estimable function. A more precise definition, which also provides an approach for the identification of an estimable function of β, is given below.

Definition 4.3.1. A linear parametric function $\mathbf{c}'\beta$ is said to be an estimable function of β if there exists an N-dimensional vector $\mathbf{t} = (t_1, \cdots, t_N)'$ such that the expectation (with respect to the distribution of $\mathbf{y}$) of the linear combination $\mathbf{t}'\mathbf{y} = t_1 Y_1 + \cdots + t_N Y_N$ is equal to $\mathbf{c}'\beta$, i.e.,

$$E(\mathbf{t}'\mathbf{y}) = \mathbf{c}'\beta. \tag{4.3.1}$$

In other words, $\mathbf{c}'\beta$ is estimable if there exists a linear function of $\mathbf{y}$ whose expected value is identically equal to $\mathbf{c}'\beta$. Note that for a particular linear function $\mathbf{c}'\beta$, the vector $\mathbf{t}$ is not required to be uniquely defined in any sense; the existence of such a vector $\mathbf{t}$ suffices. Usually, there may exist several linear functions of $\mathbf{y}$, each of whose expectations is equal to $\mathbf{c}'\beta$. For establishing estimability, it is sufficient to verify the existence of any one of these functions. If $r(\mathbf{X}) = p$, i.e., if we have a full rank linear model, then any linear function of β is a linear estimable function, which implies that we may estimate and carry out inference for any linear function of β. This, however, is not the case for the less than full rank model, and we must first check whether a function of interest is an estimable function. Only then, we can estimate it and proceed with further inference. Note also that the definition of estimability does not depend on the error variance specification. We state and prove some properties of estimable functions of β; these results are trivially true for the full rank case.

Result 4.3.1.

1. The expected value of any observation is estimable.

2. Any linear combination of estimable functions is estimable.

3. The function $\mathbf{c}'\beta$ is estimable if and only if

$$\mathbf{c}' = \mathbf{t}'\mathbf{X} \tag{4.3.2}$$

   for some vector $\mathbf{t}$.

4. The function $\mathbf{c}'\beta$ is estimable if and only if

$$\mathbf{c}' = \mathbf{c}'\mathbf{H} \tag{4.3.3}$$

   where $\mathbf{H} = \mathbf{G}\mathbf{X}'\mathbf{X}$.

5. Given an estimable function $\mathbf{c}'\beta$, the quantity $\mathbf{c}'\beta^0$ is invariant to the least squares solution β^0. That is, if (and only if) $\mathbf{c}'\beta$ is estimable, $\mathbf{c}'\beta^0$ is the (unique) least squares estimator of $\mathbf{c}'\beta$.

Proof. To prove property 1 for the ith response, consider an N-dimensional vector $\mathbf{t} = (t_1, \cdots, t_N)'$ where, for $j = 1, \cdots, N$, $t_j = 1$ if $j = i$, and $t_j = 0$ otherwise. By Definition 4.3.1, $\mathbf{t}'E(\mathbf{y})$ is an estimable function of β and is the ith element of the vector $E(\mathbf{y})$. To prove property 2, we see that by Definition 4.3.1, every estimable function of β is a linear combination of the elements of $E(\mathbf{y})$, and so is any linear combination of such estimable functions. This is therefore estimable. Alternatively, let $\mathbf{c}_1'\beta$ and $\mathbf{c}_2'\beta$ be any two estimable functions of β. This implies that for some N-dimensional vectors $\mathbf{t}_1$ and $\mathbf{t}_2$,

$$\mathbf{c}_1'\beta = E(\mathbf{t}_1'\mathbf{y}) \quad \text{and} \quad \mathbf{c}_2'\beta = E(\mathbf{t}_2'\mathbf{y}).$$

For constants a_1 and a_2,

$$a_1\mathbf{c}_1'\beta + a_2\mathbf{c}_2'\beta = (a_1\mathbf{t}_1' + a_2\mathbf{t}_2')E(\mathbf{y})$$

is a linear combination of $E(\mathbf{y})$, which proves property 2. Next, since $E(\mathbf{y}) = \mathbf{X}\beta$, we see from Definition 4.3.1. that

$$\mathbf{c}'\beta = \mathbf{t}'E(\mathbf{y}) = \mathbf{t}'\mathbf{X}\beta,$$

which holds for *all* values of β. This in turn implies that

$$\mathbf{c}' = \mathbf{t}'\mathbf{X}$$

for some N-dimensional vector $\mathbf{t}$ if and only if $\mathbf{c}'\beta$ is an estimable function, proving property 3. Property 3 thus gives a *necessary and sufficient condition* for estimability. We may also state the necessary and sufficient condition for estimability in terms of (4.3.3). To prove this, first assume that $\mathbf{c}'\beta$ is estimable. Then, from (4.3.2) and property 2 of Result 3.1.8,

$$\mathbf{c}'\mathbf{H} = \mathbf{t}'\mathbf{X}\mathbf{H} = \mathbf{t}'\mathbf{X}\mathbf{G}\mathbf{X}'\mathbf{X} = \mathbf{t}'\mathbf{X} = \mathbf{c}'.$$

To show the converse, suppose $\mathbf{c}'\mathbf{H} = \mathbf{c}'$ holds. Then,

$$\mathbf{c}' = \mathbf{c}'\mathbf{G}\mathbf{X}'\mathbf{X} = \mathbf{t}'\mathbf{X},$$

say, where $\mathbf{t}' = \mathbf{c}'\mathbf{G}\mathbf{X}'$, so that by (4.3.2), $\mathbf{c}'\beta$ is estimable. To prove property 5, we must show that $\mathbf{c}'\beta^0$ is invariant to the solution β^0 we obtain to the normal equations. We see that

$$\mathbf{c}'\beta^0 = \mathbf{t}'\mathbf{X}\beta^0 = \mathbf{t}'\mathbf{X}\mathbf{G}\mathbf{X}'\mathbf{y},$$

which is invariant to the choice of g-inverse $\mathbf{G}$ (by property 3 of Result 3.1.8) and hence to the choice of β^0.   ∎

Example 4.3.1.   In the model

$$
\begin{aligned}
E(Y_1) &= \beta_1 + \beta_2 \\
E(Y_2) &= \beta_1 + \beta_3 \\
E(Y_3) &= \beta_1 + \beta_2,
\end{aligned}
$$

we find a necessary and sufficient condition for estimability of $c_1\beta_1 + c_2\beta_2 + c_3\beta_3$, for real constants c_i, $i = 1, \cdots, 3$. $\sum_{i=1}^{3} c_i\beta_i$ is estimable if and only if there exist t_i, $i = 1, \cdots, 3$ such that $E(\sum_{i=1}^{3} t_i Y_i) = \sum_{i=1}^{3} c_i\beta_i$, i.e., if and only if c_1, c_2 and c_3 satisfy the conditions $c_1 = \sum_{i=1}^{3} t_i$, $c_2 = t_1 + t_3$, and $c_3 = t_2$, i.e., if and only if $c_1 = c_2 + c_3$. While $\beta_1 + \beta_2/2 + \beta_3/2$ is estimable, the function $\beta_1 - \beta_2/2 - \beta_3/2$ is not estimable. $\square$

If $\mathbf{c}'\beta$ is estimable, then $\mathbf{c}$ lies in the estimation space, and is orthogonal to any vector $\mathbf{d}$, where $\mathbf{d}'\mathbf{y}$ is in $\mathcal{C}^{\perp}(\mathbf{X})$. The following result is an immediate consequence of the previous result, and we leave its proof as an exercise.

Result 4.3.2.

1. $\mathbf{X}\beta$ is estimable, and any linear function of $\mathbf{X}\beta$ is also estimable.

2. $\mathbf{X}'\mathbf{X}\beta$ is estimable, and any linear function of $\mathbf{X}'\mathbf{X}\beta$ is also estimable. ∎

Note that in general, there could exist an infinite number of linear parametric estimable functions of β corresponding to a given linear model. The following result characterizes the exact number of LIN estimable functions.

Result 4.3.3. There exist exactly r LIN estimable functions of β, where $r = r(\mathbf{X})$.

Proof. By (4.3.2), $\mathbf{c}'\beta$ is estimable if $\mathbf{c}' = \mathbf{t}'\mathbf{X}$ for some vector $\mathbf{t}$. Let $\mathbf{T}$ be an $N \times N$ matrix of rank N, and let $\mathbf{C}' = \mathbf{T}'\mathbf{X}$, so that $\mathbf{C}'\beta$ denotes N estimable functions. By property 5 of Result 1.2.12, $r(\mathbf{C}) = r$, so that there are exactly r LIN rows in $\mathbf{C}'$, which implies that exactly r of the N estimable functions are LIN.   ∎

Although $\mathbf{T}$ need not be unique, its orthogonal projection onto $\mathcal{C}(\mathbf{X})$ is unique. For, if $\mathbf{T}_1$ and $\mathbf{T}_2$ are such that $\mathbf{C}' = \mathbf{T}_1'\mathbf{X} = \mathbf{T}_2'\mathbf{X}$, then

$$\mathbf{PT}_1 = \mathbf{X}(\mathbf{X}'\mathbf{X})^-\mathbf{X}'\mathbf{T}_1 = \mathbf{X}(\mathbf{X}'\mathbf{X})^-\mathbf{C} = \mathbf{X}(\mathbf{X}'\mathbf{X})^-\mathbf{X}'\mathbf{T}_2 = \mathbf{PT}_2.$$

The only linear functions of β with unique least squares estimates are estimable functions.

Result 4.3.4. The least squares estimate of $\mathbf{c}'\beta$ is unique if and only if $\mathbf{c}'\beta$ is estimable.

Proof. Suppose β_1^0 and β_2^0 satisfy $\mathbf{X}\beta_1^0 = \mathbf{X}\beta_2^0 = \mathbf{Py}$. To prove sufficiency, suppose $\mathbf{c}' = \mathbf{t}'\mathbf{X}$. Then

$$\mathbf{c}'\beta_1^0 = \mathbf{t}'\mathbf{X}\beta_1^0 = \mathbf{t}'\mathbf{Py} = \mathbf{t}'\mathbf{X}\beta_2^0 = \mathbf{c}'\beta_2^0. \blacksquare$$

Example 4.3.2. Consider the model $\mathbf{y} = \mathbf{X}\beta + \varepsilon$, where

$$\begin{pmatrix} Y_{11} \\ Y_{12} \\ Y_{13} \\ Y_{21} \\ Y_{22} \\ Y_{31} \end{pmatrix} \quad \mathbf{X} = \begin{pmatrix} 1 & 1 & 0 & 0 \\ 1 & 1 & 0 & 0 \\ 1 & 1 & 0 & 0 \\ 1 & 0 & 1 & 0 \\ 1 & 0 & 1 & 0 \\ 1 & 0 & 0 & 1 \end{pmatrix}, \quad \beta = \begin{pmatrix} \mu \\ \tau_1 \\ \tau_2 \\ \tau_3 \end{pmatrix}, \quad \varepsilon = \begin{pmatrix} \varepsilon_{11} \\ \varepsilon_{12} \\ \varepsilon_{13} \\ \varepsilon_{21} \\ \varepsilon_{22} \\ \varepsilon_{31} \end{pmatrix}.$$

Since $E(Y_{ij}) = \mu + \tau_i$, for $j = 1, \cdots, n_i$, $i = 1, \cdots, 3$, we have

$$E(Y_{1j} - Y_{2k}) = \mu + \tau_1 - \mu - \tau_2 = \tau_1 - \tau_2 = (\begin{array}{cccc} 0 & 1 & -1 & 0 \end{array})\beta,$$

so that there exists a vector $\mathbf{t} = (\begin{array}{cccccc} 1 & 0 & 0 & -1 & 0 & 0 \end{array})'$ such that $\mathbf{t}'E(\mathbf{y}) = \tau_1 - \tau_2$, which implies that $\tau_1 - \tau_2$ is an estimable function of β. Similarly, since $E(\mathbf{t}'\mathbf{y}) = \mu + \tau_1$ for $\mathbf{t} = (\begin{array}{cccccc} 1 & 0 & 0 & 0 & 0 & 0 \end{array})'$, we see that $\mu + \tau_1$ is an estimable function. To generalize, $\mu + \tau_i$, $i = 1, \cdots, 3$, and $\tau_i - \tau_k$, $i \neq k, i, k = 1, \cdots, 3$ are estimable, as are all linear combinations of such functions. In this model, $r(\mathbf{X}) = 3$, so that one set of LIN estimable functions consists of $\{\tau_1 - \tau_2, \tau_1 - \tau_3, \tau_2 - \tau_3\}$. $\quad\square$

Definition 4.3.2. Contrast. A contrast in the p-dimensional parameter vector β is a linear function $\mathbf{c}'\beta$ such that $\mathbf{c}'\mathbf{1}_p = \sum_{i=1}^{p} c_i = 0$.

Definition 4.3.3. Orthogonal contrasts. Two contrasts $\mathbf{c}_j'\beta$ and $\mathbf{c}_l'\beta$ are orthogonal if $\mathbf{c}_j'\mathbf{G}\mathbf{c}_l = 0$ in an unbalanced model. In the balanced case, the condition for orthogonality is $\mathbf{c}_j'\mathbf{c}_l = 0$.

Example 4.3.3. The normal equations that lead to the least squares solutions in the one-way model were given in Example 4.1.3. From these, it follows that $\mu + \tau_i$, $i = 1, \cdots, a$ form a set of LIN estimable functions, so that all estimable functions must be linear combinations of these functions. Estimable functions of the parameters μ, and $\tau_i, i = 1, \cdots, a$ are given below:

1. For $i = 1, \cdots, a$, $\mu + \tau_i$ is estimable; its estimate is $\overline{Y}_{i\cdot}$, with variance σ^2/n_i. The set of functions $\{\mu + \tau_i, i = 1, \cdots, a\}$ is a basis of the estimation space.

2. The function $\sum_{i=1}^{a} c_i(\mu + \tau_i)$ is estimable; its estimate is $\sum_{i=1}^{a} c_i \overline{Y}_{i\cdot}$, with variance $\sum_{i=1}^{a} c_i^2 \sigma^2/n_i$.

3. The function $\sum_{i=1}^{a} c_i \tau_i$ is estimable if and only if $\sum_{i=1}^{a} c_i = 0$; i.e., only contrasts in τ_i's are estimable.

4. μ is not estimable, and neither is τ_i, for any i.

Verification of these results follows directly from the definition of estimability. Since the expected value of any observation is estimable (see Definition 4.2.1), it follows that $\mu + \tau_i$ is estimable, being the expectation of Y_{ij}. Since $\beta^0 = (\overline{Y}_{\cdot\cdot}, \overline{Y}_{1\cdot} - \overline{Y}_{\cdot\cdot}, \cdots, \overline{Y}_{a\cdot} - \overline{Y}_{\cdot\cdot})'$ under the constraint $\sum_{i=1}^{a} \tau_i = 0$, it follows that

$$\widehat{\mu + \tau_i} = \overline{Y}_{i\cdot}, \quad i = 1, \cdots, a,$$

with variance σ^2/n_i. To obtain these results, we may write $\mu + \tau_i$ as $\mathbf{c}_i'\beta$, where $\mathbf{c}_i$ is an $(a+1)$-dimensional vector with 1 in the first and $(i+1)$th positions, and zero elsewhere. That $\{\mu + \tau_i, i = 1, \cdots, a\}$ is a set of LIN estimable functions follows directly from the form of the normal equations in Example 4.1.3, so that all estimable functions must be linear combinations of this basis. This proves properties 1 and 2. Clearly, the estimate of $\sum_{i=1}^{a} c_i(\mu + \tau_i)$ is equal to $\sum_{i=1}^{a} c_i(\widehat{\mu + \tau_i}) = \sum_{i=1}^{a} c_i \overline{Y}_{i\cdot}$, and its variance is $\sum_{i=1}^{a} c_i^2 \sigma^2/n_i$. Property 3 is a special case of property 2. We prove property 4 by contradiction. Suppose that μ is in fact estimable. Since $\{\mu + \tau_i, i = 1, \cdots, a\}$ is a basis set, there must exist constants $c_i, i = 1, \cdots, a$ such that $\mu = \sum_{i=1}^{a} c_i(\mu + \tau_i) = \mu \sum_{i=1}^{a} c_i + \sum_{i=1}^{a} c_i \tau_i$; this implies that $\sum_{i=1}^{a} c_i = 1$, and $\sum_{i=1}^{a} c_i \tau_i = 0$ for all τ_i, which in turn implies that c_i must be equal to zero for $i = 1, \cdots, a$, which is a contradiction! Hence, μ is not estimable. We leave the proof of the property that τ_i is not estimable for any i as an exercise (Exercise 4.13).

In the one-way ANOVA model, the function $\gamma = \sum_{i=1}^{a} c_i \tau_i$ such that $\sum_{i=1}^{a} c_i = 0$ is a contrast in the treatment effects τ_i, $i = 1, \cdots, a$. The functions $\tau_j - \tau_l$, for $j \neq l$ are elementary contrasts since they represent simple comparisons of two effects or groups. Other functions like $\tau_1 + \tau_2 - 2\tau_3$ or $\sum_{i=1}^{a} c_i \tau_i$, with $\sum_{i=1}^{a} c_i = 0$ are called general contrasts. General contrasts can be expressed as linear combinations of elementary contrasts. For instance, we can write $\tau_1 + \tau_2 - 2\tau_3 = (\tau_1 - \tau_3) + (\tau_2 - \tau_3)$, and $c_1\tau_1 + c_2\tau_2 + \cdots + c_a\tau_a = c_1(\tau_1 - \tau_a) + c_2(\tau_2 - \tau_a) + \cdots + c_{a-1}(\tau_{a-1} - \tau_a)$, since $\sum_{i=1}^{a} c_i = 0$. The vector $\mathbf{c}' = (c_1, \cdots, c_a)$ such that $\sum_{i=1}^{a} c_i = \mathbf{c}'\mathbf{1} = 0$ is called a contrast vector. There exists at most $a-1$ linearly independent (LIN) contrasts and $a - 1$ corresponding contrast vectors. One such contrast vector set is $(1, -1, 0, \cdots, 0), (1, 0, -1, \cdots, 0), \cdots, (1, 0, 0, \cdots, -1)$ which corresponds to contrasts $\tau_1 - \tau_2, \tau_1 - \tau_3, \cdots, \tau_1 - \tau_a$. Another set is defined by $\mathbf{c}_l' = \frac{1}{\sqrt{l(l+1)}} (\underbrace{1, 1, \cdots, 1}_{l \text{ times}}, -l, 0, \cdots, 0)$, for $l = 1, \cdots, a - 1$, and the corresponding contrasts are $(\tau_1 + \tau_2 + \cdots + \tau_l - l\tau_{l+1}) \big/ \sqrt{l(l + 1)}$, $l = 1, \cdots, a-1$. Note that $\mathbf{c}_l'\mathbf{c}_l = 1$ and $\mathbf{c}_l'\mathbf{c}_h = 0$, $l \neq h$, i.e., these are $a - 1$ mutually orthogonal contrasts. In general, two contrasts $\sum_{i=1}^{a} c_i \tau_i$ and $\sum_{i=1}^{a} d_i \tau_i$ are said to be orthogonal if $\sum_{i=1}^{a} c_i d_i = 0$ for a balanced design, and if $\sum_{i=1}^{a} n_i c_i d_i = 0$ for an unbalanced design. $\square$

4.4   Gauss-Markov theorem

We now state one of the most fundamental results in linear model theory, which gives an optimality result for linear estimates of estimable functions of β without any distributional assumption.

Result 4.4.1.   Let $\mathbf{c}'\beta$ be an estimable function of β, and let β^0 denote any solution to the normal equations (4.2.2). Then, $\mathbf{c}'\beta^0$ is the best linear unbiased estimator (b.l.u.e.) of $\mathbf{c}'\beta$, with variance $Var(\mathbf{c}'\beta^0) = \mathbf{c}'\mathbf{G}\mathbf{c}\sigma^2$.

Proof. Clearly, $c'\beta^0 = c'GX'y$ is a linear function of y. As we mentioned earlier, $c'\beta^0$ is invariant to G, and hence to β^0, and can therefore be regarded as a unique estimator of $c'\beta$. Now,

$$E(c'\beta^0) = c'E(\beta^0) = c'GX'X\beta = c'H\beta, \qquad (4.4.1)$$

where $H = GX'X$. Estimability of $c'\beta$ implies that $c' = t'X$ for some N-dimensional vector t, so that, using property 2 of Result 3.1.8

$$E(c'\beta^0) = t'XGX'X\beta = t'X\beta = c'\beta. \qquad (4.4.2)$$

This proves that $c'\beta^0$ is an unbiased estimator of $c'\beta$. Further, since $c' = t'X$, and $X'XG'X' = X'$ (see Exercise 3.4), we have

$$
\begin{aligned}
Var(c'\beta^0) &= \sigma^2 c'GX'XG'c = \sigma^2 c'GX'XG'X't \\
&= \sigma^2 c'GX't = \sigma^2 c'Gc. \qquad (4.4.3)
\end{aligned}
$$

We now show that $c'\beta^0$ has minimum variance among the class of linear unbiased estimators of $c'\beta$. Let $d'y$ denote any linear unbiased estimator of $c'\beta$ other than $c'\beta^0$. Then, we must have $E(d'y) = d'X\beta = c'\beta$, which implies that

$$d'X = c'. \qquad (4.4.4)$$

The covariance between $c'\beta^0$ and $d'y$ is

$$
\begin{aligned}
Cov(c'\beta^0, d'y) &= Cov(c'GX'y, d'y) \\
&= \sigma^2 c'GX'd = \sigma^2 c'Gc, \qquad (4.4.5)
\end{aligned}
$$

where the last equality follows from (4.4.4). Using (4.4.3) and (4.4.5), we see that

$$
\begin{aligned}
0 &\le Var(c'\beta^0 - d'y) = Var(c'\beta^0) + Var(d'y) - 2Cov(c'\beta^0, d'y) \\
&= \sigma^2 c'Gc + Var(d'y) - 2\sigma^2 c'Gc \\
&= Var(d'y) - \sigma^2 c'Gc = Var(d'y) - Var(c'\beta^0), \qquad (4.4.6)
\end{aligned}
$$

with equality holding if and only if $d'y = c'\beta^0$. We have shown that $c'\beta^0$ has the smallest variance among all linear unbiased estimators of $c'\beta$; it is the b.l.u.e. of $c'\beta$. ■

Consider a projection approach for constructing the b.l.u.e. of an estimable function $c'\beta$. Since $c'\beta$ is estimable, there exists at least one vector $t'y$ whose expectation is $c'\beta$. We can decompose the vector t into two orthogonal components as $t' = t'P + t'(I - P)$. Hence,

$$t'y = t'Py + t'(I - P)y,$$

where, from (4.2.2) and (4.3.2)

$$
\begin{aligned}
t'Py &= t'XGX'y \\
&= t'X\beta^0 = c'\beta^0.
\end{aligned}
$$

So, $\mathbf{t'Py}$ is the b.l.u.e. of $\mathbf{c'}\beta$, while $\mathbf{t'(I-P)y}$ belongs to the error space. Thus, $\mathbf{t'P}$ is the projection of $\mathbf{t'}$ onto the estimation space.

Corollary 4.4.1. In the full rank model, the Gauss-Markov theorem states that the b.l.u.e. of $\mathbf{c'}\beta$ is $\mathbf{c'}\widehat{\beta} = \mathbf{c'(X'X)^{-1}X'y}$, with variance $\sigma^2\mathbf{c'(X'X)^{-1}c}$.

Result 4.4.2. Let $\mathbf{c_1'}\beta$ and $\mathbf{c_2'}\beta$ be two estimable functions of β. Then

$$Cov(\mathbf{c_1'}\beta^0, \mathbf{c_2'}\beta^0) = \sigma^2\mathbf{c_1'Gc_2}.$$

Proof. By definition,

$$Cov(\mathbf{c_1'}\beta^0, \mathbf{c_2'}\beta^0) = \sigma^2\mathbf{c_1'}Cov(\beta^0)\mathbf{c_2} = \sigma^2\mathbf{c_1'Gc_2}. \quad \blacksquare$$

Example 4.4.1. For the simple linear regression in Example 4.1.1, we have

$$E(\widehat{\beta}_0) = \beta_0, \text{ and } Var(\widehat{\beta}_0) = \sigma^2 \sum_{i=1}^N X_i^2 \Big/ N\sum_{i=1}^N (X_i - \overline{X})^2,$$
$$E(\widehat{\beta}_1) = \beta_1 \text{ and } Var(\widehat{\beta}_1) = \sigma^2 \Big/ \sum_{i=1}^N (X_i - \overline{X})^2.$$

These results follow directly from Corollary 4.2.2. Further,

$$Cov(\widehat{\beta}_0, \widehat{\beta}_1) = -\sigma^2\overline{X} \Big/ \sum_{i=1}^N (X_i - \overline{X})^2.$$

The estimators $\widehat{\beta}_0$ and $\widehat{\beta}_1$ are clearly unbiased. When $\overline{X} = 0$, $\widehat{\beta}_0$ and $\widehat{\beta}_1$ are uncorrelated. Intuitively, we may see that this is so because when $\overline{X} = 0$, $\widehat{\beta}_0 = \overline{Y}$, while $\widehat{\beta}_1$ is unaffected by a shift in location of the Y variable, i.e., it is uncorrelated with $\overline{Y}$. That $E(\widehat{Y}_i) = \beta_0 + \beta_1 X_i$, and

$$\begin{aligned} Var(\widehat{Y}_i) &= Var(\widehat{\beta}_0) + X_i^2 Var(\widehat{\beta}_1) + 2X_i Cov(\widehat{\beta}_0, \widehat{\beta}_1) \\ &= \sigma^2/N + \sigma^2(X_i - \overline{X})^2 \Big/ \sum_{i=1}^N (X_i - \overline{X})^2 \end{aligned}$$

follow directly from property 2 of Result 4.2.4. $\square$

We will show in Chapter 7 that the vector of fitted values $\widehat{\mathbf{y}} = (\widehat{Y}_1, \cdots, \widehat{Y}_N)$ has a (singular) multivariate normal distribution. It may be verified that the residuals are uncorrelated with the fitted values, whereas they are correlated with the observed responses; the slope of the straight line fit of $\widehat{\varepsilon}_i$ on $\widehat{Y}_i$ is zero, while that of the fit on Y_i is equal to $1 - r^2$, where r denotes the sample correlation coefficient between X and Y defined by

$$r^2 = [\sum_{i=1}^N (X_i - \overline{X})(Y_i - \overline{Y})]^2 \Big/ \sum_{i=1}^N (X_i - \overline{X})^2 \sum_{i=1}^N (Y_i - \overline{Y})^2.$$

There are several situations that arise in practice where it is known that $\beta_0 = 0$, corresponding to a straight line through the origin, i.e., a simple linear regression without intercept. In this case, it is easily shown that

$$\widehat{\beta}_1 = \sum_{i=1}^{N} X_i Y_i / \sum_{i=1}^{N} X_i^2, \quad \text{and } Var(\widehat{\beta}_1) = \sigma^2 / \sum_{i=1}^{N} X_i^2. \quad \square$$

Example 4.4.2. In the two-way fixed-effects cross-classified additive model with $n = 1$, the following functions are estimable.

1. $\mu + \tau_i + \beta_j$ is estimable with b.l.u.e. $\overline{Y}_{i\cdot} + \overline{Y}_{\cdot j} - \overline{Y}_{\cdot\cdot}$;

2. $\tau_i - \tau_h$ is estimable, for $i \neq h$, with b.l.u.e. $\overline{Y}_{i\cdot} - \overline{Y}_{h\cdot}$;

3. $\beta_j - \beta_l$ is estimable, for $j \neq l$, with b.l.u.e. $\overline{Y}_{\cdot j} - \overline{Y}_{\cdot l}$;

estimability of these functions is directly verified since they are in turn $E(Y_{ij})$, $E(Y_{ij}) - E(Y_{hj})$, and $E(Y_{ij}) - E(Y_{il})$. The b.l.u.e. of $\mu + \tau_i + \beta_j$ is $\mu^0 + \tau_i^0 + \beta_j^0 = \overline{Y}_{\cdot\cdot} + \overline{Y}_{i\cdot} - \overline{Y}_{\cdot\cdot} + \overline{Y}_{\cdot j} - \overline{Y}_{\cdot\cdot} = \overline{Y}_{i\cdot} + \overline{Y}_{\cdot j} - \overline{Y}_{\cdot\cdot}$. The b.l.u.e. of $\tau_i - \tau_h$ is $\tau_i^0 - \tau_h^0 = (\overline{Y}_{i\cdot} - \overline{Y}_{\cdot\cdot}) - (\overline{Y}_{h\cdot} - \overline{Y}_{\cdot\cdot})$, with estimated variance $2\widehat{\sigma}^2 / b$. To verify the variance estimate, we may see that $Var(\overline{Y}_{i\cdot}) = Var(\sum_{j=1}^{b} Y_{ij}/b) = Var(\sum_{j=1}^{b} Y_{ij})/b^2 = b\widehat{\sigma}^2 / b^2 = \widehat{\sigma}^2 / b$. The b.l.u.e. of $\beta_j - \beta_l$ is $\beta_j^0 - \beta_l^0 = (\overline{Y}_{\cdot j} - \overline{Y}_{\cdot\cdot}) - (\overline{Y}_{\cdot l} - \overline{Y}_{\cdot\cdot})$, with estimated variance $2\widehat{\sigma}^2 / a$. $\square$

We conclude this section with a result on optimal estimation of the error variance σ^2.

Result 4.4.3. Optimal estimator of σ^2.   Consider the linear model (4.1.1), where the second, third and fourth central moments of Y_i exist and are respectively equal to σ^2, μ_3, and μ_4. Then $(N - r)\widehat{\sigma}^2$ is the unique nonnegative quadratic unbiased estimator of $(N - r)\sigma^2$, with minimum variance when $\mu_4 = 3\sigma^4$, or when the nonzero diagonal elements of the projection matrix $\mathbf{P}$ are equal (Atiqullah, 1962).

Proof.   Since $\sigma^2 \geq 0$, Rao (1952) proposed the class $\mathcal{A}$ of nonnegative quadratic unbiased estimates $\mathbf{y}'\mathbf{A}\mathbf{y}$ of $(N - r)\sigma^2$. Let $\mathbf{a}$ denote the vector of diagonal elements of $\mathbf{A}$. We will state sufficient conditions for $\mathbf{y}'(\mathbf{I}-\mathbf{P})\mathbf{y}$ to have minimum variance in $\mathcal{A}$. If $\mathbf{y}'\mathbf{A}\mathbf{y} \in \mathcal{A}$, by Result 4.2.3, $(N - r)\sigma^2 = E(\mathbf{y}'\mathbf{A}\mathbf{y}) = \sigma^2 tr(\mathbf{A}) + \beta'\mathbf{X}'\mathbf{A}\mathbf{X}\beta$ for all β. In particular, setting $\beta = \mathbf{0}$, $tr(\mathbf{A}) = (N - r)$, then $\beta'\mathbf{X}'\mathbf{A}\mathbf{X}\beta = 0$ for all β, implying that $\mathbf{X}'\mathbf{A}\mathbf{X} = \mathbf{0}$, which in turn implies that $\mathbf{A}\mathbf{X} = \mathbf{0}$ (see Exercise 2.26). It follows that $\mathbf{A}\mathbf{X}(\mathbf{X}'\mathbf{X})^-\mathbf{X}' = \mathbf{A}\mathbf{P} = \mathbf{0}$. Then

$$\begin{aligned} Var(\mathbf{y}'\mathbf{A}\mathbf{y}) &= (\mu_4 - 3\sigma^4)\mathbf{a}'\mathbf{a} + 2\sigma^4 tr(\mathbf{A}^2) + 4\sigma^2 \beta'\mathbf{X}'\mathbf{A}^2\mathbf{X}\beta + 4\mu_3\beta'\mathbf{X}'\mathbf{A}\mathbf{a} \\ &= (\mu_4 - 3\sigma^4)\mathbf{a}'\mathbf{a} + 2\sigma^4 tr(\mathbf{A}^2) \end{aligned} \qquad (4.4.7)$$

(for proof see Seber, 1977, Theorem 1.8). From (4.2.27), $(N - r)\widehat{\sigma}^2 = \mathbf{y}'(\mathbf{I} - \mathbf{P})\mathbf{y} \in \mathcal{A}$, and

$$Var[\mathbf{y}'(\mathbf{I} - \mathbf{P})\mathbf{y}] = (\mu_4 - 3\sigma^4)\mathbf{q}'\mathbf{q} + 2\sigma^4(N - r), \qquad (4.4.8)$$

where $\mathbf{q}$ is the vector of diagonal elements of $\mathbf{I}-\mathbf{P}$. Suppose $\mathbf{A} = (\mathbf{I}-\mathbf{P})+\mathbf{R}$, and similarly, $\mathbf{a} = \mathbf{q}+\mathbf{r}$. It follows that $\mathbf{R}$ is symmetric, with $tr(\mathbf{R}) = tr(\mathbf{A})-tr(\mathbf{I}-$

$\mathbf{P}) = 0$. Since $\mathbf{0} = \mathbf{AP} = (\mathbf{I}-\mathbf{P})\mathbf{P}+\mathbf{RP} = \mathbf{RP}$, we get $\mathbf{R}(\mathbf{I}-\mathbf{P}) = \mathbf{R}$; it follows using Result 4.2.1 that $tr(\mathbf{A}^2) = tr(\mathbf{I}-\mathbf{P})+tr(\mathbf{R}^2)+2tr(\mathbf{R}) = (N-r)+tr(\mathbf{R}^2)$. Substitute $\mathbf{a} = \mathbf{q}+\mathbf{r}$ in (4.4.7) and use (4.4.8) to get

$$
\begin{aligned}
Var(\mathbf{y}'\mathbf{Ay}) &= (\mu_4 - 3\sigma^4)\mathbf{a}'\mathbf{a} + 2\sigma^4[(N-r) + tr(\mathbf{R}^2)] \\
&= (\mu_4 - 3\sigma^4)(\mathbf{q}'\mathbf{q} + 2\mathbf{q}'\mathbf{r} + \mathbf{r}'\mathbf{r}) + 2\sigma^4[(N-r) + tr(\mathbf{R}^2)] \\
&= (\mu_4 - 3\sigma^4)\mathbf{q}'\mathbf{q} + 2\sigma^4(N-r) \\
&\quad + 2\sigma^4[(\mu_4 - 3\sigma^4)(\mathbf{q}'\mathbf{r} + \frac{1}{2}\mathbf{r}'\mathbf{r}) + tr(\mathbf{R}^2)] \\
&= Var(\mathbf{y}'(\mathbf{I} - \mathbf{P})\mathbf{y}) + \\
&\quad 2\sigma^4[(\mu_4 - 3\sigma^4)(\sum_{i=1}^{N} q_{ii} r_{ii} + \frac{1}{2}\sum_{i=1}^{N} r_{ii}^2) + \sum_{i=1}^{N}\sum_{j=1}^{N} r_{ij}^2].
\end{aligned}
$$

Although minimization of $Var(\mathbf{y}'\mathbf{Ay})$ subject to $tr(\mathbf{R}) = 0$ and $\mathbf{R}(\mathbf{I} - \mathbf{P}) = \mathbf{R}$ is difficult in general, we can consider two special cases. First, when $\mu_4 = 3\sigma^4$, $Var(\mathbf{y}'\mathbf{Ay}) = Var(\mathbf{y}'(\mathbf{I} - \mathbf{P})\mathbf{y}) + 2\sigma^4 \sum_{i=1}^{N}\sum_{j=1}^{N} r_{ij}^2$, which is minimum when $r_{ij} = 0$ for $i, j = 1, \cdots, N$, i.e., when $\mathbf{A} = \mathbf{I} - \mathbf{P}$. As a second case, suppose that each nonzero diagonal element of $(\mathbf{I} - \mathbf{P})$ is equal to $(N-r)/N$. The proof that $Var(\mathbf{y}'\mathbf{Ay})$ attains a minimum is left as an exercise (see Exercise 4.15). ∎

4.5 Generalized least squares

Consider the linear model

$$
\mathbf{y} = \mathbf{X}\beta + \varepsilon, \quad Var(\varepsilon) = \sigma^2\mathbf{V}, \tag{4.5.1}
$$

where $\mathbf{V}$ is a known $N \times N$ p.d. matrix. The other assumptions of the general linear model still hold. We show that the least squares procedure produces optimal estimates (in the sense of the Gauss-Markov theorem). Since $\mathbf{V}$ is p.d., it follows from Result 2.4.5 that there exists an $N \times N$ matrix $\mathbf{K}$ with $r(\mathbf{K}) = N$, such that $\mathbf{V} = \mathbf{KK}'$. Let

$$
\mathbf{z} = \mathbf{K}^{-1}\mathbf{y}, \quad \mathbf{B} = \mathbf{K}^{-1}\mathbf{X}, \quad \text{and} \quad \eta = \mathbf{K}^{-1}\varepsilon. \tag{4.5.2}
$$

Since $r(\mathbf{X}) = r \le p$, it follows from property 5 of Result 1.2.12 that $r(\mathbf{B}) = r$. It may also be verified that

$$
E(\eta) = \mathbf{0}, \quad \text{and} \quad Var(\eta) = \mathbf{K}^{-1}(\sigma^2\mathbf{V})\mathbf{K}^{-1\prime} = \sigma^2\mathbf{K}^{-1}\mathbf{KK}'\mathbf{K}^{-1\prime} = \sigma^2\mathbf{I}_N.
$$

Consider the "transformed" linear model

$$
\mathbf{z} = \mathbf{B}\beta + \eta, \quad Var(\eta) = \sigma^2\mathbf{I}_N, \tag{4.5.3}
$$

which resembles the general linear model in (4.1.1) with $r(\mathbf{B}) = r \le p$. Minimizing $\eta'\eta = (\mathbf{z} - \mathbf{B}\beta)'(\mathbf{z} - \mathbf{B}\beta)$ with respect to β, we obtain the generalized least squares (GLS) solution to the normal equations as

$$
\begin{aligned}
\beta_{GLS}^0 &= (\mathbf{B'B})^-\mathbf{B'z} \\
&= (\mathbf{X'K}^{-1'}\mathbf{K}^{-1}\mathbf{X})^-\mathbf{X'K}^{-1'}\mathbf{K}^{-1}\mathbf{y} \\
&= [\mathbf{X'}(\mathbf{KK'})^{-1}\mathbf{X}]^-\mathbf{X'}(\mathbf{KK'})^{-1}\mathbf{y} \\
&= (\mathbf{X'V}^{-1}\mathbf{X})^-\mathbf{X'V}^{-1}\mathbf{y}, \quad (4.5.4)
\end{aligned}
$$

where $(\mathbf{X'V}^{-1}\mathbf{X})^-$ is a g-inverse of the $p \times p$ matrix $\mathbf{X'V}^{-1}\mathbf{X}$ (since $\mathbf{V}$ is p.d., and $r(\mathbf{X}) = r$, it follows that $r(\mathbf{X'V}^{-1}\mathbf{X}) = r$). Notice that $\mathbf{X}\beta_{GLS}^0$ denotes a projection of $\mathbf{y}$ onto $\mathcal{C}(\mathbf{X})$, but it is not an orthogonal projection. Let $\mathbf{W} = \mathbf{X}(\mathbf{X'V}^{-1}\mathbf{X})^-\mathbf{X'V}^{-1}$; then $\mathbf{Wy} = \mathbf{X}\beta_{GLS}^0$, and $\mathcal{C}(\mathbf{W}) = \mathcal{C}(\mathbf{X})$. The matrix W is a projection matrix onto $\mathcal{C}(\mathbf{X})$, and if the inner product between two vectors $\mathbf{u}$ and $\mathbf{v}$ is defined as $\mathbf{u'V}^{-1}\mathbf{v}$, then $\mathbf{W}$ denotes the orthogonal projection onto $\mathcal{C}(\mathbf{X})$. If $r = p$, i.e., if we have a full rank model, then $(\mathbf{X'V}^{-1}\mathbf{X})^{-1}$ exists and the solution vector (4.5.4) is the unique generalized least squares (GLS) estimator of β given by

$$
\widehat{\beta}_{GLS} = (\mathbf{X'V}^{-1}\mathbf{X})^{-1}\mathbf{X'V}^{-1}\mathbf{y}. \quad (4.5.5)
$$

There is an alternate way to obtain the solution β_{GLS}^0. Write

$$
\begin{aligned}
\eta'\eta &= \varepsilon'\mathbf{V}^{-1}\varepsilon \\
&= (\mathbf{y} - \mathbf{X}\beta)'\mathbf{V}^{-1}(\mathbf{y} - \mathbf{X}\beta) \\
&= \mathbf{y'y} - 2\beta'\mathbf{X'V}^{-1}\mathbf{y} + \beta'\mathbf{X'V}^{-1}\mathbf{X}\beta.
\end{aligned}
$$

Differentiating with respect to β and setting equal to zero, i.e.,

$$
\partial\eta'\eta/\partial\beta = -2\mathbf{X'V}^{-1}\mathbf{y} + 2\mathbf{X'V}^{-1}\mathbf{X}\beta \equiv 0
$$

gives β_{GLS}^0 in (4.5.4). The unbiased GLS estimator of σ^2 is given by

$$
\begin{aligned}
\widehat{\sigma}_{GLS}^2 &= \frac{1}{(N-r)}(\mathbf{z} - \mathbf{B}\beta_{GLS}^0)'(\mathbf{z} - \mathbf{B}\beta_{GLS}^0) \\
&= \frac{1}{(N-r)}(\mathbf{y} - \mathbf{X}\beta_{GLS}^0)'(\mathbf{KK'})^{-1}(\mathbf{y} - \mathbf{X}\beta_{GLS}^0) \\
&= \frac{1}{(N-r)}(\mathbf{y} - \mathbf{X}\beta_{GLS}^0)'\mathbf{V}^{-1}(\mathbf{y} - \mathbf{X}\beta_{GLS}^0) \\
&= \frac{1}{(N-r)}SSE_{GLS}. \quad (4.5.6)
\end{aligned}
$$

A function $\mathbf{c}'\beta$ is estimable in model (4.5.1) if and only if it is estimable in the transformed model (4.5.3) (see Exercise 4.18); also see Exercise 4.19.

Result 4.5.1. Suppose $r(\mathbf{X}) = r < p$. Provided $\mathbf{c}'\beta$ is an estimable function of β, the statistic $\mathbf{c}'\beta_{GLS}^0$ is the unique best linear unbiased estimator (b.l.u.e.) of $\mathbf{c}'\beta$.

Proof. The proof mimics the proof of Result 4.4.1 for the transformed model (4.5.3). If $\mathbf{c}'\beta$ is estimable, then

$$Var(\mathbf{c}'\beta^0_{GLS}) = \sigma^2 \mathbf{c}'(\mathbf{X}'\mathbf{V}^{-1}\mathbf{X})^{-}\mathbf{c}.$$

For two estimable functions $\mathbf{c}'_1\beta$ and $\mathbf{c}'_2\beta$,

$$Cov(\mathbf{c}'_1\beta^0_{GLS}, \mathbf{c}'_2\beta^0_{GLS}) = \sigma^2 \mathbf{c}'_1(\mathbf{X}'\mathbf{V}^{-1}\mathbf{X})^{-}\mathbf{c}_2. \quad \blacksquare$$

Corollary 4.5.1.   For the full rank model with $r(\mathbf{X}) = p$, the GLS estimator $\widehat{\beta}_{GLS}$ has the following properties:

1. $\widehat{\beta}_{GLS}$ is an unbiased estimator of β.

2. The variance-covariance matrix of $\widehat{\beta}_{GLS}$ is $Var(\widehat{\beta}_{GLS}) = \sigma^2(\mathbf{X}'\mathbf{V}^{-1}\mathbf{X})^{-1}$.

3. The error sum of squares is $SSE_{GLS} = (\mathbf{y} - \mathbf{X}\widehat{\beta}_{GLS})'\mathbf{V}^{-1}(\mathbf{y} - \mathbf{X}\widehat{\beta}_{GLS})$.

4. $\mathbf{c}'\widehat{\beta}_{GLS}$ is the best linear unbiased estimator (b.l.u.e.) of $\mathbf{c}'\beta$, with variance $\sigma^2\mathbf{c}'(\mathbf{X}'\mathbf{V}^{-1}\mathbf{X})^{-1}\mathbf{c}$.

Proof.

$$E(\widehat{\beta}_{GLS}) = (\mathbf{X}'\mathbf{V}^{-1}\mathbf{X})^{-1}\mathbf{X}'\mathbf{V}^{-1}\mathbf{X}\beta = \beta,$$

which proves property 1. Property 2 follows directly by seeing that

$$
\begin{aligned}
Var(\widehat{\beta}_{GLS}) &= Var[(\mathbf{X}'\mathbf{V}^{-1}\mathbf{X})^{-1}\mathbf{X}'\mathbf{V}^{-1}\mathbf{y}] \\
&= \sigma^2(\mathbf{X}'\mathbf{V}^{-1}\mathbf{X})^{-1}\mathbf{X}'\mathbf{V}^{-1}\mathbf{V}\mathbf{V}^{-1}\mathbf{X}(\mathbf{X}'\mathbf{V}^{-1}\mathbf{X})^{-1} \\
&= \sigma^2(\mathbf{X}'\mathbf{V}^{-1}\mathbf{X})^{-1}.
\end{aligned}
$$

The error sum of squares is first computed for the transformed model; substituting the original variables gives

$$
\begin{aligned}
SSE_{GLS} &= \widehat{\eta}'\widehat{\eta} = (\mathbf{z} - \mathbf{B}\widehat{\beta}_{GLS})'(\mathbf{z} - \mathbf{B}\widehat{\beta}_{GLS}) \\
&= (\mathbf{y} - \mathbf{X}\widehat{\beta}_{GLS})'(\mathbf{KK}')^{-1}(\mathbf{y} - \mathbf{X}\widehat{\beta}_{GLS}) \\
&= (\mathbf{y} - \mathbf{X}\widehat{\beta}_{GLS})'\mathbf{V}^{-1}(\mathbf{y} - \mathbf{X}\widehat{\beta}_{GLS}).
\end{aligned}
$$

To prove property 4, we see that

$$\mathbf{c}'\widehat{\beta}_{GLS} = \mathbf{c}'(\mathbf{X}'\mathbf{V}^{-1}\mathbf{X})^{-1}\mathbf{X}'\mathbf{V}^{-1}\mathbf{y} = \mathbf{b}'_1\mathbf{y},$$

say, is a linear function of $\mathbf{y}$ which is an unbiased estimator of $\mathbf{c}'\beta$ since

$$E(\mathbf{c}'\widehat{\beta}_{GLS}) = E[\mathbf{c}'(\mathbf{X}'\mathbf{V}^{-1}\mathbf{X})^{-1}\mathbf{X}'\mathbf{V}^{-1}\mathbf{X}\beta] = \mathbf{c}'\beta.$$

Suppose $\mathbf{b}'_2\mathbf{y}$ denotes any other linear unbiased estimator of $\mathbf{c}'\beta$. In terms of the transformed variables, we can write

$$\mathbf{c}'\widehat{\beta}_{GLS} = \mathbf{c}'(\mathbf{B}'\mathbf{B})^{-1}\mathbf{B}'\mathbf{z} \quad \text{and} \quad \mathbf{b}'_2\mathbf{y} = \mathbf{b}'_2\mathbf{KK}^{-1}\mathbf{y} = (\mathbf{K}'\mathbf{b}_2)'\mathbf{z}.$$

Then,

$$Var[\mathbf{c}'\widehat{\beta}_{GLS}] \leq Var[(\mathbf{K}'\mathbf{b}_2)'\mathbf{z},$$

using reasoning similar to that in the proof of Result 4.4.1. ∎

Example 4.5.1. Consider the model

$$Y_i = \beta X_i + \varepsilon_i, \quad i = 1, \cdots, N,$$

where ε_i are normal random variables with $E(\varepsilon_i) = 0$, and $Cov(\varepsilon_i, \varepsilon_j) = \sigma^2 \rho^{|j-i|}$, $i, j = 1, \cdots, N$, $|\rho| < 1$. We can write this in the form (4.5.1) with $\mathbf{y} = (Y_1, \cdots, Y_N)'$, $\varepsilon = (\varepsilon_1, \cdots, \varepsilon_N)'$, $\mathbf{x} = (X_1, \cdots, X_N)'$, β is a scalar parameter, and

$$\mathbf{V} = \begin{pmatrix} 1 & \rho & \rho^2 & \cdots & \rho^{N-1} \\ \rho & 1 & \rho & \cdots & \rho^{N-2} \\ \vdots & \vdots & \vdots & \ddots & \vdots \\ \rho^{N-1} & \rho^{N-2} & \rho^{N-3} & \cdots & 1 \end{pmatrix}.$$

This is a linear regression model with autoregressive order 1 (AR(1)) errors, i.e., a serially correlated simple regression model. We can verify that

$$\{\mathbf{V}^{-1}\}_{i,j} = \begin{cases} 1/(1-\rho^2), & \text{if } i = j = 1, N \\ (1+\rho^2)/(1-\rho^2), & \text{if } i = j = 2, \cdots, N-1 \\ -\rho/(1-\rho^2), & \text{if } |j-i| = 1 \\ 0, & \text{otherwise}, \end{cases}$$

$$(\mathbf{x}'\mathbf{V}^{-1}\mathbf{x}) = \frac{1}{1-\rho^2} \left\{ \sum_{i=1}^{N} X_i^2 + \rho^2 \sum_{i=2}^{N-1} X_i^2 - 2\rho \sum_{i=2}^{N} X_i X_{i-1} \right\}, \text{ and}$$

$$\mathbf{x}'\mathbf{V}^{-1}\mathbf{y} = \frac{1}{1-\rho^2} \left\{ \sum_{i=1}^{N} X_i Y_i + \rho^2 \sum_{i=2}^{N-1} X_i Y_i - 2\rho \sum_{i=2}^{N} (X_i Y_{i-1} + Y_i X_{i-1}) \right\}.$$

Then, $\widehat{\beta}_{GLS} = (\mathbf{x}'\mathbf{V}^{-1}\mathbf{x})^{-1}\mathbf{x}'\mathbf{V}^{-1}\mathbf{y}$ is the b.l.u.e. of β with variance given by $\sigma^2(\mathbf{x}'\mathbf{V}^{-1}\mathbf{x})^{-1}$ (see Corollary 4.5.1). By substituting an estimate of σ^2, viz., $\widehat{\sigma}_{GLS}^2 = (\mathbf{y} - \mathbf{x}\widehat{\beta}_{GLS})'\mathbf{V}^{-1}(\mathbf{y} - \mathbf{x}\widehat{\beta}_{GLS})$, we obtain the estimated variance of the GLS estimator of β. The variance of the OLS estimator of β is $Var(\widehat{\beta}) = \sigma^2(\mathbf{x}'\mathbf{x})^{-1}\mathbf{x}'\mathbf{V}\mathbf{x}(\mathbf{x}'\mathbf{x})^{-1}$. Therefore,

$$\begin{aligned} Var(\widehat{\beta}) - Var(\widehat{\beta}_{GLS}) &= \sigma^2(\mathbf{x}'\mathbf{x})^{-1}\mathbf{x}'\mathbf{V}\mathbf{x}(\mathbf{x}'\mathbf{x})^{-1} \\ &- \sigma^2(\mathbf{x}'\mathbf{V}^{-1}\mathbf{x})^{-1}\mathbf{x}'\mathbf{V}^{-1}\mathbf{V}\mathbf{V}^{-1}\mathbf{x}(\mathbf{x}'\mathbf{V}^{-1}\mathbf{x})^{-1} \\ &= \sigma^2\mathbf{s}\mathbf{V}\mathbf{s}', \text{ say,} \end{aligned}$$

where $\mathbf{s} = (\mathbf{x}'\mathbf{x})^{-1}\mathbf{x}' - (\mathbf{x}'\mathbf{V}^{-1}\mathbf{x})^{-1}\mathbf{x}'\mathbf{V}^{-1}$. This expression is p.s.d. since $\mathbf{V}$ is p.d., verifying that $Var(\widehat{\beta}) \geq Var(\widehat{\beta}_{GLS})$; equality holds when $\mathbf{V} = \mathbf{I}_N$. □

Under certain conditions, the OLS estimator and the GLS estimator of β coincide, as shown in the next example. We then present a result due to McElroy

(1967) which gives a necessary and sufficient condition for this to happen in the full rank linear model.

Example 4.5.2.   Let $\mathbf{y} = (Y_1, \cdots, Y_N)'$ be a random vector with mean $\theta \mathbf{1}_N$ and variance covariance matrix $\sigma^2 \mathbf{V}$, where $\mathbf{V}$ is the equicorrelation matrix with $V_{ii} = 1, V_{ij} = \rho$, $i \neq j$, $i, j = 1, \cdots, N$ (see Example 1.2.8). We write this in the form (4.5.1) with $\mathbf{x} = \mathbf{1}_N$, $\beta = \theta$, and $\varepsilon = (\varepsilon_1, \cdots, \varepsilon_N)'$. Using the form of the inverse of $\sigma^2 \mathbf{V}$ derived in Example 1.2.8, we obtain $(\mathbf{x}'\mathbf{V}^{-1}\mathbf{x})^{-1} = \{1 + (N-1)\rho\}/N$, and $\mathbf{x}'\mathbf{V}^{-1}\mathbf{y} = N\overline{Y}/\{1 + (N-1)\rho\}$. From (4.5.5), the GLS estimate of θ is $\widehat{\theta}_{GLS} = \overline{Y}$. The GLS estimate of θ coincides with its OLS estimate. $\square$

Result 4.5.2.   In the full rank linear model, $\widehat{\beta}$ and $\widehat{\beta}_{GLS}$ are identical if and only if $\mathcal{C}(\mathbf{V}^{-1}\mathbf{X}) = \mathcal{C}(\mathbf{X})$.

Proof. $\widehat{\beta}$ and $\widehat{\beta}_{GLS}$ are identical if and only if

$$(\mathbf{X}'\mathbf{V}^{-1}\mathbf{X})^{-1}\mathbf{X}'\mathbf{V}^{-1}\mathbf{y} = (\mathbf{X}'\mathbf{X})^{-1}\mathbf{X}'\mathbf{y},$$

or, equivalently, if and only if

$$\mathbf{X}'\mathbf{V}^{-1}\mathbf{y} = (\mathbf{X}'\mathbf{V}^{-1}\mathbf{X})(\mathbf{X}'\mathbf{X})^{-1}\mathbf{X}'\mathbf{y}$$

for all $\mathbf{y} \in \mathcal{R}^N$. Recall that we can write $\mathbf{y} = \mathbf{y}_1 + \mathbf{y}_2$, where $\mathbf{y}_1 \in \mathcal{C}(\mathbf{X})$, and $\mathbf{y}_2 \in \mathcal{C}^{\perp}(\mathbf{X})$. This completes the proof.   ∎

The GLS estimate of β also coincides with its OLS estimate if $\mathbf{y}$ is in $\mathcal{C}(\mathbf{X})$, i.e., if $\mathbf{y} = \mathbf{Xz}$ for some vector $\mathbf{z}$. Another situation when these estimates coincide is when $\mathbf{X}'\mathbf{y} = \mathbf{0}$ and $Var(\mathbf{y}) = (1 - \rho)\mathbf{I} + \rho \mathbf{J}$ (see Exercise 4.17).

Consider the linear model (4.5.1) where $\mathbf{V} = \text{diag}(\sigma_1^2, \cdots, \sigma_N^2)$ is an $N \times N$ diagonal matrix. We refer to β_{GLS}^0 as the weighted least squares solution vector in the less than full rank case, and to $\widehat{\beta}_{GLS}$ as the WLS estimator of β in the full rank situation. When $\mathbf{V}$ is diagonal, the effect of the generalized least squares analysis is to "weight" the original observations by the corresponding diagonal entries of $\mathbf{V}$.

Example 4.5.3. Let $Y_1, \cdots, Y_N$ denote independent observations, where $Y_i \sim N(i\theta, i^2\sigma^2)$, $i = 1, \cdots, N$. We will estimate θ by the method of least squares and obtain the variance of this estimate. First, write this in the form (4.5.1) with $\mathbf{y} = (Y_1, \cdots, Y_N)'$, $\mathbf{x} = (1, 2, \cdots, N)'$, $\beta = \theta$, $\varepsilon = (\varepsilon_1, \cdots, \varepsilon_N)'$ and $\mathbf{V} = Var(\varepsilon) = \sigma^2 \text{diag}(1^2, 2^2, \cdots, N^2)$. It follows that the weighted least squares (WLS) estimate of θ and its variance are $\widehat{\theta}_{WLS} = (\mathbf{x}'\mathbf{V}^{-1}\mathbf{x})^{-1}\mathbf{x}'\mathbf{V}^{-1}\mathbf{y} = \frac{1}{N}\sum_{i=1}^{N} Y_i/i$, and $Var(\widehat{\theta}_{WLS}) = \sigma^2/N$. $\square$

Numerical Example 4.3.   Weighted least squares.   In a study of industrial establishments of varying size, the number of supervised workers, X, and the number of supervisors, Y, were recorded for 27 firms (Chatterjee and

Price, 1991). A plot of Y versus X in the following figure suggests that the variance of Y tends to increase with the magnitude of X. We show results from an OLS estimation as well as a WLS estimation, the latter with weights $1/X_i^2$.

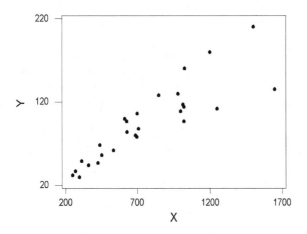

Weighted least squares.

OLS estimates for Numerical Example 4.3.

Predictor	Estimate	s.e.	t-value	$\Pr > T$
Constant	14.448	9.562	1.51	0.143
X	0.105	0.011	9.30	< 0.0001

WLS estimates for Numerical Example 4.3.

Predictor	Estimate	s.e.	t-value	$\Pr > T$
Constant	3.803	4.570	0.832	0.413
X	0.121	0.009	13.45	< 0.0001

Note that the R^2 value is respectively 0.767 and 0.879 in the two fits, while $\hat{\sigma}$ is 21.73 and 0.023 respectively. As mentioned in the earlier numerical example, the last two columns in each table will become clear after we discuss inference based on normality in Chapter 7. ▲

So far, we assumed that the matrix $\mathbf{V}$ is p.d. In some models, however, this assumption is untenable (see section 10.2). For situations where $\mathbf{V}$ is a known symmetric n.n.d. matrix, the following result, called the generalized Gauss-Markov theorem, describes optimal estimation of estimable functions of β. Let

$\mathbf{N}$ be any matrix whose column space $\mathcal{C}(\mathbf{N})$ is the same as the null space of $\mathbf{X}'$. Let Ω_V denote the class of generalized inverses $\mathbf{V}^{\sharp}$ of $\mathbf{V}$ that satisfy

$$r(\mathbf{X}'\mathbf{V}^{\sharp}\mathbf{X}) = r(\mathbf{X}), \text{ and}$$
$$\mathbf{X}'\mathbf{V}^{\sharp}\mathbf{V}\mathbf{N} = 0. \tag{4.5.7}$$

Result 4.5.3.   Let β^0 be any solution to the general normal equations

$$\mathbf{X}'\mathbf{V}^{\sharp}\mathbf{X}\beta^0 = \mathbf{X}'\mathbf{V}^{\sharp}\mathbf{y}. \tag{4.5.8}$$

Let $\mathbf{c}'\beta$ be estimable. A generalized version of the Gauss-Markov theorem states that Ω_V is nonempty and the linear system (4.5.8) is consistent. Further, $\mathbf{c}'\beta^0$ is an essentially-unique b.l.u.e. of $\mathbf{c}'\beta$ in the sense that if $d_0 + \mathbf{d}'\mathbf{y}$ is any other linear, unbiased estimator of $\mathbf{c}'\beta$, then $Var(\mathbf{c}'\beta^0) \leq Var(d_0 + \mathbf{d}'\mathbf{y})$, with equality holding if and only if $d_0 + \mathbf{d}'\mathbf{y} = \mathbf{c}'\beta^0$ with probability 1.

Proof.   Suppose $r(\mathbf{X}) = r$, $r(\mathbf{V}) = v$ and $\dim\{\mathcal{C}(\mathbf{V}) \cap \mathcal{C}(\mathbf{X})\} = s$. Then,

$$\mathbf{V} = \mathbf{P}\begin{pmatrix} \mathbf{D}_v & 0 \\ 0 & 0 \end{pmatrix}\mathbf{P}',$$

where $\mathbf{D}_v$ is a diagonal matrix of positive eigenvalues, $\mathbf{P} = (\mathbf{P}_1, \mathbf{P}_2)$ is an orthogonal matrix of eigenvectors of $\mathbf{V}$ such that the columns of $\mathbf{P}_1$ form an orthonormal basis of $\mathcal{C}(\mathbf{V})$ and the columns of $\mathbf{P}_2$ form an orthonormal basis of $\mathcal{C}^{\perp}(\mathbf{V})$. $\mathbf{V}^-$ is a g-inverse of $\mathbf{V}$ if and only if for arbitrary $\mathbf{M}$ and $\mathbf{W}$,

$$\mathbf{V}^- = \mathbf{P}\begin{pmatrix} \mathbf{D}_v^{-1} & \mathbf{L} \\ \mathbf{M} & \mathbf{W} \end{pmatrix}\mathbf{P}'.$$

Also,

$$\mathbf{V}\mathbf{V}^- = \mathbf{P}\begin{pmatrix} \mathbf{I}_v & \mathbf{D}_v\mathbf{L} \\ 0 & 0 \end{pmatrix}\mathbf{P}';$$

if $\mathbf{L} = 0$, the idempotent matrix $\mathbf{V}\mathbf{V}^-$ is a projection operator onto $\mathcal{C}(\mathbf{V})$, with the path of projection solely determined by $\mathbf{L}$. The construction of $\Omega_{\mathbf{V}}$ requires a choice of $\mathbf{L}$ by which any vector in $\mathcal{C}(\mathbf{X})$ is projected by $\mathbf{V}\mathbf{V}^-$ onto $\mathcal{C}(\mathbf{X}) \cap \mathcal{C}(\mathbf{V})$.

Let the $N \times s$ matrix $\mathbf{S}$ be a basis for $\mathcal{C}(\mathbf{X}) \cap \mathcal{C}(\mathbf{V})$, and the $N \times (r - s)$ matrix $\mathbf{R}$ be any extension of $\mathbf{S}$ to a basis of $\mathcal{C}(\mathbf{X})$, i.e., for any $v \times s$ matrix $\mathbf{A}$,

$$\mathbf{S} = \mathbf{P}_1\mathbf{A}, \text{ and } (\mathbf{S}, \mathbf{R}) = \mathbf{P}\begin{pmatrix} \mathbf{A} & \mathbf{Q}_1 \\ 0 & \mathbf{Q}_2 \end{pmatrix}.$$

$\mathbf{Q}_1$ and $\mathbf{Q}_2$ are respectively $v \times (r - s)$ and $(N - v) \times (r - s)$ matrices, and $r(\mathbf{Q}_2) = r - s$. $\mathbf{V}\mathbf{V}^{\sharp'}$ is a projection along $\mathcal{C}(\mathbf{X})$ if $\mathbf{V}\mathbf{V}^{\sharp'}\mathbf{R} = 0$, which after some simplification implies $\mathbf{Q}_1 = \mathbf{K}\mathbf{Q}_2$. This system of equations always has a solution since the columns of $\mathbf{Q}_2$ are LIN. Then $\Omega_{\mathbf{V}}$ consists of g-inverses of $\mathbf{V}$ of the form

$$\mathbf{V}^{\#\prime} = \mathbf{P} \begin{pmatrix} \mathbf{D}_v^{-1} & -\mathbf{D}_v^{-1}\mathbf{K} \\ \mathbf{M} & \mathbf{W} \end{pmatrix} \mathbf{P}',$$

where $\mathbf{M}$ and $\mathbf{W}$ are arbitrary, and is therefore nonempty. Estimability of $\mathbf{c}'\beta$ follows from the condition in (4.5.7) (for further details, see Zyskind and Martin, 1969; or Rao, 1973b). ∎

4.6 Estimation subject to linear restrictions

Suppose we wish to estimate the parameters in the linear model (4.1.1) subject to the linear restrictions imposed by $\mathbf{A}'\beta = \mathbf{b}$, where $\mathbf{A}$ is a known $p \times q$ matrix of rank q, and $\mathbf{b}$ is a known q-dimensional vector. There are many examples where a "natural restriction" on the parameters is an integral part of the model specification; we do not refer to the constraints we had to impose in order to solve the normal equations when $r(\mathbf{X}) < p$, as for instance, in the one-way ANOVA example in section 4.2. The linear model without the imposed restriction will be referred to as the *unrestricted model*. We discuss two approaches, viz., the method of Lagrangian multipliers, which is an algebraic approach, and the method of orthogonal projections, a geometrical approach.

4.6.1 Method of Lagrangian multipliers

We obtain the least squares solution of β under the restriction $\mathbf{A}'\beta = \mathbf{b}$ using the method of Lagrangian multipliers (see section 2.9). Let 2λ denote a q-dimensional vector of Lagrange multipliers. We minimize

$$S_r(\beta, \lambda) = (\mathbf{y} - \mathbf{X}\beta)'(\mathbf{y} - \mathbf{X}\beta) + 2\lambda'(\mathbf{A}'\beta - \mathbf{b}) \tag{4.6.1}$$

with respect to β and λ. Setting equal to zero the first partial derivatives of $S_r(\beta, \lambda)$ with respect to β and λ results in the following set of normal equations:

$$\frac{\partial}{\partial \beta} S_r(\beta, \lambda) = \mathbf{0} \Rightarrow \mathbf{X}'\mathbf{X}\beta_r^0 + \mathbf{A}\lambda_r^0 = \mathbf{X}'\mathbf{y}, \tag{4.6.2}$$

$$\frac{\partial}{\partial \lambda} S_r(\beta, \lambda) = \mathbf{0} \Rightarrow \mathbf{A}'\beta_r^0 = \mathbf{b}. \tag{4.6.3}$$

We will distinguish between the cases when $\mathbf{A}'\beta$ is estimable, and when it is not. First, assume that $\mathbf{A}'\beta$ is estimable. We solve (4.6.2) and (4.6.3) simultaneously for β_r^0 and λ_r^0. From (4.6.2) we see that

$$\begin{aligned} \beta_r^0 &= \mathbf{G}(\mathbf{X}'\mathbf{y} - \mathbf{A}\lambda_r^0) \\ &= \mathbf{G}\mathbf{X}'\mathbf{y} - \mathbf{G}\mathbf{A}\lambda_r^0 \\ &= \beta^0 - \mathbf{G}\mathbf{A}\lambda_r^0, \end{aligned} \tag{4.6.4}$$

while from (4.6.3) and (4.6.4) we get

$$\mathbf{A}'\beta_r^0 = \mathbf{b} = \mathbf{A}'\beta^0 - \mathbf{A}'\mathbf{G}\mathbf{A}\lambda_r^0,$$

so that

$$\lambda_r^0 = (\mathbf{A'GA})^{-1}(\mathbf{A'}\beta^0 - \mathbf{b}) \tag{4.6.5}$$

(see Exercise 4.20). It follows from (4.6.4) and (4.6.5) that

$$\beta_r^0 = \beta^0 - \mathbf{GA}(\mathbf{A'GA})^{-1}(\mathbf{A'}\beta^0 - \mathbf{b}). \tag{4.6.6}$$

We refer to β_r^0 as the restricted least squares solution of β in the linear model $\mathbf{y} = \mathbf{X}\beta + \varepsilon$ subject to the linear restriction $\mathbf{A'}\beta = \mathbf{b}$. Let $\hat{\mathbf{y}}_r = \mathbf{X}\beta_r^0$.

If $\mathbf{A'}\beta$ is not estimable, it can be shown that $\beta_r^0 = \beta^0 + (\mathbf{H} - \mathbf{I})\mathbf{z}$, where $\mathbf{z}$ satisfies $\mathbf{A'}(\mathbf{H}-\mathbf{I})\mathbf{z} = \mathbf{b} - \mathbf{A'GX'y}$, i.e., β_r^0 is merely one solution to the normal equations $\mathbf{X'X}\beta = \mathbf{X'y}$. Further, $SSE_r = SSE$ in this case (see section 7.4.3 for more details).

Result 4.6.1.   The properties of the restricted least squares solution are shown below.

1. $E(\beta_r^0) = \mathbf{H}\beta$.

2. $Cov(\beta_r^0) = \sigma^2 \mathbf{G}[\mathbf{X'X} - \mathbf{A}(\mathbf{A'GA})^{-1}\mathbf{A'}]\mathbf{G'}$.

3. $E(SSE_r) = (N - r + q)\sigma^2$, where SSE_r is the restricted error sum of squares.

Proof.   Since $\mathbf{A'}\beta$ is estimable, $\mathbf{A'H} = \mathbf{A'}$ (see (4.3.3)). Further $E(\beta^0) = \mathbf{H}\beta$, so that,

$$E(\beta_r^0) = \mathbf{H}\beta - \mathbf{GA}(\mathbf{A'GA})^{-1}(\mathbf{A'H}\beta - \mathbf{b}) = \mathbf{H}\beta,$$

proving property 1. Next,

$$Cov(\beta_r^0) = Cov\{[\mathbf{I} - \mathbf{GA}(\mathbf{A'GA})^{-1}\mathbf{A'}]\beta^0\}$$

which, after some simplification, and using (4.2.23) gives property 2. Property 3 follows directly by using Result 4.2.3, since

$$\begin{aligned} SSE_r &= (\mathbf{y} - \mathbf{X}\beta_r^0)'(\mathbf{y} - \mathbf{X}\beta_r^0) \\ &= [\mathbf{y} - \mathbf{X}\beta^0 + \mathbf{X}(\beta^0 - \beta_r^0)]'[\mathbf{y} - \mathbf{X}\beta^0 + \mathbf{X}(\beta^0 - \beta_r^0)] \\ &= (\mathbf{y} - \mathbf{X}\beta^0)'(\mathbf{y} - \mathbf{X}\beta^0) + (\beta^0 - \beta_r^0)'\mathbf{X'X}(\beta^0 - \beta_r^0) \\ &= SSE + (\mathbf{A'}\beta^0 - \mathbf{b})'(\mathbf{A'GA})^{-1}(\mathbf{A'}\beta^0 - \mathbf{b}), \end{aligned}$$

$\mathbf{X'}(\mathbf{y} - \mathbf{X}\beta^0) = \mathbf{0}$, and $\mathbf{A'} = \mathbf{T'X}$ (since $\mathbf{A'}\beta$ is estimable). ∎

Example 4.6.1.   Suppose $Y_i = \theta_i + \varepsilon_i$, $i = 1, \cdots, 5$, ε_i are iid $N(0, \sigma^2)$ variables, and θ_i are unknown real values subject to the restriction $\sum_{i=1}^5 \theta_i = 100$. We write $\mathbf{y} = \mathbf{X}\beta + \varepsilon$, where, $\mathbf{y} = (Y_1, \cdots, Y_5)'$, $\mathbf{X} = \mathbf{I}_5$, and $\beta = (\theta_1, \cdots, \theta_5)'$, subject to the restriction $\mathbf{A'}\beta = \mathbf{b}$, with $\mathbf{A} = \mathbf{1}_5$, and $b = 100$. The unrestricted least squares estimate of β is $\mathbf{y}$, while the restricted estimate (see (4.6.6)) is $\widehat{\beta}'_r = (Y_1 - \overline{Y} + 20, \cdots, Y_5 - \overline{Y} + 20)$ with $Cov(\widehat{\beta}_r) = \sigma^2(\mathbf{I} - \mathbf{J}/5)$, and $SSE_r = (\sum_{i=1}^{5} Y_i - 100)^2/5$. $\square$

Example 4.6.2. Let $Y_{ij} = \mu + \tau_i + \varepsilon_{ij}$, with $E(\varepsilon_{ij}) = 0$, $i = 1, \cdots, a$, $j = 1, \cdots, n$, and suppose that we impose the constraint $\sum_{i=1}^{a} c_i \tau_i = 0$, with $\sum_{i=1}^{a} c_i \neq 0$. We obtain the least squares solutions for μ and $\tau = (\tau_1, \cdots, \tau_a)'$ using the method of Lagrangian multipliers. Minimizing

$$S_r(\mu, \tau) = \sum_{i=1}^{a} \sum_{j=1}^{n} (Y_{ij} - \mu - \tau_i)^2 + 2\lambda' \sum_{i=1}^{a} c_i \tau_i$$

with respect to μ, τ and λ leads to the solutions $\mu^0 = \sum_{i=1}^{a} c_i \overline{Y}_i. / \sum_{i=1}^{a} c_i$, and $\tau_i^0 = \overline{Y}_i. - \mu^0$, $i = 1, \cdots, a$. $\square$

4.6.2 Method of orthogonal projections

We describe the method of orthogonal projections for the full rank case. Under the restriction $\mathbf{A}'\beta = \mathbf{b}$, let ω denote the $(p - q)$-dimensional subspace of the p-dimensional estimation space Ω. Let us denote the projection matrix $\mathbf{P} = \mathbf{X}(\mathbf{X}'\mathbf{X})^{-1}\mathbf{X}'$ in Ω by $\mathbf{P}_\Omega$, so that $\mathbf{P}_\Omega \mathbf{y} = \mathbf{X}\widehat{\beta}$. It is useful to temporarily eliminate $\mathbf{b}$ which represents an origin choice in ω. To do this, suppose β^* satisfies $\mathbf{A}'\beta = \mathbf{b}$. Since the projection onto Ω of a vector already in Ω leaves it untouched,

$$\mathbf{P}_\Omega \mathbf{X}\beta^* = \mathbf{X}\beta^* = \mathbf{b}. \tag{4.6.7}$$

Subtracting $\mathbf{X}\beta^*$ from both sides of (4.1.1), we can write

$$\mathbf{y} - \mathbf{X}\beta^* = \mathbf{X}(\beta - \beta^*) + \varepsilon = \mathbf{X}\theta + \varepsilon.$$

The vector $\theta = \beta - \beta^*$ represents the new parameter vector for which

$$\mathbf{A}'\theta = \mathbf{A}'\beta - \mathbf{A}'\beta^* = \mathbf{A}'\beta - \mathbf{b} = \mathbf{0}.$$

The columns of the $N \times q$ matrix $\mathbf{V} = \mathbf{X}(\mathbf{X}'\mathbf{X})^{-1}\mathbf{A}$ span a subspace $\omega^\perp = \Omega - \omega$ of the estimation space Ω, which is orthogonal to ω. This is obvious because $\mathbf{A}'\theta = \mathbf{0}$ implies that $\mathbf{A}'(\mathbf{X}'\mathbf{X})^{-1}\mathbf{X}'(\mathbf{X}\theta) = \mathbf{0}$. The unique projection matrix in $\omega^\perp$ is

$$\mathbf{P}_{\omega^\perp} = \mathbf{V}(\mathbf{V}'\mathbf{V})^{-1}\mathbf{V}' = \mathbf{X}(\mathbf{X}'\mathbf{X})^{-1}\mathbf{A}[\mathbf{A}'(\mathbf{X}'\mathbf{X})^{-1}\mathbf{A}]^{-1}\mathbf{A}'(\mathbf{X}'\mathbf{X})^{-1}\mathbf{X}',$$

and the projection matrix for ω is therefore

$$\mathbf{P}_\omega = \mathbf{P}_\Omega - \mathbf{P}_{\omega^\perp}.$$

Then,

$$\mathbf{P}_\omega \mathbf{y} - \mathbf{P}_\omega \mathbf{X}\beta^* = \mathbf{P}_\Omega \mathbf{y} - \mathbf{P}_\Omega \mathbf{X}\beta^* - \mathbf{P}_{\omega^\perp}(\mathbf{y} - \mathbf{X}\beta^*) \tag{4.6.8}$$

denotes the projection of $\mathbf{y} - \mathbf{X}\beta^*$ onto ω. If $\widehat{\beta}_r$ denotes the least squares estimate of β in the restricted space ω, it is clear that

$$\mathbf{P}_\omega \mathbf{y} = \mathbf{X}\widehat{\beta}_r. \tag{4.6.9}$$

Similar to (4.6.7), we have

$$\mathbf{P}_\omega \mathbf{X}\beta^* = \mathbf{X}\beta^* = \mathbf{b}, \tag{4.6.10}$$

and further,

$$\mathbf{P}_{\omega^\perp}(\mathbf{y} - \mathbf{X}\beta^*) = \mathbf{X}(\mathbf{X}'\mathbf{X})^{-1}\mathbf{A}[\mathbf{A}'(\mathbf{X}'\mathbf{X})^{-1}\mathbf{A}]^{-1}(\mathbf{A}'\widehat{\beta} - \mathbf{b}). \tag{4.6.11}$$

Simplifying (4.6.8) using (4.6.7), (4.6.10), and (4.6.11), we see that the restricted least squares estimate of β adjusts $\widehat{\beta}$ by an amount that depends on $\mathbf{X}$, $\mathbf{A}$, and the distance $||\mathbf{A}'\widehat{\beta} - \mathbf{b}||$ and has the form

$$\widehat{\beta}_r = \widehat{\beta} - (\mathbf{X}'\mathbf{X})^{-1}\mathbf{A}[\mathbf{A}'(\mathbf{X}'\mathbf{X})^{-1}\mathbf{A}]^{-1}(\mathbf{A}'\widehat{\beta} - \mathbf{b}). \tag{4.6.12}$$

This is illustrated geometrically in Figure 4.6.1. We end this chapter with an example.

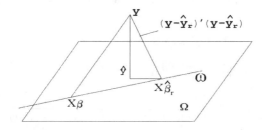

Figure 4.6.1.   Geometry of restricted least squares.

Let $\mathbf{A}$ and $\mathbf{B}$ denote two $n \times n$ n.n.d. matrices. The inequality $\mathbf{A} \leq \mathbf{B}$ implies the usual nonnegative partial ordering of matrices, i.e., $\mathbf{B} - \mathbf{A}$ is n.n.d. The following example shows that projection (under the usual inner product in Definition 1.2.1) onto any subspace of $\mathcal{S} \subset \mathcal{R}^n$ is at most the projection onto $\mathcal{S}$ (Mathew and Nordstrom, 1997).

Example 4.6.3.   Let $\mathbf{X}$ be an $n \times m$ matrix, and let $\mathbf{P} = \mathbf{X}(\mathbf{X}'\mathbf{X})^-\mathbf{X}'$ denote the orthogonal projection matrix onto the column space $\mathcal{C}(\mathbf{X})$. For a $k \times n$ matrix $\mathbf{A}$ such that $\mathbf{A}\mathbf{X} = \mathbf{0}$, we will show that

$$\mathbf{A}'(\mathbf{A}\mathbf{A}')^-\mathbf{A} \leq (\mathbf{I}_n - \mathbf{P}). \tag{4.6.13}$$

From Result 2.6.3, $\mathcal{C}(\mathbf{I}_n - \mathbf{P})$ is orthogonal to $\mathcal{C}(\mathbf{X})$. By assumption, $\mathcal{C}(\mathbf{A}')$ is orthogonal to $\mathcal{C}(\mathbf{X})$ as well. Hence, $\mathcal{C}(\mathbf{A}') \subset \mathcal{C}(\mathbf{I}_n - \mathbf{P})$. The matrix $\mathbf{A}'(\mathbf{A}\mathbf{A}')^-\mathbf{A}$

denotes the orthogonal projection onto $C(\mathbf{A}')$, so that $(\mathbf{I}_n - \mathbf{P}) - \mathbf{A}'(\mathbf{A}\mathbf{A}')^{-}\mathbf{A}$ is also a projection matrix, which is n.n.d. (see Result 2.6.7), yielding (4.6.13)). Note that equality is achieved in (4.6.13) if and only if $C(\mathbf{A}') = C(\mathbf{I}_n - \mathbf{P})$. Notice also that for $k \times n$ matrices $\mathbf{A}_1$ and $\mathbf{A}_2$ satisfying $\mathbf{A}_1\mathbf{X} = \mathbf{A}_2\mathbf{X}$, we have

$$(\mathbf{A}_1 - \mathbf{A}_2)'[(\mathbf{A}_1 - \mathbf{A}_2)(\mathbf{A}_1 - \mathbf{A}_2)']^{-}(\mathbf{A}_1 - \mathbf{A}_2) \le (\mathbf{I}_n - \mathbf{P}).$$

This is seen by setting $\mathbf{A} = \mathbf{A}_1 - \mathbf{A}_2$ in (4.6.13). □

Exercises

4.1. Verify the consistency condition for existence of a least squares solution, i.e., $r(\mathbf{X}'\mathbf{X}, \mathbf{X}'\mathbf{y}) = r(\mathbf{X}'\mathbf{X})$.

4.2. Show that

(a) $\mathbf{X}'\mathbf{X}\mathbf{H} = \mathbf{X}'\mathbf{X}$, where $\mathbf{H} = \mathbf{G}\mathbf{X}'\mathbf{X}$.

(b) $\mathbf{I}_N - \mathbf{X}\mathbf{G}\mathbf{X}'$ is symmetric and idempotent.

4.3. When an object of unit mass is subjected to an unknown force θ for a length of time t, its position changes to $t^2\theta/2$. Observed positions $Y_1, \cdots, Y_N$ are measured at known times $t_1, \cdots, t_N$. Assume the linear model $Y_i = t_i^2\theta/2 + \varepsilon_i$, $i = 1, \cdots, N$ and that the measurement errors ε_i have $E(\varepsilon_i) = 0$ and $Var(\varepsilon_i) = \sigma^2$. Obtain the least squares estimator of the unknown force θ, and derive the variance of the estimator.

4.4. The displacement S_i of the ith object at time t_i is given by the formula

$$S_i = vt_i + \varepsilon_i, \quad i = 1, \cdots, N,$$

where all the N objects are subjected to an equal velocity. Assume that $E(\varepsilon_i) = 0$, and $Var(\varepsilon_i) = \sigma^2$. Find the least squares estimate of the unknown velocity v and estimate the variance of this estimate.

4.5. Let $\mathbf{y} = \mathbf{X}\beta + \varepsilon$, where $\varepsilon \sim N(\mathbf{0}, \sigma^2\mathbf{I}_N)$, and β is a p-dimensional vector, with $N = 10$ and $p = 3$. Given $\mathbf{y}'\mathbf{y} = 58$, and given the following normal equations,

$$
\begin{aligned}
4\widehat{\beta}_1 + 2\widehat{\beta}_2 - 2\widehat{\beta}_3 &= 4 \\
2\widehat{\beta}_1 + 2\widehat{\beta}_2 + \widehat{\beta}_3 &= 7 \\
-2\widehat{\beta}_1 + \widehat{\beta}_2 + 6\widehat{\beta}_3 &= 9,
\end{aligned}
$$

find the least squares estimates of β and σ^2. What are the estimates of β_1, β_2, β_3, $\beta_1 - \beta_2$, and $\beta_1 + \beta_3$?

4.6. Suppose we have $Y_{1j} = \beta_1 + \varepsilon_{ij}$, $j = 1, \cdots, n_1$, $Y_{2j} = \beta_1 + \beta_2 + \varepsilon_{ij}$, $j = 1, \cdots, n_1$, and $Y_{3j} = \beta_1 - 2\beta_2 + \varepsilon_{ij}$, $j = 1, \cdots, n_2$, where ε_{ij} are iid $N(0, \sigma^2)$ variables. Under what condition on n_1 and n_2 are the least squares estimates of β_1 and β_2 uncorrelated?

4.7. (Rao, 1973a, p. 236). Let $\mathbf{X} = [\mathbf{x}_0, \mathbf{x}_1, \cdots, \mathbf{x}_{k-1}, \mathbf{x}_k] = [\mathbf{W}, \mathbf{x}_k]$, and let $r(\mathbf{X}) = k + 1$.

(a) Show that $|\mathbf{X}'\mathbf{X}| = |\mathbf{W}'\mathbf{W}|(\mathbf{x}_k'\mathbf{x}_k - \mathbf{x}_k'\mathbf{W}(\mathbf{W}'\mathbf{W})^{-1}\mathbf{W}'\mathbf{x}_k)$.

(b) From (a), deduce that $|\mathbf{W}'\mathbf{W}|/|\mathbf{X}'\mathbf{X}| \geq 1/\mathbf{x}_k'\mathbf{x}_k$. Use this to show that in the usual linear model $\mathbf{y} = \mathbf{X}\beta + \varepsilon$, $Var(\widehat{\beta}_k) \geq \sigma^2(\mathbf{x}_k'\mathbf{x}_k)^{-1}$, with equality holding if and only if $\mathbf{x}_k'\mathbf{x}_j = 0$, $j = 0, 1, \cdots, k - 1$.

4.8. Consider least squares estimation in the simple linear regression model (4.1.6).

(a) Prove that $Var(\widehat{\beta}_0)$ is a minimum if the observations on the predictor variable X_i, $i = 1, \cdots, N$ are chosen such that $\overline{X} = 0$.

(b) If the X_i's can be selected anywhere in the interval $[a, b]$, and if N is an even integer, show that $Var(\widehat{\beta}_1)$ is minimized if $N/2$ values of the predictor are selected equal to a and the remaining $N/2$ values are chosen to equal b.

4.9. Let $Y_1, \cdots, Y_6$ denote the yield of a production process on six consecutive days. Machine A was used on days 1, 3, and 5, while Machine B was used on days 2, 4, and 6. Consider the models

(i) $Y_i = \beta_0 + (-1)^i \beta_1 + \varepsilon_i$,

(ii) $Y_i = \beta_0 + (-1)^i \beta_1 + i\beta_2 + \varepsilon_i$.

In each case, assume that $E(\varepsilon_i) = 0$, and $Var(\varepsilon_i) = \sigma^2$. Obtain the least squares estimate of β_1 under each model, and show that the ratio of $Var(\widehat{\beta}_1)$ under Model (i) to $Var(\widehat{\beta}_1)$ under Model (ii) is 32/35.

4.10. In (4.2.32) with $n = 1$, show that it is not possible to carry out inference on the effects, although it is possible to obtain point estimates.

4.11. Prove Result 4.3.2.

4.12. In the general linear model (4.1.1), prove that all linear functions $\mathbf{c}'\beta$ are estimable if and only if the columns of $\mathbf{X}$ are LIN.

4.13. In the model (4.1.7), show that τ_i is not estimable for any i.

4.14. In the model (4.2.31), show that $\sum_{i=1}^a c_i \tau_i$ is estimable if and only if $\sum_{i=1}^a c_i = 0$.

4.15. In Result 4.4.3, show that $(N - r)\widehat{\sigma}^2$ is the unique nonnegative quadratic unbiased estimator of $(N-r)\sigma^2$, with minimum variance when the nonzero diagonal elements of the projection matrix $\mathbf{P}$ are equal.

4.16. Suppose Y_{i1} denotes a pre-treatment score and Y_{i2} denotes a post-treatment score on the ith individual, $i = 1, \cdots, N$. For $i = 1, \cdots, N$ and $j = 1, 2$, let $E(Y_{ij}) = \tau_j$, $Var(Y_{ij}) = \sigma^2$, and $Corr(Y_{i1}, Y_{k2}) = \rho$ if $i = k$, and 0 if $i \neq k$.

   (a) Estimate the parameters τ_1 and τ_2 in this linear model.

   (b) How will you obtain the estimated standard errors of the estimates in (a)?

4.17. In the model (4.5.1), show that $\widehat{\beta}_{GLS}$ and $\widehat{\beta}$ coincide when

   (a) $\mathbf{y} \in \mathcal{C}(\mathbf{X})$, or

   (b) $V = (1 - \rho)\mathbf{I} + \rho \mathbf{J}$ and $\mathbf{y}$ is orthogonal to $\mathbf{X}$, the first column of $\mathbf{X}$ being $\mathbf{1}_N$.

4.18. Show that $\mathbf{c}'\beta$ is estimable in the model (4.5.1) if and only if it is estimable in the model (4.5.3).

4.19. In the model (4.5.1), show that

   (a) $(\mathbf{X}'\mathbf{V}^{-1}\mathbf{X})\beta$ is estimable.

   (b) $\mathbf{c}'\beta$ is estimable if $\mathbf{c}(\mathbf{X}'\mathbf{V}^{-1}\mathbf{X})^-(\mathbf{X}'\mathbf{V}^{-1}\mathbf{X}) = \mathbf{c}'$.

4.20. In (4.6.5), show that $(\mathbf{A}'\mathbf{GA})^{-1}$ exists.

4.21. Suppose Y_1, Y_2, and Y_3 are measurements of the angles of a triangle subject to error. The information is given as a linear model $Y_i = \theta_i + \varepsilon_i$, where θ_i are the true angles, $i = 1, 2, 3$. Assume that $E(\varepsilon_i) = 0$, and $Var(\varepsilon_i) = \sigma^2$. Obtain the least squares estimates of θ_i (subject to the constraint $\theta_1 + \theta_2 + \theta_3 = 180°$).

4.22. Consider the model $Y_{ij} = \mu + \tau_i + \varepsilon_{ij}$, $j = 1, \cdots, n$, $i = 1, \cdots, a$. Construct a set of $(a - 1)$ orthogonal contrasts in $(\tau_1, \cdots, \tau_a)$. What is the relationship between $SSR_c = n \sum_{i=1}^{a} (\overline{Y}_{i\cdot} - \overline{Y}_{\cdot\cdot})^2$ and the sums of squares due to these contrasts?

4.23. In the model $Y_i = \beta_0 + \beta_1 X_i + \varepsilon_i$, $i = 1, \cdots, N$, suppose the X_i's are restricted to lie in the interval $[-10, 15]$. Choose the X_i's to minimize (a) $Var(\widehat{\beta}_0)$, and (b) $Var(\widehat{\beta}_1)$. Repeat the exercise assuming that the X_i's are restricted to lie in the interval $[-10, 10]$.

4.24. Consider the model $\mathbf{y} = \beta + \varepsilon$, $\varepsilon \sim N(\mathbf{0}, \sigma^2 \mathbf{V})$, where $\mathbf{V}$ is an $N \times N$ p.d. matrix. If $\mathbf{z} = \mathbf{By}$, and $\eta = \mathbf{B}\varepsilon$, where $\mathbf{B} = \mathbf{V}^{-1/2}$, show that the linear model can be expressed as $\mathbf{z} = \mathbf{B}\beta + \eta$, with $\eta \sim N(\mathbf{0}, \sigma^2 \mathbf{I}_N)$. Obtain the least squares estimate of β. Also obtain the estimate of β under the restriction $\mathbf{C}'\beta = \mathbf{0}$, where $\mathbf{C}$ is a $q \times N$ matrix of rank $q < N$.

4.25. Consider the model $\mathbf{y} = \mathbf{X}\beta + \varepsilon$, where

$$\mathbf{y} = \begin{pmatrix} Y_1 \\ Y_2 \\ Y_3 \\ Y_4 \end{pmatrix}, \quad \mathbf{X} = \begin{pmatrix} 0 & 1 & 0 \\ 1 & 0 & 1 \\ -1 & 1 & -1 \\ 1 & -1 & 1 \end{pmatrix}, \quad \beta = \begin{pmatrix} \beta_1 \\ \beta_2 \\ \beta_3 \end{pmatrix},$$

and $\varepsilon \sim N(0, \sigma^2 \mathbf{I})$. If possible, obtain the b.l.u.e.'s of (i) $\beta_1 + \beta_3$, and (ii) β_2, and compute their variances.

4.26. Show that $\parallel \mathbf{y} - \widehat{\mathbf{y}}_r \parallel^2 = \parallel \mathbf{y} - \widehat{\mathbf{y}} \parallel^2 + \parallel \widehat{\mathbf{y}} - \widehat{\mathbf{y}}_r \parallel^2$, where $\widehat{\mathbf{y}} = \mathbf{X}\beta^0$ and $\widehat{\mathbf{y}}_r = \mathbf{X}\beta_r^0$.

Chapter 5

Multivariate Normal and Related Distributions

This chapter describes distributions that are at the heart of linear model theory. We begin with the definition and properties of the multivariate normal distribution, and then define various distributions such as the chi-square, F, and t distributions that are derived from the normal distribution. Using these, we are able to describe the distributions of functions of quadratic forms in normal random vectors, which form the backbone of statistical inference in linear model theory. In section 5.5, we highlight some distributions that are useful as alternatives to the multivariate normal distribution in a contemporary treatment of linear models. These distributions accommodate anomalous observations better than the normal distributions. We begin with a brief review of basic concepts of distributions of random vectors in section 5.1.

5.1 Multivariate probability distributions

Consider n random variables $X_1, X_2, \cdots, X_n$ with realized values $x_1, x_2, \cdots, x_n$. The cumulative distribution function (cdf) of the n-dimensional random vector $\mathbf{x} = (X_1, X_2, \cdots, X_n)'$ is

$$F(\mathbf{x}) = F(x_1, x_2, \cdots, x_n) = P(X_1 \leq x_1, X_2 \leq x_2, \cdots, X_n \leq x_n) \qquad (5.1.1)$$

and the joint probability density function (pdf), provided it exists, is

$$f(\mathbf{x}) = f(x_1, x_2, \cdots, x_n) = \frac{\partial^n}{\partial x_1 \cdots \partial x_n} F(x_1, x_2, \cdots, x_n), \qquad (5.1.2)$$

where $f(x_1, x_2, \cdots, x_n) \geq 0$, for $-\infty < x_i < \infty$, $i = 1, \cdots, n$, and

$$\int\limits_{-\infty}^{\infty} \cdots \int\limits_{-\infty}^{\infty} f(x_1, x_2, \cdots, x_n) dx_1 \cdots dx_n = 1.$$

The marginal pdf of the subvector $(X_{k+1}, \cdots, X_n)'$ of $\mathbf{x}$ is obtained from the joint pdf $f(x_1, \cdots, x_n)$ by integrating out $(X_1, \cdots, X_k)$ as

$$f_{k+1,\cdots,n}(x_{k+1}, \cdots, x_n) = \int\limits_{-\infty}^{\infty} \cdots \int\limits_{-\infty}^{\infty} f(x_1, \cdots, x_k, x_{k+1}, \cdots, x_n) dx_1 \cdots dx_k.$$

(5.1.3)

The marginal pdf of the subvector $(X_1, \cdots, X_k)$ is defined similarly and denoted by $f_{1,\cdots,k}(x_1, \cdots, x_k)$. Note that we can use this definition to obtain the marginal pdf of single components of the vector $\mathbf{x}$; we will use the notation $f_i(x_i)$, $i = 1, \cdots, n$ to denote these marginal densities. The conditional pdf of $(X_1, \cdots, X_k)$ given $(X_{k+1} = x_{k+1}, \cdots, X_n = x_n)$ is defined as

$$g_{(1,\cdots,k|k+1,\cdots,n)}(x_1, \cdots, x_k | x_{k+1}, \cdots, x_n) = \frac{f(x_1, x_2, \cdots, x_n)}{f_{k+1,\cdots,n}(x_{k+1}, \cdots, x_n)}. \quad (5.1.4)$$

The conditional density function of $(x_{k+1}, \cdots, x_n | x_1, \cdots, x_k)$ is defined similarly.

The moment generating function (mgf) $M_{\mathbf{x}}(\mathbf{t})$ of a random vector $\mathbf{x}$ with pdf $f(\mathbf{x})$ is defined as

$$M_{\mathbf{x}}(\mathbf{t}) = E[\exp(\mathbf{t}'\mathbf{x})] = \int\limits_{-\infty}^{\infty} \cdots \int\limits_{-\infty}^{\infty} \exp(\mathbf{t}'\mathbf{x}) f(x_1, \cdots, x_n) dx_1 \cdots dx_n \quad (5.1.5)$$

for $\mathbf{t}' = (t_1, \cdots, t_n)$, $-h < t_i < h$, $i = 1, \cdots, n$, and for some positive real number h, provided the integral on the right side of (5.1.5) exists. For two cdfs all of whose moments exist, we have $F_{\mathbf{x}_1}(\mathbf{u}) = F_{\mathbf{x}_2}(\mathbf{u})$ if and only if $M_{\mathbf{x}_1}(\mathbf{t}) = M_{\mathbf{x}_2}(\mathbf{t})$, which shows how a distribution can be characterized. This leads to the well-known moment generating function technique for determining the distribution of a "new" random variable, which we use in various places throughout this chapter. Given the mgf about the origin of $\mathbf{x}$, the cumulant generating function (cgf) is defined as

$$K_{\mathbf{x}}(\mathbf{t}) = \log[M_{\mathbf{x}}(\mathbf{t})].$$

We say that $(X_1, \cdots, X_n)$ are mutually independent if and only if

$$F(\mathbf{x}) = \prod_{i=1}^{n} F_i(x_i) \quad (5.1.6)$$

for all $\mathbf{x} \in \mathcal{R}^n$, where $F_i(x_i)$ denotes the ith marginal cdf, or equivalently, if

$$M_{\mathbf{x}}(\mathbf{t}) = \prod_{i=1}^{n} M_{X_i}(t_i) \quad (5.1.7)$$

for all $\mathbf{t}$ in an open rectangle in $\mathcal{R}^n$ which includes the origin. Note that functions of independent random vectors are themselves independent.

If $M_{\mathbf{x}}(\mathbf{t})$ exists, then moments of all orders exist. The rth moment of X_i whose marginal pdf is $f_i(x_i)$ is given by

$$\mu_i^{(r)} = E(X_i^r) = \int\limits_{-\infty}^{\infty} x_i^r \, f_i(x_i)dx_i = \int\limits_{-\infty}^{\infty} \cdots \int\limits_{-\infty}^{\infty} x_i^r \, f(x_1, \cdots, x_n)dx_1 \cdots dx_n.$$

(5.1.8)

The mean of X_i is the first moment,

$$\mu_i = \mu_i^{(1)} = E(X_i).$$

(5.1.9)

We let $\mu' = (\mu_1, \cdots, \mu_n)$ denote the mean of the random vector $\mathbf{x}$, i.e., $\mu = E(\mathbf{x})$. The variance of X_i is

$$\sigma_i^2 = \mu_i^{(2)} - \mu_i^2 = Var(X_i)$$

(5.1.10)

and the standard deviation of X_i is the positive square root of the variance and is denoted by σ_i. The covariance $Cov(X_i, X_j)$ between X_i and X_j, for $i \neq j$ is

$$
\begin{aligned}
\sigma_{ij} &= E[(X_i - \mu_i)(X_j - \mu_j)] \\
&= \int\limits_{-\infty}^{\infty}\int\limits_{-\infty}^{\infty} (x_i - \mu_i)(x_j - \mu_j)f_{ij}(x_i, x_j)dx_i dx_j \\
&= \int\limits_{-\infty}^{\infty} \cdots \int\limits_{-\infty}^{\infty} (x_i - \mu_i)(x_j - \mu_j)f(x_1, \cdots, x_n)dx_1 \cdots dx_n.
\end{aligned}
$$

(5.1.11)

The variance-covariance matrix of $\mathbf{x} = (X_1, \cdots, X_n)'$ is defined by $\Sigma = \{\sigma_{ij}\}$ where the elements σ_{ij} for $i, j = 1, \cdots, n$ are given by (5.1.11). The ith diagonal element of Σ is $Var(X_i)$, and the (i, j)th off-diagonal element is $Cov(X_i, X_j)$. The variance-covariance matrix Σ is a nonnegative definite matrix, since for nonzero $\mathbf{t}$, $\mathbf{t}'\Sigma\mathbf{t} = \sum_{i=1}^n \sum_{j=1}^n t_{ij}\sigma_i\sigma_j = Var(\mathbf{t}'\mathbf{x}) \geq 0$, with equality only if $\mathbf{t}'\mathbf{x} = 0$. Clearly,

$$\Sigma = Cov(\mathbf{x}) = E\{[\mathbf{x} - E(\mathbf{x})][\mathbf{x} - E(\mathbf{x})]'\} = E(\mathbf{xx}') - E(\mathbf{x})E(\mathbf{x}').$$

(5.1.12)

The correlation between X_i and X_j is $\sigma_{ij} / \sigma_i\sigma_j$ for $i, j = 1, \cdots, n$; the correlation matrix of $\mathbf{x}$ is

$$\mathbf{R} = \left\{ \frac{\sigma_{ij}}{\sigma_i\sigma_j} \right\} = \mathbf{D}^{-1}\Sigma\mathbf{D}^{-1},$$

(5.1.13)

where $\mathbf{D} = \text{diag}(\sigma_1, \cdots, \sigma_n)$. The correlation matrix $\mathbf{R}$ is a symmetric, nonnegative definite matrix with unit diagonal elements. Suppose $\mathbf{x}$ is partitioned as

$$\mathbf{x}' = (\mathbf{x}_1', \mathbf{x}_2', \cdots, \mathbf{x}_M'),$$

where $\mathbf{x}_i$ is a q_i-dimensional vector, $q_i > 0$, and $\sum_{i=1}^{M} q_i = n$. Suppose the mean vector μ and the variance-covariance matrix Σ of $\mathbf{x}$ are partitioned conformably, so that $E(\mathbf{x}_i)$ is the q_i-dimensional vector μ_i, and $Cov(\mathbf{x}_i, \mathbf{x}_j) = \Sigma_{ij}$, which is a $(q_i \times q_j)$ matrix. We say $\mathbf{x}_i$ and $\mathbf{x}_j$ are uncorrelated if and only if $Cov(\mathbf{x}_i, \mathbf{x}_j) = \mathbf{0}$.

Result 5.1.1. Transformation. Let $\mathbf{x} = (X_1, \cdots, X_n)'$ be an n-dimensional continuous random vector with pdf $f(\mathbf{x})$, which is positive in a domain $\mathcal{D}_{\mathbf{x}} \subset \mathcal{R}^n$. Let $\mathbf{y} = (Y_1, \cdots, Y_n)'$ denote another n-dimensional vector. Let

$$Y_i = g_i(X_1, \cdots, X_n), \quad i = 1, \cdots, n$$

denote n real-valued one-one transformations of the n variables $X_1, \cdots, X_n$ with inverse transformation

$$X_i = g_i^*(Y_1, \cdots, Y_n), \quad i = 1, \cdots, n.$$

Assuming that the functions are differentiable, the pdf of $\mathbf{y}$ is given by

$$f(\mathbf{y}) = f(\mathbf{x})J(\mathbf{y}),$$

where $J(\mathbf{y}) = |\det(\mathbf{J})|$ denotes the absolute value of the Jacobian of the transformation, with

$$\mathbf{J} = \begin{pmatrix} \frac{\partial X_1}{\partial Y_1} & \frac{\partial X_1}{\partial Y_2} & \cdots & \frac{\partial X_1}{\partial Y_n} \\ \frac{\partial X_2}{\partial Y_1} & \frac{\partial X_2}{\partial Y_2} & \cdots & \frac{\partial X_2}{\partial Y_n} \\ \vdots & \vdots & \ddots & \vdots \\ \frac{\partial X_n}{\partial Y_1} & \frac{\partial X_n}{\partial Y_2} & \cdots & \frac{\partial X_n}{\partial Y_n} \end{pmatrix}$$

and $\det(\mathbf{J})$ denotes the determinant of the matrix $\mathbf{J}$.

Proof. Let $\mathcal{A}$ and $\mathcal{B}$ be some subsets of $\mathcal{R}^n$. We know that $P(\mathbf{x} \in \mathcal{A}) = \int_{\mathcal{A}} f(\mathbf{x})d\mathbf{x}$. Suppose that each $\mathbf{x} \in \mathcal{A}$ is mapped by the transformation into a vector $\mathbf{y} \in \mathcal{B}$, and the inverse transformation maps each $\mathbf{y} \in \mathcal{B}$ back into $\mathbf{x} \in \mathcal{A}$. Using results on multiple integrals, we see that

$$\int_{\mathcal{A}} f(\mathbf{x})d\mathbf{x} = \int_{\mathcal{B}} f[g_1^*(Y_1, \cdots, Y_n), \cdots, g_n^*(Y_1, \cdots, Y_n)]J(\mathbf{y})d\mathbf{y}.$$

This holds for all $\mathcal{A} \subset \mathcal{R}^n$; the right side of the above equation is the pdf of $\mathbf{y}$, which completes the proof. ∎

The class of nonsingular linear transformations, which is a simple case of Result 5.1.1, plays a special role in the theory of linear models. Next, let us define linear transformations of a random vector $\mathbf{x}$ with pdf $f(\mathbf{x})$. Let $\mathbf{T}$ be a nonsingular matrix and suppose

$$\mathbf{y} = \mathbf{T}\mathbf{x} \tag{5.1.14}$$

where $\mathbf{y} = (Y_1, \cdots, Y_n)'$. Then, $\mathbf{x} = \mathbf{T}^{-1}\mathbf{y}$, and the Jacobian of the transformation is $|\mathbf{J}| = 1/|\det(\mathbf{T})|$. The pdf of $\mathbf{y}$ is

$$h(\mathbf{y}) = f(\mathbf{T}^{-1}\mathbf{y})|\mathbf{J}|. \tag{5.1.15}$$

Now, let $\mathbf{x}$ and $\mathbf{y}$ be respectively n-dimensional and m-dimensional random vectors. The covariance matrix of $\mathbf{x}$ and $\mathbf{y}$ is defined as

$$Cov(\mathbf{x}, \mathbf{y}) = E\{[\mathbf{x} - E(\mathbf{x})][\mathbf{y} - E(\mathbf{y})]'\} = \{Cov(\mathbf{y}, \mathbf{x})\}'. \tag{5.1.16}$$

Let $\mathbf{A}$ and $\mathbf{B}$ be $p \times n$ and $q \times m$ matrices respectively. Then,

$$
\begin{aligned}
Cov(\mathbf{Ax}, \mathbf{By}) &= E\{[\mathbf{Ax} - E(\mathbf{Ax})][\mathbf{By} - E(\mathbf{By})]'\} \\
&= \mathbf{A}E\{[\mathbf{x} - E(\mathbf{x})][\mathbf{y} - E(\mathbf{y})]'\}\mathbf{B}' \\
&= \mathbf{A}Cov(\mathbf{x}, \mathbf{y})\mathbf{B}'. \tag{5.1.17}
\end{aligned}
$$

For further details and examples, the reader is referred to Casella and Berger (1990) or Mukhopadhyay (2000).

If $\mathbf{x}_1, \cdots, \mathbf{x}_n$ are independent k-dimensional random vectors with a common variance-covariance matrix Σ, then the "rolled out" vector of the $\mathbf{x}_i$'s, viz., $\mathbf{y} = (\mathbf{x}_1', \cdots, \mathbf{x}_n')' = vec(\mathbf{x}_1, \cdots, \mathbf{x}_n)$ (see section 2.8) has variance-covariance matrix

$$Cov(\mathbf{y}) = \begin{pmatrix} \Sigma & \mathbf{0} & \cdots & \mathbf{0} \\ \mathbf{0} & \Sigma & \cdots & \mathbf{0} \\ \vdots & \vdots & \vdots & \vdots \\ \mathbf{0} & \mathbf{0} & \cdots & \Sigma \end{pmatrix}.$$

This vectorized version is useful in a discussion of multivariate linear model theory, including multivariate time series.

We conclude this section with two results useful for evaluating integrals that arise in the context of multivariate normal distributions (see section 5.2). From integral calculus, we recall that for a scalar variable x,

$$
\begin{aligned}
\int_{-\infty}^{\infty} \exp\{-\frac{1}{2}x^2\}dx &= \sqrt{2\pi}, \\
\int_{-\infty}^{\infty} x\exp\{-\frac{1}{2}x^2\}dx &= 0, \text{ and} \\
\int_{-\infty}^{\infty} x^2 \exp\{-\frac{1}{2}x^2\}dx &= \sqrt{2\pi}. \tag{5.1.18}
\end{aligned}
$$

Result 5.1.2. Aitken's integral.   Let $\mathbf{A}$ be an $n \times n$ p.d. symmetric matrix and let $\mathbf{x} = (X_1, \cdots, X_n)'$ be an n-dimensional vector. Then

$$\int_{-\infty}^{\infty} \cdots \int_{-\infty}^{\infty} \exp\{-\frac{1}{2}\mathbf{x}'\mathbf{A}\mathbf{x}\}dx = (2\pi)^{n/2}|\mathbf{A}|^{-1/2}. \qquad (5.1.19)$$

Proof. Since $\mathbf{A}$ is p.d., by Result 2.4.5, there exists a nonsingular matrix $\mathbf{P}$ satisfying $\mathbf{A} = \mathbf{P}\mathbf{P}'$. Letting $\mathbf{Q} = \mathbf{P}^{-1}$, we see that $\mathbf{Q}\mathbf{A}\mathbf{Q}' = \mathbf{I}_n$, so that $|\mathbf{Q}\mathbf{A}\mathbf{Q}'| = |\mathbf{Q}|^2|\mathbf{A}| = 1$, and hence $|\mathbf{Q}| = |\mathbf{A}|^{-1/2}$. Under the transformation $\mathbf{y} = \mathbf{P}'\mathbf{x}$, we have $\mathbf{x}'\mathbf{A}\mathbf{x} = \mathbf{y}'\mathbf{Q}\mathbf{A}\mathbf{Q}'\mathbf{y} = \mathbf{y}'\mathbf{y}$ and

$$
\begin{aligned}
\int_{-\infty}^{\infty} \cdots \int_{-\infty}^{\infty} \exp\{-\frac{1}{2}\mathbf{x}'\mathbf{A}\mathbf{x}\}dx &= \int_{-\infty}^{\infty} \cdots \int_{-\infty}^{\infty} |\mathbf{Q}| \exp\{-\frac{1}{2}\mathbf{y}'\mathbf{y}\}dy \\
&= |\mathbf{A}|^{-1/2} \int_{-\infty}^{\infty} \cdots \int_{-\infty}^{\infty} \exp\{-\frac{1}{2}\sum_{i=1}^{n}y_i^2\}dy_1 \cdots dy_n \\
&= |\mathbf{A}|^{-1/2} \prod_{i=1}^{n} \int_{-\infty}^{\infty} \exp\{-\frac{1}{2}y_i^2\}dy_i \\
&= (2\pi)^{n/2}|\mathbf{A}|^{-1/2}
\end{aligned}
$$

using (5.1.18).   ∎

Result 5.1.3. General integral evaluation theorem.   Let a_0 and b_0 denote scalars, let $\mathbf{a}$ and $\mathbf{b}$ denote n-dimensional vectors of constants, let $\mathbf{A}$ be an $n \times n$ symmetric matrix of constants, and let $\mathbf{B}$ be a p.d. matrix of constants. For an n-dimensional vector $\mathbf{x} = (X_1, \cdots, X_n)'$, the integral

$$I = \int_{-\infty}^{\infty} \cdots \int_{-\infty}^{\infty} (\mathbf{x}'\mathbf{A}\mathbf{x} + \mathbf{x}'\mathbf{a} + a_0) \exp\{-(\mathbf{x}'\mathbf{B}\mathbf{x} + \mathbf{x}'\mathbf{b} + b_0)\}dx \qquad (5.1.20)$$

is evaluated as

$$
\begin{aligned}
I &= \frac{1}{2}\pi^{n/2}|\mathbf{B}|^{-1/2}\{tr(\mathbf{A}\mathbf{B}^{-1}) - \mathbf{b}'\mathbf{B}^{-1}\mathbf{a} + \frac{1}{2}\mathbf{b}'\mathbf{B}^{-1}\mathbf{A}\mathbf{B}^{-1}\mathbf{b} + 2a_0\} \\
&\quad \times \ \exp\{\frac{1}{4}\mathbf{b}'\mathbf{B}^{-1}\mathbf{b} - b_0\}. \qquad (5.1.21)
\end{aligned}
$$

Proof.   It is easily verified (by expanding the right side in each case and simplifying to the expression on the left) that the exponent in (5.1.20) can be written as

$$\mathbf{x}'\mathbf{B}\mathbf{x} + \mathbf{x}'\mathbf{b} + b_0 = \frac{1}{2}(\mathbf{x} + \frac{1}{2}\mathbf{B}^{-1}\mathbf{b})'(2\mathbf{B})(\mathbf{x} + \frac{1}{2}\mathbf{B}^{-1}\mathbf{b}) - \frac{1}{4}\mathbf{b}'\mathbf{B}^1\mathbf{b} + b_0,$$
$$\qquad (5.1.22)$$

while the nonexponent can be written as

$$
\begin{aligned}
\mathbf{x}'\mathbf{A}\mathbf{x} + \mathbf{x}'\mathbf{a} + a_0 \;=\;& (\mathbf{x} + \tfrac{1}{2}\mathbf{B}^{-1}\mathbf{b})'\mathbf{A}(\mathbf{x} + \tfrac{1}{2}\mathbf{B}^{-1}\mathbf{b}) \\
+\;& \mathbf{x}'(\mathbf{a} - \mathbf{A}\mathbf{B}^{-1}\mathbf{b}) - \tfrac{1}{4}\mathbf{b}'\mathbf{B}^{-1}\mathbf{A}\mathbf{B}^{-1}\mathbf{b} + a_0. \ (5.1.23)
\end{aligned}
$$

Substituting (5.1.22) and (5.1.23) into (5.1.20), we see that

$$
\begin{aligned}
I \;=\;& [\exp\{\tfrac{1}{4}\mathbf{b}'\mathbf{B}^{-1}\mathbf{b} - b_0\}] \\
&\times [\int_{-\infty}^{\infty} \cdots \int_{-\infty}^{\infty} (\mathbf{x} - \mathbf{c})'\mathbf{A}(\mathbf{x} - \mathbf{c}) \exp\{-\tfrac{1}{2}(\mathbf{x} - \mathbf{c})'\mathbf{R}(\mathbf{x} - \mathbf{c})dx_1 dx_2 \cdots dx_n \\
&+ \int_{-\infty}^{\infty} \cdots \int_{-\infty}^{\infty} \mathbf{x}'\mathbf{d} \exp\{-\tfrac{1}{2}(\mathbf{x} - \mathbf{c})'\mathbf{R}(\mathbf{x} - \mathbf{c})\}dx_1 dx_2 \cdots dx_n \\
&+ \int_{-\infty}^{\infty} \cdots \int_{-\infty}^{\infty} (-\tfrac{1}{4}\mathbf{b}'\mathbf{B}^{-1}\mathbf{A}\mathbf{B}^{-1}\mathbf{b} + a_0) \exp\{-\tfrac{1}{2}(\mathbf{x} - \mathbf{c})'\mathbf{R}(\mathbf{x} - \mathbf{c})\}dx_1 dx_2 \cdots dx_n] \\
\;=\;& [\exp\{\tfrac{1}{4}\mathbf{b}'\mathbf{B}^{-1}\mathbf{b} - b_0\}][I_1 + I_2 + I_3], \text{ say} \qquad (5.1.24)
\end{aligned}
$$

where we define $\mathbf{c} = -\tfrac{1}{2}\mathbf{B}^{-1}\mathbf{b}$, $\mathbf{d} = \mathbf{a} - \mathbf{A}\mathbf{B}^{-1}\mathbf{b}$, and $\mathbf{R} = 2\mathbf{B}$; note that $\mathbf{R}$ is p.d., since $\mathbf{B}$ is. Then,

$$
I_1 = \int_{-\infty}^{\infty} \cdots \int_{-\infty}^{\infty} (\mathbf{x} - \mathbf{c})'\mathbf{A}(\mathbf{x} - \mathbf{c}) \exp\{-\tfrac{1}{2}(\mathbf{x} - \mathbf{c})'\mathbf{R}(\mathbf{x} - \mathbf{c})\}d\mathbf{x}.
$$

Since $\mathbf{R}$ is p.d., there exists an $n \times n$ nonsingular matrix $\mathbf{P}$ such that $\mathbf{R} = \mathbf{P}\mathbf{P}'$. Let $\mathbf{z} = \mathbf{P}'(\mathbf{x} - \mathbf{c})$, so that $\mathbf{x} = (\mathbf{P}')^{-1}\mathbf{z} + \mathbf{c}$, and the Jacobian is

$$
J = |\mathbf{P}^{-1}| = |\mathbf{P}|^{-1} = |\mathbf{R}|^{-1/2}.
$$

We see that

$$
\begin{aligned}
I_1 \;=\;& \int_{-\infty}^{\infty} \cdots \int_{-\infty}^{\infty} \{\mathbf{z}'\mathbf{P}^{-1}\mathbf{A}(\mathbf{P}')^{-1}\mathbf{z}\} \exp[-\tfrac{1}{2}\mathbf{z}'\mathbf{z}]|J|d\mathbf{z} \\
\;=\;& |\mathbf{R}|^{-1/2}\sum_{i,j} w_{ij} \int_{-\infty}^{\infty} \cdots \int_{-\infty}^{\infty} z_i z_j \exp\{-\tfrac{1}{2}\mathbf{z}'\mathbf{z}\}d\mathbf{z},
\end{aligned}
$$

and further simplification yields

$$
\begin{aligned}
I_1 &= |\mathbf{R}|^{-1/2}\sum_i w_{ii} \int_{-\infty}^{\infty} z_i^2 \exp\{-\frac{1}{2}z_i^2\}dz_i \prod_{s\neq i}\int_{-\infty}^{\infty} \exp\{-\frac{1}{2}z_s^2\}dz_s \\
&+ |\mathbf{R}|^{-1/2}\sum_{i,j\neq i} w_{ij} \int_{-\infty}^{\infty} z_i \exp\{-\frac{1}{2}z_i^2\}dz_i \int_{-\infty}^{\infty} z_j \exp\{-\frac{1}{2}z_j^2\}dz_j \\
&\times \prod_{s\neq i,j}\int_{-\infty}^{\infty} \exp\{-\frac{1}{2}z_s^2\}dz_s.
\end{aligned}
$$

Finally, we simplify this expression to get

$$
\begin{aligned}
I_1 &= |\mathbf{R}|^{-1/2}\sum_i w_{ii}(2\pi)^{1/2}(2\pi)^{(n-1)/2} = (2\pi)^{n/2}|\mathbf{R}|^{-1/2}tr\{\mathbf{P}^{-1}\mathbf{A}(\mathbf{P}')^{-1}\} \\
&= (2\pi)^{n/2}|\mathbf{R}|^{-1/2}tr\{\mathbf{A}(\mathbf{P}')^{-1}\mathbf{P}^{-1}\} = (2\pi)^{n/2}|\mathbf{R}|^{-1/2}tr\{\mathbf{A}\mathbf{R}^{-1}\} \\
&= \frac{1}{2}\pi^{n/2}|\mathbf{B}|^{-1/2}tr(\mathbf{A}\mathbf{B}^{-1}).
\end{aligned}
\tag{5.1.25}
$$

Since $\mathbf{x}'\mathbf{d} = \sum_{i=1}^{n} x_i d_i$, I_2 can be written as the sum of n integrals, so that,

$$
\begin{aligned}
I_2 &= \mathbf{d}'\mathbf{c} \int_{-\infty}^{\infty} \cdots \int_{-\infty}^{\infty} \exp\{-\frac{1}{2}(\mathbf{x}-\mathbf{c})'\mathbf{R}(\mathbf{x}-\mathbf{c})\}d\mathbf{x} \\
&+ \int_{-\infty}^{\infty} \cdots \int_{-\infty}^{\infty} \mathbf{d}'(\mathbf{x}-\mathbf{c})\exp\{-\frac{1}{2}(\mathbf{x}-\mathbf{c})'\mathbf{R}(\mathbf{x}-\mathbf{c})\}d\mathbf{x}.
\end{aligned}
$$

Simplifying further, we see that

$$
\begin{aligned}
I_2 &= (\mathbf{d}'\mathbf{c}) \int_{-\infty}^{\infty} \cdots \int_{-\infty}^{\infty} \exp[-\frac{1}{2}\mathbf{z}'\mathbf{z}]|J|d\mathbf{z} \\
&+ \int_{-\infty}^{\infty} \cdots \int_{-\infty}^{\infty} \{\mathbf{d}'(\mathbf{P}')^{-1}\mathbf{z}\}\exp\{-\frac{1}{2}\mathbf{z}'\mathbf{z}\}|J|d\mathbf{z} \\
&= (\mathbf{d}'\mathbf{c})|\mathbf{R}|^{-1/2}\prod_{i=1}^{n}\int_{-\infty}^{\infty} \exp\{-\frac{1}{2}z_i^2\}dz_i \\
&+ |R|^{-1/2}\sum_{i=1}^{n} v_i \int_{-\infty}^{\infty} z_i \exp\{-\frac{1}{2}z_i^2\}dz_i \prod_{s\neq i}\int_{-\infty}^{\infty} \exp\{-\frac{1}{2}z_s^2\}dz_s \\
&= (\mathbf{d}'\mathbf{c})|\mathbf{R}|^{-1/2}(2\pi)^{n/2} = \frac{1}{2}\pi^{n/2}|\mathbf{B}|^{-1/2}\mathbf{b}'\mathbf{B}^{-1}(\mathbf{A}\mathbf{B}^{-1}\mathbf{b}-\mathbf{a}).
\end{aligned}
$$

We evaluate

$$
\begin{aligned}
I_3 &= (-\frac{1}{4}\mathbf{b}'\mathbf{B}^{-1}\mathbf{A}\mathbf{B}^{-1}\mathbf{b} + a_0)(2\pi)^{n/2}|\mathbf{R}|^{-1/2} \\
&= \pi^{n/2}|\mathbf{B}|^{-1/2}(a_0 - \frac{1}{4}\mathbf{b}'\mathbf{B}^{-1}\mathbf{A}\mathbf{B}^{-1}\mathbf{b}).
\end{aligned}
$$

Substituting these expressions for I_1, I_2, and I_3 into (5.1.24), we get the required expression for I. ∎

5.2 Multivariate normal distribution and properties

The multivariate normal distribution is the most widely used distribution to characterize the probabilistic behavior of a k-dimensional random vector $\mathbf{x} = (X_1, \cdots, X_k)'$. In this section, we define this distribution, and describe some important properties associated with this distribution. The normal distribution forms the basis for the development of the classical theory of linear models and multivariate analysis. We begin with the definition of the standard multivariate normal distribution.

Definition 5.2.1. $N_k(\mathbf{0}, \mathbf{I})$.   A random vector $\mathbf{z} = (Z_1, \cdots, Z_k)'$ defined on $\mathcal{R}^k$ has a multivariate standard normal distribution if and only if

$$
f(\mathbf{z}) = \frac{1}{(2\pi)^{k/2}} \exp\left\{-\frac{1}{2}\mathbf{z}'\mathbf{z}\right\}, \tag{5.2.1}
$$

and we say $\mathbf{z} \sim N_k(\mathbf{0}, \mathbf{I})$.

The mean of this distribution is $E(\mathbf{z}) = \mathbf{0}$, and its variance-covariance matrix is $Cov(\mathbf{z}) = \mathbf{I}_k$. It is easily verified that $f(\mathbf{z}) \geq 0$ for all $\mathbf{z} \in \mathcal{R}^k$, and using Aitken's integral in Result 5.1.2, we can easily see that $\int_{-\infty}^{\infty} \cdots \int_{-\infty}^{\infty} f(\mathbf{z})d\mathbf{z} = 1$, so (5.2.1) is a proper pdf.

Result 5.2.1. Let $\mathbf{z} \sim N_k(\mathbf{0}, \mathbf{I})$. The mgf of $\mathbf{z}$ is

$$
M_{\mathbf{z}}(\mathbf{t}) = \exp\{\frac{1}{2}\mathbf{t}'\mathbf{t}\} \tag{5.2.2}
$$

for $\mathbf{t} = (t_1, \cdots, t_k)$ in $\mathcal{R}^k$.

Proof. From (5.1.5),

$$
\begin{aligned}
M_{\mathbf{z}}(\mathbf{t}) &= E\{\exp(\mathbf{t}'\mathbf{z})\} = \int_{-\infty}^{\infty} \cdots \int_{-\infty}^{\infty} \exp(\mathbf{t}'\mathbf{z})f(\mathbf{z})d\mathbf{z} \\
&= \frac{1}{(2\pi)^{k/2}} \int_{-\infty}^{\infty} \cdots \int_{-\infty}^{\infty} \exp\{\mathbf{t}'\mathbf{z} - \frac{1}{2}\mathbf{z}'\mathbf{z}\}d\mathbf{z}.
\end{aligned}
$$

By application of Aitken's integral (see (5.1.19)),

$$
\begin{aligned}
M_{\mathbf{z}}(\mathbf{t}) &= \frac{1}{(2\pi)^{k/2}} \int_{-\infty}^{\infty} \cdots \int_{-\infty}^{\infty} \exp\{-\frac{1}{2}[(\mathbf{z}-\mathbf{t})'(\mathbf{z}-\mathbf{t})] + \frac{1}{2}\mathbf{t}'\mathbf{t}\}d\mathbf{z} \\
&= \exp\{\frac{1}{2}\mathbf{t}'\mathbf{t}\}, \quad \mathbf{t} \in \mathcal{R}^k
\end{aligned}
\tag{5.2.3}
$$

follows directly. ∎

It can be shown that if $X_1, \cdots, X_k$ are mutually independent normal random variables with respective means $\mu_1, \cdots, \mu_k$, and a common variance σ^2, then $\mathbf{x} = (X_1, \cdots, X_k) \sim N_k(\mu, \sigma^2\mathbf{I})$, where $\mu = (\mu_1, \cdots, \mu_k)'$.

Result 5.2.2. Let $\mathbf{z} \sim N_k(\mathbf{0}, \mathbf{I})$, let $\gamma = (\gamma_1, \cdots, \gamma_k)'$ be a nonzero vector of constants and let γ_0 be a scalar constant. Then the univariate linear function of $\mathbf{z}$ defined by $X = \gamma'\mathbf{z} + \gamma_0 = \sum_{i=1}^{k}\gamma_i Z_i + \gamma_0$ has a $N(\gamma_0, \gamma'\gamma)$ distribution. That is, any linear function of a standard multivariate normal vector itself has a normal distribution.

Proof. The mgf of X is given by $M_X(t) = E[\exp\{tX\}] = E[\exp\{t(\gamma'\mathbf{z}+\gamma_0)\}]$, which we evaluate using Aitken's integral as

$$
\begin{aligned}
M_X(t) &= \frac{\exp\{\gamma_0 t\}}{(2\pi)^{k/2}} \int_{-\infty}^{\infty} \cdots \int_{-\infty}^{\infty} \exp\{t\gamma'\mathbf{z} - \frac{1}{2}\mathbf{z}'\mathbf{z}\}d\mathbf{z} \\
&= \exp\{\gamma_0 t + \frac{1}{2}\gamma'\gamma t^2\}.
\end{aligned}
\tag{5.2.4}
$$

From (A4), this is seen to be the mgf of a $N(\gamma_0, \gamma'\gamma)$ random variable. ∎

In general, let $\mathbf{x} = (X_1, \cdots, X_k)'$, $\mu' = E(X_1, \cdots, X_k) = (\mu_1, \cdots, \mu_k)$, and the n.n.d. matrix $\Sigma = E\{(\mathbf{x}-\mu)(\mathbf{x}-\mu)'\} = Cov(\mathbf{x})$ with $r(\Sigma) = r < k$. Suppose Σ is factored as $\Sigma = \Gamma'\Gamma$, where Γ' is a $k \times r$ matrix of rank r (see Result 2.2.1). Then $\mathbf{x} \sim N_k(\mu, \Sigma)$ if and only if the cdf of $\mathbf{x}$ is the same as the cdf of $\Gamma'\mathbf{z} + \mu$, where $\mathbf{z} \sim N_r(\mathbf{0}, \mathbf{I})$. This result holds since, if $\mathbf{x}$ is to have the same cdf as $\Gamma'\mathbf{z} + \mu$, then $E(\Gamma'\mathbf{z} + \mu)$ must coincide with $E(\mathbf{x})$ and $Cov(\Gamma'\mathbf{z} + \mu)$ with $Cov(\mathbf{x})$. We can verify that these are in fact true, i.e.,

$$
E(\Gamma'\mathbf{z} + \mu) = \Gamma'E(\mathbf{z}) + \mu = \mu = E(\mathbf{x})
\tag{5.2.5}
$$

and

$$
\begin{aligned}
Cov(\Gamma'\mathbf{z} + \mu) &= E[\Gamma'\mathbf{z} + \mu - E(\Gamma'\mathbf{z} + \mu)][\Gamma'\mathbf{z} + \mu - E(\Gamma'\mathbf{z} + \mu)]' \\
&= E[(\Gamma'\mathbf{z})(\Gamma'\mathbf{z})'] = \Gamma'E(\mathbf{z}\mathbf{z}')\Gamma = \Gamma'\Gamma = \Sigma = Cov(\mathbf{x}).
\end{aligned}
\tag{5.2.6}
$$

Result 5.2.3. Let $x \sim N_k(\mu, \Sigma)$ with $r(\Sigma) = r < k$. Then

$$M_{\mathbf{x}}(\mathbf{t}) = \exp\{\mathbf{t}'\mu + \frac{1}{2}\mathbf{t}'\Sigma\mathbf{t}\}, \quad \mathbf{t} \in \mathcal{R}^k. \tag{5.2.7}$$

Proof. From the discussion above this result, we see that both $\mathbf{x}$ and $\Gamma'\mathbf{z} + \mu$ have the same cdf, and hence the same mgf. Therefore, $M_{\mathbf{x}}(\mathbf{t}) = M_{\Gamma'\mathbf{z}+\mu}(\mathbf{t}) = E[\exp\{\mathbf{t}'(\Gamma'\mathbf{z} + \mu)\}]$, so that

$$
\begin{aligned}
M_{\mathbf{x}}(\mathbf{t}) &= \int_{-\infty}^{\infty} \cdots \int_{-\infty}^{\infty} \frac{\exp\{\mathbf{t}'\mu\}}{(2\pi)^{k/2}} \exp\{\mathbf{t}'\Gamma'\mathbf{z} - \frac{1}{2}\mathbf{z}'\mathbf{z}\}d\mathbf{z} \tag{5.2.8} \\
&= \frac{\exp\{\mathbf{t}'\mu\}}{(2\pi)^{k/2}} \int_{-\infty}^{\infty} \cdots \int_{-\infty}^{\infty} \exp\{-\frac{1}{2}(\mathbf{z} - \Gamma\mathbf{t})'(\mathbf{z} - \Gamma\mathbf{t}) + \frac{1}{2}\mathbf{t}'\Gamma'\Gamma\mathbf{t}\}d\mathbf{z}
\end{aligned}
$$

from which the result follows using Aitken's integral. ∎

Definition 5.2.2. $N_k(\mu, \Sigma)$. A random vector $\mathbf{x} = (X_1, \cdots, X_k)'$ in $\mathcal{R}^k$ is said to have a multivariate normal distribution if and only if, for a p.d. covariance matrix Σ, and for $\mu \in \mathcal{R}^k$, the pdf of $\mathbf{x}$ (with respect to Lebesgue measure) is given by

$$f(\mathbf{x}; \mu, \Sigma) = \frac{1}{(2\pi)^{k/2}|\Sigma|^{1/2}} \exp\{-\frac{1}{2}(\mathbf{x} - \mu)'\Sigma^{-1}(\mathbf{x} - \mu)\}, \quad \mathbf{x} \in \mathcal{R}^k. \tag{5.2.9}$$

The mean of this distribution is $E(\mathbf{x}) = \mu$, and its variance-covariance matrix is $Cov(\mathbf{x}) = \Sigma$. It is easy to verify that $f(\mathbf{x}; \mu, \Sigma) \geq 0$ for all $\mathbf{x} \in \mathcal{R}^k$, and that $\int_{-\infty}^{\infty} \cdots \int_{-\infty}^{\infty} f(\mathbf{x}; \mu, \Sigma)d\mathbf{x} = 1$ (using Result 5.1.2). We directly derive the mgf $M_{\mathbf{x}}(\mathbf{t})$ from $f(\mathbf{x}; \mu, \Sigma)$ as follows:

$$
\begin{aligned}
M_{\mathbf{x}}(\mathbf{t}) &= \int_{-\infty}^{\infty} \cdots \int_{-\infty}^{\infty} \exp\{\mathbf{t}'\mathbf{x}\}\frac{1}{(2\pi)^{k/2}|\Sigma|^{1/2}} \exp\{-\frac{1}{2}(\mathbf{x} - \mu)'\Sigma^{-1}(\mathbf{x} - \mu)\}d\mathbf{x} \\
&= (2\pi)^{-k/2}|\Sigma|^{-1/2} \int_{-\infty}^{\infty} \cdots \int_{-\infty}^{\infty} \exp\{-\frac{1}{2}\mathbf{x}'\Sigma^{-1}\mathbf{x} + (\Sigma^{-1}\mu + \mathbf{t})'\mathbf{x} \\
&\quad - \frac{1}{2}\mu'\Sigma^{-1}\mu\}d\mathbf{x} \\
&= (2\pi)^{-k/2}|\Sigma|^{-1/2} \int_{-\infty}^{\infty} \cdots \int_{-\infty}^{\infty} \exp\{-[\frac{1}{2}(\mathbf{x} - \mu - \Sigma\mathbf{t})'\Sigma^{-1}(\mathbf{x} - \mu - \Sigma\mathbf{t})] \\
&\quad + \mathbf{t}'\mu + \frac{1}{2}\mathbf{t}'\Sigma\mathbf{t}\}d\mathbf{x}. \tag{5.2.10}
\end{aligned}
$$

Let $\mathbf{y} = \mathbf{x} - \mu - \Sigma\mathbf{t}$. From Result 5.1.2, we see that

$$M_{\mathbf{x}}(\mathbf{t}) = \exp\{\mathbf{t}'\mu + \frac{1}{2}\mathbf{t}'\Sigma\mathbf{t}\}, \quad \mathbf{t} \in \mathcal{R}^k.$$

The cumulant generating function (cgf) $K_{\mathbf{x}}(\mathbf{t})$ of $\mathbf{x}$ is

$$\log\{M_{\mathbf{x}}(\mathbf{t})\} = \mathbf{t}'\mu + \frac{1}{2}\mathbf{t}'\Sigma\mathbf{t} = \sum_{i=1}^{k}\mu_i t_i + \frac{1}{2}\sum_{i=1}^{k}\sum_{j=1}^{k}t_i t_j \sigma_{ij}, \qquad (5.2.11)$$

so that $K_{r_1,\cdots,r_k} = 0$, when $\sum_{i=1}^{k} r_i > 2$. In particular, $K_{1,0,\cdots,0} = \mu_1, \cdots,$ $K_{0,\cdots,0,1} = \mu_k$, $K_{2,0,\cdots,0} = \sigma_{11}, \cdots,$ $K_{0,\cdots,0,2} = \sigma_{kk}$, etc.

Example 5.2.1. Bivariate normal distribution.   Let $\mathbf{x} = (X_1, X_2)'$, $\mu' = (\mu_1, \mu_2)$, and $\Sigma = \begin{pmatrix} \sigma_1^2 & \rho\sigma_1\sigma_2 \\ \rho\sigma_1\sigma_2 & \sigma_2^2 \end{pmatrix}$, where $-\infty < X_i < \infty$, $-\infty < \mu_i < \infty$, $\sigma_i > 0$, for $i = 1, 2$, and $|\rho| < 1$. Then, $|\Sigma| = \sigma_1^2\sigma_2^2(1 - \rho^2)$ and

$$\Sigma^{-1} = \frac{1}{\sigma_1^2\sigma_2^2(1-\rho^2)}\begin{pmatrix} \sigma_2^2 & -\rho\sigma_1\sigma_2 \\ -\rho\sigma_1\sigma_2 & \sigma_1^2 \end{pmatrix} = \frac{1}{1-\rho^2}\begin{pmatrix} \frac{1}{\sigma_1^2} & -\frac{\rho}{\sigma_1\sigma_2} \\ -\frac{\rho}{\sigma_1\sigma_2} & \frac{1}{\sigma_2^2} \end{pmatrix}.$$

We will obtain the form of the pdf of $\mathbf{x}$ starting from two iid $N(0,1)$ variables Z_1 and Z_2. Note that Σ is p.d. since $\rho \neq 1$. Hence, by Result 2.4.5, there exists a nonsingular matrix $\mathbf{P}$ such that $\mathbf{PP}' = \Sigma$. The matrix $\mathbf{P}$ is not unique, however. Let $\mathbf{P} = \begin{pmatrix} p_{11} & p_{12} \\ p_{21} & p_{22} \end{pmatrix}$, so that $\mathbf{PP}' = \begin{pmatrix} p_{11}^2 + p_{12}^2 & p_{11}p_{21} + p_{12}p_{22} \\ p_{21}p_{11} + p_{22}p_{12} & p_{21}^2 + p_{22}^2 \end{pmatrix}$. One choice of $\mathbf{P}$ is: $p_{11}^2 = \sigma_1^2$, $p_{12} = 0$, $p_{21} = \rho\sigma_2$, $p_{22}^2 = \sigma_2^2 - \rho^2\sigma_2^2$. Another choice of $\mathbf{P}$ is: $p_{22}^2 = \sigma_2^2$, $p_{21} = 0$, $p_{12} = \rho\sigma_1$, $p_{11}^2 = \sigma_1^2 - \rho^2\sigma_1^2$. Consider the transformation $\mathbf{x} = \mu + \mathbf{Pz}$, i.e.,

$$\begin{pmatrix} X_1 \\ X_2 \end{pmatrix} = \begin{pmatrix} \mu_1 \\ \mu_2 \end{pmatrix} + \mathbf{P}\begin{pmatrix} Z_1 \\ Z_2 \end{pmatrix}.$$

The inverse transformation is $\mathbf{z} = \mathbf{P}^{-1}(\mathbf{x} - \mu)$, with Jacobian $J = |\mathbf{P}^{-1}| = |\Sigma|^{-1/2}$. The joint pdf of Z_1 and Z_2 is for $\mathbf{z} \in \mathcal{R}^k$,

$$f(z_1, z_2) = \tfrac{1}{2\pi}\exp\{-\tfrac{1}{2}(z_1^2 + z_2^2)\} = \tfrac{1}{2\pi}\exp\{-\tfrac{1}{2}\mathbf{z}'\mathbf{z}\}$$

so that the joint pdf of X_1 and X_2 for $-\infty < X_1 < \infty$, $-\infty < X_2 < \infty$ is

$$\begin{aligned} f(x_1, x_2) &= \frac{1}{2\pi|\Sigma|^{1/2}}\exp\left\{-\frac{1}{2}(x_1 - \mu_1, \ x_2 - \mu_2)\Sigma^{-1}\begin{pmatrix} x_1 - \mu_1 \\ x_2 - \mu_2 \end{pmatrix}\right\} \\ &= \frac{1}{2\pi\sigma_1\sigma_2(1-\rho^2)^{1/2}}\exp[-\frac{1}{2(1-\rho^2)}\{(\frac{x_1-\mu_1}{\sigma_1})^2 + (\frac{x_2-\mu_2}{\sigma_2})^2 \\ &\quad -2\rho(\frac{x_1-\mu_1}{\sigma_1})(\frac{x_2-\mu_2}{\sigma_2})\}]. \end{aligned} \qquad (5.2.12)$$

We sometimes denote this bivariate normal distribution for (X_1, X_2) by $N_2(\mu_1, \mu_2, \sigma_1^2, \sigma_2^2, \rho)$.   □

The multivariate normal pdf is constant on ellipsoids in k-dimensional Euclidean space, i.e., $(\mathbf{x} - \mu)'\Sigma^{-1}(\mathbf{x} - \mu) = c^2$, for all $c > 0$. The center of this ellipsoid is μ, its shape and orientation are determined by Σ, while c determines its size. From the expression in (5.2.12) for the bivariate case, it is evident that the paths of $\mathbf{x}$ values yielding a constant height for the density (called contours) are ellipsoids. In general, the multivariate normal pdf assumes a constant value on surfaces where the squared distance $(\mathbf{x} - \mu)'\Sigma^{-1}(\mathbf{x} - \mu)$ is constant, i.e.,

$$(\mathbf{x} - \mu)'\Sigma^{-1}(\mathbf{x} - \mu) = c^2. \tag{5.2.13}$$

The ellipsoid can be characterized in terms of the eigenvalues and eigenvectors of Σ^{-1}, or in terms of the eigenvalues and eigenvectors of the p.d. matrix Σ (see Result 2.3.5). Let $\lambda_1 \geq \cdots \geq \lambda_k > 0$ denote the eigenvalues of Σ and let $\mathbf{v}_1, \cdots, \mathbf{v}_k$ denote the corresponding normalized eigenvectors. If the multiplicity m_j of λ_j is 1, then $\mathbf{v}_j$ determines the direction of the jth principal axis, i.e., the jth principal axis is in the direction of the jth eigenvector of Σ, and its length is $2c\sqrt{\lambda_j}$, $j = 1, \cdots, k$. However, if $m_j > 1$, then the corresponding eigenvectors and hence the corresponding principal axes are not uniquely defined. The center of this ellipsoid is at μ and its volume is proportional to $c^k|\Sigma^{-1}|$. For a fixed c, if Σ^{-1} is a constant diagonal matrix, i.e., $\Sigma^{-1} = \text{diag}(1/\sigma, \cdots, 1/\sigma)$, then (5.2.13) represents a k-dimensional sphere with radius $c/\sqrt{\sigma}$, while if $\Sigma^{-1} = \mathbf{I}_k$, (5.2.13) reduces to $(\mathbf{x} - \mu)'(\mathbf{x} - \mu) = c^2$, so that $c = \| \mathbf{x} - \mu \|$. If we choose $c^2 = \chi^2_{k,\alpha}$, which is the upper (100α)th percentile from a chi-square distribution with k degrees of freedom (d.f.), we obtain contours that contain $100(1 - \alpha)\%$ of the probability.

Example 5.2.2. We discuss contours of the bivariate normal density defined in (5.2.12), assuming that $\sigma_1^2 = \sigma_2^2$ (Johnson and Wichern, 1988). It is easy to verify that the eigenvalues and corresponding eigenvectors of Σ are

$$\lambda_1 = \sigma_1^2(1 + \rho), \quad \lambda_2 = \sigma_1^2(1 - \rho), \text{ and}$$

$$\mathbf{v}_1 = \begin{pmatrix} 1/\sqrt{2} \\ 1/\sqrt{2} \end{pmatrix}, \quad \mathbf{v}_2 = \begin{pmatrix} 1/\sqrt{2} \\ -1/\sqrt{2} \end{pmatrix}.$$

When $\rho > 0$, λ_1 is the largest eigenvalue and $\mathbf{v}_1$ lies along the $45°$ line through the point (μ_1, μ_2); the major axis is associated with λ_1. When $\rho < 0$, then λ_2 is the largest eigenvalue and the major axis of the constant density ellipse will lie along a straight line at right angles to the $45°$ line through (μ_1, μ_2). $\square$

Example 5.2.3. Suppose $\mathbf{x}$ has a bivariate normal distribution with mean and covariance respectively given by

$$\mu = \begin{pmatrix} 2 \\ 5 \end{pmatrix}, \text{ and } \Sigma = \begin{pmatrix} 2 & 1 \\ 1 & 1 \end{pmatrix},$$

so that we identify $\mu_1 = 2$, $\mu_2 = 5$, $\sigma_1 = \sqrt{2}$, $\sigma_2 = 1$, and $\rho = 1/\sqrt{2}$. We will find an ellipse which contains $\mathbf{x}$ with probability α, $0 < \alpha < 1$. For the bivariate normal distribution, we can write $(\mathbf{x} - \mu)'\Sigma^{-1}(\mathbf{x} - \mu)$ as

$$\left[\left(\tfrac{X_1-\mu_1}{\sigma_1}\right)^2 - 2\rho\left(\tfrac{X_1-\mu_1}{\sigma_1}\right)\left(\tfrac{X_2-\mu_2}{\sigma_2}\right) + \left(\tfrac{X_2-\mu_2}{\sigma_2}\right)^2\right]/(1-\rho^2),$$

so that, in this example, contours of equal density have the form

$$2\{\tfrac{1}{2}(X_1-2)^2 - (X_1-2)(X_2-5) + (X_2-5)^2\} = c^2.$$

The value of c corresponds to the upper (100α)th percentile of the chi-square distribution with 2 degrees of freedom (see (A6)) which is given as the value of u such that the chi-square cdf $F(u)$ is equal to α, i.e.,

$$c = -2\ln(1-\alpha).$$

By computing the contour for different α values, we generate the elliptical contours of the bivariate normal pdf. □

The pdf in (5.2.9) involves k parameters of location, and $k(k+1)/2$ distinct parameters that characterize Σ. Thus, for $k > 2$, tabulation of its distribution function is a formidable task! Tables corresponding to selected values of ρ for a bivariate normal distribution are found in Pearson's *Tables for Statisticians and Biometricians, Part 2*. The evaluation of the k-variate normal integral when $X_j > 0$, $j = 1, \cdots, k$ is of interest in some problems (see Gupta, 1963). Although simple analytical results do not exist when $k > 3$, it is possible to obtain a simple form of the solution in the special case when all the correlations are equal.

The existence of the pdf $f(\mathbf{x}; \mu, \Sigma)$ of $\mathbf{x}$ with respect to Lebesgue measure in $\mathcal{R}^k$ depends on the nature of Σ. In general, we distinguish between two cases with respect to the multivariate normal distribution. If Σ is p.d., then $r(\Sigma) = k$, and the density of $\mathbf{x}$ exists in $\mathcal{R}^k$. Note that $\mathbf{x} \sim N_k(\mu, \Sigma)$ if and only if $\mathbf{x} = \Gamma'\mathbf{z} + \mu$, where $\mathbf{z} \sim N_k(\mathbf{0}, \mathbf{I})$ and where $r(\Gamma') = k$. The inverse transformation, viz., $\mathbf{z} = (\Gamma')^{-1}(\mathbf{x} - \mu)$ exists, the Jacobian of the transformation being $|J| = |\Gamma'| = |\Sigma|^{-1/2}$ (since $\Sigma = \Gamma\Gamma'$). In this case, $f(\mathbf{x}; \mu, \Sigma)$ which we defined in (5.2.9) is the pdf of $\mathbf{x}$ with respect to Lebesgue measure in $\mathcal{R}^k$. If, on the other hand, Σ is not p.d., so that $r(\Sigma) = r < k$, then the inverse transformation $\mathbf{z} = (\Gamma')^{-1}(\mathbf{x} - \mu)$ does not exist and no explicit determination of the pdf of $\mathbf{x}$ with respect to Lebesgue measure in $\mathcal{R}^k$ exists. However, the pdf of $\mathbf{x}$ is concentrated on an r-dimensional hyperplane, and we say $\mathbf{x}$ has a singular normal distribution. We describe this in the following result and then give some examples of singular multivariate normal distributions.

Result 5.2.4. Let $E(\mathbf{x}) = \mu$, and $Var(\mathbf{x}) = \Sigma$, where Σ is a n.n.d. matrix of rank $r < k$. The following definitions of a singular normal distribution are equivalent.

(i) $\mathbf{x}$ is said to have a (singular) $N_k(\mu, \Sigma)$ distribution of rank r if it can be expressed as $\mathbf{x} \overset{d}{=} \mu + \mathbf{Bz}$, where $\mathbf{B}$ is a $k \times r$ matrix satisfying $\mathbf{BB}' = \Sigma$, and $\mathbf{z} \sim N_r(\mathbf{0}, \mathbf{I})$.

(ii) $\mathbf{x}$ is said to have a $N_k(\mu, \Sigma)$ distribution of rank r if

$$M_{\mathbf{x}}(\mathbf{t}) = \exp\{\mathbf{t}'\mu + \tfrac{1}{2}\mathbf{t}'\Sigma\mathbf{t}\}.$$

(iii) $\mathbf{x}$ is said to have a $N_k(\mu, \Sigma)$ distribution of rank r if every linear combination $\mathbf{c}'\mathbf{x}$, $(\mathbf{c} \neq \mathbf{0})$, has a $N(\mathbf{c}'\mu, \mathbf{c}'\Sigma\mathbf{c})$ distribution.

Proof. We first show that (i) implies (ii). Letting $\mathbf{a}' = \mathbf{t}'\mathbf{B}$, we see that

$$
\begin{aligned}
M_{\mathbf{x}}(\mathbf{t}) &= E\{\exp(\mathbf{t}'\mathbf{x})\} = E[\exp\{\mathbf{t}'(\mu + \mathbf{B}\mathbf{z})\}] \\
&= \exp(\mathbf{t}'\mu)E\{\exp(\mathbf{a}'\mathbf{z})\} = \exp\{\mathbf{t}'\mu + \frac{1}{2}\mathbf{a}'\mathbf{a}\} \\
&= \exp\{\mathbf{t}'\mu + \frac{1}{2}\mathbf{t}'\mathbf{B}\mathbf{B}'\mathbf{t}\} = \exp\{\mathbf{t}'\mu + \mathbf{t}'\Sigma\mathbf{t}\}.
\end{aligned}
$$

Next, it follows that (ii) implies (iii) since, setting $\mathbf{d}' = b\mathbf{a}'$, we see that

$$
\begin{aligned}
E\{\exp(b\mathbf{a}'\mathbf{x})\} &= E\{\exp(\mathbf{d}'\mathbf{x})\} = \exp(\mathbf{d}'\mu + \frac{1}{2}\mathbf{d}'\Sigma\mathbf{d}) \\
&= \exp\{b(\mathbf{a}'\mu) + \frac{1}{2}b^2(\mathbf{a}'\Sigma\mathbf{a})\}
\end{aligned}
$$

which implies that the univariate linear combination $\mathbf{a}'\mathbf{x}$ has a $N(\mathbf{a}'\mu, \mathbf{a}'\Sigma\mathbf{a})$ distribution. We see that (iii) implies (ii) since

$$E[\exp\{\mathbf{t}'\mathbf{x}\}] = E[\exp\{1.\mathbf{t}'\mathbf{x}\}] = \exp\{\mathbf{t}'\mu + \tfrac{1}{2}\mathbf{t}'\Sigma\mathbf{t}\}.$$

Again, (ii) implies (i) since

$$E\{\exp(\mathbf{t}'\mathbf{x})\} = \exp(\mathbf{t}'\mu + \tfrac{1}{2}\mathbf{t}'\Sigma\mathbf{t}) = \exp(\mathbf{t}'\mu + \tfrac{1}{2}\mathbf{t}'\mathbf{B}\mathbf{B}'\mathbf{t}).$$

Letting $\mathbf{a}' = \mathbf{t}'\mathbf{B}$, and since $\mathbf{z} \sim N_r(\mathbf{0}, \mathbf{I})$, we see that $E\{\exp(\mathbf{t}'\mathbf{x})\} = \exp\{\mathbf{t}'\mu\} \times \exp\{\tfrac{1}{2}\mathbf{a}'\mathbf{a}\} = \exp\{\mathbf{t}'\mu\}E\{\exp(\mathbf{t}'\mathbf{z})\} = E\{\exp(\mathbf{t}'\mu + \mathbf{a}'\mathbf{z})\} = E\{\exp(\mathbf{t}'\mu + \mathbf{t}'\mathbf{B}\mathbf{z})\} = E\{\exp[\mathbf{t}'(\mu + \mathbf{B}\mathbf{z})]\}$, which implies that $\mathbf{x} \overset{d}{=} \mu + \mathbf{B}\mathbf{z}$. For example, the bivariate normal distribution with $\rho = 1$ is singular. In this case, $X_1 = a + bX_2$, and the distribution is concentrated on a straight line. ∎

Example 5.2.4. When $k = 1$, Σ corresponds to a scalar, and a singular (univariate) normal distribution is obtained only if the variance is zero. The mgf of the normal random variable X is $M_X(t) = \exp(\mu t)$, which is the mgf of a random variable Y which is degenerate at μ, i.e., $P(Y = \mu) = 1$. That is, the singular normal distribution when $k = 1$ is a discrete distribution degenerate at a single value. When $k = 2$, we can verify that $\Sigma = \begin{pmatrix} \sigma_{11} & \sigma_{12} \\ \sigma_{12} & \sigma_{22} \end{pmatrix} > 0$ if and only if $\sigma_{11} > 0, \sigma_{22} > 0$, and $\sigma_{11}\sigma_{22} - \sigma_{12}^2 > 0$ (see the proof of Result 2.4.2). Bivariate singular normal distributions occur under the following four scenarios:

(i) $\sigma_{11} = \sigma_{22} = 0$ (so that $\sigma_{12} = 0$). Then, $\mathbf{x} \sim N_2(\mu, \mathbf{0})$, so that $\mathbf{x}$ is degenerate at $\mu = (\mu_1, \mu_2)'$.

(ii) $\sigma_{11} = 0, \sigma_{22} > 0$ (so that $\sigma_{12} = 0$). Then, $X_1 \sim N(\mu_1, 0)$, and is degenerate, while $X_2 \sim N(\mu_2, \sigma_{22})$ and is nondegenerate. Since a degenerate random variable is independent of any other random variable, X_1 and X_2 are independent.

(iii) $\sigma_{11} > 0, \sigma_{22} = 0$ (so that $\sigma_{12} = 0$). This case is similar to (ii), with the roles of X_1 and X_2 reversed.

(iv) $\sigma_{11} > 0, \sigma_{22} > 0$, and $\sigma_{11}\sigma_{22} = \sigma_{12}^2$. In this case, both X_1 and X_2 have nondegenerate distributions. However, we can verify that all the probability lies on a line $\sigma_{22}X_1 - \sigma_{12}X_2 = \sigma_{22}\mu_1 - \sigma_{12}\mu_2$, since $Var(\sigma_{22}X_1 - \sigma_{12}X_2) = 0$, from which it follows that $P(\sigma_{22}X_1 - \sigma_{12}X_2 = \sigma_{22}\mu_1 - \sigma_{12}\mu_2) = 1$.

An extension of the discussion for the bivariate case to $k = 3$ implies that all the probability lies either at a point, or on a line, or a plane, each of which is a subset of $\mathcal{R}^3$. For the general k-variate case, all the probability lies in any one of the lower-dimensional subspaces (sometimes called affine subspaces) of $\mathcal{R}^k$. In these cases, it is not possible to write down the pdf of $\mathbf{x}$.   □

In the proofs of many of the following results, we will use the mgf of the normal vector $\mathbf{x}$. There are two reasons for this, the first being that if Σ is not p.d., then there is no density function defined on $\mathcal{R}^k$, while the mgf exists. The second reason is that the mgf is a natural tool to use for derivation of the distributional results that we require. The next result states that a linear combination of multivariate normal vectors also has a multivariate normal distribution.

Result 5.2.5. Reproductive property. Suppose $\mathbf{x}_j$, $j = 1, \cdots, p$ are independently distributed as $N_k(\mu_j, \Sigma_j)$. Then

$$\sum_{j=1}^p a_j\mathbf{x}_j \sim N_k(\sum_{j=1}^p a_j\mu_j, \sum_{j=1}^p a_j^2\Sigma_j),$$

where a_j, $j = 1, \cdots, p$ are constants.

Proof. The mgf of $\mathbf{y} = \sum_{j=1}^p a_j\mathbf{x}_j$ is

$$M_{\mathbf{y}}(\mathbf{t}) = E\left[\exp\left\{\mathbf{t}'\sum_{j=1}^p a_j\mathbf{x}_j\right\}\right] = \prod_{j=1}^p E[\exp\{a_j\mathbf{t}'\mathbf{x}_j\}]$$

$$= \prod_{j=1}^p \exp\{\mathbf{t}'a_j\mu_j + \frac{1}{2}a_j^2\mathbf{t}'\Sigma_j\mathbf{t}\}$$

$$= \exp\{\mathbf{t}'(\sum_{j=1}^p a_j\mu_j) + \frac{1}{2}\sum_{j=1}^p \mathbf{t}'(a_j^2\Sigma_j)\mathbf{t}\}$$

from which the result follows by noting the form of the mgf of a normal vector in (5.2.7). ■

The following two results are widely used in linear model theory. They state that if a k-variate normal random vector is subject to a linear transformation, then the resulting vector also has a multivariate normal distribution of appropriate dimension. The usefulness of these results may be appreciated by recalling that in linear model theory, the least squares estimates (which correspond to the maximum likelihood estimates under normality) of the model parameters are linear functions of the response vector $\mathbf{y}$. The distributions of such estimators will be derived in Chapter 7 using the following results.

Result 5.2.6. Let $\mathbf{x} \sim N_k(\mu, \Sigma)$ where $r(\Sigma) = r \leq k$. For a given $q \times k$ matrix $\mathbf{B}$ of constants and a q-dimensional vector $\mathbf{b}$ of constants,

$$\mathbf{y} = \mathbf{B}\mathbf{x} + \mathbf{b} \sim N_q(\mathbf{B}\mu + \mathbf{b}, \mathbf{B}\Sigma\mathbf{B}'). \tag{5.2.14}$$

Proof. Let $\mathbf{t}' = (t_1, \cdots, t_q) \in \mathcal{R}^q$. Then

$$
\begin{aligned}
M_\mathbf{y}(\mathbf{t}) &= E\{\exp(\mathbf{t}'\mathbf{y})\} = E[\exp\{\mathbf{t}'(\mathbf{B}\mathbf{x} + \mathbf{b})\}] \\
&= \exp\{\mathbf{t}'\mathbf{b}\}E[\exp\{\mathbf{t}'\mathbf{B}\mathbf{x}\}] = \exp\{\mathbf{t}'\mathbf{b}\}M_\mathbf{x}(\mathbf{B}'\mathbf{t}) \\
&= \exp\{\mathbf{t}'(\mathbf{B}\mu + \mathbf{b}) + \tfrac{1}{2}\mathbf{t}'\mathbf{B}\Sigma\mathbf{B}'\mathbf{t}\},
\end{aligned}
\tag{5.2.15}
$$

which is the mgf of a normal random vector with mean $\mathbf{B}\mu + \mathbf{b}$ and variance-covariance matrix $\mathbf{B}\Sigma\mathbf{B}'$. ∎

An immediate consequence is that if $\mathbf{x} \sim N_k(\mu, \Sigma)$, then $\mathbf{x} - \mu \sim N_k(\mathbf{0}, \Sigma)$.

Result 5.2.7. The random vector $\mathbf{x} \sim N_k(\mu, \Sigma)$ if and only if every linear combination $\mathbf{c}'\mathbf{x}$ has a univariate $N(\mathbf{c}'\mu, \mathbf{c}'\Sigma\mathbf{c})$ distribution, where $\mathbf{c} \neq \mathbf{0}$ is a real vector. This technique of reducing a multivariate normal distribution into a univariate distribution is known as the Cramer-Wold technique.

Proof. Let $\mathbf{c}' = (c_1, \cdots, c_k)$, $\mathbf{P}\mathbf{P}' = \Sigma$, $\mathbf{z} \sim N_k(\mathbf{0}, \mathbf{I})$, and $\mathbf{d}' = t\mathbf{c}'\mathbf{P}$. Then $E[\exp\{t\mathbf{c}'\mathbf{x}\}] = E[\exp\{t\mathbf{c}'(\mu + \mathbf{P}\mathbf{z})\}] = \exp\{t\mathbf{c}'\mu\}E[\exp\{\mathbf{d}'\mathbf{z}\}] = \exp\{t\mathbf{c}'\mu + \tfrac{1}{2}\mathbf{d}'\mathbf{d}\}$ $= \exp\{t\mathbf{c}'\mu + \tfrac{1}{2}t^2\mathbf{c}'\mathbf{P}\mathbf{P}'\mathbf{c}\} = \exp\{t\mathbf{c}'\mu + \tfrac{1}{2}t^2\mathbf{c}'\Sigma\mathbf{c}\}$ so that $\mathbf{c}'\mathbf{x} \sim N(\mathbf{c}'\mu, \mathbf{c}'\Sigma\mathbf{c})$. To show the converse, we assume that every linear combination of $\mathbf{x}$ has a univariate normal distribution; in particular, let $\mathbf{c}' = \mathbf{t}' = (t_1, \cdots, t_k)$. Then,

$$E[\exp\{\mathbf{t}'\mathbf{x}\}] = E[\exp\{1.\mathbf{t}'\mathbf{x}\}] = \exp\{\mathbf{t}'\mu + \tfrac{1}{2}\mathbf{t}'\Sigma\mathbf{t}\},$$

which completes the proof. ∎

Example 5.2.5. Let $\mathbf{x} = (X_1, X_2, X_3)' \sim N_3(\mu, \Sigma)$. We use Result 5.2.6 to find the distribution of

$$\mathbf{B}\mathbf{x} = \begin{pmatrix} X_1 - X_2 \\ X_2 - X_3 \end{pmatrix} = \begin{pmatrix} 1 & -1 & 0 \\ 0 & 1 & -1 \end{pmatrix} \begin{pmatrix} X_1 \\ X_2 \\ X_3 \end{pmatrix}.$$

This vector clearly has a bivariate normal distribution with mean

$$\mathbf{B}\mu = \begin{pmatrix} 1 & -1 & 0 \\ 0 & 1 & -1 \end{pmatrix} \begin{pmatrix} \mu_1 \\ \mu_2 \\ \mu_3 \end{pmatrix} = \begin{pmatrix} \mu_1 - \mu_2 \\ \mu_2 - \mu_3 \end{pmatrix}$$

and covariance matrix

$$\mathbf{B}\Sigma\mathbf{B}' = \begin{pmatrix} 1 & -1 & 0 \\ 0 & 1 & -1 \end{pmatrix} \begin{pmatrix} \sigma_{11} & \sigma_{12} & \sigma_{13} \\ \sigma_{12} & \sigma_{22} & \sigma_{23} \\ \sigma_{13} & \sigma_{23} & \sigma_{33} \end{pmatrix} \begin{pmatrix} 1 & 0 \\ -1 & 1 \\ 0 & -1 \end{pmatrix}. \quad \Box$$

Example 5.2.6. Let $\mathbf{x} = (X_1, \cdots, X_n)' \sim N_n(\mu\mathbf{1}_n, \sigma^2\mathbf{I}_n)$. Note that $\mathbf{x}$ represents a "random sample" of size n from a normal population with mean μ and variance σ^2. Then $\overline{X} = \sum_{i=1}^n X_i/n = \mathbf{c}'\mathbf{x}$, whére $\mathbf{c}' = \mathbf{1}'/n$. It is easily verified that $\mathbf{c}'\mu = \sum_{i=1}^n \mu/n = \mu$, and $\mathbf{c}'\Sigma\mathbf{c} = \sigma^2/n$. By Result 5.2.7, $\overline{X}$ is a linear function of $\mathbf{x}$, and has a $N(\mu, \sigma^2/n)$ distribution. $\Box$

Definition 5.2.3.   Let $\mathbf{y}_1 = \mathbf{A}_1\mathbf{x}$ and $\mathbf{y}_2 = \mathbf{A}_2\mathbf{x}$ denote two linear functions of a random vector $\mathbf{x} \sim N_k(\mu, \Sigma)$. The covariance between $\mathbf{y}_1$ and $\mathbf{y}_2$ is given by

$$Cov(\mathbf{y}_1, \mathbf{y}_2) = \mathbf{A}_1\Sigma\mathbf{A}_2'.$$

Definition 5.2.3 enables us to obtain conditions under which linear forms in a normal random vector are independently distributed. For example, let $\mathbf{x} \sim N_k(\mu, \sigma^2\mathbf{I})$. We can verify that a necessary and sufficient condition for nonzero linear forms $\mathbf{a}'\mathbf{x}$ and $\mathbf{b}'\mathbf{x}$ to be independently distributed is $\mathbf{a}'\mathbf{b} = 0$.

Example 5.2.7. Let $\mathbf{x} \sim N_k(\mathbf{0}, \sigma^2\mathbf{I})$. We show that $\mathbf{y}_1 = \mathbf{A}\mathbf{x}$ and $\mathbf{y}_2 = (\mathbf{I} - \mathbf{A}^-\mathbf{A})'\mathbf{x}$ are independently normally distributed, where $\mathbf{A}^-$ denotes a g-inverse of the $q \times k$ matrix $\mathbf{A}$. That $\mathbf{y}_1$ and $\mathbf{y}_2$ have normal distributions is immediate from Result 5.2.6. We see that $\mathbf{A}\mathbf{x} \sim N_q(\mathbf{0}, \sigma^2\mathbf{A}\mathbf{A}')$, while $\mathbf{y}_2 \sim N_k(\mathbf{0}, \sigma^2(\mathbf{I} - \mathbf{A}^-\mathbf{A})'(\mathbf{I} - \mathbf{A}^-\mathbf{A}))$. Also,

$$Cov\{\mathbf{A}\mathbf{x}, (\mathbf{I} - \mathbf{A}^-\mathbf{A})'\mathbf{x}\} = \sigma^2\mathbf{A}(\mathbf{I} - \mathbf{A}^-\mathbf{A}) = \mathbf{0}$$

using Definition 3.1.1. $\Box$

Result 5.2.8. Let $\mathbf{x} \sim N_k(\mu, \Sigma)$. Suppose we partition $\mathbf{x}$ as $\mathbf{x}' = (\mathbf{x}_1', \mathbf{x}_2')'$ where $\mathbf{x}_1' = (X_1, \cdots, X_q)$ is a q-dimensional vector, and $\mathbf{x}_2' = (X_{q+1}, \cdots, X_k)$ is a $(k - q)$-dimensional vector. We partition μ and Σ conformably. That is, let $\mu' = (\mu_1', \mu_2')$ where $\mu_1' = (\mu_1, \cdots, \mu_q)$ is a q-dimensional vector, and $\mu_2' = (\mu_{q+1}, \cdots, \mu_k)$ is a $(k - q)$-dimensional vector. We let $\Sigma = \begin{pmatrix} \Sigma_{11} & \Sigma_{12} \\ \Sigma_{21} & \Sigma_{22} \end{pmatrix}$ where Σ_{11}, Σ_{12}, Σ_{21}, and Σ_{22} are respectively $q \times q$, $q \times (k - q)$, $(k - q) \times q$, and $(k - q) \times (k - q)$ submatrices. The marginal distribution of the subvector $\mathbf{x}_1$ is $N_q(\mu_1, \Sigma_{11})$, while the marginal distribution of the subvector $\mathbf{x}_2$ is $N_{k-q}(\mu_2, \Sigma_{22})$.

Proof. We first derive the marginal distribution of $\mathbf{x}_1$. Since $\mathbf{x}$ has a $N_k(\mu, \Sigma)$ distribution, applying Result 5.2.6 with the $q \times k$ matrix $\mathbf{B} = \begin{pmatrix} \mathbf{I}_q & \mathbf{0} \end{pmatrix}$ and the q-dimensional vector $\mathbf{b} = \mathbf{0}$, we see that $\mathbf{B}\mu = \mu_1$, and $\mathbf{B}\Sigma\mathbf{B}' = \Sigma_{11}$. It directly follows that $\mathbf{x}_1$ has a $N_q(\mu_1, \Sigma_{11})$ distribution. The marginal distribution of $\mathbf{x}_2$ follows similarly by setting the $(k - q) \times k$ matrix $\mathbf{B} = \begin{pmatrix} \mathbf{0} & \mathbf{I}_{k-q} \end{pmatrix}$ and the $(k - q)$-dimensional vector $\mathbf{b} = \mathbf{0}$. ∎

It is clear from Result 5.2.8 that all subsets of a multivariate normal random vector themselves have normal distributions. The mean and variance of the normal distribution of a particular subvector of $\mathbf{x}$ is, in fact, obtained by simply selecting appropriate elements from μ and Σ.

Example 5.2.8. Let $\mathbf{x} \sim N_4(\mu, \Sigma)$, where

$$\mu' = \begin{pmatrix} 2 & 3 & 0 & -1 \end{pmatrix} \text{ and } \Sigma = \begin{pmatrix} 4 & 1 & 0 & -1 \\ 1 & 3 & 0 & 2 \\ 0 & 0 & 2 & 0 \\ -1 & 2 & 0 & 5 \end{pmatrix}.$$

We first note that Σ is p.d., since all its principal minors are positive. We will find the distribution of $\mathbf{x}_1 = (X_2, X_4)'$. By Result 5.2.8, we see that $\mathbf{x}_1$ has a bivariate normal distribution with $\mu_1' = \begin{pmatrix} 3 & -1 \end{pmatrix}$ and $\Sigma_{11} = \begin{pmatrix} 3 & 2 \\ 2 & 5 \end{pmatrix}$. Since the off-diagonal elements of Σ_{11} are nonzero, the random variables X_2 and X_4 are dependent. □

Result 5.2.9. Suppose $\mathbf{x} \sim N_k(\mu, \Sigma)$, which we partition as $\mathbf{x}' = (\mathbf{x}_1', \cdots, \mathbf{x}_m')'$, $\mathbf{x}_j$ being a q_j-dimensional subvector, for $j = 1, \cdots, m$, and $\sum_{j=1}^{m} q_j = k$. Suppose we partition μ and Σ conformably. Then, $\mathbf{x}_1, \cdots, \mathbf{x}_m$ are jointly independently distributed if and only if $\Sigma_{ij} = \mathbf{0}$, for $i \neq j$, $i, j = 1, \cdots, m$.

Proof. First, suppose $\Sigma_{ij} = \mathbf{0}$, for $i \neq j$, $i, j = 1, \cdots, m$. Then,

$$
\begin{aligned}
M_{\mathbf{x}}(\mathbf{t}) &= \exp\{\mathbf{t}'\mu + \frac{1}{2}\mathbf{t}'\Sigma\mathbf{t}\} \\
&= \exp\{\sum_{j=1}^{m}\mathbf{t}_j'\mu_j + \frac{1}{2}\sum_{i=1}^{m}\sum_{j=1}^{m}\mathbf{t}_i'\Sigma_{ij}\mathbf{t}_j\} \\
&= \prod_{j=1}^{m}\exp\{\mathbf{t}_j'\mu_j + \frac{1}{2}\mathbf{t}_j'\Sigma_{jj}\mathbf{t}_j\} \\
&= \prod_{j=1}^{m}M_{\mathbf{x}_j}(\mathbf{t}_j), \quad\quad\quad (5.2.16)
\end{aligned}
$$

so that, by (5.1.7), $\mathbf{x}_1, \cdots, \mathbf{x}_m$ are jointly independently distributed. To prove the converse, if we assume that $\mathbf{x}_1, \cdots, \mathbf{x}_m$ are jointly independently distributed, then

$$\Sigma_{ij} = E[(\mathbf{x}_i - \mu_i)(\mathbf{x}_j - \mu_j)'] = [E(\mathbf{x}_i - \mu_i)][E(\mathbf{x}_j - \mu_j)'] = \mathbf{0}, \quad (5.2.17)$$

which proves the result.   ■

Example 5.2.8. (continued).   We will verify that $\mathbf{x}_1 = (X_1, X_2)'$ and $\mathbf{x}_2 = X_3$ are independently distributed. Once again, from Result 5.2.8, we see that the distribution of $\mathbf{x}_{(1)} = (X_1, X_2, X_3)'$ is a trivariate normal with mean and covariance given by

$$\mu_{(1)} = \begin{pmatrix} 2 \\ 3 \\ 0 \end{pmatrix}, \text{ and } \Sigma_{(1)} = \begin{pmatrix} 4 & 1 & 0 \\ 1 & 3 & 0 \\ 0 & 0 & 2 \end{pmatrix}.$$

In the notation of Result 5.2.9, this gives $\Sigma_{12} = \begin{pmatrix} 0 \\ 0 \end{pmatrix}$, so that $\mathbf{x}_1$ and $\mathbf{x}_2$ are independent.   □

Result 5.2.10. Let $\mathbf{x} \sim N_k(\mu, \Sigma)$ with $r(\Sigma) = k$. Suppose we partition $\mathbf{x}$ as $\mathbf{x}' = (\mathbf{x}_1', \mathbf{x}_2')$, where $\mathbf{x}_1$ is a q-dimensional subvector, $0 < q < k$, $\mathbf{x}_2$ is $(k - q)$-dimensional, and suppose that μ and Σ are partitioned conformably. The conditional distribution of $\mathbf{x}_1$ given that $\mathbf{x}_2 = \mathbf{c}_2$ is multivariate normal with mean vector

$$\mu_{1.2} = \mu_1 + \Sigma_{12}\Sigma_{22}^{-1}(\mathbf{c}_2 - \mu_2) \qquad (5.2.18)$$

and variance-covariance matrix

$$\Sigma_{11.2} = \Sigma_{11} - \Sigma_{12}\Sigma_{22}^{-1}\Sigma_{21}. \qquad (5.2.19)$$

Proof. Let $f(\mathbf{x}_1, \mathbf{x}_2)$ denote the joint pdf of $\mathbf{x}$, and $f_1(\mathbf{x}_1)$ and $f_2(\mathbf{x}_2)$ denote the marginal pdfs of $\mathbf{x}_1$ and $\mathbf{x}_2$ respectively. The conditional pdf of $\mathbf{x}_1$ given $\mathbf{x}_2 = \mathbf{c}_2$, provided $f_2(\mathbf{c}_2) > 0$ is

$$g(\mathbf{x}_1 | \mathbf{x}_2 = \mathbf{c}_2) = \frac{f(\mathbf{x}_1, \mathbf{c}_2)}{f_2(\mathbf{c}_2)}$$

$$= \frac{(2\pi)^{-k/2}|\Sigma|^{-1/2} \exp\left[-\frac{1}{2}\begin{pmatrix} \mathbf{x}_1 - \mu_1 \\ \mathbf{c}_2 - \mu_2 \end{pmatrix}' \begin{pmatrix} \Sigma_{11} & \Sigma_{12} \\ \Sigma_{21} & \Sigma_{22} \end{pmatrix}^{-1} \begin{pmatrix} \mathbf{x}_1 - \mu_1 \\ \mathbf{c}_2 - \mu_2 \end{pmatrix}\right]}{(2\pi)^{-(k-q)/2}|\Sigma_{22}|^{-1/2} \exp[-\frac{1}{2}(\mathbf{c}_2 - \mu_2)'\Sigma_{22}^{-1}(\mathbf{c}_2 - \mu_2)]}$$

Substituting for Σ^{-1} using Result 2.1.3 as

$$\begin{pmatrix} \Sigma_{11} & \Sigma_{12} \\ \Sigma_{21} & \Sigma_{22} \end{pmatrix}^{-1} = \begin{pmatrix} \Sigma_{11.2}^{-1} & -\Sigma_{11.2}^{-1}\Sigma_{12}\Sigma_{22}^{-1} \\ -\Sigma_{22}^{-1}\Sigma_{21}\Sigma_{11.2}^{-1} & \Sigma_{22.1}^{-1} \end{pmatrix}$$

$$= \begin{pmatrix} \Sigma_{11.2}^{-1} & -\Sigma_{11}^{-1}\Sigma_{12}\Sigma_{22.1}^{-1} \\ -\Sigma_{22.1}^{-1}\Sigma_{21}\Sigma_{11}^{-1} & \Sigma_{22.1}^{-1} \end{pmatrix}$$

where $\Sigma_{11.2} = \Sigma_{11} - \Sigma_{12}\Sigma_{22}^{-1}\Sigma_{21}$ and $\Sigma_{22.1} = \Sigma_{22} - \Sigma_{21}\Sigma_{11}^{-1}\Sigma_{12}$. We obtain

$$g(\mathbf{x}_1 | \mathbf{x}_2 = \mathbf{c}_2) = (2\pi)^{-q/2}|\Sigma_{22}|^{1/2}|\Sigma|^{-1/2} \exp\{-\frac{1}{2}(Q - Q_2)\}$$

where

$$Q = (\mathbf{x}_1 - \mu_1)'\Sigma_{11\cdot2}^{-1}(\mathbf{x}_1 - \mu_1) - (\mathbf{x}_1 - \mu_1)'\Sigma_{11\cdot2}^{-1}\Sigma_{12}\Sigma_{22}^{-1}(\mathbf{c}_2 - \mu_2)$$
$$-(\mathbf{c}_2 - \mu_2)'\Sigma_{22}^{-1}\Sigma_{21}\Sigma_{11\cdot2}^{-1}(\mathbf{x}_1 - \mu_1) + (\mathbf{c}_2 - \mu_2)'\Sigma_{22\cdot1}^{-1}(\mathbf{c}_2 - \mu_2)$$

and

$$Q_2 = (\mathbf{c}_2 - \mu_2)'\Sigma_{22}^{-1}(\mathbf{c}_2 - \mu_2)$$

so that

$$Q - Q_2 = [(\mathbf{x}_1 - \mu_1) - \Sigma_{12}\Sigma_{22}^{-1}(\mathbf{c}_2 - \mu_2)]'\Sigma_{11\cdot2}^{-1}[(\mathbf{x}_1 - \mu_1) - \Sigma_{12}\Sigma_{22}^{-1}(\mathbf{c}_2 - \mu_2)].$$

From Result 2.1.2, $|\Sigma| = |\Sigma_{22}||\Sigma_{11\cdot2}|$, so that

$$g(\mathbf{x}_1|\mathbf{x}_2 = \mathbf{c}_2) = (2\pi)^{-q/2}|\Sigma_{11\cdot2}|^{-1/2}\exp\{-\tfrac{1}{2}(\mathbf{x}_1 - \mu_{1\cdot2})'\Sigma_{11\cdot2}^{-1}(\mathbf{x}_1 - \mu_{1\cdot2})\}.$$

By (5.2.9), this is a normal pdf with mean $\mu_{1\cdot2}$ and covariance $\Sigma_{11\cdot2}$, which completes the proof. ∎

Example 5.2.9. Let $\mathbf{x} = (X_1, X_2, X_3)' \sim N_3(\mathbf{0}, \Sigma)$, where

$$\Sigma = \begin{pmatrix} 4 & 1 & 0 \\ 1 & 2 & 1 \\ 0 & 1 & 3 \end{pmatrix}.$$

We illustrate the computation of marginal and conditional distributions as well as distributions of a linear combination of the components of $\mathbf{x}$. By Result 5.2.8, we see that $X_1 \sim N(0, 4)$, $X_2 \sim N(0, 2)$, and $X_3 \sim N(0, 3)$. The marginal distribution of the vector $(X_2, X_3)'$ is bivariate normal with mean vector and covariance matrix given respectively by

$$\begin{pmatrix} 0 \\ 0 \end{pmatrix} \text{ and } \begin{pmatrix} 2 & 1 \\ 1 & 3 \end{pmatrix}.$$

From Result 5.2.10, we see that the conditional distribution of $(X_1|X_2 = x_2, X_3 = x_3)$ is univariate normal with mean and variance given respectively by (see (5.2.18) and (5.2.19)):

$$E(X_1|X_2 = x_2, X_3 = x_3) = (3x_2 - x_3)/5, \text{ and}$$
$$Var(X_1|X_2 = x_2, X_3 = x_3) = 17/5.$$

To find the distribution of a linear function of $\mathbf{x}$, viz., $Y = 4X_1 - 6X_2 + X_3 - 18$, we use Result 5.2.6 with $q = 1$, $\mathbf{B} = (4, -6, 1)$, and $b = -18$. Then, $Y \sim N(-18, 79)$. □

Definition 5.2.4. Simple correlation coefficient. Suppose the random vector $\mathbf{x} = (X_1, \cdots, X_k)'$ has a $N_k(\mu, \Sigma)$ distribution. The simple correlation between any two random variables X_i and X_j is defined by

$$\rho_{ij} = \frac{Cov(X_i, X_j)}{[Var(X_i)Var(X_j)]^{1/2}} = \frac{\sigma_{ij}}{\sqrt{\sigma_{ii}\sigma_{jj}}}, \tag{5.2.20}$$

provided $\sigma_{ii} > 0$ and $\sigma_{jj} > 0$. If either term in the denominator is zero, then ρ_{ij} is undefined.

For a collection of algebraic, geometric, and trigonometric interpretations of the simple correlation coefficient, see Rodgers and Nicewander (1988).

Result 5.2.11. The simple correlation coefficient satisfies the inequality $-1 \leq \rho_{ij} \leq 1$, with $|\rho_{ij}| = 1$ if and only if there exist constants $a \neq 0$ and b such that $P(X_j = aX_i + b) = 1$. If $\rho_{ij} = 1$, then $a > 0$, and if $\rho_{ij} = -1$, then $a < 0$.

Proof. For every real constant c, we have $E[(X_j - \mu_j) - c(X_i - \mu_i)]^2 \geq 0$, which implies that the discriminant of the nonnegative quadratic function $Var(X_j) - 2cCov(X_i, X_j) + c^2 Var(X_i)$ is nonpositive, i.e., $4[Cov(X_i, X_j)]^2 - 4Var(X_i)Var(X_j) \leq 0$. This implies that $[Cov(X_i, X_j)]^2 / Var(X_i)Var(X_j) \leq 1$, or $\rho_{ij}^2 \leq 1$, from which it follows that $-1 \leq \rho_{ij} \leq 1$. This result may also be proved as a direct consequence of the Cauchy-Schwarz inequality which we defined in Result 1.2.1. Also, $|\rho_{ij}| = 1$ if and only if the discriminant is equal to zero, i.e., the quadratic function $E[(X_j - \mu_j) - c(X_i - \mu_i)]^2$ has a single root. Since $[(X_j - \mu_j) - c(X_i - \mu_i)] \geq 0$, the expected value $E[(X_j - \mu_j) - c(X_i - \mu_i)]^2 = 0$ if and only if

$$P\{[(X_j - \mu_j) - c(X_i - \mu_i)]^2 = 0\} = 1,$$

which is equivalent to

$$P\{[(X_j - \mu_j) - c(X_i - \mu_i)] = 0\} = 1.$$

That is, $P(X_j = aX_i + b) = 1$ with $a = c$, and $b = \mu_j - c\mu_i$. The single root of the quadratic function is $c = Cov(X_i, X_j) / Var(X_i)$, so that if $\rho_{ij} = 1$, then $a > 0$, while if $\rho_{ij} = -1$, then $a < 0$. ■

Result 5.2.12. If X_i and X_j are independent random variables, then $\rho_{ij} = 0$.

Proof. If X_i and X_j are independent, $E(X_i X_j) = E(X_i)E(X_j)$. Hence,

$$Cov(X_i, X_j) = E(X_i X_j) - E(X_i)E(X_j) = 0,$$

and using (5.2.20), it follows that $\rho_{ij} = 0$. ■

Note that if X_i and X_j are uncorrelated, they need not necessarily be independent. The covariance and correlation measure only a particular kind of *linear* relationship between X_i and X_j. In Example 5.2.10, we present two dependent random variables with zero correlation. In Example 5.2.1, we defined the bivariate normal distribution of $\mathbf{x} = (X_1, X_2)$ with correlation ρ between X_1 and X_2. In Example 5.2.11, we show that for this normal case, $\rho = 0$ does indeed imply independence of X_1 and X_2. ■

Example 5.2.10. Let the joint pdf of X_1 and X_2 be uniform on the square with vertices $(-1, 0)$, $(0, 1)$, $(1, 0)$, and $(0, -1)$. By symmetry of the marginal distributions, we see that $E(X_1) = E(X_2) = 0$. Since the contributions from the domains with $x_1 x_2 > 0$ and $x_1 x_2 < 0$ cancel each other in the integral $\int_{-\infty}^{\infty} \int_{-\infty}^{\infty} x_1 x_2 f(x_1, x_2) dx_1 dx_2$, we see that $E(X_1 X_2) = 0$, and hence $\rho_{12} = 0$. Yet, these two random variables are dependent. $\square$

Example 5.2.11. (a) In the definition of the bivariate normal distribution for $\mathbf{x} = (X_1, X_2)'$ given in Example 5.2.1, let $\rho = 0$. Then, $\Sigma = \begin{pmatrix} \sigma_1^2 & 0 \\ 0 & \sigma_2^2 \end{pmatrix}$, $|\Sigma| = \sigma_1^2 \sigma_2^2$, and $\Sigma^{-1} = \begin{pmatrix} 1/\sigma_1^2 & 0 \\ 0 & 1/\sigma_2^2 \end{pmatrix}$, so that (5.2.12) becomes

$$f(x_1, x_2) = (2\pi \sigma_1 \sigma_2)^{-1} \exp\left\{-(x_1 - \mu_1)^2 / 2\sigma_1^2\right\} \exp\left\{-(x_2 - \mu_2)^2 / 2\sigma_2^2\right\}$$

for $-\infty < x_1 < \infty$, and $-\infty < x_2 < \infty$, which is the product of two univariate normal pdfs (see (A1)), indicating independence of X_1 and X_2.

(b) Let $\mathbf{x}$ have a k-variate normal distribution with mean vector μ and covariance matrix $\mathbf{I}_k$. Consider $Y_1 = \mathbf{a}'\mathbf{x}$, $Y_2 = \mathbf{b}'\mathbf{x}$, with $\mathbf{a}'\mathbf{b} = 0$. By Result 5.2.7, $\mathbf{y} = (Y_1, Y_2)'$ has a bivariate normal distribution with mean vector $(\mathbf{a}'\mu, \mathbf{b}'\mu)'$, and covariance matrix $\Sigma = \begin{pmatrix} \mathbf{a}'\mathbf{a} & 0 \\ 0 & \mathbf{b}'\mathbf{b} \end{pmatrix}$, since $\mathbf{a}'\mathbf{b} = 0$. The joint distribution of $\mathbf{y}$ factors into the marginal distributions of Y_1 and Y_2, so that Y_1 and Y_2 are independent. $\square$

Result 5.2.13. For any two random variables X_i and X_j with respective means μ_i and μ_j and correlation ρ_{ij},

$$Var(aX_i + bX_j) = a^2 Var(X_i) + b^2 Var(X_j) + 2ab\rho_{ij}\sqrt{Var(X_i)Var(X_j)}.$$
$$(5.2.21)$$

If X_i and X_j are independent, then

$$Var(aX_i + bX_j) = a^2 Var(X_i) + b^2 Var(X_j). \qquad (5.2.22)$$

Proof. Since $E(aX_i + bX_j) = a\mu_i + b\mu_j$, we see that

$$\begin{aligned}
Var(aX_i + bX_j) &= E[\{(aX_i + bX_j) - (a\mu_i + b\mu_j)\}^2] \\
&= E[\{a(X_i - \mu_i) + b(X_j - \mu_j)\}^2] \\
&= a^2 E(X_i - \mu_i)^2 + b^2 E(X_j - \mu_j)^2 + 2ab E(X_i - \mu_i)(X_j - \mu_j) \\
&= a^2 Var(X_i) + b^2 Var(X_j) + 2ab Cov(X_i, X_j)
\end{aligned}$$

and we get (5.2.21) using the definition in (5.2.20). Equation (5.2.22) follows directly from Result 5.2.12. ∎

Definition 5.2.5. Correlation matrix. Let $\mathbf{x} = (X_1, \cdots, X_k)'$ be a random vector with componentwise means μ_i, $i = 1, \cdots, k$, and pairwise correlations ρ_{ij},

$i, j = 1, \cdots, k$. The $k \times k$ symmetric matrix $\mathbf{R} = \{\rho_{ij}\}$ is called the correlation matrix of $\mathbf{x}$. Each diagonal element of $\mathbf{R}$ is equal to 1, while each off-diagonal element lies between -1 and 1.

Result 5.2.14. The correlation matrix $\mathbf{R}$ is nonnegative definite.

Proof. The variance covariance matrix Σ of $\mathbf{x}$ is nonnegative definite. Let $\mathbf{D}$ be a diagonal matrix with ith diagonal element $\sigma_{ii}^{-1/2}$, $i = 1, \cdots k$, where $\sigma_{ii} = Var(X_i)$. We can write $\mathbf{R} = \mathbf{D}'\Sigma\mathbf{D}$, from which it follows that $\mathbf{R}$ too is n.n.d. ∎

Example 5.2.12.   Let $\mathbf{x} = (X_1, X_2, X_3, X_4)' \sim N_4(\mu, \Sigma)$ where

$$\mu = \begin{pmatrix} 1 \\ 2 \\ -1 \\ 3 \end{pmatrix} \text{ and } \Sigma = \begin{pmatrix} 2 & 0 & 1 & -1 \\ 0 & 3 & 0 & 2 \\ 1 & 0 & 5 & 0 \\ -1 & 2 & 0 & 3 \end{pmatrix}.$$

It is easy to verify that $\rho_{11} = \rho_{22} = \rho_{33} = \rho_{44} = 1$, $\rho_{12} = \rho_{23} = \rho_{34} = 0$, $\rho_{13} = 1/\sqrt{10}$, $\rho_{14} = -1/\sqrt{6}$, and $\rho_{24} = 2/3$. The correlation matrix is

$$\mathbf{R} = \begin{pmatrix} 1 & 0 & 1/\sqrt{10} & -1/\sqrt{6} \\ 0 & 1 & 0 & 2/3 \\ 1/\sqrt{10} & 0 & 1 & 0 \\ -1/\sqrt{6} & 2/3 & 0 & 1 \end{pmatrix}. \quad \square$$

Definition 5.2.6. Fisher's z-transformation of ρ_{ij}.   The z-transformation or the arctanh transformation of ρ_{ij} is

$$\delta_{ij} = \tfrac{1}{2}\log_e\left[(1 + \rho_{ij})/(1 - \rho_{ij})\right] = \operatorname{arctanh}(\rho_{ij}).$$

In Chapter 6, we describe sampling from a multivariate normal distribution and properties of various sample statistics that arise in this context. In particular, we will consider Fisher's z-transformation of the sample correlation coefficient and derive its distribution. This finds use in linear model theory for conducting inference on ρ_{ij}.

Definition 5.2.7. Partial correlation coefficient.   Suppose the random vector $\mathbf{x} = (X_1, \cdots, X_k)'$ has a $N_k(\mu, \Sigma)$ distribution, and suppose we partition $\mathbf{x}$ as $\mathbf{x}' = (\mathbf{x}_1', \mathbf{x}_2')'$ where $\mathbf{x}_1' = (X_1, \cdots, X_q)$ is a q-dimensional vector, and $\mathbf{x}_2' = (X_{q+1}, \cdots, X_k)$ is a $(k - q)$-dimensional vector. We partition μ and Σ conformably, as in Result 5.2.8. Let X_j and X_l be components of the subvector $\mathbf{x}_1$. The partial correlation coefficient of X_j and X_l given $\mathbf{x}_2 = \mathbf{c}_2$ is defined by

$$\rho_{jl|(q+1,\cdots,k)} = \frac{\sigma_{jl|(q+1,\cdots,k)}}{\{\sigma_{jj|(q+1,\cdots,k)}\sigma_{ll|(q+1,\cdots,k)}\}^{1/2}}, \qquad (5.2.23)$$

provided the expressions in the denominator are nonzero, and where $\sigma_{jl|(q+1,\cdots,k)}$ is the (j, l)th element in $\Sigma_{11.2} = \Sigma_{11} - \Sigma_{12}\Sigma_{22}^{-1}\Sigma_{21}$.

Result 5.2.15. A partial correlation coefficient defined by (5.2.23) satisfies

$$-1 \leq \rho_{ij|(q+1,\cdots,k)} \leq 1. \tag{5.2.24}$$

Proof. This follows directly from the Cauchy-Schwarz inequality (see Result 1.2.1). ∎

Example 5.2.13. Continuing with Example 5.2.12, we compute the partial correlations between components of $\mathbf{x}$. To compute $\rho_{12(3,4)}$ given Σ, we first compute the conditional covariance matrix of $(X_1, X_2|X_3, X_4)$ as

$$\begin{pmatrix} 2 & 0 \\ 0 & 3 \end{pmatrix} - \begin{pmatrix} 1 & -1 \\ 0 & 2 \end{pmatrix} \begin{pmatrix} 5 & 0 \\ 0 & 3 \end{pmatrix}^{-1} \begin{pmatrix} 1 & 0 \\ -1 & 2 \end{pmatrix} = \begin{pmatrix} 22/15 & 2/3 \\ 2/3 & 5/3 \end{pmatrix}.$$

Hence, $\rho_{12(3,4)} = \dfrac{2/3}{\sqrt{22/15}\sqrt{5/3}} = \sqrt{\frac{2}{11}}$. The other partial correlations may be computed similarly. □

Definition 5.2.8. Multiple correlation coefficient. Suppose the random vector $(X_0, X_1, \cdots, X_k)'$ has a $N_{k+1}(\mu, \Sigma)$ distribution, and suppose

$$\mathbf{x} = \begin{pmatrix} X_0 \\ \mathbf{x}^{(1)} \end{pmatrix}, \quad \mu = \begin{pmatrix} \mu_0 \\ \mu^{(1)} \end{pmatrix}, \quad \text{and } \Sigma = \begin{pmatrix} \sigma_{00} & \sigma_{01} \\ \sigma_{10} & \Sigma^{(1)} \end{pmatrix},$$

where $\mathbf{x}^{(1)} = (X_1, \cdots, X_k)'$, $\mu^{(1)} = (\mu_1, \cdots, \mu_k)'$, $\Sigma^{(1)}$ is the lower $k \times k$ submatrix of Σ, $\sigma_{10} = (\sigma_{10}, \cdots \sigma_{k0})'$ is a k-dimensional vector consisting of covariances between X_0 and $X_1, \cdots, X_k$, and $\sigma_{01} = \sigma'_{10}$. The multiple correlation coefficient of X_0 and $\mathbf{x}^{(1)}$ is

$$\rho_{0(1,\cdots,k)} = \frac{Cov(W, X_0)}{\{Var(W)Var(X_0)\}^{1/2}}, \tag{5.2.25}$$

where $W = \mu_0 + \sigma_{01}[\Sigma^{(1)}]^{-1}(\mathbf{x}^{(1)} - \mu^{(1)})$. A computationally simple formula is given by

$$\rho_{0(1,\cdots,k)} = \{\frac{\sigma_{01}[\Sigma^{(1)}]^{-1}\sigma_{10}}{\sigma_{00}}\}^{1/2}. \tag{5.2.26}$$

Example 5.2.14. We continue with Example 5.2.12, and compute $\rho_{1(2,3)}$, the multiple correlation coefficient of X_1 and (X_2, X_3) using (5.2.26). First, we find the marginal distribution of (X_1, X_2, X_3). From Result 5.2.8, this distribution is normal with mean and variance given by

$$\begin{pmatrix} 1 \\ 2 \\ -1 \end{pmatrix} \quad \text{and} \quad \begin{pmatrix} 2 & 0 & 1 \\ 0 & 3 & 0 \\ 1 & 0 & 5 \end{pmatrix}.$$

Further, $\sigma_{11} = Var(X_1) = 2$, $\sigma_{12} = (\sigma_{12}, \sigma_{13})' = (0,1)$, and $\Sigma^{(1)} = \begin{pmatrix} 3 & 0 \\ 0 & 5 \end{pmatrix}$. Therefore, $\rho_{1(2,3)} = 0$. Next, using (5.2.26), we compute

$$\rho_{1(2,3,4)} = \sqrt{3/5}. \quad \square$$

Result 5.2.16. Suppose $(X_0, X_1, \cdots, X_k)$ has a $N_{k+1}(\mu, \Sigma)$ distribution, and suppose it is partitioned as in Definition 5.2.8. Let $\sigma^2 = \sigma_{00} - \sigma_{01}[\Sigma^{(1)}]^{-1}\sigma_{10}$ denote the conditional variance $Var(X_0|X_1 = x_1, \cdots, X_k = x_k)$. Then, the multiple correlation coefficient can be computed as

$$\rho_{0(1,\cdots,k)} = (\sigma_{00} - \sigma^2)^{1/2}/\sigma_{00}^{1/2}.$$

Proof. By definition,

$$
\begin{aligned}
Var(X_0) &= E[(X_0 - \mu_0)^2] = \sigma_{00} \\
Var(W) &= E\{\sigma_{01}[\Sigma^{(1)}]^{-1}(\mathbf{x}^{(1)} - \mu^{(1)})\}^2 \\
&= \sigma_{01}[\Sigma^{(1)}]^{-1}E[(\mathbf{x}^{(1)} - \mu^{(1)})(\mathbf{x}^{(1)} - \mu^{(1)})'][\Sigma^{(1)}]^{-1}\sigma_{10} \\
&= \sigma_{01}[\Sigma^{(1)}]^{-1}\sigma_{10}, \text{ and} \\
Cov(X_0, W) &= E[(X_0 - \mu_0)\{\mu_0 + \sigma_{01}[\Sigma^{(1)}]^{-1}(\mathbf{x}^{(1)} - \mu^{(1)}) - \mu_0\}'] \\
&= E\{(X_0 - \mu_0)(\mathbf{x}^{(1)} - \mu^{(1)})'[\Sigma^{(1)}]^{-1}\sigma_{10}\} = \sigma_{01}[\Sigma^{(1)}]^{-1}\sigma_{10}.
\end{aligned}
$$

The proof follows from substituting into (5.2.25) and simplifying.   ■

Result 5.2.17. The multiple correlation coefficient in Definition 5.2.8 satisfies $0 \le \rho_{0(1,\cdots,k)} \le 1$.

Proof. The expression $Cov(X_0, W)$ in the proof of Result 5.2.16 is nonnegative, from which it follows that $\rho_{0(1,2,\cdots,k)} \ge 0$. That $\rho_{0(1,2,\cdots,k)} \le 1$ follows from observing that $\sigma^2 \le \sigma_{00}$ (since $\sigma_{00} - \sigma^2 = \sigma_{01}[\Sigma^{(1)}]^{-1}\sigma_{10} \ge 0$, being equal to $Var(W)$).   ■

Result 5.2.18. Let $\mathbf{y} = (X_0, X_1, \cdots, X_k) \sim N_{k+1}(\mu_y, \Sigma_y)$. The following equation relates the multiple and partial correlation coefficients and holds for $q = 2, 3, \cdots, k$:

$$\rho_{0(1,2,\cdots,q)}^2 = \rho_{0(1,2,\cdots,q-1)}^2 + [1 - \rho_{0(1,2,\cdots,q-1)}^2]\rho_{0q|(1,2,\cdots,q-1)}^2. \qquad (5.2.27)$$

Proof. Let $\mathbf{y}^* = (X_0, X_1, \cdots, X_q)'$ denote a $(q+1)$-dimensional subvector of $\mathbf{y}$. By Result 5.2.8, $\mathbf{y}^*$ has a $(q+1)$-variate normal distribution with mean and covariance given by

$$\mu^* = (\mu_0, \mu_1, \cdots, \mu_q)', \text{ and } \Sigma^* = \begin{pmatrix} \sigma_{00} & \sigma_{01}^* \\ \sigma_{10}^* & \Sigma^{*(1)} \end{pmatrix},$$

where $\sigma_{10}^* = (\sigma_{10}, \cdots \sigma_{q0})'$, $\sigma_{01}^* = \sigma_{10}^{*\,\prime}$, and $\Sigma^{*(1)}$ is the $q \times q$ covariance matrix of $(X_1, \cdots, X_q)'$. We partition Σ^* and its inverse Δ^* as

$$\Sigma^* = \begin{pmatrix} \sigma_{00} & \sigma_{01} & \sigma_{0q} \\ \sigma_{10} & \Sigma & \sigma_{1q} \\ \sigma_{q0} & \sigma_{q1} & \sigma_{qq} \end{pmatrix} \text{ and } \Delta^* = \begin{pmatrix} \delta_{00} & \delta_{01} & \delta_{0q} \\ \delta_{10} & \Delta & \delta_{1q} \\ \delta_{q0} & \delta_{q1} & \delta_{qq} \end{pmatrix},$$

where σ_{00}, σ_{0q}, σ_{q0}, and σ_{qq} are scalars, σ_{01} and σ_{q1} have dimension $1 \times (q-1)$, σ_{10}, and σ_{1q} have dimension $(q-1) \times 1$, and Σ is a $(q-1) \times (q-1)$ matrix. Entries in corresponding locations in Δ^* have dimensions similar to components of Σ^*. We consider the conditional distribution of $(X_0, X_q | X_1 = x_1, \cdots, X_{q-1} = x_{q-1})$; by Result 5.2.10, this distribution is bivariate normal with covariance

$$\begin{pmatrix} \delta_{00} & \delta_{0q} \\ \delta_{q0} & \delta_{qq} \end{pmatrix}^{-1} = \frac{1}{(\delta_{00}\delta_{qq} - \delta_{0q}^2)} \begin{pmatrix} \delta_{qq} & -\delta_{q0} \\ -\delta_{0q} & \delta_{00} \end{pmatrix}$$

$$= \begin{pmatrix} \sigma_{00|(1,2,\cdots,q-1)} & \sigma_{0q|(1,2,\cdots,q-1)} \\ \sigma_{q0|(1,2,\cdots,q-1)} & \sigma_{qq|(1,2,\cdots,q-1)} \end{pmatrix}, \text{ say.}$$

By Definition 5.2.7,

$$\begin{aligned} \rho_{0q|(1,2,\cdots,q-1)}^2 &= \sigma_{0q|(1,2,\cdots,q-1)}^2 / [\sigma_{00|(1,2,\cdots,q-1)}\sigma_{qq|(1,2,\cdots,q-1)}] \\ &= (-\delta_{0q})^2 / [\delta_{00}\delta_{qq}]. \end{aligned}$$

From Result 5.2.16, we see that

$$\rho_{0(1,2,\cdots,q)}^2 = (\sigma_{00} - \delta_{00}^{-1})/\sigma_{00},$$

and that

$$\begin{aligned} \rho_{0(1,2,\cdots,q-1)}^2 &= [\sigma_{00} - \sigma_{00|(1,\cdots,q-1)}]/\sigma_{00} \\ &= [\sigma_{00} - \delta_{qq}(\delta_{00}\delta_{qq} - \delta_{0q}^2)^{-1}]/\sigma_{00}. \end{aligned}$$

Hence,

$$\begin{aligned} [1 - \rho_{0(1,2,\cdots,q-1)}^2][1 - \rho_{0q|(1,2,\cdots,q-1)}^2] &= [\delta_{qq}(\delta_{00}\delta_{qq} - \delta_{0q}^2)^{-1}\sigma_{00}^{-1}] \\ &\quad \times [1 - \frac{\delta_{0q}^2}{\delta_{00}\delta_{qq}}] \qquad (5.2.28) \\ &= \frac{1}{\sigma_{00}\delta_{00}} = 1 - \rho_{0(1,2,\cdots,q)}^2. \end{aligned}$$

After simplification of (5.2.28), we get the required result. ∎

Result 5.2.19. Given any positive integer q, $1 \le q \le k$, the following inequality holds:

$$\rho_{0(1)}^2 \le \rho_{0(1,2)}^2 \le \cdots \le \rho_{0(1,2,\cdots,q)}^2.$$

Proof. From the proof of Result 5.2.18, we see that $1 - \rho_{0(1,2,\cdots,q-1)}^2 = \delta_{qq}(\delta_{00}\delta_{qq} - \delta_{0q}^2)^{-1}\sigma_{00}^{-1} \ge 0$, and $\rho_{0q|(1,2,\cdots,q-1)}^2 = \frac{(-\delta_{0q})^2}{\delta_{00}\delta_{qq}} \ge 0$. From (5.2.27), it follows that $\rho_{0(1,2,\cdots,q)}^2 \ge \rho_{0(1,2,\cdots,q-1)}^2$, for $q = 2, 3, \cdots, k$. ∎

We conclude this section with a look at another geometrical property associated with the multivariate normal distribution.

Result 5.2.20. Concentration ellipse. Let $\mathbf{x} = (X_1, \cdots, X_k)'$ be a k-variate random vector with $E(\mathbf{x}) = \mu$, and $Var(\mathbf{x}) = \Sigma$. Suppose the vector $\xi = (\xi_1, \cdots, \xi_k)'$ has a uniform distribution on the ellipsoid $(\mathbf{x} - \mu)'\mathbf{A}(\mathbf{x} - \mu) = c^2$, where $\mathbf{A}$ is a p.d. matrix. Such an ellipse with $E(\xi) = \mu$, and $Var(\xi) = \Sigma$ is called the *concentration ellipse* and is written as

$$(\mathbf{x} - \mu)'\Sigma^{-1}(\mathbf{x} - \mu) = k + 2. \tag{5.2.29}$$

Proof. The joint distribution of $\xi = (\xi_1, \cdots, \xi_k)'$ is $f(\xi_1, \cdots, \xi_k) = const$, if $(\mathbf{x} - \mu)'\mathbf{A}(\mathbf{x} - \mu) \leq c^2$. Consider the transformation $\mathbf{y} = \mathbf{B}(\mathbf{x} - \mu)/c$, where $\mathbf{A} = \mathbf{B}'\mathbf{B}$ is the decomposition of the p.d. matrix $\mathbf{A}$. Then,

$$\mathbf{I}/(k + 2) = Var(\mathbf{y}) = \mathbf{B}\Sigma\mathbf{B}'/c^2,$$

so that $\mathbf{B}\Sigma\mathbf{B}' = c^2\mathbf{I}/(k + 2)$, and $\Sigma = c^2\mathbf{A}^{-1}/(k + 2)$, which implies that $\mathbf{A} = c^2\Sigma^{-1}/(k + 2)$. The equation of the concentration ellipse is therefore the expression in (5.2.29). ∎

5.3　Some noncentral distributions

The noncentral chi-square, noncentral F, and noncentral t-distributions are derived from the multivariate normal distribution and are useful for a discussion of inference for linear models. In general, these distributions arise as the sampling distributions of statistics when a null hypothesis of interest is not true. The pdf of the central chi-square and the noncentral chi-square distributions have been variously derived in the literature. For instance, Kendall and Stuart (1958, Sec. 11.2) give a geometrical derivation of the central chi-square pdf using spherical (or polar) coordinates while Guenther (1964) extended this approach to the noncentral chi-square distribution. In this section, we present derivations that are based on the moment generating function method. We begin with the derivation of the central chi-square distribution, starting from the $N_k(\mathbf{0}, \mathbf{I})$ distribution.

Result 5.3.1. Let $\mathbf{z} \sim N_k(\mathbf{0}, \mathbf{I})$, and let $U = \mathbf{z}'\mathbf{z} = \sum_{i=1}^{k} Z_i^2$. Then, $U \sim \chi_k^2$, i.e., U has a (central) chi-square distribution with k degrees of freedom (d.f.) and pdf given by

$$f(u) = \frac{1}{2^{k/2}\Gamma(k/2)} u^{(k-2)/2} \exp(-u/2), \quad u > 0. \tag{5.3.1}$$

Proof. Since U is a function of a multivariate standard normal random vector $\mathbf{z}$, we have

$$M_U(t) = E[\exp\{tU\}] = \int_{-\infty}^{\infty} \cdots \int_{-\infty}^{\infty} \frac{1}{(2\pi)^{k/2}} \exp\{t\sum_{i=1}^{k} z_i^2 - \frac{1}{2}\sum_{i=1}^{k} z_i^2\}d\mathbf{z}$$

$$= \frac{1}{(2\pi)^{k/2}} \int_{-\infty}^{\infty} \cdots \int_{-\infty}^{\infty} \exp\{-\frac{1}{2}(1 - 2t)\sum_{i=1}^{k} z_i^2\}d\mathbf{z} = (1 - 2t)^{-k/2},$$

$$\tag{5.3.2}$$

which follows from the use of an integral evaluation theorem, either Result 5.1.2 or Result 5.1.3. Comparing (5.3.2) with (A7), we see that (5.3.2) is the mgf of a χ_k^2 random variable. The pdf of U follows from (A6). ∎

In particular, if $Z \sim N(0,1)$, then $U = Z_1^2 \sim \chi_1^2$. However, $U \sim \chi_k^2$ does not imply that $Y = \sqrt{U}$ has a standard normal distribution. Properties of the central chi-square distribution are given in the appendix. It is useful to recall that the χ_k^2 distribution, where k is an integer, is a special case of the Gamma(α, β) distribution with $\alpha = k/2$ and $\beta = 2$. The chi-square distribution plays an important role in statistical inference, especially when sampling from a normal population. In tests for the variance of a single normal population using information from a random sample of size n, it is well known that under the null hypothesis, the test statistic follows a central chi-square distribution with $(n - 1)$ degrees of freedom. Critical values from the corresponding central chi-square distribution enables us to construct the rejection region for the test. When the mean of a normal random vector $\mathbf{x}$ is nonzero, the distribution of the quadratic form $\mathbf{x}'\mathbf{x}$ no longer has a central chi-square distribution. Result 5.3.2 generalizes this to the case where $E(\mathbf{x}) = \mu \neq \mathbf{0}$. The next example shows a property of the central chi-square distribution.

Example 5.3.1. If $m > n$, both being integers, we show that $P(\chi_m^2 > c) > P(\chi_n^2 > c)$, where c is a known constant. This result is obvious since clearly $P(\sum_{j=1}^{m} X_j^2 > c) > P(\sum_{j=1}^{n} X_j^2 > c)$ where X_j's are iid $N(0,1)$ variables. □

Result 5.3.2. Let $\mathbf{x} \sim N_k(\mu, \mathbf{I})$, where $\mu' = (\mu_1, \cdots, \mu_k) \neq \mathbf{0}$, and let $U = \mathbf{x}'\mathbf{x}$. The pdf of U is

$$f(u) = \sum_{j=0}^{\infty} \frac{\exp(-\lambda)\lambda^j}{j!} \frac{u^{(k+2j-2)/2} \exp\{-u/2\}}{2^{j+\frac{k}{2}}\Gamma(\frac{1}{2}(k+2j))}, \quad u > 0, \tag{5.3.3}$$

where $\lambda = \frac{1}{2}\mu'\mu = \frac{1}{2}\sum_{j=1}^{k}\mu_j^2$. We say $U \sim \chi^2(k, \lambda)$, i.e., U has a noncentral chi-square distribution with k degrees of freedom and noncentrality parameter equal to λ.

Proof. We derive the mgf of $U = \mathbf{x}'\mathbf{x}$, where $\mathbf{x} \sim N_k(\mu, \mathbf{I})$, and show that this coincides with the mgf of a random variable with pdf (5.3.3). Since $\mathbf{x} \sim N_k(\mu, \mathbf{I})$, we have

$$M_{\mathbf{x}'\mathbf{x}}(t) = \int_{-\infty}^{\infty} \cdots \int_{-\infty}^{\infty} \frac{1}{(2\pi)^{k/2}} \exp\{t\mathbf{x}'\mathbf{x} - \frac{1}{2}(\mathbf{x}-\mu)'(\mathbf{x}-\mu)\}d\mathbf{x}$$

$$= (1-2t)^{-k/2}\exp\{2t\lambda/(1-2t)\}, \quad t < 1/2, \tag{5.3.4}$$

which follows directly from Result 5.1.3, with $\mathbf{B} = \text{diag}\{(1-2t)/2\}$, $\mathbf{b} = -\mu$, $b_0 = \mu'\mu/2$, $\mathbf{A} = \mathbf{0}$, $\mathbf{a} = \mathbf{0}$, and $a_0 = 1$. Alternately, we can write the mgf in the form $M_{\mathbf{x}'\mathbf{x}}(t) = (1-2t)^{-k/2}\exp\{-\lambda[1-(1-2t)^{-1}]\}$, for $t < 1/2$. Next, we evaluate the mgf of a random variable U with pdf (5.3.3) as $M_U(t) = E[\exp(Ut)]$, i.e.,

$$
\begin{aligned}
M_U(t) &= \int_0^\infty \exp\{ut\} \sum_{j=0}^\infty \frac{e^{-\lambda}\lambda^j}{j!} \frac{u^{(k+2j-2)/2}\exp\{-u/2\}}{2^{j+\frac{k}{2}}\Gamma(\frac{1}{2}(k+2j))} du \\
&= (1-2t)^{-k/2} \sum_{j=0}^\infty \frac{e^{-\lambda}\lambda^j}{j!(1-2t)^j} \\
&= (1-2t)^{-k/2} \exp\{2\lambda t/(1-2t)\}, \quad t < 1/2 \\
&= (1-2t)^{-k/2} \exp\{-\lambda[1-(1-2t)^{-1}]\}, \quad t < 1/2. \quad (5.3.5)
\end{aligned}
$$

Therefore, $U = \mathbf{x}'\mathbf{x} \sim \chi^2(k,\lambda)$ distribution.   ∎

Note that $\lambda = 0$ if and only if $\mu = \mathbf{0}$, in which case, the distribution of U is a central chi-square. The noncentral chi-square distribution is the distribution of a quadratic form $\mathbf{x}'\mathbf{x}$ when $\mathbf{x}$ has a nonzero mean. The jth term in (5.3.3) is the product of the Poisson pmf with mean λ at count j and a central chi-square density with $k + 2j$ degrees of freedom. In other words, the noncentral chi-square distribution defined in Result 5.3.2 is an example of a *mixture distribution* involving central chi-square and Poisson distributions. The hierarchy is (see Casella and Berger, 1990, Chapter 4):

$$U|Y \sim \chi^2_{k+2Y} \text{ and } Y \sim Poisson(\lambda). \quad (5.3.6)$$

Example 5.3.2.   Suppose $X_1, \cdots, X_k$ are independently distributed random variables, with $X_j \sim N(\mu_j, \sigma_j^2)$, $j = 1, \cdots, k$. We obtain the distribution of $\sum_{j=1}^k X_j^2/\sigma_j^2$. Note that if we set $Z_j = X_j/\sigma_j$, $j = 1, \cdots, k$, then $Z_1, \cdots, Z_k$ are independently distributed, with $Z_j \sim N(\mu_j/\sigma_j, 1)$, $j = 1, \cdots, k$. Hence, by Result 5.3.2, $\sum_{j=1}^k Z_j^2 = \sum_{j=1}^k X_j^2/\sigma_j^2$ has a $\chi^2(k,\lambda)$ distribution, where $\lambda = \sum_{j=1}^k \mu_j^2/2\sigma_j^2$.   □

Example 5.3.3.   Suppose $U \sim \chi^2(k,\lambda)$ and $V \sim \chi^2_k$. We show that $P(U > c) \geq P(V > c)$, for some constant c. We have

$$
\begin{aligned}
P(U > c) &= \sum_{j=0}^\infty P(U > c|J = j)P(J = j), \quad \text{where } J \sim Poisson(\frac{\lambda}{2}) \\
&= \sum_{j=0}^\infty P(\chi^2_{2j+k} > c)P(J = j) \\
&\geq \sum_{j=0}^\infty P(\chi^2_k > c)P(J = j) \quad \text{(see Example 5.3.1)} \\
&= P(\chi^2_k > c)\sum_{j=0}^\infty P(J = j) \\
&= P(\chi^2_k > c). \quad \square
\end{aligned}
$$

Example 5.3.4. Let $U \sim \chi^2(k, \lambda)$. For a given constant c, we show that a property of the noncentral chi-square distribution is that $P(U > c)$ is an increasing function of λ. Again,

$$h(\lambda) = P(U > c) = \sum_{j=0}^{\infty} P(\chi^2_{2j+k} > c) \frac{1}{j!} \exp(-\frac{\lambda}{2})(\frac{\lambda}{2})^j,$$

so that the first derivative of $h(\lambda)$ is

$$
\begin{aligned}
h'(\lambda) &= \sum_{j=1}^{\infty} P(\chi^2_{2j+k} > c)[-\frac{1}{2j!} \exp(-\frac{\lambda}{2})(\frac{\lambda}{2})^j \\
&\quad + \frac{1}{2(j-1)!} \exp(-\frac{\lambda}{2})(\frac{\lambda}{2})^{j-1}] - \frac{1}{2} \exp(-\frac{\lambda}{2}) P(\chi^2_k > c) \\
&= \frac{1}{2} \sum_{j=0}^{\infty} P(\chi^2_{2j+2+k} > c) \frac{1}{j!} \exp(-\frac{\lambda}{2})(\frac{\lambda}{2})^j \\
&\quad - \frac{1}{2} \sum_{j=0}^{\infty} P(\chi^2_{2j+k} > c) \frac{1}{j!} \exp(-\frac{\lambda}{2})(\frac{\lambda}{2})^j \\
&\geq 0,
\end{aligned}
$$

which shows that $P(U > c)$ is an increasing function of λ. $\square$

Result 5.3.3. Let $\mathbf{x} \sim N_k(\mu, \Sigma)$, with $r(\Sigma) = k$. Then

$$
\begin{aligned}
U_1 &= (\mathbf{x} - \mu)'\Sigma^{-1}(\mathbf{x} - \mu) \sim \chi^2_k, \text{ and} \\
U_2 &= \mathbf{x}'\Sigma^{-1}\mathbf{x} \sim \chi^2(k, \lambda),
\end{aligned}
$$

where $\lambda = \frac{1}{2}\mu'\Sigma^{-1}\mu$.

Proof. Let $\Sigma = \Gamma\Gamma'$, with $r(\Gamma) = k$, and let $\mathbf{z}_1 = (\Gamma')^{-1}(\mathbf{x} - \mu)$. From Result 5.2.6, $\mathbf{z}_1 \sim N_k(\mathbf{0}, \mathbf{I})$. Using Result 5.3.1, we see that $\mathbf{z}_1'\mathbf{z}_1 \sim \chi^2_k$. But

$$\mathbf{z}_1'\mathbf{z}_1 = (\mathbf{x} - \mu)'\Gamma^{-1}\Gamma'^{-1}(\mathbf{x} - \mu) = (\mathbf{x} - \mu)'\Sigma^{-1}(\mathbf{x} - \mu) = U_1,$$

which proves the first result. To derive the distribution of U_2, we see again that $\mathbf{z}_2 = (\Gamma')^{-1}\mathbf{x} \sim N_k(\Gamma'^{-1}\mu, \mathbf{I})$, so that using Result 5.3.2, we see that $\mathbf{z}_2'\mathbf{z}_2 \sim \chi^2(k, \lambda)$. Again,

$$\mathbf{z}_2'\mathbf{z}_2 = \mathbf{x}'\Gamma^{-1}\Gamma'^{-1}\mathbf{x} = \mathbf{x}'\Sigma^{-1}\mathbf{x} = U_2,$$

which proves the second result. ∎

Result 5.3.4. Let $U \sim \chi^2(k, \lambda)$. Then $E(U) = k + 2\lambda$ and $Var(U) = 2(k + 4\lambda)$.

Proof. Using the hierarchical setup given in (5.3.6), we have

$$
\begin{aligned}
E(U) &= E[E(U|Y)] = E[k + 2Y] = k + 2\lambda, \text{ and} && (5.3.7) \\
Var(U) &= E[Var(U|Y)] + Var[E(U|Y)] \\
&= E(2k + 4Y) + Var(k + 2Y) \\
&= 2k + 4\lambda + 4\lambda \\
&= 2(k + 4\lambda). && (5.3.8)
\end{aligned}
$$

Alternatively, we can derive these expressions using

$$E(U^j) = \frac{\partial^j}{\partial t^j} M_U(t)|_{t=0}, \quad j = 1, 2, \tag{5.3.9}$$

and $Var(U) = E(U^2) - [E(U)]^2$. Note that all moments of the pdf (5.3.3) exist and we may interchange summation and integration in order to compute these moments. ∎

Result 5.3.5. Let $U_i \sim \chi^2(k_i, \lambda_i)$, $i = 1, \cdots, K$, and suppose the U_i's are all independent. Then

$$U = \sum_{i=1}^{K} U_i \sim \chi^2(\sum_{i=1}^{K} k_i, \sum_{i=1}^{K} \lambda_i). \tag{5.3.10}$$

Proof.   For $t < 1/2$, the mgf of U is

$$\begin{aligned} M_U(t) &= \prod_{i=1}^{K} M_{U_i}(t) \quad \text{(by independence)} \\ &= \prod_{i=1}^{K} (1 - 2t)^{-k_i/2} \exp\{-\lambda_i[1 - (1 - 2t)^{-1}]\}, \\ &= (1 - 2t)^{-\sum_i k_i/2} \exp\{-[1 - (1 - 2t)^{-1}] \sum_i \lambda_i\}, \end{aligned}$$

which is the mgf of a $\chi^2(\sum_{i=1}^{K} k_i, \sum_{i=1}^{K} \lambda_i)$ distribution, thus establishing the additive property of the noncentral chi-square distribution. ∎

Result 5.3.6.   Let $U_1 \sim \chi^2(k_1, \lambda)$, let $U_2 \sim \chi^2_{k_2}$, and let U_1 and U_2 be independently distributed. Then

$$F = \frac{U_1 / k_1}{U_2 / k_2} \sim F(k_1, k_2, \lambda), \tag{5.3.11}$$

i.e., a noncentral F-distribution with numerator and denominator degrees of freedom equal to k_1 and k_2 respectively, noncentrality parameter λ, and with pdf

$$f(v; k_1, k_2, \lambda) = \sum_{j=0}^{\infty} \frac{e^{-\lambda}\lambda^j}{j!} \frac{k_1^{(k_1+2j)/2} k_2^{k_2/2} \Gamma(k_1/2 + k_2/2 + j) v^{k_1/2+j-1}}{\Gamma(k_1/2+j)\Gamma(k_2/2)(k_2+k_1 v)^{k_1/2+k_2/2+j}} \quad v > 0.$$

Proof.   Since U_1 and U_2 are independently distributed, we have from (5.3.1) and (5.3.3) that for $u_1 > 0$, $u_2 > 0$,

$$\begin{aligned} f(u_1, u_2) &= f(u_1)f(u_2) \\ &= \sum_{j=0}^{\infty} \frac{\exp(-\lambda)\lambda^j}{j!} \frac{u_1^{(k_1+2j-2)/2} \exp\{-u_1/2\}}{2^{(k_1+2j)/2}\Gamma((k_1+2j)/2)} \frac{u_2^{(k_2-2)/2} \exp(-u_2/2)}{2^{k_2/2}\Gamma(k_2/2)}. \end{aligned}$$

$$\tag{5.3.12}$$

Let

$$\alpha_j = \exp(-\lambda)\lambda^j/\{j!2^{(k_1+k_2+2j)/2}\Gamma((k_1+2j)/2)\Gamma(k_2/2)\}.$$

Consider the following transformation of variables:

$$F = k_2 U_1/k_1 U_2, \text{ and } Z = U_1 + U_2$$

with Jacobian

$$|J| = k_2(U_1 + U_2)/(k_1 U_2^2)$$

so that

$$
\begin{aligned}
f(v; k_1, k_2, \lambda) &= \int_0^\infty \frac{1}{|J|} f(v, z) dz \\
&= \int_0^\infty \sum_{j=0}^\infty \alpha_j \left(\frac{k_1 v z}{k_1 v + k_2} \right)^{\frac{1}{2}k_1+j-1} \left(\frac{k_2 z}{k_1 v + k_2} \right)^{\frac{1}{2}k_2-1} \\
&\quad \times \frac{k_1 k_2 z}{(k_1 v + k_2)^2} \exp(-z/2) dz \\
&= \sum_{j=0}^\infty \alpha_j k_1^{\frac{1}{2}k_1+j} k_2^{\frac{1}{2}k_2} \frac{v^{\frac{1}{2}k_1+j-1}}{(k_1 v + k_2)^{\frac{1}{2}k_1+\frac{1}{2}k_2+j}} \\
&\quad \times \int_0^\infty z^{\frac{1}{2}k_1+\frac{1}{2}k_2+j-1} \exp(-z/2) dz.
\end{aligned}
$$

Since

$$\int_0^\infty z^{\frac{1}{2}k_1+\frac{1}{2}k_2+j-1} \exp(-z/2) dz = 2^{\frac{1}{2}k_1+\frac{1}{2}k_2+j}\Gamma(\tfrac{1}{2}k_1 + \tfrac{1}{2}k_2 + j),$$

the result follows directly. ∎

The noncentral F-distribution is an extension of the central F-distribution to the case when the normal random vector $\mathbf{x}$ has nonzero mean, i.e., the quadratic form in the numerator has a noncentral chi-square distribution (see the appendix). The noncentral F-distribution is useful in order to evaluate the power of tests of hypotheses, which requires the evaluation of

$$G(\lambda) = \int_g^\infty f(v; k_1, k_2, \lambda) dv, \qquad (5.3.13)$$

where $g = F_{k_1,k_2,\alpha}(\lambda)$ denotes the 100αth percentile point of the noncentral $F(k_1, k_2, \lambda)$ distribution, and α denotes the level of significance of the test. Tang's (1938) tables may be used for evaluating $G(\lambda)$; see also Pearson and Hartley (1970). The noncentral Beta distribution, which is discussed in Result 5.3.7 is also related to a noncentral chi-square and an independent central chi-square random variable.

Result 5.3.7. Let $U_1 \sim \chi^2(k_1, \lambda)$, let $U_2 \sim \chi^2_{k_2}$, and let U_1 and U_2 be independently distributed. Then

$$G = U_1/(U_1 + U_2) \sim Beta(k_1, k_2, \lambda)$$

i.e., a noncentral *Beta* distribution with numerator and denominator degrees of freedom equal to k_1 and k_2 respectively, noncentrality parameter λ, and with pdf

$$f(w; k_1, k_2, \lambda) = \exp(-\tfrac{\lambda^2}{2}) \sum_{j=0}^{\infty} \left(\tfrac{\lambda^2}{2}\right)^j \tfrac{1}{j!} B(w; \tfrac{k_1}{2} + j, \tfrac{k_2}{2}), \quad 0 < w < 1,$$

where $B(w; \alpha, \beta)$ corresponds to the (central) Beta pdf with shape parameter α and scale parameter β (see the appendix).

Proof. We begin with the joint pdf of U_1 and U_2 which was shown in (5.3.12). Consider the change of variable

$$G = U_1/(U_1 + U_2);$$

the derivation of the noncentral Beta pdf is similar to that of the noncentral F distribution. ∎

Two other noncentral distributions that we define are the noncentral t-distribution and the doubly noncentral F-distribution. Scheffe (1959) presented an application of the doubly noncentral F-distribution and also showed a procedure for approximating it via the noncentral F-distribution.

Result 5.3.8. If $X \sim N(\mu, \sigma^2)$, $U/\sigma^2 \sim \chi^2_k$, and X is distributed independently of U, then

$$T = \frac{X}{\sqrt{U/k}} \sim t(k, \delta) \tag{5.3.14}$$

has a noncentral t-distribution with pdf (Rao 1973a, p. 172)

$$f(t; k, \delta) = \frac{k^{k/2}}{\Gamma(k/2)} \frac{\exp(-\delta^2/2)}{(k + t^2)^{(k+1)/2}} \sum_{s=0}^{\infty} \Gamma\left(\frac{k + s + 1}{2}\right) \left(\frac{\delta^s}{s!}\right) \left(\frac{2t^2}{k + t^2}\right)^{s/2} \tag{5.3.15}$$

for $-\infty < t < \infty$, where $\delta = \mu/\sigma$.

Proof. The joint distribution of X and U is

$$c_1 \exp\{-\tfrac{(x-\mu)^2}{2\sigma^2}\} \exp\{-\tfrac{u}{\sigma^2}\} u^{k/2-1}$$

where $c_1^{-1} = \sqrt{2\pi} \sigma^{k+1} 2^{k/2} \Gamma(k/2)$. Consider the transformation

$$X = R \sin \theta, \quad U = R^2 \cos^2 \theta;$$

the joint density of R and θ is equal to

$$c_2 r^k (\cos\theta)^{k-1} \exp\{-(r^2 - 2\mu r \sin\theta)/2\sigma^2\},$$

where $c_2 = c_1 \exp\{-\mu^2/2\sigma^2\} = c_1 \exp\{-\delta^2/2\}$. The joint pdf does not factor into two expressions, one involving r alone, and the other involving only θ, so R and θ are not independent. By expanding $\exp\{\mu r \sin\theta/\sigma^2\}$, we write the joint density as an infinite series

$$c_2 \exp\{-r^2/2\sigma^2\}(\cos\theta)^{k-1} \sum_j \frac{(\mu\sin\theta)^j r^{k+j}}{j!\sigma^{2j}}. \tag{5.3.16}$$

We obtain the marginal density of θ by integrating out term by term with respect to r in (5.3.16), to get

$$(c_2/2)(\cos\theta)^{k-1}\sum_j \Gamma\left(\tfrac{k+j+1}{2}\right) 2^{(j+k+1)/2} \tfrac{(\delta\sin\theta)^j}{j!}.$$

Now, transforming from θ to $T = \sqrt{k}\tan\theta$, we obtain the pdf in (5.3.15). ∎

Note also that if $Z \sim N(0,1)$, $U \sim \chi^2_k$, δ is a constant, and Z and U are independently distributed, then

$$T = (Z + \delta)/\sqrt{U/k} \sim t(k,\delta)$$

has a noncentral t-distribution. The noncentral t-distribution plays the following role in statistical inference. Suppose we consider a test $H_0 : \mu = 0$ versus $H_1 : \mu \neq 0$ on the basis of observations $\mathbf{x} = (X_1, \cdots, X_n) \sim N(\mu\mathbf{1}_n, \sigma^2\mathbf{I}_n)$, where both μ and σ^2 are unknown. The test statistic is $\sqrt{n}\overline{X}\,/\,S$ where $\overline{X} = \sum_{i=1}^n X_i/n$, and $S^2 = \sum_{i=1}^n (X_i - \overline{X})^2/(n-1)$. Under H_0, $\overline{X} \sim N(0, \sigma^2/n)$, $(n-1)S^2/\sigma^2 \sim \chi^2_{n-1}$, and they are distributed independently. Hence, $\sqrt{n}\overline{X}\,/\,S \sim t_{n-1}$, which is the central t-distribution with $(n-1)$ degrees of freedom. Under the alternative hypothesis H_1 however, $\overline{X} \sim N(\mu, \sigma^2/n)$, and $(n-1)S^2/\sigma^2$ is still distributed independently as a χ^2_{n-1} variable, so that $\sqrt{n}\overline{X}\,/\,S$ has a noncentral t-distribution with $(n-1)$ degrees of freedom and noncentrality parameter $\lambda = \mu^2/2\sigma^2$. The noncentral t-distribution is useful for power calculations.

Result 5.3.9. Let U_1 and U_2 have independent noncentral chi-square distributions; $U_1 \sim \chi^2(k_1, \lambda_1)$, and $U_2 \sim \chi^2(k_2, \lambda_2)$. Then

$$F^* = \frac{U_1/\,k_1}{U_2/\,k_2} \sim F''(k_1, k_2, \lambda_1, \lambda_2)$$

where $F''(k_1, k_2, \lambda_1, \lambda_2)$ refers to the doubly noncentral F-distribution with degrees of freedom k_1 and k_2, and noncentrality parameters λ_1 and λ_2. The doubly noncentral F-distribution is based on the ratio of two independent noncentral chi-square random variables, and for $v > 0$ has pdf

$$f(v) = \sum_{k_2=0}^{\infty} \sum_{k_1=0}^{\infty} N(k_1, k_2)/D(k_1, k_2),$$

where

$$
\begin{aligned}
N(k_1, k_2) &= \exp(-\lambda_1 - \lambda_2)\lambda_1^{k_1}\lambda_2^{k_2}\Gamma(\frac{1}{2}n_1 + \frac{1}{2}n_2 + k_1 + k_2) \\
&\times n_1^{\frac{1}{2}n_1+k_1} n_2^{\frac{1}{2}n_2+k_2} v^{\frac{1}{2}n_1+k_1-1}, \text{ and} \\
D(k_1, k_2) &= k_1! k_2! \Gamma(\frac{1}{2}n_1 + k_1)\Gamma(\frac{1}{2}n_2 + k_2) \\
&\times (n_1 v + n_2)^{\frac{1}{2}n_1 + \frac{1}{2}n_2 + k_1 + k_2}.
\end{aligned}
$$

Proof. Recall that we can write $U_1 \sim \chi^2_{2J_1+k_1}$, and $U_2 \sim \chi^2_{2J_2+k_2}$, where J_1 and J_2 are independent Poisson random variables with respective means $\lambda_1/2$ and $\lambda_2/2$. Given $J_1 = j_1$ and $J_2 = j_2$, U_1 and U_2 are independently distributed and

$$
U = U_1/U_2 \sim \{(2j_1 + k_1)/(2j_2 + k_2)\}F_{2j_1+k_1, 2j_2+k_2}
$$

i.e., conditional on J_1 and J_2, the ratio of U_1 and U_2 is proportional to a central F-distribution. The pdf of U is then

$$
\begin{aligned}
f(u) &= \sum_{j_2=0}^{\infty} \sum_{j_1=0}^{\infty} \frac{1}{j_1!}\exp(-\frac{\lambda_1}{2})\left(\frac{\lambda_1}{2}\right)^{j_1} \frac{1}{j_2!}\exp(-\frac{\lambda_2}{2})\left(\frac{\lambda_2}{2}\right)^{j_2} \\
&\times \{B[\frac{1}{2}(2j_1 + k_1), \frac{1}{2}(2j_2 + k_2)]\}^{-1}(1 + u)^{-(2j_1+2j_2+k_1+k_2)/2} \\
&\times u^{(2j_1+k_1)/2-1} u^{(2j_2+k_2)/2-1},
\end{aligned}
$$

which after some simplification yields the required result. ∎

5.4   Distributions of quadratic forms

There is a rich literature on the distribution of quadratic forms (see Graybill, 1961 and Rao, 1973a). The basic theorems dealing with distributions of quadratic forms in normal random vectors are due to Cochran (1934), Craig (1943), and Rao (1973a), while Shanbhag (1966) dealt with independence of quadratic forms. Although the discussion that we present is by no means complete, it gives the basic results that are needed for the development of linear model theory. Recent references are Driscoll (1999), Hayes and Haslett (1999), Khuri (1999) and Seely, Birkes, and Lee (1997). As before, we assume that the matrix of a quadratic form is symmetric.

Result 5.4.1. Let $\mathbf{x} \sim N_k(\mathbf{0}, \mathbf{I})$. The quadratic form $\mathbf{x}'\mathbf{Ax} \sim \chi^2_m$ if and only if the matrix of the quadratic form $\mathbf{A}$ is idempotent with $r(\mathbf{A}) = m$.

Proof. Let $\mathbf{A}$ be a symmetric and idempotent matrix of rank m. We will show that $\mathbf{x}'\mathbf{Ax} \sim \chi^2_m$ distribution. By Result 2.3.4, there exists a $k \times k$ orthogonal matrix $\mathbf{P}$ such that $\mathbf{P}'\mathbf{AP} = \begin{pmatrix} \mathbf{I}_m & \mathbf{0} \\ \mathbf{0} & \mathbf{0} \end{pmatrix}$. Define $\mathbf{z} = \mathbf{P}'\mathbf{x}$. Partition

$\mathbf{P}$ as $\mathbf{P} = (\mathbf{P}_1 \quad \mathbf{P}_2)$, where $\mathbf{P}_1'\mathbf{P}_1 = \mathbf{I}_m$, and partition $\mathbf{z}' = (\mathbf{z}_1' \quad \mathbf{z}_2')$. Then, $\mathbf{z}_1 = \mathbf{P}_1'\mathbf{x} \sim N_m(\mathbf{0}, \mathbf{I})$ and

$$
\begin{aligned}
\mathbf{x}'\mathbf{A}\mathbf{x} &= (\mathbf{P}\mathbf{z})'\mathbf{A}(\mathbf{P}\mathbf{z}) = \mathbf{z}'\mathbf{P}'\mathbf{A}\mathbf{P}\mathbf{z} \\
&= (\mathbf{z}_1' \quad \mathbf{z}_2') \begin{pmatrix} \mathbf{I}_m & \mathbf{0} \\ \mathbf{0} & \mathbf{0} \end{pmatrix} \begin{pmatrix} \mathbf{z}_1 \\ \mathbf{z}_2 \end{pmatrix} = \mathbf{z}_1'\mathbf{z}_1.
\end{aligned}
\tag{5.4.1}
$$

Since $\mathbf{z}_1 \sim \mathbf{N}_m(\mathbf{0}, \mathbf{I})$, the proof follows from Result 5.3.1. To prove the converse, assume that $\mathbf{x}'\mathbf{A}\mathbf{x} \sim \chi_m^2$. We must show that this implies that the symmetric matrix $\mathbf{A}$ is idempotent of rank m. Since $\mathbf{x}'\mathbf{A}\mathbf{x} \sim \chi_m^2$, we have by (A7),

$$
M_{\mathbf{x}'\mathbf{A}\mathbf{x}}(t) = (1 - 2t)^{-m/2}, \quad t < 1/2.
\tag{5.4.2}
$$

Since $\mathbf{x} \sim N_k(\mathbf{0}, \mathbf{I})$, we can also write down the mgf of $\mathbf{x}'\mathbf{A}\mathbf{x}$ using an integral evaluation theorem, as

$$
\begin{aligned}
M_{\mathbf{x}'\mathbf{A}\mathbf{x}}(t) &= \int_{-\infty}^{\infty} \cdots \int_{-\infty}^{\infty} \frac{1}{(2\pi)^{k/2}} \exp\{t(\mathbf{x}'\mathbf{A}\mathbf{x}) - \frac{1}{2}\mathbf{x}'\mathbf{x}\} d\mathbf{x} \\
&= |\mathbf{I}_k - 2t\mathbf{A}|^{-1/2} = \prod_{i=1}^{k}(1 - 2t\lambda_i)^{-1/2},
\end{aligned}
\tag{5.4.3}
$$

where λ_i, $i = 1, \cdots, k$ are the eigenvalues of the symmetric matrix $\mathbf{A}$. Comparing the two expressions in (5.4.2) and (5.4.3) which must be equal to one another, we should have

$$
\prod_{i=1}^{k}(1 - 2t\lambda_i)^{-1/2} = (1 - 2t)^{-m/2}
\tag{5.4.4}
$$

for every t in some neighborhood of zero. This will be true if m of the eigenvalues of $\mathbf{A}$ are equal to 1, and the remaining $k - m$ eigenvalues are equal to 0. By Result 2.3.10, this implies that $\mathbf{A}$ is an idempotent matrix of rank m. ∎

Result 5.4.2. Let $\mathbf{x} \sim N_k(\mu, \Sigma)$. The rth cumulant of the quadratic form $\mathbf{x}'\mathbf{A}\mathbf{x}$ is

$$
\kappa_r(\mathbf{x}'\mathbf{A}\mathbf{x}) = 2^{r-1}(r-1)![tr(\mathbf{A}\Sigma)^r + r\mu'\mathbf{A}(\Sigma\mathbf{A})^{r-1}\mu].
\tag{5.4.5}
$$

Proof. The mgf of $\mathbf{x}'\mathbf{A}\mathbf{x}$ is

$$
\begin{aligned}
M_{\mathbf{x}'\mathbf{A}\mathbf{x}}(t) &= \int_{-\infty}^{\infty} \cdots \int_{-\infty}^{\infty} \frac{1}{(2\pi)^{k/2}|\Sigma|^{1/2}} \exp\{t(\mathbf{x}'\mathbf{A}\mathbf{x}) - \frac{1}{2}(\mathbf{x}-\mu)'\Sigma^{-1}(\mathbf{x}-\mu)\} d\mathbf{x} \\
&= |\mathbf{I}_k - 2t\mathbf{A}\Sigma|^{-1/2} \exp\{-\frac{1}{2}\mu'[\mathbf{I} - (\mathbf{I} - 2t\mathbf{A}\Sigma)^{-1}]\Sigma^{-1}\mu\}.
\end{aligned}
\tag{5.4.6}
$$

The cumulant generating function of $\mathbf{x}'\mathbf{A}\mathbf{x}$ is

$$K_{\mathbf{x}'\mathbf{A}\mathbf{x}}(t) = \sum_{r=1}^{\infty} \kappa_r t^r / r! = \log[M_{\mathbf{x}'\mathbf{A}\mathbf{x}}(t)],$$

so that

$$\sum_{r=1}^{\infty} \frac{1}{r!} \kappa_r t^r = -\frac{1}{2} \log |\mathbf{I} - 2t\mathbf{A}\Sigma| - \frac{1}{2} \mu'[\mathbf{I} - (\mathbf{I} - 2t\mathbf{A}\Sigma)^{-1}]\Sigma^{-1}\mu. \qquad (5.4.7)$$

For sufficiently small $|t|$, suppose λ_j and δ_j, $j = 1, \cdots, k$, denote the eigenvalues of $(\mathbf{I} - 2t\mathbf{A}\Sigma)$ and $\mathbf{A}\Sigma$ respectively. Then

$$
\begin{aligned}
-\frac{1}{2} \log |\mathbf{I} - 2t\mathbf{A}\Sigma| &= -\frac{1}{2} \sum_{j=1}^{k} \log\{\lambda_j\} = -\frac{1}{2} \sum_{j=1}^{k} \log\{1 - 2t\delta_j\} \\
&= -\frac{1}{2} \sum_{j=1}^{k} \sum_{r=1}^{\infty} \frac{-(2t\delta_j)^r}{r}, \quad \text{for } |2t\delta_j| < 1 \\
&= \sum_{r=1}^{\infty} \frac{2^{r-1}t^r}{r} \sum_{j=1}^{k} \delta_j^r = \sum_{r=1}^{\infty} \frac{2^{r-1}t^r}{r} tr(\mathbf{A}\Sigma)^r. \quad (5.4.8)
\end{aligned}
$$

Also, by direct binomial expansion, we see that for sufficiently small t,

$$\mathbf{I} - (\mathbf{I} - 2t\mathbf{A}\Sigma)^{-1} = -\sum_{r=1}^{\infty} 2^r t^r (\mathbf{A}\Sigma)^r. \qquad (5.4.9)$$

Substituting from (5.4.8) and (5.4.9) into the right side of (5.4.7), and equating coefficients of like powers of t^r on both sides of that equation gives the required result for $\kappa_r(\mathbf{x}'\mathbf{A}\mathbf{x})$. ∎

From Result 5.4.2, we can show directly (see Exercise 5.23) that

$$
\begin{aligned}
E(\mathbf{x}'\mathbf{A}\mathbf{x}) &= tr(\mathbf{A}\Sigma) + \mu'\mathbf{A}\mu, \\
Var(\mathbf{x}'\mathbf{A}\mathbf{x}) &= 2tr(\mathbf{A}\Sigma)^2 + 4\mu'\mathbf{A}\Sigma\mathbf{A}\mu, \text{ and} \\
Cov(\mathbf{x}, \mathbf{x}'\mathbf{A}\mathbf{x}) &= 2\Sigma\mathbf{A}\mu.
\end{aligned}
$$

These properties are useful to characterize the first two moments of the distribution of $\mathbf{x}'\mathbf{A}\mathbf{x}$. We sometimes encounter the need to employ the following result on the moments of quadratic forms, which we state without proof (see Magnus and Neudecker, 1988).

Result 5.4.3.   Let $\mathbf{A}$, $\mathbf{B}$, and $\mathbf{C}$ be symmetric $k \times k$ matrices and let $\mathbf{x} \sim N_k(\mathbf{0}, \Sigma)$. Then

$$
\begin{aligned}
E(\mathbf{x}'\mathbf{A}\mathbf{x} \cdot \mathbf{x}'\mathbf{B}\mathbf{x}) &= tr(\mathbf{A}\Sigma)tr(\mathbf{B}\Sigma) + 2tr(\mathbf{A}\Sigma\mathbf{B}\Sigma), \\
E(\mathbf{x}'\mathbf{A}\mathbf{x} \cdot \mathbf{x}'\mathbf{B}\mathbf{x} \cdot \mathbf{x}'\mathbf{C}\mathbf{x}) &= tr(\mathbf{A}\Sigma)tr(\mathbf{B}\Sigma)tr(\mathbf{C}\Sigma) + 2[tr(\mathbf{A}\Sigma)][tr(\mathbf{B}\Sigma\mathbf{C}\Sigma)] \\
&\quad + 2[tr(\mathbf{B}\Sigma)][tr(\mathbf{A}\Sigma\mathbf{C}\Sigma)] + 2[tr(\mathbf{C}\Sigma)][tr(\mathbf{A}\Sigma\mathbf{B}\Sigma)] \\
&\quad + 8tr(\mathbf{A}\Sigma\mathbf{B}\Sigma\mathbf{C}\Sigma).
\end{aligned}
$$

We next state and prove an important result which gives a condition under which a quadratic form in a normal random vector has a noncentral chi-square distribution. This result is fundamental for a discussion of linear model inference under normality.

Result 5.4.4. Let $\mathbf{x} \sim N_k(\mu, \Sigma)$, Σ being p.d., and let $\mathbf{A}$ be a symmetric matrix of rank r. The necessary and sufficient condition for the quadratic form $U = \mathbf{x}'\mathbf{A}\mathbf{x}$ to have a noncentral chi-square distribution, i.e., $U \sim \chi^2(r, \lambda)$, with r d.f. and noncentrality parameter $\lambda = \mu'\mathbf{A}\mu/2$, is that $\mathbf{A}\Sigma$ is idempotent of rank r.

Proof. We present a proof which only uses simple calculus and matrix algebra (see Khuri, 1999; Driscoll, 1999).
Necessity. We assume that $U \sim \chi^2(r, \lambda)$, and must show that this implies $\mathbf{A}\Sigma$ is idempotent of rank r. By Result 2.4.5, we can write $\Sigma = \mathbf{PP}'$, for nonsingular $\mathbf{P}$. Let $\mathbf{y} = \mathbf{P}^{-1}\mathbf{x}$. Clearly, $\mathbf{x}'\mathbf{A}\mathbf{x} = \mathbf{y}'\mathbf{P}'\mathbf{A}\mathbf{P}\mathbf{y}$. Since $\mathbf{P}'\mathbf{A}\mathbf{P}$ is symmetric, by Result 2.3.4, there exists an orthogonal matrix $\mathbf{Q}$ such that $\mathbf{P}'\mathbf{A}\mathbf{P} = \mathbf{Q}\mathbf{D}\mathbf{Q}'$, the elements of the diagonal matrix $\mathbf{D}$ being the eigenvalues of $\mathbf{P}'\mathbf{A}\mathbf{P}$, i.e., of $\mathbf{A}\Sigma$. Let d_i denote the nonzero elements of $\mathbf{D}$, with d_i having multiplicity m_i, $i = 1, \cdots, p$. Let $\mathbf{Q}_i$ denote a matrix with m_i columns of $\mathbf{Q}$ with the orthonormal eigenvectors of $\mathbf{P}'\mathbf{A}\mathbf{P}$ corresponding to d_i. Then, $\mathbf{z} = \mathbf{Q}'\mathbf{y}$ has a $N(\mathbf{Q}'\mathbf{P}^{-1}\mu, \mathbf{I})$ distribution. Also,

$$\mathbf{x}'\mathbf{A}\mathbf{x} = \mathbf{z}'\mathbf{D}\mathbf{z} = \sum_{i=1}^{p} d_i W_i, \tag{5.4.10}$$

where the W_i's have independent $\chi^2(m_i, \theta_i)$ distributions, the noncentrality parameter being $\theta_i = \mu'\mathbf{P}'^{-1}\mathbf{Q}_i\mathbf{Q}_i'\mathbf{P}^{-1}\mu \geq 0$, $i = 1, \cdots, p$.
From (5.3.5), the mgf of W_i is

$$M_{W_i}(t) = (1 - 2t)^{-m_i/2} \exp\{-\theta_i[1 - (1 - 2t)^{-1}]\}, \quad i = 1, \cdots, p,$$

while the mgf of $U = \mathbf{x}'\mathbf{A}\mathbf{x}$ is

$$M_{\mathbf{x}'\mathbf{A}\mathbf{x}}(t) = (1 - 2t)^{-r/2} \exp\{-\lambda[1 - (1 - 2t)^{-1}]\}.$$

Equating the mgf's of the variables on both sides of (5.4.10), we obtain

$$(1 - 2t)^{-r/2} \exp\{-\lambda[1 - (1 - 2t)^{-1}]\} = \prod_{i=1}^{p} (1 - 2d_i t)^{-m_i/2}$$
$$\times \exp\{-\theta_i[1 - (1 - 2d_i t)^{-1}]\},$$

and taking natural logarithms of both sides, we get

$$-\frac{r}{2}\log(1 - 2t) - \lambda[1 - (1 - 2t)^{-1}] = \sum_{i=1}^{p} \{-\frac{m_i}{2}\log(1 - 2d_i t) - \theta_i[1 - (1 - 2d_i t)^{-1}]\}$$

$$\tag{5.4.11}$$

Using the expansions

$$\log(1-u) = -\sum_{j=1}^{\infty} u^j/j, \text{ and}$$

$$1 - (1-u)^{-1} = -\sum_{j=1}^{\infty} u^j \qquad (5.4.12)$$

in (5.4.11), we see that

$$(r/2)\sum_{j=1}^{\infty}\{(2t)^j/j\} + \lambda\sum_{j=1}^{\infty}(2t)^j = \sum_{i=1}^{p}\{(m_i/2)\sum_{j=1}^{\infty}[(2d_it)^j/j] + \theta_i\sum_{j=1}^{\infty}(2d_it)^j\}.$$

$$(5.4.13)$$

Equating coefficients of $(2t)^j$ on both sides on (5.4.13), we get

$$(r/2j) + \lambda = \sum_{i=1}^{p}\{(m_i/2j) + \theta_i\}d_i^j, \quad j = 1, 2, \cdots, \qquad (5.4.14)$$

which implies that $|d_i| \le 1$, $i = 1, \cdots, p$. We see this must be true, since, if, on the contrary, $|d_i| > 1$, then by letting $j \to \infty$, the right side of (5.4.14) tends to infinity, while the left side is equal to $\lambda < \infty$.

In fact, $|d_i| = 1$, $i = 1, \cdots, p$, as we now show. If, on the contrary, $|d_i| < 1$, by summing terms on both sides of (5.4.14) over j, we get

$$\sum_{j=1}^{\infty}\{(r/2j) + \lambda\} = \sum_{i=1}^{p}(m_i/2)\{\sum_{j=1}^{\infty}(d_i^j/j)\} + \sum_{i=1}^{p}\theta_i\sum_{j=1}^{\infty}d_i^j.$$

Using (5.4.12), this implies

$$\sum_{j=1}^{\infty}\{(r/2j) + \lambda\} = -\sum_{i=1}^{p}(m_i/2)\log(1-d_i) - \sum_{i=1}^{p}\theta_i[1 - (1-d_i)^{-1}],$$

which is impossible since the right side is finite, while the left side is infinite. Hence, we must have $|d_i| = 1$, $i = 1, \cdots, p$. The values of d_i can only be one of the following three cases. Case (i): $p = 2$, $d_1 = 1$, $d_2 = -1$; Case (ii): $p = 1$, $d_1 = -1$; and Case (iii): $p = 1$, $d_1 = 1$. We show that Case (iii) is the only valid case.

Under Case (i), choose j to be an even integer in (5.4.14). Then,

$$(r/2j) + \lambda = \sum_{i=1}^{2}\{(m_i/2j) + \theta_i\}, \quad j = 2, 4, \cdots;$$

letting $j \to \infty$ implies $\lambda = \theta_1 + \theta_2$, so that $r = m_1 + m_2$. However, choosing j to be an odd integer in (5.4.14) gives

$$(r/2j) + \lambda = (m_1/2j) + \theta_1 - (m_2/2j) + \theta_2;$$

substituting $r = m_1 + m_2$ and $\lambda = \theta_1 + \theta_2$, gives $(m_2/2j) + \theta_2 = -(m_2/2j) - \theta_2$, which is not possible since $m_i > 0$ and $\theta_i \ge 0$, $i = 1, 2$. Therefore, Case (i) is not valid. To show that Case (ii) is invalid as well, set j to be an odd integer in (5.4.14); we get

$$(r/2j) + \lambda = -(m_1/2j) - \theta_1,$$

which is invalid since the right side is negative, while the left side is positive. Hence, Case (iii) must be valid. In this case,

$$(r/2j) + \lambda = (m_1/2j) + \theta_1, \quad j = 1, 2, \cdots,$$

which implies that $m_1 = r$ and $\theta_1 = \lambda$. Therefore, $\mathbf{A\Sigma}$ has r eigenvalues equal to one, and must be an idempotent matrix of rank r.

Sufficiency. We must show that if $\mathbf{A\Sigma}$ is idempotent of rank r, then U has a $\chi^2(r, \lambda)$ distribution. Since $\mathbf{A\Sigma}$ is idempotent, in (5.4.10), $p = 1$, $d_1 = 1$, and $m_1 = r$. Hence, $\mathbf{x'Ax}$ will have a $\chi^2(r, \lambda)$ distribution, where $\lambda = \theta_1$. An alternate proof of sufficiency amounts to showing that the mgf of $\mathbf{x'Ax}$ coincides with the mgf of a $\chi^2(r, \lambda)$ random variable, which is obvious from (5.3.5) and (5.4.6). ∎

We state the following result without proof.

Result 5.4.5. Let $\mathbf{x} \sim N_k(\mu, \Sigma)$ with $r(\Sigma) = k$. The quadratic form $U = \mathbf{x'Ax} \sim \chi^2(m, \lambda)$ with $\lambda = \mu'\mathbf{A}\mu/2$ if and only if any one of the following three conditions are met:

1. $\mathbf{A\Sigma}$ is an idempotent matrix of rank m,

2. $\mathbf{\Sigma A}$ is an idempotent matrix of rank m,

3. Σ is a g-inverse of $\mathbf{A}$ with $r(\mathbf{A}) = m$.

Example 5.4.1. Suppose $\mathbf{x} \sim N_k(\mu, \Sigma)$, where Σ is p.d. We show that $\mathbf{x'Ax}$ is distributed as a linear combination of independent noncentral chi-square variables. First, since Σ is p.d, there is a nonsingular matrix $\mathbf{P}$ such that $\Sigma = \mathbf{PP'}$. Since $\mathbf{P'AP}$ is symmetric, there exists an orthogonal matrix $\mathbf{Q}$ such that $\mathbf{Q'P'APQ} = \mathbf{D} = \text{diag}(\lambda_1, \cdots, \lambda_r, 0, \cdots, 0)$, these being the distinct eigenvalues of $\mathbf{P'AP}$. Let $\mathbf{x} = \mathbf{PQz}$. From Result 5.2.6, $\mathbf{z} \sim N(\mathbf{Q'P^{-1}}\mu, \mathbf{I})$; also $\mathbf{x'Ax} = \mathbf{z'Dz} = \sum_{i=1}^{k} \lambda_i Z_i^2$. The required result follows from Result 5.3.2. □

Result 5.4.6. Let $\mathbf{x} \sim N_k(\mu, \Sigma)$. The linear form $\mathbf{Bx}$ and the quadratic form $\mathbf{x'Ax}$ are independently distributed if and only if $\mathbf{B\Sigma A} = \mathbf{0}$.

Proof. By Result 2.2.1, $\mathbf{A} = \mathbf{LL'}$ with $r(\mathbf{A}) = r(\mathbf{L})$. Let us assume first that $\mathbf{B\Sigma A} = \mathbf{0}$. This implies that $\mathbf{B\Sigma LL'} = \mathbf{0}$, and since $(\mathbf{L'L})^{-1}$ exists (see Example 2.2.1), this implies that $\mathbf{B\Sigma LL'L(L'L)^{-1}} = \mathbf{0}$, i.e., $\mathbf{B\Sigma L} = \mathbf{0}$. However, $\mathbf{B\Sigma L} = Cov(\mathbf{Bx}, \mathbf{x'L})$, and since $\mathbf{x} \sim N_k(\mu, \Sigma)$, this implies that $\mathbf{Bx}$ and $\mathbf{x'L}$ are independently distributed, and therefore $\mathbf{Bx}$ and $\mathbf{x'LL'x} = \mathbf{x'Ax}$ are independently distributed, which proves sufficiency. To prove necessity, note that independence of $\mathbf{Bx}$ and $\mathbf{x'Ax}$ implies that $Cov(\mathbf{Bx}, \mathbf{x'Ax}) = \mathbf{0}$. Using Result

5.4.2, we can show that this implies (see Exercise 5.23) $2\mathbf{B}\Sigma\mathbf{A}\mu = \mathbf{0}$ for all μ, i.e., $\mathbf{B}\Sigma\mathbf{A} = \mathbf{0}$. ∎

The following result is a generalization of Craig's theorem (Craig, 1943) and gives a necessary and sufficient condition for the independence of two quadratic forms in a normal random vector. Two random variables W_1 and W_2 that have cgf's are independent if and only if their cumulants satisfy

$$\kappa_r(aW_1 + bW_2) = \kappa_r(aW_1) + \kappa_r(bW_2)$$

for all real a and b and for all positive integers r.

Result 5.4.7.   Let $\mathbf{x} \sim N_k(\mu, \Sigma)$, where Σ is p.d. The two quadratic forms $\mathbf{x}'\mathbf{A}\mathbf{x}$ and $\mathbf{x}'\mathbf{B}\mathbf{x}$ are independently distributed if and only if

$$\mathbf{A}\Sigma\mathbf{B} = \mathbf{0}, \text{ or equivalently, } \mathbf{B}\Sigma\mathbf{A} = \mathbf{0}. \tag{5.4.15}$$

Proof.   Since Σ is p.d., we can write $\Sigma = \mathbf{T}\mathbf{T}'$ (see Result 2.4.5). The rth cumulant of the quadratic form $\mathbf{x}'\mathbf{C}\mathbf{x}$, where $\mathbf{C} = a\mathbf{A} + b\mathbf{B}$, has the form in (5.4.5):

$$\kappa_r(\mathbf{x}'\mathbf{C}\mathbf{x}) = 2^{r-1}(r-1)!\{tr(\mathbf{C}\Sigma)^r + r\mu'\mathbf{C}(\Sigma\mathbf{C})^{r-1}\mu\}.$$

Sufficiency.   Using (5.4.15) in $\kappa_r(\mathbf{x}'\mathbf{C}\mathbf{x})$, we get

$$\kappa_r(\mathbf{x}'\mathbf{C}\mathbf{x}) = \kappa_r(\mathbf{x}'(a\mathbf{A})\mathbf{x}) + \kappa_r(\mathbf{x}'(b\mathbf{B})\mathbf{x}), \tag{5.4.16}$$

for all r and real a and b, which implies that Q_1 and Q_2 are distributed independently.

Necessity. Q_1 and Q_2 are assumed to be distributed independently, so that (5.4.16) holds. For fixed, but arbitrary real values a and b, let $\lambda_1, \cdots, \lambda_p$ denote the elements in the union of three sets of eigenvalues, viz., those of $a\mathbf{A}\Sigma$, those of $b\mathbf{B}\Sigma$, and those of $(a\mathbf{A} + b\mathbf{B})\Sigma$ (so that the λ_i are nonzero and distinct). Let $\mathbf{C}$ represent one of the matrices $a\mathbf{A}$, $b\mathbf{B}$, or $a\mathbf{A} + b\mathbf{B}$. In the spectral decomposition of $\mathbf{C}\Sigma$ (see Result 2.3.4), let λ_i be an eigenvalue of $\mathbf{C}\Sigma$ with multiplicity $m_{i,\mathbf{C}}$, and let $\mathbf{P}_{i,\mathbf{C}}$ denote the matrix associated with λ_i in the decomposition. If λ_i is not an eigenvalue of $a\mathbf{A}$, take $m_{i,a\mathbf{A}}$ to be 0, and $\mathbf{P}_{i,a\mathbf{A}}$ to be the zero matrix. Let $\mu_{i,\mathbf{C}}$ denote $\mu'\mathbf{C}\mathbf{P}_{i,\mathbf{C}}\mu$. Then, $(\mathbf{C}\Sigma)^r = \sum_i^p \lambda_i^r \mathbf{P}_{i,\mathbf{C}}$, and

$$\kappa_r(\mathbf{x}'\mathbf{C}\mathbf{x}) = 2^{r-1}(r-1)!\sum_{i=1}^p \{\lambda_i^r m_{i,\mathbf{C}} + r\lambda_i^{r-1}\mu_{i,\mathbf{C}}\}.$$

Using (5.4.16), this implies that for any positive integer r,

$$\sum_{i=1}^p \lambda_i^r \{m_{i,a\mathbf{A}+b\mathbf{B}} - m_{i,a\mathbf{A}} - m_{i,b\mathbf{B}}\}$$

$$+ \sum_{i=1}^p r\lambda_i^{r-1}\{\mu_{i,a\mathbf{A}+b\mathbf{B}} - \mu_{i,a\mathbf{A}} - \mu_{i,b\mathbf{B}}\} = 0.$$

Write the first $2p$ of these equations in the matrix form

$$\Lambda\nu = \mathbf{0}, \qquad (5.4.17)$$

where Λ is a $2p \times 2p$ matrix with elements $\Lambda_{i,j} = \lambda_j^i$, and $\Lambda_{i,p+j} = i\lambda_j^{i-1}$ for $i = 1, \cdots, 2p$ and $j = 1, \cdots, p$. Also, ν is a $2p$-dimensional vector with elements $\nu_i = m_{i,a\mathbf{A}+b\mathbf{B}} - m_{i,a\mathbf{A}} - m_{i,b\mathbf{B}}$, and $\nu_{p+i} = \mu_{i,a\mathbf{A}+b\mathbf{B}} - \mu_{i,a\mathbf{A}} - \mu_{i,b\mathbf{B}}$ for $i = 1, \cdots, p$. Since the matrix Λ is nonsingular (see Exercise 5.34), (5.4.17) implies that for $i = 1, \cdots, p$,

$$m_{i,a\mathbf{A}+b\mathbf{B}} - m_{i,a\mathbf{A}} - m_{i,b\mathbf{B}} = 0, \quad \text{and} \quad \mu_{i,a\mathbf{A}+b\mathbf{B}} - \mu_{i,a\mathbf{A}} - \mu_{i,b\mathbf{B}} = 0.$$

Therefore,

$$tr\{(a\mathbf{A} + b\mathbf{B})\Sigma\}^r = a^r tr(\mathbf{A}\Sigma)^r + b^r tr(\mathbf{B}\Sigma)^r \qquad (5.4.18)$$

$$\mu'(a\mathbf{A} + b\mathbf{B})\{\Sigma(a\mathbf{A} + b\mathbf{B})\}^{r-1}\mu = a^r \mu'\mathbf{A}(\Sigma\mathbf{A})^{r-1}\mu + b^r \mu'\mathbf{B}(\Sigma\mathbf{B})^{r-1}\mu \qquad (5.4.19)$$

for all positive integers r and for all real a and b (since these were arbitrary choices). Setting $r = 4$ in (5.4.18), expanding the left side and equating coefficients of $a^2 b^2$, and using property 4 of Result 1.2.8, we get

$$tr(\mathbf{T}'\mathbf{A}\Sigma\mathbf{B}\mathbf{T} + \mathbf{T}'\mathbf{B}\Sigma\mathbf{A}\mathbf{T})^2 + 2tr(\mathbf{T}'\mathbf{A}\Sigma\mathbf{B}\mathbf{T})(\mathbf{T}'\mathbf{A}\Sigma\mathbf{B}\mathbf{T})' = 0.$$

Since each of these terms is of the form $tr(\mathbf{C}\mathbf{C}')$, it is nonnegative. This implies then that $2tr(\mathbf{T}'\mathbf{A}\Sigma\mathbf{B}\mathbf{T})(\mathbf{T}'\mathbf{A}\Sigma\mathbf{B}\mathbf{T})' = 0$, so that $\mathbf{T}'\mathbf{A}\Sigma\mathbf{B}\mathbf{T} = \mathbf{0}$, i.e., $\Sigma\mathbf{A}\Sigma\mathbf{B}\Sigma = \mathbf{0}$. This together with (5.4.19) when $r = 4$ gives

$$(\mathbf{T}'\mathbf{A}\Sigma\mathbf{B}\mu)'(\mathbf{T}'\mathbf{A}\Sigma\mathbf{B}\mu) + (\mathbf{T}'\mathbf{B}\Sigma\mathbf{A}\mu)'(\mathbf{T}'\mathbf{B}\Sigma\mathbf{A}\mu) = \mathbf{0},$$

which implies that $\Sigma\mathbf{A}\Sigma\mathbf{B}\mu$ and $\Sigma\mathbf{B}\Sigma\mathbf{A}\mu$ must be zero vectors. If we set $r = 2$ in (5.4.19) and equate like coefficients in ab, we obtain $\mu'\mathbf{A}\Sigma\mathbf{B}\mu = 0$. ∎

For more details, see Ogawa (1950, 1993), Laha (1956), and Reid and Driscoll (1988). Using only linear algebra and calculus, Driscoll and Krasnicka (1995) proved the general case where Σ may be singular. In this case, they showed that a necessary and sufficient condition for $\mathbf{x}'\mathbf{A}\mathbf{x}$ and $\mathbf{x}'\mathbf{B}\mathbf{x}$ to be independently distributed is that

$$\Sigma\mathbf{A}\Sigma\mathbf{B}\Sigma = \mathbf{0}, \Sigma\mathbf{A}\Sigma\mathbf{B}\mu = \mathbf{0}, \Sigma\mathbf{B}\Sigma\mathbf{A}\mu = \mathbf{0}, \quad \text{and} \quad \mu'\mathbf{A}\Sigma\mathbf{B}\mu = \mathbf{0}.$$

Example 5.4.2. We show independence between the mean and sum of squares. Let $\mathbf{x} = (X_1, \cdots, X_n)' \sim N_n(\mathbf{0}, \mathbf{I})$ so that we can think of $X_1, \cdots, X_n$ as a random sample from a $N(0, 1)$ population. The sample mean $\overline{X} = \mathbf{1}'\mathbf{x}/n$ has a $N(0, 1/n)$ distribution (using Result 5.2.7), and the sample sum of squares $\sum_{i=1}^{n}(X_i - \overline{X})^2$ has a central chi-square distribution with $(n-1)$ degrees of freedom (by Result 5.4.1). It is easily verified by expressing $\overline{X}^2$ and $\sum_{i=1}^{n}(X_i - \overline{X})^2$ as quadratic forms in $\mathbf{x}$ that $\overline{X}^2$, and hence $\overline{X}$ is independent of $\sum_{i=1}^{n}(X_i - \overline{X})^2$. □

Example 5.4.3.   Let $\mathbf{x} \sim N_k(\mu, \mathbf{I})$ and suppose a $k \times k$ orthogonal matrix $\mathbf{T}$ is partitioned as $\mathbf{T} = (\mathbf{T}_1', \mathbf{T}_2')'$, where $\mathbf{T}_i$ is a $k \times k_i$ matrix, $i = 1, 2$, such that $k_1 + k_2 = k$. It is easy to verify that $\mathbf{T}_1 \mathbf{T}_1' = \mathbf{I}_{k_1}$, $\mathbf{T}_2 \mathbf{T}_2' = \mathbf{I}_{k_2}$, $\mathbf{T}_1 \mathbf{T}_2' = \mathbf{0}$, $\mathbf{T}_2 \mathbf{T}_1' = \mathbf{0}$, and $\mathbf{T}'\mathbf{T} = \mathbf{I}_k$. Also, $\mathbf{T}_i' \mathbf{T}_i$ is idempotent of rank k_i, $i = 1, 2$. By Result 5.4.5, $\mathbf{x}' \mathbf{T}_i' \mathbf{T}_i \mathbf{x} \sim \chi^2(k_i, \mu' \mathbf{T}_i' \mathbf{T}_i \mu)$, $i = 1, 2$. By Result 5.4.7, these two quadratic forms are independently distributed.   □

Note that Result 5.4.6 and Result 5.4.7 apply whether or not the quadratic forms $\mathbf{x}'\mathbf{A}\mathbf{x}$ and $\mathbf{x}'\mathbf{B}\mathbf{x}$ have chi-square distributions. A related result, called Craig's Theorem (Shanbhag, 1966) is given in Exercise 5.31. We next discuss without proof a more general theorem dealing with quadratic forms in normal random vectors. The basic result is due to Cochran (1934), which was later modified by James (1952).

Result 5.4.8 Let $\mathbf{x} \sim N_k(\mu, \Sigma)$, $\mathbf{A}_i$ be $k \times k$ symmetric matrices with $r(\mathbf{A}_i) = r_i$, $i = 1, \cdots, n$, and let $\mathbf{A} = \sum_{i=1}^{n} \mathbf{A}_i$ with $r(\mathbf{A}) = r$. Then

   (i) $\mathbf{x}' \mathbf{A}_i \mathbf{x} \sim \chi^2(r_i, \frac{1}{2}\mu' \mathbf{A}_i \mu)$,

   (ii) $\mathbf{x}' \mathbf{A}_i \mathbf{x}$ are pairwise independent, and

   (iii) $\mathbf{x}' \mathbf{A} \mathbf{x} \sim \chi^2(r, \frac{1}{2}\mu' \mathbf{A} \mu)$

if and only if

   I. any two of the following statements are true:

      (a) $\mathbf{A}_i \Sigma$ is idempotent for $i = 1, \cdots, n$,

      (b) $\mathbf{A}_i \Sigma \mathbf{A}_j = 0$ for all $i < j$,

      (c) $\mathbf{A}\Sigma$ is idempotent, or

   II. (c) is true and (d) $r = \sum_{i=1}^{n} r_i$ holds, or

   III. (c) is true and so is (e) each of the matrices $\mathbf{A}_1 \Sigma, \cdots, \mathbf{A}_{n-1} \Sigma$ is idempotent and $\mathbf{A}_n \Sigma$ is n.n.d.

There are many other results in the literature that summarize properties of quadratic forms in normal random vectors. We present two more results. For a proof of these results, see Rao (1973a, section 3b.4).

Result 5.4.9.   Fisher-Cochran theorem.   Let $\mathbf{x} \sim N_k(\mu, \mathbf{I})$. Let $Q_1, \cdots, Q_L$ denote L quadratic forms in $\mathbf{x}$ with respective ranks $r_1, \cdots, r_L$ such that $\mathbf{x}'\mathbf{x} = \sum_{j=1}^{L} Q_j$. Then, Q_j's are independently distributed as $\chi^2(r_j, \lambda_j)$ variables if and only if $\sum_{j=1}^{L} r_j = k$; then $\lambda_j = \mu' \mathbf{A} \mu$ if $Q_j = \mathbf{x}' \mathbf{A}_j \mathbf{x}$.

Result 5.4.10.   Let $\mathbf{x} \sim N_k(\mu, \Sigma)$. The quadratic form $(\mathbf{x} - \mu)' \mathbf{A}(\mathbf{x} - \mu)$ has a χ^2_p distribution if and only if $\Sigma \mathbf{A} \Sigma \mathbf{A} \Sigma = \Sigma \mathbf{A} \Sigma$, where $p = r(\mathbf{A}\Sigma)$ (Ogasawara and Takahashi, 1951).

Result 5.4.11. Let $\mathbf{x} \sim N_k(\mu, \Sigma)$, where Σ is p.d. Then $Q_1 = \mathbf{x}'\mathbf{A}\mathbf{x} + \mathbf{a}'\mathbf{x}$ and $Q_2 = \mathbf{x}'\mathbf{B}\mathbf{x} + \mathbf{b}'\mathbf{x}$ are independently distributed if and only if (i) $\mathbf{A}\Sigma\mathbf{B} = \mathbf{0}$, (ii) $\mathbf{a}'\Sigma\mathbf{B} = \mathbf{0}$, (iii) $\mathbf{b}'\Sigma\mathbf{A} = \mathbf{0}$, and (iv) $\mathbf{a}'\Sigma\mathbf{b} = \mathbf{0}$. This is often referred to as Laha's theorem (Laha, 1956).

5.5 Alternatives to multivariate normal distribution

The multivariate normal distributions constitute a very useful family of symmetric distributions that have found widespread use in the classical theory of linear models and multivariate analysis. However, the normal distribution is not the only choice to characterize the response variable in many situations. Particularly, in robustness studies, where interest lies in assessing sensitivity of procedures to the assumption of normality, interest has centered on a more general class of multivariate distributions (see Johnson and Kotz, 1972). Of special interest are distributions whose contours of equal density have elliptical shapes (see section 5.2), and whose tail behavior differs from that of the normal. It is also possible to incorporate skewness to obtain a richer family of distributions. We begin the discussion by introducing a finite mixture distribution of multivariate normal distributions, as well as scale mixtures of multivariate normals. We then extend these to a more general class of spherically symmetric distributions, and finally to the class of elliptically symmetric distributions.

5.5.1 Mixture of normals distribution

A finite parametric mixture of normal distributions is useful in several practical applications. We give a definition and some examples.

Definition 5.5.1. We say that $\mathbf{x}$ has an L-component mixture of k-variate normal distributions if its pdf is

$$f(\mathbf{x}; \mu_1, \Sigma_1, p_1, \cdots, \mu_L, \Sigma_L, p_L) = \sum_{j=1}^{L} p_j (2\pi)^{-k/2} |\Sigma_j|^{-1/2}$$

$$\times \exp\left\{ -\frac{1}{2} (\mathbf{x} - \mu_j)' \Sigma_j^{-1} (\mathbf{x} - \mu_j) \right\}, \quad \mathbf{x} \in \mathcal{R}^k.$$

This pdf exhibits multimodality with up to L distinct peaks.

Example 5.5.1. We saw the form of the bivariate normal pdf in Example 5.2.1. Mixtures of L bivariate normal distributions enable us to generate a rich class of bivariate densities which have up to L distinct peaks. Let $\mu_1 = \mu_2 = \mathbf{0}$, $\sigma_{1,j}^2 = \sigma_{2,j}^2 = 1$, for $j = 1, 2$, $\rho_1 = 1/2$, and $\rho_2 = -1/2$. With mixing proportions $p_1 = p_2 = 1/2$, the mixture pdf of $\mathbf{x} = (X_1, X_2)$ is

$$f(\mathbf{x}, \mu_1, \Sigma_1, p_1, \mu_2, \Sigma_2, p_2) = \sum_{j=1}^{2} \tfrac{1}{2\pi\sqrt{3}} \exp\{-\tfrac{2}{3}(X_1^2 - X_1 X_2 + X_2^2)\}, \quad \mathbf{x} \in \mathcal{R}^2.$$

A plot of this pdf reveals regions where one of the two components dominates, and there are also regions of transition where the pdf does not appear to be "normal". A well known property of a bivariate normal mixture is that all conditional and marginal distributions are univariate normal mixtures.   □

Example 5.5.2.   Consider the following ϵ-contaminated normal distribution which is a mixture of a $N(\mathbf{0}, \mathbf{I})$ and a $N(\mathbf{0}, \sigma^2 \mathbf{I})$, with $0 \le \epsilon \le 1$. Its pdf is

$$f(\mathbf{x}; \sigma^2, \epsilon) = (1 - \varepsilon)(2\pi)^{-k/2} \exp\{-\tfrac{1}{2}\mathbf{x}'\mathbf{x}\} + \epsilon(2\pi)^{-k/2}\sigma^{-k} \exp\{-\tfrac{1}{2\sigma^2}\mathbf{x}'\mathbf{x}\}. \quad □$$

The mixture of normals accommodates modeling in situations where the data exhibits multimodality. Suppose λ denotes a discrete random variable, assuming two distinct positive values λ_1 and λ_2, with respective probabilities p_1 and p_2, where $p_1 + p_2 = 1$. Let $\mathbf{x}$ be a k-dimensional random vector which is defined as follows: conditionally on $\lambda = \lambda_j$, $\mathbf{x} \sim N_k(\mathbf{0}, \lambda_j \mathbf{I})$, $j = 1, 2$. The "conditional" pdf of $\mathbf{x}$ (conditional on λ) is

$$f(\mathbf{x}|\lambda_j) = (2\pi)^{-k/2}\lambda_j^{-k/2} \exp\{-\mathbf{x}'\mathbf{x}/2\lambda_j\}, \quad \mathbf{x} \in \mathcal{R}^k.$$

The unconditional distribution of $\mathbf{x}$ has the mixture pdf

$$f(\mathbf{x}) = (2\pi)^{-k/2}\{p_1\lambda_1^{-k/2} \exp(-\mathbf{x}'\mathbf{x}/2\lambda_1) + p_2\lambda_2^{-k/2} \exp(-\mathbf{x}'\mathbf{x}/2\lambda_2)\} .$$

This distribution is called a scale mixture of multivariate normals. In general, we can include L mixands, $L \ge 2$. By varying the mixing proportions p_j and the values λ_j, we can generate a flexible class of distributions that are useful in modeling a variety of multivariate data. It can be shown that all marginal distributions of this scale distribution mixture are themselves scale mixtures of normals of appropriate dimensions, a property which this distribution shares with the multivariate normal (see Result 5.2.8). Suppose we wish to maintain unimodality while allowing for heavy-tailed behavior, we would assume that the mixing random variable λ has a continuous distribution with pdf $\pi(\lambda)$. We define the resulting flexible class of distributions and show several examples which have useful applications in modeling multivariate data.

Definition 5.5.2. Multivariate scale mixture of normals (SMN) distribution.   A k-dimensional random vector $\mathbf{x}$ has a multivariate SMN distribution with mean vector θ and covariance matrix Σ if its pdf has a "mixture" form

$$f(\mathbf{x}; \theta, \Sigma) = \int_{\mathcal{R}^+} N_k(\mathbf{x}; \theta, \kappa(\lambda)\Sigma)\pi(\lambda)d\lambda \qquad (5.5.1)$$

where $\kappa(.)$ is a positive function defined on $\mathcal{R}^+$, and $\pi(.)$ is a probability function, which may be either discrete or continuous. The scalar λ is called the mixing parameter, and $\pi(.)$ is the mixing density.

Example 5.5.3. Suppose we set $\kappa(\lambda) = 1/\lambda$ in (5.5.1), and assume that the parameter $\lambda \sim \text{Gamma}(\nu/2, \nu/2)$, i.e.,

$$\pi(\lambda) = \frac{1}{\Gamma(\nu/2)}(\nu/2)^{\nu/2}\lambda^{\nu/2-1}\exp\{-\nu\lambda/2\}, \quad -\infty < \lambda < \infty.$$

The resulting multivariate t-distribution is a special example of the scale mixtures of normals family with ν degrees of freedom and pdf

$$f(\mathbf{x}; \theta, \Sigma, \nu) = \frac{\Gamma\{\frac{1}{2}(k+\nu)\}}{\Gamma(\nu/2)(\nu\pi)^{k/2}|\Sigma|^{1/2}}\left(1 + \frac{1}{\nu}(\mathbf{x}-\theta)'\Sigma^{-1}(\mathbf{x}-\theta)\right)^{-(\nu+k)/2},$$

$$(5.5.2)$$

for $\mathbf{x} \in \mathcal{R}^k$. When $\nu \to \infty$, the multivariate t-distribution approaches the multivariate normal distribution. By setting $\theta = \mathbf{0}$, and $\Sigma = \mathbf{I}_k$ in (5.5.2), we get the standard distribution, usually denoted by $f(\mathbf{z})$. When $\nu = 1$, the distribution corresponds to a k-variate Cauchy distribution. In particular, when $k = 2$, let $\mathbf{z} = (Z_1, Z_2)$ denote a random vector with a Cauchy distribution. The pdf of $\mathbf{z}$ is

$$f(\mathbf{z}) = \tfrac{1}{2\pi}(1 + \mathbf{z}'\mathbf{z})^{-3/2}, \quad \mathbf{z} \in \mathcal{R}^2,$$

and corresponds to a (standard) bivariate Cauchy distribution, which is a simple example of a bivariate scale mixture of normals distribution. □

Example 5.5.4. If we assume $\kappa(\lambda) = 4\lambda^2$, where λ follows an asymptotic Kolmogorov distribution with pdf

$$\pi(\lambda) = 8\sum_{j=1}^{\infty}(-1)^{j+1}j^2\lambda\exp\{-2j^2\lambda^2\},$$

the resulting multivariate logistic distribution is a special case of the scale mixture of normals family. This distribution finds use in modeling multivariate binary data. □

Example 5.5.5. If we set $\kappa(\lambda) = 2\lambda$, and assume that $\pi(\lambda)$ is a positive stable pdf $S^P(\alpha, 1)$ (see the appendix) whose polar form of the pdf is given by (Samorodnitsky and Taqqu, 1994)

$$\pi_{SP}(\lambda; \alpha, 1) = \{\alpha/(1-\alpha)\}\lambda^{-\{\alpha/(1-\alpha)+1\}}\int_0^1 s(u)\exp\{-s(u)/\lambda^{\alpha/(1-\alpha)}\}du,$$

for $0 < \alpha < 1$, and

$$s(u) = \{\sin(\alpha\pi u)/\sin(\pi u)\}^{\alpha/(1-\alpha)}\{\sin[(1-\alpha)\pi u]/\sin(\pi u)\}.$$

The resulting scale mixture of normals distributions is called the multivariate symmetric stable distribution. □

5.5.2   Spherical distributions

In this section, we define the class of spherical (or radial) distributions.

Definition 5.5.3.   A k-dimensional random vector $\mathbf{z} = (Z_1, \cdots, Z_k)'$ is said to have a spherical (or spherically symmetric) distribution if its distribution does not change under rotations of the coordinate system, i.e., if the distribution of the vector $\mathbf{Az}$ is the same as the distribution of $\mathbf{z}$ for any orthogonal $k \times k$ matrix $\mathbf{A}$. If the pdf of $\mathbf{z}$ exists in $\mathcal{R}^k$, it depends on $\mathbf{z}$ only through $\mathbf{z}'\mathbf{z} = \sum_{i=1}^{k} Z_i^2$; for any function h (called the density generator function),

$$f(\mathbf{z}) \propto h(\mathbf{z}'\mathbf{z}) = c_k h(\mathbf{z}'\mathbf{z}), \tag{5.5.3}$$

where c_k is a constant. The mean and covariance of $\mathbf{z}$, provided they exist, are

$$E(\mathbf{z}) = \mathbf{0}, \quad \text{and} \quad Cov(\mathbf{z}) = c\mathbf{I}_k,$$

where $c \geq 0$ is some constant.

Different choices of the function h gives rise to different examples of the spherical distributions (Muirhead, 1982; Fang, Kotz and Ng, 1990). Contours of constant density of a spherical random vector $\mathbf{z}$ are circles when $k = 2$, or spheres for $k > 2$, which are centered at the origin. The spherical normal distribution shown in the following example is a popular member of this class.

Example 5.5.6.   Let $\mathbf{z}$ have a k-variate normal distribution with mean $\mathbf{0}$ and covariance $\sigma^2 \mathbf{I}_k$. We say $\mathbf{z}$ has a spherical normal distribution with pdf

$$
\begin{aligned}
f(\mathbf{z}; \sigma^2) &= \frac{1}{(2\pi)^{k/2}\sigma^k} \exp\{-\frac{1}{2\sigma^2} \parallel \mathbf{z} \parallel^2\}, \quad \mathbf{z} \in \mathcal{R}^k \\
&= \frac{1}{(2\pi)^{k/2}\sigma^k} \exp\{-\frac{1}{2\sigma^2}\mathbf{z}'\mathbf{z}\}, \quad \mathbf{z} \in \mathcal{R}^k.
\end{aligned}
$$

The density generator function is clearly $h(u) = c \exp\{-u/2\}, u \geq 0$.   □

The ϵ-contaminated normal distribution shown in Example 5.5.2. is also an example of a spherical distribution, as is the standard multivariate t-distribution defined in Example 5.5.3. The following example generalizes the well-known double-exponential (Laplace) distribution to the multivariate case; this distribution is useful for modeling data with outliers.

Example 5.5.7.   Consider the bivariate generalization of the standard double-exponential distribution to a vector $\mathbf{z} = (Z_1, Z_2)$ with pdf

$$f(\mathbf{z}) = \tfrac{1}{2\pi} \exp\{-(\mathbf{z}'\mathbf{z})^{1/2}\}, \quad \mathbf{z} \in \mathcal{R}^2.$$

This is an example of a spherical distribution; notice the similarity of this pdf to that of the bivariate standard normal vector.   □

Definition 5.5.4. The squared radial random variable $T =\parallel \mathbf{z} \parallel$ has pdf

$$\frac{\pi^{k/2}}{\Gamma(k/2)} t^{(k/2)-1} h(t), \quad t > 0. \tag{5.5.4}$$

We say T has a radial-squared distribution with k d.f. and density generator h, i.e., $T \sim R_k^2(h)$.

The main appeal of spherical distributions lies in the fact that many results that we have seen for the multivariate normal hold for the general class of spherical distributions. For example, if $\mathbf{z} = (Z_1, Z_2)'$ is a bivariate spherically distributed random vector, the ratio $V = Z_1/Z_2$ has a Cauchy distribution provided $P(Z_2 = 0) = 0$. If $\mathbf{z} = (Z_1, \cdots, Z_k)'$ has a k-variate spherical distribution, $k \geq 2$, with $P(\mathbf{z} = \mathbf{0}) = 0$, we can show that

$$V = Z_1/\{(Z_2^2 + \cdots + Z_k^2)^{1/2}/(k-1)\} \sim t_{k-1}.$$

In many cases, we wish to extend the definition of a spherical distribution to include random vectors with a nonzero mean μ and a general covariance matrix Σ. This generalization leads us from spherical distributions to elliptical (or elliptically contoured distributions), which form the topic of the next subsection.

5.5.3 Elliptical distributions

The family of elliptical or elliptically contoured distributions is the most general family that we will consider as alternatives to the multivariate normal distribution. We derive results on the forms of the corresponding marginal and conditional distributions, and also give some useful results on distributions of quadratic forms in elliptical random vectors. There is a vast literature on spherical and elliptical distributions (Kelker, 1970; Devlin, Gnanadesikan and Ketternring, 1976; Chmielewski, 1981; Fang, Kotz and Ng, 1990; and Fang and Anderson, 1990) and the reader is referred to these for more details on this interesting and useful class of distributions.

Definition 5.5.5. Let the k-dimensional random vector $\mathbf{z}$ follow a spherical distribution, μ be a fixed k-dimensional vector, and Γ be a $k \times k$ matrix. The random vector $\mathbf{x} = \mu + \Gamma\mathbf{z}$ is said to have an elliptical, or elliptically contoured, or elliptically symmetric distribution. Provided they exist, the mean and covariance of $\mathbf{x}$ are

$$E(\mathbf{x}) = \mu, \quad \text{and} \quad Cov(\mathbf{x}) = c\Gamma\Gamma' = c\mathbf{V}$$

where $c \geq 0$ is a constant. The mgf of the distribution, if it exists, has the form

$$M_{\mathbf{x}}(\mathbf{t}) = \psi(\mathbf{t}'\mathbf{V}\mathbf{t}) \exp\{\mathbf{t}'\mu\}$$

for some function ψ. In case the mgf does not exist, we invoke the characteristic function of the distribution for proof of distributional properties.

In order for an elliptically contoured random vector to admit a density (with respect to Lebesgue measure), the matrix $\mathbf{V}$ must be p.d, and the density generator function $h(.)$ in (5.5.3) must satisfy the condition

$$\int_0^\infty \frac{\pi^{k/2}}{\Gamma(k/2)} t^{(k/2)-1} h(t) dt = 1, \quad t \geq 0.$$

If the pdf of $\mathbf{x}$ exists, it will be a function only of the norm $\| \mathbf{x} \| = (\mathbf{x}'\mathbf{x})^{1/2}$ (see Definition 1.2.36). We denote the class of elliptical distributions by $E_k(\mu, \mathbf{V}, h)$. If a random vector $\mathbf{x} \sim E_k(\mathbf{0}, \mathbf{I}_k, h)$, then $\mathbf{x}$ has a spherical distribution. Suppose μ is a fixed k-dimensional vector, and $\mathbf{y} = \mu + \mathbf{Px}$, where $\mathbf{P}$ is a nonsingular $k \times k$ matrix. Then, $\mathbf{y} \sim E_k(\mu, \mathbf{V}, h)$, with $\mathbf{V} = \mathbf{PP}'$.

Result 5.5.1. Let $\mathbf{z}$ denote a spherically distributed random vector with pdf $f(\mathbf{z})$, and let $\mathbf{x} = \mu + \Gamma\mathbf{z}$ have an elliptical distribution, where Γ is a $k \times k$ nonsingular matrix. Let $\mathbf{V} = \Gamma\Gamma'$, and note that $\mathbf{z} = \Gamma^{-1}(\mathbf{x} - \mu)$. Then the pdf of $\mathbf{x}$ has the form

$$f(\mathbf{x}) = c_k |\mathbf{V}|^{-1/2} h[(\mathbf{x} - \mu)'\mathbf{V}^{-1}(\mathbf{x} - \mu)], \quad \mathbf{x} \in \mathcal{R}^k \qquad (5.5.5)$$

for some function $h(.)$ which can be independent of k, and such that $r^{k-1}h(r^2)$ is integrable over $[0, \infty)$.

Proof. The transformation from $\mathbf{z}$ to $\mathbf{x} = \mu + \Gamma\mathbf{z}$ has Jacobian $J = |\Gamma^{-1}|$. By Result 5.1.1, we have for $\mathbf{x} \in \mathcal{R}^k$,

$$\begin{aligned} f(\mathbf{x}) &= c_k |\Gamma|^{-1} f\{\Gamma^{-1}(\mathbf{x} - \mu)\} \\ &= c_k [|\Gamma|^{-1}|\Gamma|^{-1}]^{1/2} h[(\mathbf{x} - \mu)'\Gamma'^{-1}\Gamma^{-1}(\mathbf{x} - \mu)] \\ &= c_k |\mathbf{V}|^{-1/2} h[(\mathbf{x} - \mu)'\mathbf{V}^{-1}(\mathbf{x} - \mu)]. \end{aligned}$$

Note that the same steps are used in the derivation of the multivariate normal pdf in section 5.2. The relation between the spherical distribution and the (corresponding) elliptical distribution is the same as the relationship between the multivariate standard normal distribution (Definition 5.2.1) and the corresponding normal distribution with nonzero mean and covariance Σ (Definition 5.2.2). ■

The distribution of $\mathbf{x}$ will have m moments provided the function $r^{m+k-1}h(r^2)$ is integrable on $[0, \infty)$. We show two examples.

Example 5.5.8. Let $\mathbf{x}$ have a k-variate normal distribution with mean μ and covariance $\sigma^2\mathbf{I}$. Then $\mathbf{x}$ has an elliptical distribution. A rotation about μ is given by $\mathbf{y} = \mathbf{P}(\mathbf{x} - \mu) + \mu$, where $\mathbf{P}$ is an orthogonal matrix. We see that $\mathbf{y} \sim N_k(\mu, \sigma^2\mathbf{I})$ (see Exercise 5.9), so that the distribution is unchanged under rotations about μ. We say that the distribution is spherically symmetric about μ. In fact, the normal distribution is the only multivariate distribution with independent components $X_j, j = 1, \cdots, k$, that is spherically symmetric. □

Example 5.5.9. Suppose $\mathbf{x} = \mu + \Gamma \mathbf{z}$, where $\mathbf{z}$ was defined in Example 5.5.3, $\mu = (\mu_1, \mu_2)'$ is a fixed vector, and Γ is a nonsingular 2×2 matrix. Let $\mathbf{A} = \Gamma\Gamma'$; the pdf of $\mathbf{x} = (X_1, X_2)'$ is

$$f(\mathbf{x}; \mu, \mathbf{A}) = (2\pi)^{-1}|\mathbf{A}|^{-1/2} \left[1 + (\mathbf{x} - \mu)'\mathbf{A}^{-1}(\mathbf{x} - \mu)\right]^{-3/2}, \quad \mathbf{x} \in \mathcal{R}^2.$$

This is the multivariate Cauchy distribution, which is a special case of the multivariate t-distribution. The density generator for the k-variate Cauchy distribution is $h(u) = c\{1 + u\}^{-(k+1)/2}$, while the density generator for the k-variate t-distribution with ν degrees of freedom is $h(u) = c\{1 + u/\nu\}^{-(k+\nu)/2}$. In terms of its use in linear model theory, the Cauchy distribution and the Student's t-distribution with small ν are considered useful as robust alternatives to the multivariate normal distribution in terms of error distribution specification. □

Example 5.5.10. Let $\mathbf{z}$ be the standard double exponential variable specified in Example 5.5.7, and suppose we define $\mathbf{x} = \mu + \Gamma \mathbf{z}$ where $\mu = (\mu_1, \mu_2)'$ is a fixed vector, and Γ is a nonsingular 2×2 matrix. Let $\mathbf{A} = \Gamma\Gamma'$; the pdf of $\mathbf{x} = (X_1, X_2)'$ is

$$f(\mathbf{x}; \mu, \mathbf{A}) = (2\pi)^{-1}|\mathbf{A}|^{-1/2} \exp\{-[(\mathbf{x} - \mu)'\mathbf{A}^{-1}(\mathbf{x} - \mu)]^{1/2}\}, \quad \mathbf{x} \in \mathcal{R}^2.$$

A comparison of the contours of this distribution with those of a bivariate normal distribution having the same location and spread shows that this distribution is more peaked at the center and has heavier tails. □

The next result specifies the marginal distributions and the conditional distributions. Result 5.5.3 characterizes the class of normal distributions within the family of elliptically symmetric distributions. Let $\mathbf{x} = (X_1, \cdots, X_k)' \sim E_k(\mu, \mathbf{V}, h)$.

Result 5.5.2. Suppose we partition $\mathbf{x}$ as $\mathbf{x} = (\mathbf{x}_1', \mathbf{x}_2')'$, where $\mathbf{x}_1$ and $\mathbf{x}_2$ are respectively q-dimensional and $(k - q)$-dimensional vectors. Suppose μ and $\mathbf{V}$ are partitioned conformably (similar to Result 5.2.8).

1. The marginal distribution of $\mathbf{x}_i$ is elliptical, i.e., $\mathbf{x}_1 \sim E_q(\mu_1, \mathbf{V}_{11})$ and $\mathbf{x}_2 \sim E_{k-q}(\mu_2, \mathbf{V}_{22})$. Unless $f(\mathbf{x})$ has an atom of weight at the origin, the pdf of each marginal distribution exists.

2. The conditional distribution of $\mathbf{x}_1$ given $\mathbf{x}_2 = \mathbf{c}_2$ is q-variate elliptical with mean

$$E(\mathbf{x}_1|\mathbf{x}_2 = \mathbf{c}_2) = \mu_1 + \mathbf{V}_{12}\mathbf{V}_{22}^{-1}(\mathbf{c}_2 - \mu_2), \tag{5.5.6}$$

while the conditional covariance of $\mathbf{x}_1$ given $\mathbf{x}_2 = \mathbf{c}_2$ only depends on $\mathbf{c}_2$ through the quadratic form $(\mathbf{x}_2 - \mathbf{c}_2)'\mathbf{V}_{22}^{-1}(\mathbf{x}_2 - \mathbf{c}_2)$. The distribution of $\mathbf{x}_2$ given $\mathbf{x}_1 = \mathbf{c}_1$ is derived similarly.

Proof.   The mgf of x_1 is $\psi(t_1' V_{11} t_1) \exp\{t_1' \mu_1\}$, and that of x_2 is $\psi(t_2' V_{22} t_2)$ $\exp\{t_2' \mu_2\}$, so that $x_1 \sim E_q(\mu_1, V_{11})$ and $x_2 \sim E_{k-q}(\mu_2, V_{22})$. The pdf of x_1, if it exists, has the form

$$f_1(x_1) = c_q |V_{11}|^{-1/2} h_q[(x_1 - \mu_1)' V_{11}^{-1}(x_1 - \mu_1)],$$

where the function h_q depends only on h and q, and is independent of μ and V. To show property 2, we see that by definition, the conditional mean is

$$E(x_1|x_2 = c_2) = \int x_1 dF_{x_1|c_2}(x_1).$$

Substituting $y = x_1 - \mu_1 - V_{12} V_{22}^{-1}(c_2 - \mu_2)$ and simplifying, we get

$$E(x_1|x_2 = c_2) = \int y dF_{y|c_2}(y) + \mu_1 + V_{12} V_{22}^{-1}(c_2 - \mu_2).$$

Since it can be verified that the joint mgf of y and x_2, when it exists, satisfies $M_{y,x_2}(-t_1, t_2) = M_{y,x_2}(t_1, t_2)$, we see that $\int y dF_{y|c_2}(y) = 0$, proving (5.5.6). The conditional covariance is

$$Cov(x_1|x_2 = c_2) = \int [x_1 - E(x_1|x_2 = c_2)][x_1 - E(x_1|x_2 = c_2)]' f_{x_1|x_2}(x_1) dx_1$$

$$= \frac{c_k}{|V|^{1/2}} \int zz' \frac{h[z'V_{11.2}z + (c_2 - \mu_2)'V_{22}^{-1}(c_2 - \mu_2)]}{f_{x_2}(c_2)} dz,$$

where $V_{11.2} = V_{11} - V_{12} V_{22}^{-1} V_{21}$. The result follows since $f_{x_2}(c_2)$ is a function of the quadratic form $(x_2 - c_2)' V_{22}^{-1}(x_2 - c_2)$. ∎

Result 5.5.3.   Suppose x, μ and V are partitioned as in Result 5.5.2.

1. If any marginal pdf of a random vector x which has an $E_k(\mu, V, h)$ distribution is normal, then x must have a normal distribution.

2. If the conditional distribution of x_1 given $x_2 = c_2$ is normal for any q, $q = 1, \cdots, k-1$, then x has a normal distribution.

3. Let $k > 2$, and assume that the pdf of x exists. The conditional covariance of x_1 given $x_2 = c_2$ is independent of x_2 only if x has a normal distribution.

4. If $x \sim E_k(\mu, V, h)$, and V is diagonal, then the components of x are independent only if the distribution of x is normal.

Proof.   By Result 5.5.2, the mgf (or characteristic function) of x has the same form as the mgf (or characteristic function) of x_1, from which property 1 follows. Without loss of generality, let $\mu = 0$ and $V = I$, so that by Result 5.5.2, the conditional mean of x_1 given $x_2 = c_2 = 0$, and its conditional covariance has the form $\phi(c_2) I_{k-q}$. Also, $g(x_1|x_2 = c_2) = c_k h(x_1' x_1 + x_2' x_2)/f_2(c_2)$ is a function of $x_1' x_1$. If the conditional distribution is normal,

$$c_k h(x_1' x_1 + x_2' x_2) = \{2\pi\sigma(c_2)\}^{-(k-q)/2} f_2(c_2) \exp\{-\tfrac{1}{2} x_1' x_1/\sigma(c_2)\},$$

so that

$$c_k h(\mathbf{x}_1'\mathbf{x}_1) = \{2\pi\sigma(\mathbf{c}_2)\}^{-(k-q)/2} f_2(\mathbf{c}_2) \exp\{\tfrac{1}{2}\mathbf{x}_2'\mathbf{x}_2/\sigma(\mathbf{c}_2)\} \exp\{-\tfrac{1}{2}\mathbf{x}_1'\mathbf{x}_1/\sigma(\mathbf{c}_2)\}.$$

This implies that $f(\mathbf{x}) = c_k h(\mathbf{x}'\mathbf{x})$, i.e., $\mathbf{x}$ has a normal distribution, proving property 2. The proof of properties 3 and 4 is left as an exercise. ∎

We end this subsection with results on distributions of quadratic forms in elliptical random vectors, some of which are analogous to the theory for normal distributions. Note that if a random vector $\mathbf{y}$ has pdf $f(\mathbf{y}) = c_k h(\mathbf{y}'\mathbf{y})$, then the pdf of $\| \mathbf{y} \|$ is

$$f_{\|\mathbf{y}\|}(w) = \frac{2c_k \pi^{k/2}}{\Gamma(k/2)} w^{k-1} h(w^2) \tag{5.5.7}$$

(see Kelker, 1970).

Result 5.5.4. Let $\mathbf{x} \sim E_k(\mathbf{0}, \mathbf{V}, h)$ with pdf $f(\mathbf{x}) = c_k |\mathbf{V}|^{-1/2} h(\mathbf{x}'\mathbf{V}^{-1}\mathbf{x})$, and let $Q = \mathbf{x}'\mathbf{V}^{-1}\mathbf{x}$. Then

$$f_Q(w) = \frac{\pi^{k/2}}{\Gamma(k/2)} c_k w^{k/2-1} h(w). \tag{5.5.8}$$

Proof. Let $\mathbf{y} = \mathbf{V}^{-1/2}\mathbf{x}$, and $f(\mathbf{y}) = c_k h(\mathbf{y}'\mathbf{y})$. The distributions of Q and $\mathbf{y}'\mathbf{y}$ coincide. ∎

For $q < k$,

$$g_q(w) = \frac{\pi^{q/2}}{\Gamma(q/2)} c_q w^{q/2-1} h_q(w) \tag{5.5.9}$$

is the pdf of $\sum_{i=1}^q Y_i^2$, for $\mathbf{y} = (Y_1, \cdots, Y_k)'$.

Result 5.5.5. Let $\mathbf{x} \sim E_k(\mathbf{0}, \mathbf{V}, h)$ with finite fourth moment, and let $\mathbf{A}$ be a symmetric matrix of rank r. Then $\mathbf{x}'\mathbf{A}\mathbf{x} \sim g_r(.)$ if and only if

1. $r + r(\mathbf{V}^{-1} - \mathbf{A}) = k$, or

2. $\mathbf{A} = \mathbf{A}\mathbf{V}\mathbf{A}$.

Proof. To prove property 1, assume first that $r + r(\mathbf{V}^{-1} - \mathbf{A}) = k$. By Result 2.4.5, there exists a nonsingular matrix $\mathbf{P}$ such that $\mathbf{V} = \mathbf{P}\mathbf{P}'$. Let $\mathbf{y} = \mathbf{P}^{-1}\mathbf{x}$; $f(\mathbf{y}) = c_k h(\mathbf{y}'\mathbf{y})$. Now, $\mathbf{x}'\mathbf{V}^{-1}\mathbf{x} = \mathbf{x}'\mathbf{A}\mathbf{x} + \mathbf{x}'(\mathbf{V}^{-1} - \mathbf{A})\mathbf{x}$, i.e., $\mathbf{y}'\mathbf{y} = \mathbf{y}'\mathbf{P}'\mathbf{A}\mathbf{P}\mathbf{y} + \mathbf{y}'(\mathbf{I} - \mathbf{P}'\mathbf{A}\mathbf{P})\mathbf{y}$. The rank condition ensures the existence of an orthogonal transformation $\mathbf{z} = \mathbf{B}\mathbf{y}$ such that $f(\mathbf{z}) = f(Z_1, \cdots, Z_k) = c_k h(\mathbf{z}'\mathbf{z})$. Now, $\mathbf{x}'\mathbf{A}\mathbf{x} = \mathbf{y}'\mathbf{P}'\mathbf{A}\mathbf{P}\mathbf{y} = \sum_{i=1}^r Z_i^2 \sim g_r(w)$. To prove the converse, suppose $\mathbf{x}'\mathbf{A}\mathbf{x} \sim g_r(w)$, where $r = r(\mathbf{A})$. There exists a nonsingular matrix $\mathbf{P}$ such that $\mathbf{V} = \mathbf{P}\mathbf{P}'$, and an orthogonal matrix $\mathbf{Q}$ such that $\mathbf{Q}'\mathbf{A}\mathbf{Q} = \mathbf{D} = \text{diag}(\lambda_1, \cdots, \lambda_r, 0, \cdots, 0)$. If $\mathbf{x} = \mathbf{Q}\mathbf{P}\mathbf{z}$, it follows that $\mathbf{x}'\mathbf{A}\mathbf{x} = \mathbf{z}'\mathbf{P}'\mathbf{Q}'\mathbf{A}\mathbf{Q}\mathbf{P}\mathbf{z} =$

$\sum_{i=1}^{r} \lambda_i Z_i^2$. Using the second and fourth moments of $\mathbf{z}$, it can be shown that $\sum_{i=1}^{r} \lambda_i = \sum_{i=1}^{r} \lambda_i^2 = r$, so that $\lambda_i = 1$, $i = 1, \cdots, r$. We can therefore write $\mathbf{x}'\mathbf{V}^{-1}\mathbf{x} = \mathbf{x}'\mathbf{A}\mathbf{x} + \mathbf{x}'(\mathbf{V}^{-1} - \mathbf{A})\mathbf{x}$ as $\mathbf{z}'\mathbf{z} = \sum_{i=1}^{r} Z_i^2 + \sum_{i=r+1}^{k} Z_i^2$. This implies that $r(\mathbf{A}) + r(\mathbf{V}^{-1} - \mathbf{A}) = k$, proving property 1. The proof of property 2 is similar to the proof of property 2 of Result 5.4.5. ∎

Anderson and Fang (1987) discuss Cochran's theorem for elliptical distributions. Matrix variate elliptically contoured distributions extend the elliptical distributions from the vector to the matrix case and an excellent discussion can be seen in Gupta and Varga (1993). Azzalini and Dalla Valle (1996) have discussed the multivariate skew-normal distributions which extend the class of normal distributions by the inclusion of a shape parameter. They described different methods to generate skew-normal distributions. Branco and Dey (2001) used a conditioning method to generate multivariate skew-elliptical distributions.

Exercises

5.1. Let $\mathbf{x} = (X_1, \cdots, X_k) \sim N_k(\mu, \Sigma)$, with $r(\Sigma) = k$.

(a) Show that

$$
\begin{aligned}
I &= \int_{-\infty}^{\infty} \cdots \int_{-\infty}^{\infty} \exp\{-\frac{1}{2}(\mathbf{x} - \mu)'\Sigma^{-1}(\mathbf{x} - \mu)\} dx_1 \cdots dx_k \\
&= (2\pi)^{k/2}|\Sigma|^{1/2}.
\end{aligned}
$$

(b) Evaluate $\int_{-\infty}^{\infty} \cdots \int_{-\infty}^{\infty} \exp\{-(x_1^2 + 2x_1 x_2 + 4x_2^2)\} dx_1 dx_2$.

5.2. [Graybill, 1961]. Let $\mathbf{x} = (X_1, X_2)$ have a bivariate normal distribution with pdf

$$
f(\mathbf{x}; \mu, \Sigma) = \frac{1}{k} \exp(-Q/2)
$$

where $Q = 2x_1^2 - x_1 x_2 + 4x_2^2 - 11x_1 - 5x_2 + 19$, and k is a constant. Find a constant a such that $P(3X_1 - X_2 < a) = 0.01$.

5.3. Let X_1 and X_2 be random variables such that $X_1 + X_2$ and $X_1 - X_2$ have independent standard normal distributions. Show that $\mathbf{x} = (X_1, X_2)$ has a bivariate normal distribution.

5.4. The logarithm of the mgf of a trivariate random vector $\mathbf{x} = (X_1, X_2, X_3)'$ is given by

$$
\ln M_{\mathbf{x}}(\mathbf{t}) = 5t_1^2 + 3t_2^2 + 6t_3^2 - 2t_1 t_2 + 4t_1 t_3 + 2t_2 t_3 + 4t_1 - 2t_2 + t_3.
$$

Show that **x** has a trivariate normal distribution. Identify the mean and variance-covariance matrix of the distribution.

5.5. (a) Show that (X_1, X_2) has a bivariate normal distribution with means μ_1, μ_2, variances σ_1^2 and σ_2^2, and correlation coefficient ρ if and only if every linear combination $c_1 X_1 + c_2 X_2$ has a univariate normal distribution with mean $c_1 \mu_1 + c_2 \mu_2$, and variance $c_1^2 \sigma_1^2 + c_2^2 \sigma_2^2 + 2 c_1 c_2 \rho \sigma_{12}$, where c_1 and c_2 are real constants, not both equal to zero.

(b) Let $Y_i = X_i / \sigma_i$, $i = 1, 2$. Show that $Var(Y_1 - Y_2) = 2(1 - \rho)$.

5.6. (a) Let $(X_1, X_2) \sim N_2(\mu_1, \mu_2, \sigma_1^2, \sigma_2^2, \rho)$ where $\mu_1 = \mu_2 = 0$, and $\rho \neq 1$. The polar coordinate transformation is defined by $X_1 = R \cos \Theta$, $X_2 = R \sin \Theta$. Show that the joint pdf of R and Θ is given by

$$r(2\pi)^{-1}(1 - \rho^2)^{-1/2} \exp\left\{ -\frac{1}{2(1-\rho^2)} r^2 (1 - \rho \sin 2\theta) \right\},$$

$0 \le r < \infty$, and $0 \le \theta \le 2\pi$, and that the marginal pdf of Θ is

$$(2\pi)^{-1}(1 - \rho^2)^{1/2}(1 - \rho \sin 2\theta)^{-1}, \quad 0 \le \theta \le 2\pi.$$

(b) Suppose (X_1, X_2) has a bivariate normal distribution $N_2(0, 0, \sigma_1^2, \sigma_2^2, \rho)$, $|\rho| \neq 1$. Show that

$$P(X_1 > 0, X_2 > 0) = \tfrac{1}{4} + \tfrac{1}{2\pi} \sin^{-1}(\rho).$$

5.7. The random vector $\mathbf{x} = (X_1, X_2, \cdots, X_k)'$ is said to have a symmetric multivariate normal distribution if $\mathbf{x} \sim N_k(\mu, \Sigma)$ where $\mu = \mu \mathbf{1}_k$, i.e., the mean of each X_j is equal to the same constant μ, and Σ is the equicorrelation dispersion matrix, i.e.,

$$\Sigma = \sigma^2 \begin{pmatrix} 1 & \rho & \cdots & \rho \\ \rho & 1 & \cdots & \rho \\ \vdots & \vdots & \ddots & \vdots \\ \rho & \rho & \cdots & 1 \end{pmatrix}.$$

When $k = 3$, $\mu = 0$, $\sigma^2 = 2$ and $\rho = 1/2$, find the probability that $X_3 = \min(X_1, X_2, X_3)$.

Hint: Recall that if $\mathbf{x} = (X_1, \cdots, X_k)'$ has a continuous symmetric distribution, then all possible permutations of $X_1, \cdots, X_k$ are equally likely, each having probability $P(X_{i_1} < \cdots < X_{i_k}) = 1/k!$ for any permutation $(i_1, \cdots, i_k)$ of the first k positive integers.

5.8. Let $\mathbf{x} \sim N_k(\mathbf{0}, \Sigma)$ with pdf $f(\mathbf{x})$ where $\Sigma = \{\Sigma_{ij}\}$. The entropy $h(\mathbf{x})$ is defined as

$$h(\mathbf{x}) = -\int f(\mathbf{x}) \ln f(\mathbf{x})$$

(a) Show that $h(\mathbf{x}) = \tfrac{1}{2} \ln(2\pi e)^k |\Sigma|$.

(b) Hence, or otherwise, show that $|\Sigma| \leq \prod_{i=1}^{k} \Sigma_{ii}$, with equality holding if and only if $\Sigma_{ij} = 0$, for $i \neq j$ [Hadamard's inequality].

5.9. Let $\mathbf{x} \sim N_k(\mathbf{0}, \sigma^2 \mathbf{I})$ and let $\mathbf{y} = \mathbf{P}\mathbf{x}$, where $\mathbf{P}$ is a $k \times k$ orthogonal matrix. Show that $\mathbf{y}$ has a $N_k(\mathbf{0}, \sigma^2 \mathbf{I})$ distribution.

5.10. Let $\mathbf{x} \sim N_k(\mu, \Sigma)$, where $r(\Sigma) = r \leq k$. Show that there exists an $r \times k$ matrix $\mathbf{B}$ and an r-dimensional vector $\mathbf{b}$ such that the vector $\mathbf{z} = \mathbf{B}\mathbf{x} + \mathbf{b}$ has a $N_r(\mathbf{0}, \mathbf{I})$ distribution.

5.11. Let $\mathbf{x} \sim N_k(\mu, \Sigma)$, where $\mu = (\mu_1, \cdots, \mu_k)'$ and $\Sigma = \{\sigma_{ij}\}$, $i, j = 1, \cdots, k$. Show that $X_i \sim N(\mu_i, \sigma_{ii})$.

5.12. Let $\mathbf{x} \sim N_k(\mu, \Sigma)$ and suppose that $\mathbf{x} = (\mathbf{x}_1', \mathbf{x}_2', \mathbf{x}_3')'$, where $\mathbf{x}_i$ is a k_i-dimensional vector, and $\sum_{i=1}^{3} k_i = k$. Assume that μ and Σ are partitioned conformably. Derive the conditional distribution of $\mathbf{x}_3$ given $\mathbf{x}_1 = \mathbf{c}_1$, and $\mathbf{x}_2 = \mathbf{c}_2$.

5.13. Let $\mathbf{x} = (X_1, X_2, X_3)' \sim N_3(\mu, \Sigma)$, where $\mu = (\mu_1, \mu_2, \mu_3)'$ and $\Sigma = \sigma^2 \begin{pmatrix} 1 & \rho & 0 \\ \rho & 1 & \rho \\ 0 & \rho & 1 \end{pmatrix}$.

(a) What are the marginal distributions of X_2 and X_3?

(b) Write down the conditional distribution of X_1 given X_2 and X_3. Under what condition does this distribution coincide with the marginal distribution of X_1?

(c) For what value of ρ are the two random variables $X_1 + X_2 + X_3$ and $X_1 - X_2 - X_3$ independently distributed?

5.14. Let $\mathbf{x} = (X_1, X_2, X_3)' \sim N_3(\mathbf{0}, \Sigma)$, where $\Sigma = \begin{pmatrix} 1 & \rho & \rho \\ \rho & 1 & \rho \\ \rho & \rho & 1 \end{pmatrix}$. Show that

(a) $Corr(X_1^2, X_2^2) = \rho^2$

(b) $\rho_{12|3} = \rho/(1 + \rho)$

(c) $\rho_{1(2,3)} = 2\rho^2/(1 + \rho)$.

5.15. For any distribution, let $E(X_2|X_1 = x_1) = \alpha + \beta x_1$. Show that $Corr(X_1, X_2) = \beta \sigma_1/\sigma_2$, where σ_1 and σ_2 denote the respective standard deviations of X_1 and X_2.

5.16. Show that $\chi^2(k, \lambda) = \chi^2(1, \lambda) + \chi^2_{k-1}$.

5.17. Let $U \sim \chi^2(k, \lambda)$. Show that $P(U \leq u) = P(X_1 - X_2 \geq k/2)$ where X_1 and X_2 are independent Poisson random variables with respective means $u/2$ and λ.

5.18. Suppose $X_1, \cdots, X_k$ are iid $\chi^2(1, \lambda/k)$. Show that $Y = \sum_{i=1}^{k} X_i$ has a $\chi^2(k, \lambda)$ distribution.

5.19. Let $(X_1, X_2) \sim N_2(\mu_1, \mu_2, \sigma_1^2, \sigma_2^2, \rho)$, $|\rho| \neq 1$. Show that

$$T = \tfrac{1}{(1-\rho^2)} \left[\left(\tfrac{X_1-\mu_1}{\sigma_1} \right)^2 - 2\rho \left(\tfrac{X_1-\mu_1}{\sigma_1} \right) \left(\tfrac{X_2-\mu_2}{\sigma_2} \right) + \left(\tfrac{X_2-\mu_2}{\sigma_2} \right)^2 \right]$$

has a χ^2 distribution. What are its parameters?

5.20. (a) Let $\mathbf{x} \sim N_k(\mu, \mathbf{I})$. Show that $U = \mathbf{x}'\mathbf{x}$ has a $\chi^2(k, \lambda)$ distribution, with $\lambda = \mu'\mu/2$.

(b) Let $\mathbf{x} \sim N_k(\mu, \sigma^2\mathbf{I})$. Show that $\mathbf{x}'\mathbf{x}/\sigma^2 \sim \chi^2(k, \mu'\mu/2\sigma^2)$.

5.21. (a) Let $\mathbf{x} \sim N_k(\mu, \mathbf{D})$, where $\mathbf{D} = \text{diag}(\sigma_1^2, \cdots, \sigma_k^2)$, $r(\mathbf{D}) = k$. Find the mean and variance of the random variable $U = \mathbf{x}'\mathbf{D}^{-1}\mathbf{x}$.

(b) Let $\mathbf{x} \sim N_k(\mu, \Sigma)$, with $r(\Sigma) = k$. What is the distribution of $U = (\mathbf{x} - \mu)'\Sigma^{-1}(\mathbf{x} - \mu)$?

(c) Suppose $\mathbf{A} = \mathbf{D}^{-1} - (\mathbf{D}^{-1}\mathbf{1}\mathbf{1}'\mathbf{D}^{-1})/\mathbf{1}'\mathbf{D}^{-1}\mathbf{1}$. Assume that $\mathbf{x} \sim N_k(\mu, \mathbf{D})$ distribution. Find the distribution of $\mathbf{x}'\mathbf{A}\mathbf{x}$.

5.22. Let $V \sim F(k_1, k_2, \lambda)$. Show that

$$E(V) = \tfrac{k_2}{k_2-2}(1 + \tfrac{2\lambda}{k_1})$$

and

$$Var(V) = \tfrac{2k_2^2}{k_1^2(k_2-2)} \left[\tfrac{(k_1+2\lambda)^2}{(k_2-2)(k_2-4)} + \tfrac{k_1+4\lambda}{k_2-4} \right]$$

5.23. If $\mathbf{x} \sim N_k(\mu, \Sigma)$, show that

(a) $E(\mathbf{x}'\mathbf{A}\mathbf{x}) = tr(\mathbf{A}\Sigma) + \mu'\mathbf{A}\mu$.

(b) $Var(\mathbf{x}'\mathbf{A}\mathbf{x}) = 2tr(\mathbf{A}\Sigma)^2 + 4\mu'\mathbf{A}\Sigma\mathbf{A}\mu$.

(c) $Cov(\mathbf{x}, \mathbf{x}'\mathbf{A}\mathbf{x}) = 2\Sigma\mathbf{A}\mu$.

5.24. Let $\mathbf{x} \sim N_k(\mu, \mathbf{I})$. Show that $\mathbf{x}'\mathbf{A}\mathbf{x} \sim \chi^2(k, \tfrac{1}{2}\mu'\mathbf{A}\mu)$ if and only if $\mathbf{A}$ is idempotent of rank m.

5.25. Let $\mathbf{x} \sim N_k(\mathbf{0}, \Sigma)$. Show that $\mathbf{x}'\mathbf{A}\mathbf{x} \sim \chi_m^2$ if and only if $\mathbf{A}\Sigma$ is an idempotent matrix with $r(\mathbf{A}) = m$.

5.26. Let $\mathbf{x} \sim N_k(\mu, \mathbf{Q}\mathbf{A})$, where $\mathbf{A}$ is a positive definite matrix, and $\mathbf{Q}$ is symmetric and idempotent with $tr(Q) = m$. What is the distribution of $U = \mathbf{x}'\mathbf{A}^{-1}\mathbf{x}$?

5.27. Suppose $\mathbf{x} = (X_1, X_2, X_3)'$ is distributed as $N_3(\mathbf{0}, \mathbf{I})$. Let $Q = \tfrac{1}{6}(X_1^2 + 4X_2^2 + X_3^2 - 4X_1X_2 + 2X_1X_3 - 4X_2X_3)$. Find the distribution of Q.

5.28. Let $\mathbf{x} \sim N_k(\mathbf{0}, \Sigma)$, where $\Sigma = \sigma^2[(1 - \rho)\mathbf{I}_k + \rho\mathbf{J}_k]$, $0 \leq \rho < 1$.

   (a) Show that the distinct eigenvalues of Σ are $\lambda_1 = 1 - \rho$, with multiplicity $g_1 = k - 1$, and $\lambda_2 = 1 + (k - 1)\rho$ with multiplicity $g_2 = 1$.

   (b) Define $\mathbf{A}_1 = \mathbf{I}_k - \mathbf{J}_k/k$, and $\mathbf{A}_2 = \mathbf{J}_k/k$. Show that $\mathbf{A}_1$ and $\mathbf{A}_2$ are
idempotent, $\mathbf{A}_1\mathbf{A}_2 = \mathbf{0}$, and that $\Sigma = \lambda_1\mathbf{A}_1 + \lambda_2\mathbf{A}_2$.

   (c) Let $Q_i = \mathbf{x}'\mathbf{A}_i\mathbf{x}/\lambda_i$, $i = 1, 2$. Show that Q_1 and Q_2 have independent
chi-square distributions. Find the parameters of these distributions.

5.29. Let $\mathbf{x} \sim N_k(\mu, \Sigma)$, where $\mu = \mu\mathbf{1}_k$ and $\Sigma = \sigma^2[(1 - \rho)\mathbf{I}_k + \rho\mathbf{1}_k\mathbf{1}_k']$, $0 \leq \rho < 1$.

   (a) Derive the distributions of $\overline{X} = \sum_{i=1}^{k} X_i/k$ and $Q = \sum_{i=1}^{k}(X_i - \overline{X})^2/[\sigma^2(1 - \rho)]$.

   (b) Verify that $\overline{X}$ is distributed independently of Q.

5.30. Let $\mathbf{x} \sim N_k(\Sigma\mu, \sigma^2\Sigma)$, where Σ is a symmetric matrix of rank k, $\sigma^2 > 0$, and μ is a fixed vector. Let $\mathbf{B} = \Sigma^{-1} - \Sigma^{-1}\mathbf{1}_k(\mathbf{1}_k'\Sigma^{-1}\mathbf{1}_k)^{-1}\mathbf{1}_k'\Sigma^{-1}$.

   (a) Derive the distribution of $\mathbf{y} = \mathbf{B}\mathbf{x}$.

   (b) Derive the distribution of $\mathbf{y}'\Sigma\mathbf{y}$ when (i) $\mu = \mathbf{0}$, and (ii) $\mu \neq \mathbf{0}$.

   Hint: Show that $\mathbf{B}$ is symmetric and $\mathbf{B}\Sigma$ is idempotent.

5.31. (a) Show that two quadratic forms $\mathbf{x}'\mathbf{A}\mathbf{x}$ and $\mathbf{x}'\mathbf{B}\mathbf{x}$ in $\mathbf{x} \sim N_k(\mathbf{0}, \sigma^2\mathbf{I})$ are
independently distributed if and only if $\mathbf{A}\mathbf{B} = \mathbf{0}$ (Craig's Thoerem).

   (b) If further, $\mathbf{A}$ and $\mathbf{B}$ are idempotent matrices, show that $\mathbf{x}'\mathbf{A}\mathbf{x}/\sigma^2$
and $\mathbf{x}'\mathbf{B}\mathbf{x}/\sigma^2$ are independent chi-square variables.

5.32. Let $\mathbf{x} = (X_1, X_2)' \sim N_2(\mu\mathbf{1}, \Sigma)$, where $\Sigma = (1 - \rho)\mathbf{I}_2 + \rho\mathbf{J}_2$. Let $Q_1 = (X_1 - X_2)^2$ and $Q_2 = (X_1 + X_2)^2$. Show that $Q_1/2(1 - \rho)$ has a χ^2 distribution and that Q_1 and Q_2 are distributed independently.

5.33. Let $\mathbf{x} \sim N_k(\mu, \Sigma)$. Show that a necessary and sufficient condition for $(\mathbf{x} - \mu)'\mathbf{A}(\mathbf{x} - \mu)$ and $(\mathbf{x} - \mu)'\mathbf{B}(\mathbf{x} - \mu)$ to be independently distributed is $\Sigma\mathbf{A}\Sigma\mathbf{B}\Sigma = \mathbf{0}$.

5.34. [Driscoll and Krasnicka, 1995]. Show that the matrix Λ in (5.4.17) is nonsingular.

5.35. Prove properties 3 and 4 in Result 5.5.3.

Chapter 6

Sampling from the Multivariate Normal Distribution

Let $\mathbf{x}_1, \cdots, \mathbf{x}_N$ denote a random sample from a k-variate normal distribution with mean vector μ and variance-covariance matrix Σ, where we write $\mathbf{x}_i = (X_{i,1}, \cdots, X_{i,k})'$, $i = 1, \cdots, N$. Let $\mathbf{X}' = (\mathbf{x}_1, \cdots, \mathbf{x}_N)$. The joint density of this random sample is obtained as the product of N multivariate normal densities. Let us denote the parameter space by $\Omega = \{\mu, \Sigma; \mu \in \mathcal{R}^k, \Sigma \text{ p.d.}\}$. In the following sections, we describe estimation of the parameters from a multivariate normal distribution and describe properties of these estimates. We also describe inference for the simple, multiple, and partial correlation coefficients based on the normal random sample. In practice, we must of course assess whether the random sample does indeed come from a normal distribution. We present some methods for assessing normality and also describe suitable transformations to normality.

6.1 Distribution of sample mean and covariance

The mean of the random sample $\mathbf{x}_1, \cdots, \mathbf{x}_N$ is defined as the k-dimensional vector

$$\overline{\mathbf{x}}_N = \frac{1}{N} \sum_{i=1}^{N} \mathbf{x}_i, \tag{6.1.1}$$

and the sample covariance matrix is the $k \times k$ matrix $\mathbf{S}_N/(N-1)$, where

$$\mathbf{S}_N = \sum_{i=1}^{N} (\mathbf{x}_i - \overline{\mathbf{x}}_N)(\mathbf{x}_i - \overline{\mathbf{x}}_N)' = \sum_{i=1}^{N} \mathbf{x}_i \mathbf{x}_i' - N\overline{\mathbf{x}}_N \overline{\mathbf{x}}_N'. \tag{6.1.2}$$

We can write $\mathbf{S}_N/(N-1) = \{S_{jl}\}$, $j, l = 1, \cdots, k$, with

$$S_{jl} = \sum_{i=1}^{N}(X_{i,j} - \overline{X}_j)(X_{i,l} - \overline{X}_l)/(N-1),$$

where $\overline{X}_j = \sum_{i=1}^{N} X_{i,j}/N$. The sample covariance matrix has k variances $S_{jj}, j = 1, \cdots, k$ and $k(k-1)/2$ possibly distinct covariances, $S_{jl}, j < l, j, l = 1, \cdots, k$. The generalized sample variance is the scalar quantity $|\mathbf{S}_N/(N-1)|$, which determines the degree of "peakedness" of the joint density of $\mathbf{x}_1, \cdots, \mathbf{x}_N$, and is a natural summary measure of variability in the sample.

Given a univariate random sample $X_1, \cdots, X_N$ from a $N(\mu, \sigma^2)$ population, we know that the sample mean $\overline{X}$ has a normal distribution with mean μ and variance σ^2/N, the statistic $(N-1)S^2/\sigma^2$ is distributed as a χ^2_{N-1} variable, and the two distributions are independent (Casella and Berger, 1990; Mukhopadhyay, 2000). The corresponding distributional result for the k-variate situation is given in Result 6.1.1. We first define a multivariate distribution called the Wishart distribution, which is derived from the multivariate normal distribution as the sampling distribution of the sample statistic $\sum_{i=1}^{N}(\mathbf{x}_i - \overline{\mathbf{x}}_N)(\mathbf{x}_i - \overline{\mathbf{x}}_N)'$. The Wishart distribution is a multivariate extension of the chi-square distribution.

Definition 6.1.1. Wishart distribution.   A random $k \times k$ matrix $\mathbf{W}$ is said to follow a k-dimensional (noncentral) Wishart distribution, $(W_k(\Sigma, m, \lambda))$, with m degrees of freedom, parameter Σ, and noncentrality parameter $\lambda = \mu'\Sigma^{-1}\mu/2$ if $\mathbf{W}$ can be represented as $\mathbf{W} = \sum_{j=1}^{m}\mathbf{x}_j\mathbf{x}_j'$, where $\mathbf{x}_j$, $j = 1, \cdots, m$ are iid $N_k(\mu, \Sigma)$ vectors. Provided $m > k$, the density function of $\mathbf{W}$ is

$$f(\mathbf{W}; \mu, \Sigma) = \frac{|\mathbf{W}|^{(m-k-1)/2}\exp\{tr(-\Sigma^{-1}\mathbf{W}/2)\}}{2^{km/2}|\Sigma|^{m/2}\Gamma_k(m/2)}, \qquad (6.1.3)$$

where $\Gamma_k(m/2) = \pi^{k(k-1)/4}\prod_{j=1}^{k}\Gamma(\frac{1}{2}(m+1-j))$ is the multivariate Gamma function. If $\lambda = 0$, we say that $\mathbf{W}$ follows a central Wishart distribution $W_k(\Sigma, m)$; since Σ is p.d., it is clear that $\lambda = 0$ if and only if $\mu = \mathbf{0}$. The additivity property of Wishart matrices states that if $\mathbf{W}_j \overset{\text{ind}}{\sim} W_k(\Sigma, m_j)$, $j = 1, \cdots, J$, then $\sum_{j=1}^{J}\mathbf{W}_j \sim W_k(\Sigma, \sum_{j=1}^{J} m_j)$.

Result 6.1.1.   Distribution of $\overline{\mathbf{x}}_N$ and $\mathbf{S}_N$.   Let $\mathbf{x}_1, \cdots, \mathbf{x}_N$ denote a random sample from a $N_k(\mu, \Sigma)$ population. Then

1. the distribution of $\overline{\mathbf{x}}_N$ is $N_k(\mu, \Sigma/N)$,

2. for $N \geq 2$, $\mathbf{S}_N$ follows a Wishart $W_k(\Sigma, N-1)$ distribution, and

3. $\overline{\mathbf{x}}_N$ and $\mathbf{S}_N$ are independently distributed.

Proof. From (5.2.7), $M_{\mathbf{x}_j}(\mathbf{t}) = \exp\{\mathbf{t}'\mu + \frac{1}{2}\mathbf{t}'\Sigma\mathbf{t}\}$, so that

$$M_{\bar{\mathbf{x}}_N}(\mathbf{t}) = \prod_{j=1}^{N} M_{\mathbf{x}_j}(\mathbf{t}/N) = \exp\{\mathbf{t}'\mu + \tfrac{1}{2}\mathbf{t}'(\Sigma/N)\mathbf{t}\},$$

which proves property 1. We prove property 2 by induction on N (see Ghosh, 1996). For $N = 2$, it follows from (6.1.2) that

$$
\begin{aligned}
\mathbf{S}_2 &= [\mathbf{x}_1 - \frac{1}{2}(\mathbf{x}_1 + \mathbf{x}_2)][\mathbf{x}_1 - \frac{1}{2}(\mathbf{x}_1 + \mathbf{x}_2)]' \\
&= \frac{1}{2}(\mathbf{x}_1 - \mathbf{x}_2)(\mathbf{x}_1 - \mathbf{x}_2)',
\end{aligned}
$$

while from Result 5.2.5 and Result 5.2.6, we see that $(\mathbf{x}_1 - \mathbf{x}_2)/\sqrt{2} \sim N_k(\mathbf{0}, \Sigma)$. By Definition 6.1.1, $\mathbf{S}_2 \sim W_k(\Sigma, 1)$. To use the induction argument, assume that property 2 holds for $N = m$. We leave as an exercise the verification of the following identities:

$$
\begin{aligned}
\bar{\mathbf{x}}_{m+1} &= \frac{1}{m+1}(m\bar{\mathbf{x}}_m + \mathbf{x}_{m+1}), \text{ and} \\
\mathbf{S}_{m+1} &= \mathbf{S}_m + \frac{m}{m+1}(\mathbf{x}_{m+1} - \bar{\mathbf{x}}_m)(\mathbf{x}_{m+1} - \bar{\mathbf{x}}_m)'. \quad (6.1.4)
\end{aligned}
$$

Since $\mathbf{x}_i$, $i = 1, \cdots, m+1$ are mutually independent, and since $(\bar{\mathbf{x}}_m, \mathbf{S}_m)$ is a function only of $\mathbf{x}_i$, $i = 1, \cdots, m$, it follows that $(\bar{\mathbf{x}}_{m+1}, \mathbf{S}_m)$ is independent of $\mathbf{x}_{m+1}$. By the induction hypothesis, we also have independence of $\bar{\mathbf{x}}_m$ and $\mathbf{S}_m$. It follows that $\bar{\mathbf{x}}_m$, $\mathbf{S}_m$, and $\mathbf{x}_{m+1}$ are mutually independent. Thus, $\mathbf{S}_m$ is independent of $(\bar{\mathbf{x}}_m, \mathbf{x}_{m+1})$, and hence independent of $\mathbf{x}_{m+1} - \bar{\mathbf{x}}_m$ which follows a $N_k(\mathbf{0}, \frac{m+1}{m}\Sigma)$. By Definition 6.1.1, $\frac{m}{m+1}(\mathbf{x}_{m+1} - \bar{\mathbf{x}}_m)(\mathbf{x}_{m+1} - \bar{\mathbf{x}}_m)' \sim W_k(\Sigma, 1)$. By assumption, $\mathbf{S}_m \sim W_k(\Sigma, m-1)$. The proof of property 2 follows from the additivity property of Wishart matrices. To prove property 3, note that

$$Cov(\mathbf{x}_i - \bar{\mathbf{x}}_N, \bar{\mathbf{x}}_N) = \tfrac{1}{N}\Sigma - \tfrac{1}{N}\Sigma = \mathbf{0}, \quad i = 1, \cdots, N,$$

which implies that $[(\mathbf{x}_1 - \bar{\mathbf{x}}_N)', \cdots, (\mathbf{x}_N - \bar{\mathbf{x}}_N)']'$ is uncorrelated with, and therefore independent of, $\bar{\mathbf{x}}_N$. It follows directly that $\mathbf{S}_N$ is distributed independently of $\bar{\mathbf{x}}_N$. ∎

Example 6.1.1. For any vector $\mathbf{a} = (a_1, \cdots, a_k)'$, we show that the statistic $\mathbf{a}'\mathbf{S}_N\mathbf{a}/\mathbf{a}'\Sigma\mathbf{a} \sim \chi^2_{N-1}$. Decomposing $\mathbf{S}_N$ as in (6.1.2), $\mathbf{a}'\mathbf{S}_N\mathbf{a} = \sum_{i=1}^{N} \mathbf{a}'(\mathbf{x}_i - \bar{\mathbf{x}}_N)(\mathbf{x}_i - \bar{\mathbf{x}}_N)'\mathbf{a}$. That $\mathbf{a}'\mathbf{S}_N\mathbf{a}$ is a scaled chi-square is an immediate consequence. □

Anderson (1984) gives an alternate proof using the Helmert transformation, while Mardia, Kent and Bibby (1979) use a multivariate version of Cochran's theorem. A *sufficient statistic* for a parameter is a function of the sample observations that captures all the information about that parameter. Additional information in the sample, beyond that contained in the sufficient statistic, provides no information about the parameter of interest. The conditional distribution of the sufficient statistic given the sample data does not depend on the parameter. The factorization theorem (Halmos and Savage, 1949) enables us to identify a sufficient statistic by inspecting the form of the pdf or pmf of the random sample. We give a statement of the factorization theorem and use it to identify the sufficient statistics in a random sample from a k-variate normal distribution. Let $f(x|\theta)$ denote the joint pdf or pmf of a random sample $\mathbf{X}$. A statistic $T(\mathbf{X})$ is a sufficient statistic for θ if and only if there exist functions $g(t|\theta)$ and $h(x)$ such that $f(x|\theta) = g(T(x)|\theta)h(x)$, for all sample points x and all parameter values θ.

Result 6.1.2.   The sample mean and sample variance are sufficient statistics for μ and Σ in a k-variate normal random sample $\mathbf{x}_1, \cdots, \mathbf{x}_N$.

Proof.   The joint density function of N random vectors $\mathbf{x}_1, \cdots, \mathbf{x}_N$ is a product of the marginal k-variate normal densities:

$$
\begin{aligned}
f(\mathbf{x}_1, \cdots, \mathbf{x}_N; \mu, \Sigma) &= \prod_{i=1}^{N} \frac{\exp\{-\frac{1}{2}(\mathbf{x}_i - \mu)'\Sigma^{-1}(\mathbf{x}_i - \mu)\}}{(2\pi)^{k/2}|\Sigma|^{1/2}} \\
&= \frac{\exp\{-\frac{1}{2}\sum_{i=1}^{N}(\mathbf{x}_i - \mu)'\Sigma^{-1}(\mathbf{x}_i - \mu)\}}{(2\pi)^{Nk/2}|\Sigma|^{N/2}}.
\end{aligned} \tag{6.1.5}
$$

Since $\sum_{i=1}^{N}(\mathbf{x}_i - \bar{\mathbf{x}}_N)(\bar{\mathbf{x}}_N - \mu)' = \mathbf{0}$, and $\sum_{i=1}^{N}(\bar{\mathbf{x}}_N - \mu)(\mathbf{x}_i - \bar{\mathbf{x}}_N)' = \mathbf{0}$, using Result 1.2.8, we can write $\sum_{i=1}^{N}(\mathbf{x}_i - \mu)'\Sigma^{-1}(\mathbf{x}_i - \mu) = \sum_{i=1}^{N} tr(\mathbf{x}_i - \mu)'\Sigma^{-1}(\mathbf{x}_i - \mu) = \sum_{i=1}^{N} tr[\Sigma^{-1}(\mathbf{x}_i - \mu)(\mathbf{x}_i - \mu)'] = tr[\Sigma^{-1}\sum_{i=1}^{N}\{(\mathbf{x}_i - \mu)(\mathbf{x}_i - \mu)'\}] = tr[\Sigma^{-1}\sum_{i=1}^{N}\{(\mathbf{x}_i - \bar{\mathbf{x}}_N + \bar{\mathbf{x}}_N - \mu)(\mathbf{x}_i - \bar{\mathbf{x}}_N + \bar{\mathbf{x}}_N - \mu)'\}] = tr[\Sigma^{-1}\sum_{i=1}^{N}\{(\mathbf{x}_i - \bar{\mathbf{x}}_N)(\mathbf{x}_i - \bar{\mathbf{x}}_N)'\}] + N(\bar{\mathbf{x}}_N - \mu)'\Sigma^{-1}(\bar{\mathbf{x}}_N - \mu)$. The joint density function can be written as

$$
f(\mathbf{x}_1, \cdots, \mathbf{x}_N; \mu, \Sigma) = \frac{\exp\left\{-\frac{1}{2}tr\left[(N-1)\Sigma^{-1}\mathbf{S}_N\right] - \frac{N}{2}(\bar{\mathbf{x}}_N - \mu)'\Sigma^{-1}(\bar{\mathbf{x}}_N - \mu)\right\}}{(2\pi)^{Nk/2}|\Sigma|^{N/2}},
$$

(6.1.6)

and depends on the sample observations $\mathbf{x}_1, \cdots, \mathbf{x}_N$ only through $\bar{\mathbf{x}}_N$ and $\mathbf{S}_N$. By the factorization theorem, these two sample statistics are *sufficient statistics* for μ and Σ.   ∎

Result 6.1.2 states a special property of a multivariate normal sample. Further, by Basu's theorem (Basu, 1964), $\bar{\mathbf{x}}_N$ and $\mathbf{S}_N$ are independently distributed. In general, the sample mean and variance are not sufficient statistics in nonnormal samples. Given observed values of $\mathbf{x}_1, \cdots, \mathbf{x}_N$, (6.1.6) viewed as a function of μ and Σ is the *likelihood function*, maximizing which yields the MLE's of these parameters. The MLE's of the mean vector and covariance matrix of a k-variate normal population are derived in the following result.

Result 6.1.3. Maximum likelihood estimation of μ and Σ. Based on a random sample $\mathbf{x}_1, \cdots, \mathbf{x}_N$ from a $N_k(\mu, \Sigma)$ distribution, the maximum likelihood estimates of μ and Σ are

$$\widehat{\mu}_{ML} = \frac{1}{N}\sum_{i=1}^{N}\mathbf{x}_i = \overline{\mathbf{x}}_N, \text{ and} \tag{6.1.7}$$

$$\widehat{\Sigma}_{ML} = \frac{1}{N}\sum_{i=1}^{N}(\mathbf{x}_i - \overline{\mathbf{x}}_N)(\mathbf{x}_i - \overline{\mathbf{x}}_N)' = \frac{N-1}{N}\mathbf{S}_N. \tag{6.1.8}$$

Proof. The likelihood function $L(\mu, \Sigma; \mathbf{x}_1, \cdots, \mathbf{x}_N)$ has the form shown on the right side of (6.1.5). The MLE's of μ and Σ are denoted by $\widehat{\mu}_{ML}$ and $\widehat{\Sigma}_{ML}$, and are the values that maximize $L(\mu, \Sigma; \mathbf{x}_1, \cdots, \mathbf{x}_N)$. Since Σ^{-1} is p.d. (see Definition 2.4.5), the distance $(\overline{\mathbf{x}}_\mathbf{N} - \mu)'\Sigma^{-1}(\overline{\mathbf{x}}_\mathbf{N} - \mu)$ in the exponent of the likelihood function is positive unless $\mu = \overline{\mathbf{x}}_\mathbf{N}$. The MLE of μ is then $\overline{\mathbf{x}}_\mathbf{N}$, since it is the value of μ that maximizes the likelihood function. We next maximize the following function with respect to Σ:

$$L(\widehat{\mu}_{ML}, \Sigma) = \frac{\exp\left\{-\frac{1}{2}tr\left[\Sigma^{-1}\sum_{i=1}^{N}(\mathbf{x}_i - \overline{\mathbf{x}}_N)(\mathbf{x}_i - \overline{\mathbf{x}}_N)'\right]\right\}}{(2\pi)^{Nk/2}|\Sigma|^{N/2}}. \tag{6.1.9}$$

Using Example 2.4.4 with $\mathbf{A} = \Sigma$, $\mathbf{B} = \sum_{i=1}^{N}(\mathbf{x}_i - \overline{\mathbf{x}}_N)(\mathbf{x}_i - \overline{\mathbf{x}}_N)'$, and $b = N/2$, we can show that $\widehat{\Sigma}_{ML} = \frac{1}{N}\sum_{i=1}^{N}(\mathbf{x}_i - \overline{\mathbf{x}}_N)(\mathbf{x}_i - \overline{\mathbf{x}}_N)'$ maximizes $L(\widehat{\mu}_{ML}, \Sigma)$. The maximized likelihood is

$$L(\widehat{\mu}_{ML}, \widehat{\Sigma}_{ML}) = \frac{\exp(-\frac{Nk}{2})}{(2\pi)^{Nk/2}|\widehat{\Sigma}_{ML}|^{N/2}}, \tag{6.1.10}$$

which completes the proof. ∎

Corollary 6.1.1. Using the invariance property of MLE's, which states that the MLE of a function $g(\theta)$ of a parameter θ is $g(\widehat{\theta}_{ML})$, we see that

1. the MLE of the function $\mu'\Sigma^{-1}\mu$ is $\widehat{\mu}'_{ML}\widehat{\Sigma}^{-1}_{ML}\widehat{\mu}_{ML}$,

2. the MLE of $\sqrt{\sigma_{lj}}$, the (l, j)th element of Σ is given by $\sqrt{\widehat{\sigma}_{lj}}$, the square-root of the MLE of the (l, j)th entry in $\widehat{\Sigma}_{ML}$.

Although the estimator $\widehat{\mu}_{ML}$ is a unbiased estimator of μ, $\widehat{\Sigma}_{ML}$ is a biased estimator of Σ. Analogous to the univariate case, an unbiased estimator of Σ is $\widehat{\Sigma} = \frac{1}{N-1}\mathbf{S}_N$. The unbiased estimators of μ and Σ denoted by $\widehat{\mu}$ and $\widehat{\Sigma}$ respectively are complete sufficient statistics (Seber, 1984).

6.2   Distributions related to correlation coefficients

In Chapter 5, we defined theoretical versions of simple, multiple, and partial correlations; we described properties of each type of correlation, and discussed relationships between them. In this section, we discuss estimation of these correlation coefficients, as well as distributional properties of these estimators that enable inference. We begin with the simple correlation based on iid bivariate normal samples $(X_{i,j}, X_{i,l})$, $i = 1, \cdots, N$, where X_j and X_l denote the jth and lth components of the k-dimensional vector $\mathbf{x}$. Suppose $E(X_{i,j}) = \mu_j$, $E(X_{i,l}) = \mu_l$, $Var(X_{i,j}) = \sigma_j^2$, $Var(X_{i,l}) = \sigma_l^2$, and $Corr(X_{i,j}, X_{i,l}) = \rho_{jl}$.

Result 6.2.1. Estimation of simple correlations.   Suppose we have a random multivariate normal sample $\mathbf{x}_1, \cdots, \mathbf{x}_N$.

1. The maximum likelihood estimator of the simple correlation between X_j and X_l is

$$\widehat{\rho}_{jl} = \frac{\widehat{\sigma}_{jl}}{\sqrt{\widehat{\sigma}_{jj}\widehat{\sigma}_{ll}}}, \tag{6.2.1}$$

where the quantities on the right side have been defined in property 2 of Corollary 6.1.1. The estimator $\widehat{\rho}_{jl}$ can be expressed as a function of the complete, sufficient statistics $\overline{\mathbf{x}}_N$ and $\mathbf{S}_N$.

2. When $\rho_{jl} = 0$, the pdf of $\widehat{\rho}_{jl}$ is

$$f(r) = \frac{1}{B(1/2, (N-2)/2)}(1 - r^2)^{(N-4)/2}, \quad -1 \le r \le 1. \tag{6.2.2}$$

3. When $\rho_{jl} = 0$, the random variable

$$T_{jl} = \widehat{\rho}_{jl}\sqrt{\frac{N-2}{1 - \widehat{\rho}_{jl}^2}} \tag{6.2.3}$$

has a Student's t-distribution with $(N-2)$ degrees of freedom.

Proof. The form of $\widehat{\rho}_{jl}$ follows from the invariance of the MLE (see Corollary 6.1.1). Since the correlation coefficient is invariant under change of location and scale, we can assume without loss of generality that $\mu_j = \mu_l = 0$, and $\sigma_{jj}^2 = \sigma_{ll}^2 = 1$, and for $i = 1, \cdots, N$, the pairs $(X_{i,j}, X_{i,l})$ are iid samples from a bivariate normal distribution with these means and variances, and correlation ρ_{jl}. When $\rho_{jl} = 0$,

$$f(X_{1,l}, \cdots, X_{N,l} | X_{1,j}, \cdots, X_{N,j}) \quad = \quad f(X_{1,l}, \cdots, X_{N,l})$$

$$\propto \quad \exp\{-\frac{1}{2}\sum_{i=1}^{N}X_{i,l}^2\}.$$

Consider the transformation

$$U_1 = \sum_{i=1}^N X_{i,l}/\sqrt{N}, \quad U_2 = \sum_{i=1}^N X_{i,l}(X_{i,j} - \overline{X}_j)\Big/[\sum_{i=1}^N (X_{i,j} - \overline{X}_j)^2]^{1/2},$$

and U_i, $i = 3, \cdots, N$ orthogonal to each other, and to U_1, U_2, such that the entire transformation is orthogonal, and let

$$r_{jl} = U_2/(\sum_{i=2}^N U_i^2)^{1/2}.$$

Then,

$$\sum_{i=1}^N U_i^2 = \sum_{i=1}^N X_{i,l}^2, \text{ and}$$

$$\sum_{i=2}^N U_i^2 = \sum_{i=1}^N X_{i,l}^2 - N\overline{X}_l^2 = \sum_{i=1}^N (X_{i,l} - \overline{X}_l)^2,$$

so that

$$f(U_1, \cdots, U_N | X_{1,j}, \cdots, X_{N,j}) \propto \exp\{\tfrac{1}{2}\sum_{i=1}^N U_i^2\}.$$

Let $V = \sum_{i=1}^N U_i^2$. Computing the joint distribution of r_{jl} and V, and integrating out the V, we obtain,

$$f(r|X_{1,j}, \cdots, X_{N,j}) = \{B(1/2, (N-2)/2)\}^{-1}(1 - r^2)^{(N-4)/2}, \quad -1 \le r \le 1,$$

which does not involve the conditioning variables, and is therefore the unconditional pdf of $\widehat{\rho}_{jl}$. This proves property 2. To prove property 3, note that $W = U_2(N-2)^{1/2}/(\sum_{i=3}^N U_i^2)^{1/2}$ is an increasing function of $\widehat{\rho}_{jl}$. Conditional on $X_{i,j}$, $i = 1, \cdots, N$, U_i, $i = 1, \cdots, N$ are iid $N(0,1)$ variables, and W has a t_{N-2} distribution. Further, since the distribution of W does not involve these conditioning variables, the unconditional distribution of W is also t_{N-2}. Since

$$U_2(N-2)^{1/2}/(\sum_{i=3}^N U_i^2)^{1/2} = \{U_2(N-2)^{1/2}/(\sum_{i=2}^N U_i^2)^{1/2}\}$$

$$\div \{1 - U_2^2/\sum_{i=2}^N U_i^2\}^{1/2}$$

$$= (N-2)^{1/2}\widehat{\rho}_{jl}/(1 - \widehat{\rho}_{jl}^2)^{1/2} = R^*,$$

say, which is increasing in $\widehat{\rho}_{jl}$, it follows that when $\rho_{jl} = 0$, $R^* \sim t_{N-2}$. ∎

For an alternate proof of this result, as well as for a proof of the sampling distribution of $\widehat{\rho}_{jl}$ when $\rho_{jl} \ne 0$, see Rao (1973a). Here, we present two alternate forms for the nonnull distribution of $\widehat{\rho}_{jl}$. Starting from the joint distribution of S_{jj}, S_{ll} and r_{jl} (see Exercise 6.5), it can be shown that this has the form

$$f(r) = \frac{2^{N-3}(1 - \rho_{jl}^2)^{(N-1)/2}}{\pi\Gamma(N-2)}(1 - r^2)^{(N-4)/2}\sum_{t=0}^\infty \frac{(2r\rho_{jl})^t}{t!}[\Gamma(\frac{N+t-1}{2})]^2.$$

$$(6.2.4)$$

Another form of the distribution of $\widehat{\rho}_{jl}$ is

$$
f(r) \;=\; \frac{(1 - \rho_{jl}^2)^{(N-1)/2}}{\pi} (N - 2)(1 - r^2)^{(N-4)/2}
$$

$$
\times \; \int_0^1 \frac{u^{N-2}}{(1 - u^2)^{1/2}} \frac{1}{(1 - \rho_{jl} r u)^{N-1}} du, \qquad (6.2.5)
$$

which is obtained by verifying that

$$
\int_0^1 u^{N-2}(1 - u^2)^{-1/2}(1 - ru\rho_{jl})^{-(N-1)} du = \frac{2^{N-3}}{\Gamma(N-1)} \sum_{t=0}^{\infty} \frac{(2r\rho_{jl})^t}{t!} [\Gamma(\tfrac{N+t-1}{2})]^2.
$$

It would be natural to test $H_0 : \rho_{jl} = 0$ versus $H_1 : \rho_{jl} \neq 0$ using property 2 in Result 6.2.1. Unfortunately, the critical values under this null distribution of $\widehat{\rho}_{jl}$ have not been widely tabulated. The null distribution of the transformed variable in property 3 is generally used instead. The two-sided test procedure rejects H_0 at level of significance α if $|(N - 2)^{1/2}\widehat{\rho}_{jl}/\sqrt{1 - \widehat{\rho}_{jl}}| \geq t_{N-2,\alpha/2}$. In practice, Fisher's z-transformation of $\widehat{\rho}_{jl}$ leads to simpler inference, as shown in the next result. For a proof of this result, see Kendall and Stuart (1958), section 16.33.

Result 6.2.2.   Let

$$
Z_{jl} \;=\; \frac{1}{2} \ln \left(\frac{1 + \widehat{\rho}_{jl}}{1 - \widehat{\rho}_{jl}} \right) = \tanh^{-1}(\widehat{\rho}_{jl}),
$$

$$
\delta_{jl} \;=\; \frac{1}{2} \ln \left(\frac{1 + \rho_{jl}}{1 - \rho_{jl}} \right) = \tanh^{-1}(\rho_{jl}), \quad \text{and}
$$

$$
v^2 \;=\; \frac{1}{N - 3}; \qquad\qquad\qquad\qquad (6.2.6)
$$

then, Z_{jl} has an approximate $N(\delta_{jl}, v^2)$ distribution (Fisher, 1921).

We now consider estimation of the partial correlations (see Definition 5.2.7) based on the random sample $\mathbf{x}_1, \cdots, \mathbf{x}_N$. Recall that we partitioned the random vector $\mathbf{x}_i = (X_{i,1}, \cdots, X_{i,k})'$ as $\mathbf{x}_i' = (\mathbf{x}_{i,1}', \mathbf{x}_{i,2}')'$ where $\mathbf{x}_{i,1}' = (X_{i,1}, \cdots, X_{i,q})$ is a q-dimensional vector, and $\mathbf{x}_{i,2}' = (X_{i,q+1}, \cdots, X_{i,k})$ is a $(k - q)$-dimensional vector. We partition μ, Σ, $\overline{\mathbf{x}}_N$, and $\mathbf{S}_N$ conformably (as in Result 5.2.8). In particular, suppose

$$
\mathbf{S}_N = \begin{pmatrix} \mathbf{S}_{11} & \mathbf{S}_{12} \\ \mathbf{S}_{21} & \mathbf{S}_{22} \end{pmatrix},
$$

where $\mathbf{S}_{11}$ is a $q \times q$ matrix. Define

$$
\mathbf{S}_{11.2} = \mathbf{S}_{11} - \mathbf{S}_{12}\mathbf{S}_{22}^{-1}\mathbf{S}_{21},
$$

and let $X_{i,j}$ and $X_{i,l}$ denote components of the subvector $\mathbf{x}_{i,1}$.

Result 6.2.3.   The quantity $\mathbf{S}_{11.2}$ has a $W_k(\Sigma_{11.2}, N-1-k+q)$ distribution.

Proof.   From property 2 of Result 6.1.1, $\mathbf{S}_N \sim W_k(\Sigma, N-1)$, which implies that $\mathbf{S}_N = \sum_{i=1}^{N-1} \mathbf{z}_i \mathbf{z}_i'$, where $\mathbf{z}_i$ are independent $N_k(\mathbf{0}, \Sigma)$. Let $\mathbf{z}_i' = (\mathbf{z}_{i,1}', \mathbf{z}_{i,2}')'$, where $\mathbf{z}_{i,1}$ is a q-dimensional vector. For a fixed q-dimensional vector $\mathbf{h}$,

$$\mathbf{z}_i^* = \begin{pmatrix} \mathbf{h}'\mathbf{z}_{i,1} \\ \mathbf{z}_{i,2} \end{pmatrix} \sim N_{k-q+1}(\mathbf{0}, \Sigma^*), \text{ with } \Sigma^* = \begin{pmatrix} \mathbf{h}'\Sigma_{11}\mathbf{h} & \mathbf{h}'\Sigma_{12} \\ \Sigma_{21}\mathbf{h} & \Sigma_{22} \end{pmatrix}, \text{ and}$$

$$\mathbf{S}^* = \sum_{i=1}^{N-1} \mathbf{z}_i^* \mathbf{z}_i^{*\prime} = \begin{pmatrix} \mathbf{h}'\mathbf{S}_{11}\mathbf{h} & \mathbf{h}'\mathbf{S}_{12} \\ \mathbf{S}_{21}\mathbf{h} & \mathbf{S}_{22} \end{pmatrix} \sim W_{k-q+1}(\Sigma^*, N-1).$$

It may be verified that the first diagonal elements of Σ^* and $\mathbf{S}^*$ are respectively $|\Sigma_{22}|/|\Sigma^*|$ and $|\mathbf{S}_{22}|/|\mathbf{S}^*|$, and also that $\frac{|\mathbf{S}^*|}{|\mathbf{S}_{22}|} \Big/ \frac{|\Sigma^*|}{|\Sigma_{22}|} \sim \chi^2_{N-1-k+q}$. From Result 2.1.2, $|\mathbf{S}^*|/|\mathbf{S}_{22}| = \mathbf{h}'[\mathbf{S}_{11}-\mathbf{S}_{12}\mathbf{S}_{22}^{-1}\mathbf{S}_{21}]\mathbf{h} = \mathbf{h}'\mathbf{S}_{11.2}\mathbf{h}$, and $|\Sigma^*|/|\Sigma_{22}| = \mathbf{h}'[\Sigma_{11}-\Sigma_{12}\Sigma_{22}^{-1}\Sigma_{21}]\mathbf{h} = \mathbf{h}'\Sigma_{11.2}\mathbf{h}$. Since $\mathbf{h}'\mathbf{S}_{11.2}\mathbf{h} \sim \mathbf{h}'\Sigma_{11.2}\mathbf{h}\chi^2_{N-1-k+q}$, the required result follows directly. $\blacksquare$

Result 6.2.4. Estimation of partial correlation coefficients.

1. The maximum likelihood estimator of $\rho_{jl|(q+1,\cdots,k)}$ is

$$\widehat{\rho}_{jl|(q+1,\cdots,k)} = \frac{[\mathbf{S}_{11.2}]_{j,l}}{[\mathbf{S}_{11.2}]_{j,j}^{1/2}[\mathbf{S}_{11.2}]_{l,l}^{1/2}} \tag{6.2.7}$$

where $[\mathbf{S}_{11.2}]_{m,n}$ denotes the (m,n)th element of the $q \times q$ matrix $\mathbf{S}_{11.2}$.

2. If $\rho_{jl|(q+1,\cdots,k)} = 0$, then

$$\frac{[N-(k-q)-2]^{1/2}\widehat{\rho}_{jl|(q+1,\cdots,k)}}{\{1-\widehat{\rho}_{jl|(q+1,\cdots,k)}^2\}^{1/2}} \sim t_{N-(k-q)-2}. \tag{6.2.8}$$

Proof.   The form of the estimator follows from the invariance property of the MLE. When $\rho_{jl|(q+1,\cdots,k)} = 0$, the pdf of $\widehat{\rho}_{jl|(q+1,\cdots,k)}$ has the form in (6.2.2), replacing the empirical and theoretical simple correlations by corresponding partial correlations, and replacing N by $N-(k-q)$. $\blacksquare$

We next discuss estimation of the multiple correlation coefficient based on N samples from a $(k+1)$-variate normal distribution. Using notation similar to Definition 5.2.8, let

$$\overline{\mathbf{x}}_N = \begin{pmatrix} \overline{X}_0 \\ \overline{\mathbf{x}}^{(1)} \end{pmatrix} \text{ and } \mathbf{S} = \begin{pmatrix} S_{00} & \mathbf{s}_{01} \\ \mathbf{s}_{10} & \mathbf{S}^{(1)} \end{pmatrix} \tag{6.2.9}$$

denote the sample mean and sample variance-covariance matrix of the random sample $(X_{i,0}, X_{i,1}, \cdots, X_{i,k})$, $i = 1, \cdots, N$.

Result 6.2.5. Estimation of the multiple correlation coefficient.

1. The maximum likelihood estimator of $\rho_{0(1,\cdots,k)}$ is

$$\widehat{\rho}_{0(1,\cdots,k)} = \frac{\{s_{01}[S^{(1)}]^{-1}s_{10}\}^{1/2}}{S_{00}^{1/2}}. \tag{6.2.10}$$

2. When $\rho_{0(1,\cdots,k)} = 0$,

$$\frac{(N-k-1)\widehat{\rho}_{0(1,\cdots,k)}^2}{k[1-\widehat{\rho}_{0(1,\cdots,k)}^2]} \sim F_{k,N-k-1}. \tag{6.2.11}$$

Proof. The proof of property 1 follows directly from the form of the multiple correlation coefficient and invariance of the maximum likelihood estimator. Let $S_{00.1} = S_{00} - s_{01}[S^{(1)}]^{-1}s_{10}$. Then, $1 - \widehat{\rho}_{0(1,\cdots,k)}^2 = S_{00.1}/S_{00}$, so that

$$\widehat{\rho}_{0(1,\cdots,k)}^2/(1 - \widehat{\rho}_{0(1,\cdots,k)}^2) = \{s_{01}[S^{(1)}]^{-1}s_{10}\}/S_{00.1}.$$

When $\rho_{0(1,\cdots,k)} = 0$, $\sigma_{01} = 0$ (see Definition 5.2.8), so that $S_{00.1} \sim W_1(\Sigma_{00}, N - k - 1)$, $s_{01}[S^{(1)}]^{-1}s_{10} \sim W_1(\Sigma_{00}, k)$, and they have independent distributions. The proof of property 2 follows from the definition of the F-distribution (see (A9)). ∎

When $\rho_{0(1,\cdots,k)} = 0$, the statistic $B = \widehat{\rho}_{0(1,\cdots,k)}^2/[1 - \widehat{\rho}_{0(1,\cdots,k)}^2]$ follows a Beta$(k-1, N-k)$ distribution, as we ask the reader to show in Exercise 6.8. The non-null distribution of B is a non-central Beta (see Result 5.3.7).

6.3   Assessing the normality assumption

In this section, we discuss a few procedures that enable us to detect situations where the observed data depart, to a small or large extent, from the assumption of a normal parent population. There exist several procedures in the literature for assessing the hypothesis of univariate normality, such as (a) skewness and kurtosis tests, (b) omnibus tests such as Shapiro and Wilk's W-test, (c) likelihood ratio tests with specific nonnormal alternatives, (d) goodness of fit tests such as the χ^2-test and the Kolmogorov-Smirnov test, and (e) graphical methods such as normal probability plots. Assume that we have a random sample $X_1, \cdots, X_N$ from some continuous distribution with cdf $F(.)$. We denote the empirical cdf by

$$F_N(x) = \tfrac{1}{N}(\text{Number of observations} \leq x).$$

The Kolmogorov-Smirnoff test is useful for testing $H_0 : F(x) = F_0(x) \; \forall \; x$ versus $H_1 : F(x) \neq F_0(x)$ for some x, where $F_0(.)$ corresponds to a $N(\mu, \sigma^2)$ distribution. The Kolmogorov-Smirnoff test statistic is

$$D_N = \sup_x |F_N(x) - F_0(x)|, \tag{6.3.1}$$

which will be large if the data are not consistent with H_0. The p-values can be computed based on the asymptotic null distribution of D_N given by

$$\lim_{N \to \infty} P\{\sqrt{N} D_N \le z\} = Q(z),$$

$$Q(z) = 1 - 2 \sum_{k=1}^{\infty} (-1)^{k-1} \exp(-2k^2 z^2)$$

for every $z > 0$. The function $Q(z)$ is the cdf of a continuous distribution called the *Kolmogorov distribution*. In general, the parameters μ and σ^2 are unknown, and may be replaced by their sample counterparts.

Another test for normality is due to Shapiro and Wilk and is based on a comparison of ordered sample values with their expected locations under the null hypothesis of normality. Let $Z_{(1)} \le \cdots \le Z_{(N)}$ be an ordered sample from a standard normal distribution, and let $m_i = E(Z_{(i)})$, $i = 1, \cdots, N$ be the normal scores. Under the hypothesis of normality,

$$E(X_{(i)}) = \mu + \sigma E(Z_{(i)}) = \mu + \sigma m_i,$$

i.e., we expect that the ordered observations $X_{(i)}$'s are linearly related to the m_i's. Shapiro and Wilk (1965) proposed the statistic

$$SW = (\mathbf{m}'\Omega^{-1}\mathbf{m})^{-1}(\mathbf{m}'\Omega^{-1}\mathbf{u})^2 / \sum_{i=1}^{N}(X_i - \overline{X})^2,$$

where $\mathbf{m}$ and Ω are the mean and covariance of $\mathbf{z} = (Z_{(1)}, \cdots, Z_{(N)})'$. The statistic SW may be interpreted as the ratio of an estimate of variability based on ordered statistics and normality to the usual residual mean square. Shapiro and Wilk provided extensive tables of percentage points of SW.

The well known *normal probability plot*, which is a plot of the empirical quantiles versus the theoretical quantiles from a standard normal distribution, is available with most software packages. When the points in the normal probability plot lie very nearly along a straight line, the normality assumption is reasonable. The pattern of possible deviations of the scatter points from a straight line will indicate the nature of departure from normality, such as skewness, kurtosis, outliers or multimodality.

Next, we discuss some approaches for assessing multivariate normality, including tests based on multivariate measures of skewness and kurtosis, as well as graphical procedures (Gnanadesikan, 1977). In Chapter 5, we have seen that (a) contours of the multivariate normal distribution are ellipsoids, and (b) linear combinations of normal random variables also have a normal distribution. As a first step in assessing multivariate normality, we may check to see whether the univariate marginal empirical distributions are approximately univariate normal using any of the approaches described earlier.

To assess bivariate normality, scatterplots of pairs of variables, X_j and X_l are useful. By Result 5.2.6, the vector $\mathbf{x}_2 = (X_j, X_l)$ has a bivariate normal distribution, i.e., $N_2(\mu_2, \Sigma_2)$, say. In Example 5.2.3, we showed that contours of constant density would be ellipses defined by $(\mathbf{x}_2 - \mu_2)'\Sigma_2^{-1}(\mathbf{x}_2 - \mu_2) = \chi_{2,\alpha}^2$, where, $\chi_{2,\alpha}^2$ is the upper (100α)th percentile from a chi-square distribution with

$k = 2$ degrees of freedom. If the data follows a multivariate normal distribution, the scatterplot of $X_{i,j}$ versus $X_{i,l}$, $i = 1, \cdots, N$ should exhibit a pattern that is (nearly) elliptical and roughly $100\alpha\%$ of the points should lie inside the estimated ellipse $(\mathbf{x}_2 - \bar{\mathbf{x}}_2)'\mathbf{S}_2^{-1}(\mathbf{x}_2 - \bar{\mathbf{x}}_2) \leq \chi^2_{2,\alpha}$, where $\bar{\mathbf{x}}_2$ is the mean of the bivariate sample, and $\mathbf{S}_2$ is the sample variance covariance matrix. This comparison of the empirical proportion of points within the estimated ellipse to the theoretical probability gives a rough assessment of bivariate normality. Alternately, for any $k \geq 2$, one can compute the squared generalized distances

$$d_j^2 = (N - 1)(\mathbf{x}_j - \bar{\mathbf{x}}_N)'\mathbf{S}_N^{-1}(\mathbf{x}_j - \bar{\mathbf{x}}_N), \quad j = 1, \cdots, N.$$

Provided the data follows a k-variate normal distribution, and both $N \geq 30$ and $N - k \geq 30$, $\bar{\mathbf{x}}_N$ converges in probability to μ, while $\mathbf{S}_N$ converges in probability to Σ; then, d_j^2 behaves like a chi-square random variable. The following plot, called the *chi-square plot*, or the *gamma plot* enables us to assess multivariate normality. First, order the squared generalized distances, $d_{(1)}^2 \leq \cdots \leq d_{(N)}^2$. Plot the pairs of points $(d_{(j)}^2, \chi^2_{k,\, j^*})$, where $j^* = \frac{1}{N}(j - 1/2)$, and $\chi^2_{k,\, j^*}$ denotes the upper $(100j^*)$th percentile of the chi-square distribution with k degrees of freedom. If the points lie approximately on a straight line, normality may be assumed, but not otherwise. Once again, the pattern of points may suggest the nature of departure from normality (Andrews et al., 1971; and Gnanadesikan, 1977).

Mardia (1970) proposed a test for normality based on multivariate skewness and kurtosis, arguing that these quantities provide direct measures of departure from normality. Let $\mathbf{x}$ follow a k-variate distribution with mean μ and covariance Σ, and suppose $\Sigma^{-1} = \{\sigma^{rr^*}\}$.

Definition 6.3.1.   A multivariate measure of skewness which is invariant under nonsingular transformations (such as $\mathbf{x} = \mathbf{A}\mathbf{y} + \mathbf{b}$) is defined by

$$\beta_{1,k} = \sum_{r,s,t} \sum_{r^*s^*t^*} \sigma^{rr^*}\sigma^{ss^*}\sigma^{tt^*} \mu_{111}^{(rst)}\mu_{111}^{(r^*s^*t^*)},$$

where $\mu_{111}^{(rst)} = E\{(X_r - \mu_r)(X_s - \mu_s)(X_t - \mu_t)\}$. For any symmetric distribution about μ, $\beta_{1,k} = 0$.

When $k = 1$, $\beta_{1,1} = \beta_1$, the usual univariate measure of skewness. When $k = 2$, with (r, s)th central moment $\mu_{r,s}$, $Var(X_1) = 1$, $Var(X_2) = 1$, and $Corr(X_1, X_2) = \rho = 0$, the bivariate skewness measure is

$$\beta_{1,2} = \mu_{3,0}^2 + \mu_{0,3}^2 + 3\mu_{1,2}^2 + 3\mu_{2,1}^2,$$

which is identically zero if and only if μ_{30}, $\mu_{0,3}$, $\mu_{1,2}$ and $\mu_{2,1}$ all vanish.

Definition 6.3.2.   A measure of multivariate kurtosis invariant under nonsingular transformations is

$$\beta_{2,k} = E\{(\mathbf{x} - \mu)'\Sigma^{-1}(\mathbf{x} - \mu)\}^2$$

When $\mu = \mathbf{0}$, and $\Sigma = \mathbf{I}_k$, the measure of kurtosis is invariant under orthogonal transformations and is $\beta_{2,k} = E\{(\mathbf{x}'\mathbf{x})^2\}$.

Let $\mathbf{x}_1, \cdots, \mathbf{x}_N$ denote a random sample from a k-dimensional population with mean μ and covariance matrix Σ. Let $\overline{\mathbf{x}}_N$ and $\mathbf{S}_N/(N-1) = \{S_{ij}\}$ respectively denote the sample mean and sample covariance matrix, and let $\{S^{ij}\}$ denote the inverse. A sample measure of skewness corresponding to $\beta_{1,k}$ is

$$b_{1,k} = (N-1)^3 \sum_{r,s,t} \sum_{r^*s^*t^*} S^{rr^*} S^{ss^*} S^{tt^*} M_{111}^{(rst)} M_{111}^{(r^*s^*t^*)}, \tag{6.3.2}$$

where $M_{111}^{(rst)} = \sum_{i=1}^{N}(X_{i,r} - \overline{X}_r)(X_{i,s} - \overline{X}_s)(X_{i,t} - \overline{X}_t)/N$. An alternate expression for $b_{1,k}$ is (see Mardia, 1975)

$$b_{1,k} = \frac{1}{N^2} \sum_{i=1}^{N} \sum_{j=1}^{N} r_{ij}^3 \tag{6.3.3}$$

where we define

$$r_{ij} = (N-1)(\mathbf{x}_i - \overline{\mathbf{x}}_N)' \mathbf{S}_N^{-1} (\mathbf{x}_j - \overline{\mathbf{x}}_N).$$

The sample skewness $b_{1,k}$ is also invariant under nonsingular transformations of the data. A sample measure of kurtosis is

$$b_{2,k} = \frac{N-1}{N} \sum_{i=1}^{N} \{(\mathbf{x}_i - \overline{\mathbf{x}}_N)' \mathbf{S}_N^{-1} (\mathbf{x}_i - \overline{\mathbf{x}}_N)\}^2, \tag{6.3.4}$$

which is also invariant under nonsingular transformations such as $\mathbf{x} = \mathbf{A}\mathbf{y} + \mathbf{b}$. For large samples, we can test for k-variate normality based on these measures as shown in the following result. For a proof of the result, the reader is referred to Mardia (1970).

Result 6.3.1. The following tests for multivariate normality hold in large samples.

1. The statistic $A = \frac{1}{6}Nb_{1,k}$ has a χ^2 distribution with $k(k+1)(k+2)/6$ degrees of freedom under the null hypothesis $H_0 : \beta_{1,k} = 0$. We reject the null hypothesis of normality for large values of A. We can also use the approximation that for $k > 7$, $\sqrt{2A} \sim N(\frac{1}{3}[k(k+1)(k+2) - 3], 1)$.

2. Under the null hypothesis $H_0 : \beta_{2,k} = k(k+2)$, the statistic

$$B = \sqrt{N}(b_{2,k} - \beta_{2,k})/[8k(k+2)]^{1/2}$$

has a standard normal distribution.

Geometrically, the *Mahalanobis distance* between $\mathbf{x}_i$ and $\mathbf{x}_j$ is

$$d_{ij}^2 = (N-1)(\mathbf{x}_i - \mathbf{x}_j)'\mathbf{S}_N^{-1}(\mathbf{x}_i - \mathbf{x}_j)$$

and let r_{ii} be the square of the Mahalanobis distance between $\mathbf{x}_i$ and $\overline{\mathbf{x}}_N$. It may be verified that $r_{ij} = \frac{1}{2}(r_{ii} + r_{jj} - d_{ij}^2)$. The Mahalanobis angle between the vectors $\mathbf{x}_i - \overline{\mathbf{x}}_N$ and $\mathbf{x}_j - \overline{\mathbf{x}}_N$ is defined by

$$\cos\theta_{ij} = r_{ij}/[r_{ii}r_{jj}]^{1/2}.$$

We can express the multivariate skewness and kurtosis in terms of these quantities:

$$b_{1,k} = \frac{1}{N^2}\sum_{i=1}^{N}\sum_{j=1}^{N}\{r_{ii}r_{jj}\}^{3/2}\{\cos\theta_{ij}\}^3,$$

$$b_{2,k} = \frac{1}{N}\sum_{i=1}^{N}r_{ii}^2.$$

If the sample points $\mathbf{x}_i$, $i = 1, \cdots, N$ are uniformly distributed on a k-dimensional hypersphere or ellipsoid, then $b_{1,k} \simeq 0$. If, however, the data departs from spherical symmetry, then $b_{1,k}$ will be large; this might occur for instance when there is an abnormal clustering of points. In such cases, the value of $b_{2,k}$ will also be abnormally large. Figure 6.3.1 (a) and (b) represent the symmetric and abnormal clustering cases respectively.

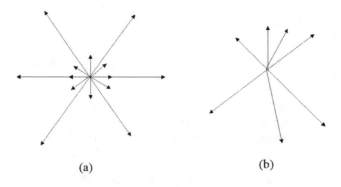

(a)   (b)

Figure 6.3.1.   Graphical representation of skewness.

6.4 Transformations to approximate normality

The normal distribution plays a central role in the classical theory of linear models. The normal general linear model is attractive because it has closed form expressions for estimators and test statistics and the distribution theory is elegant. When the assumptions of homoscedasticity, independence, or normality are violated, as often happens in practice, there are several choices. A usual remedy for the problem of heteroscedasticity is the use of generalized least squares for estimation and inference. This procedure may be carried out using the matrix and distributional tools we have described so far. When the normality assumption is violated, the data can be transformed, if possible, so that the transformed variables are approximately normal. A general family of univariate and multivariate transformations is introduced in this section. It should be kept in mind, however, that there are some drawbacks associated with these transformations. In particular, the parameters of the transformed data model may not be as meaningful as those in the original model. Alternatively, one can consider general linear models where the errors have an alternate distribution (than the normal) chosen from the general family of elliptically contoured distributions which were described in section 5.5.

6.4.1 Univariate transformations

A transformation of X is a function T which replaces X by a new "transformed" variable $T(X)$. The simplest and most widely used transformations belong to the family of power transformations, which are defined below.

Definition 6.4.1. Power transformation. The family of power transformations have the form

$$T_P(X) = \begin{cases} aX^p + b & \text{if} \quad p \neq 0 \\ c \log X + d & \text{if} \quad p = 0 \end{cases} \tag{6.4.1}$$

where a, b, c, d, and p are arbitrary real scalars.

The power transformation is useful for bringing skewed distributions of random variables closer to symmetry, and thence, to normality. The square root transformation or the logarithmic transformation, for instance, have the effect of "pulling in " one tail of the distribution. Any power transformation is either concave or convex throughout its domain of positive numbers, i.e., there is no point of inflection. This implies that a power transformation either compresses the scale for larger X values more than it does for smaller X values (for example, $T_P(X) = \log X$), or it does the reverse (for example, $T_P(X) = X^2$). We cannot however, use a power transformation to expand the scale of X for large and small values, while compressing it for values in between! Tukey (1957) considered the family of transformations

$$X^{(\lambda)} = \begin{cases} X^\lambda & \text{if} \quad \lambda \neq 0 \\ \log X & \text{if} \quad \lambda = 0, \text{ and } X > 0 \end{cases} \tag{6.4.2}$$

which is a special case of (6.4.1). This family of transformations, indexed by λ, includes the well-known square root (when $\lambda = 1/2$), logarithmic (when $\lambda = 0$), and reciprocal (when $\lambda = -1$) transformations. Notice that (6.4.2) has a discontinuity at $\lambda = 0$. The Box-Cox transformation offers a remedy to this problem and is defined below.

Definition 6.4.2. Box-Cox transformation.   Box and Cox (1964) defined the transformation

$$X^{(\lambda)} = \begin{cases} [X^\lambda - 1]/\lambda & \text{if} & \lambda \neq 0 \\ \log X & \text{if} & \lambda = 0, \text{ and } X > 0 \end{cases} \qquad (6.4.3)$$

which has been widely used in practice to achieve transformation to normality. If some of the X_i's assume negative values, a positive constant ω may be added to all the variables to make them positive. Box and Cox also proposed the shifted power transformation which is defined below.

Definition 6.4.3. Box-Cox shifted power transformation. Box and Cox also proposed the shifted power transformation

$$X^{(\lambda)} = \begin{cases} [(X + \delta)^\lambda - 1]/\lambda & \text{if} & \lambda \neq 0 \\ \log[X + \delta] & \text{if} & \lambda = 0 \end{cases} \qquad (6.4.4)$$

where the parameter δ is chosen such that $X > -\delta$.

Several modifications of the Box-Cox transformation exist in the literature, of which a few are mentioned here. Manly (1976) proposed a modification of the Box-Cox transformation which allows the incorporation of negative observations and is an effective tool to transform skewed unimodal distributions to approximate normality. This is given by

$$X^{(\lambda)} = \begin{cases} [\exp(\lambda X) - 1]/\lambda & \text{if} & \lambda \neq 0 \\ X & \text{if} & \lambda = 0. \end{cases} \qquad (6.4.5)$$

Bickel and Doksum (1981) proposed a modification which incorporates unbounded support for $X^{(\lambda)}$:

$$X^{(\lambda)} = [|X|^\lambda \text{sign}(X) - 1]/\lambda. \qquad (6.4.6)$$

With any of these transformations, it is important to note that very often the range of the transformed variable $X^{(\lambda)}$ is restricted based on the sign of λ, in turn implying that the transformed values may not cover the entire real line. Consequently, only approximate normality may result from the transformation.

Definition 6.4.4. Modulus transformation.   The following transformation was suggested by John and Draper (1980):

$$X^{(\lambda)} = \begin{cases} \text{sign}[(|X| + 1)^\lambda - 1]/\lambda & \text{if} & \lambda \neq 0 \\ \text{sign}[\log(|X| + 1)] & \text{if} & \lambda = 0, \end{cases} \qquad (6.4.7)$$

where the sign of $X^{(\lambda)}$ is that corresponding to the observation X. The modulus transformation works best to achieve approximate normality when the distribution of X is already approximately symmetric about some location. It alters each half of the distribution about this central value via the same power transformation in order to bring the distribution closer to a normal distribution. It is not difficult to see that when $X > 0$, (6.4.7) is equivalent to the power transformation. Given a random sample $X_1, \cdots, X_N$, estimation of λ using the maximum likelihood approach and the Bayesian framework was proposed by Box and Cox (1964), while Carroll and Ruppert (1988) discussed several robust adaptations. The maximum likelihood approach for estimating λ in the context of linear regression is described in section 8.1.1. A generalization of the Box-Cox transformation to symmetric distributions was considered by Hinkley (1975), while Solomon (1985) extended it to random-effects models.

6.4.2 Multivariate transformations

Andrews et al. (1971) proposed a multivariate generalization of the Box-Cox transformation. A transformation of a k-dimensional random vector $\mathbf{x}$ may be defined either with the objective of transforming each component X_j, $j = 1, \cdots, k$, marginally to normality, or to achieve joint normality. They defined the simple family of "marginal" transformations as follows.

Definition 6.4.5. Transformation to marginal normality The transformation for the jth component X_j is defined for $j = 1, \cdots, k$ by

$$X_j^{(\lambda_j)} = \begin{cases} [X_j^{\lambda_j} - 1]/\lambda_j & \text{if} \quad \lambda_j \neq 0 \\ \log X_j & \text{if} \quad \lambda_j = 0, \text{ and } X_j > 0 \end{cases} \quad (6.4.8)$$

where the λ_j are chosen to improve the marginal normality of $X_j^{(\lambda_j)}$ for $j = 1, \cdots, k$, via maximum likelihood estimation.

It is well known that marginal normality of the components does not imply multivariate normality; in using the marginal transformations in the previous section, it is hoped that the marginal normality of $X_j^{(\lambda_j)}$ might lead to a transformed $\mathbf{x}$ vector which is more amenable to procedures assuming multivariate normality. The following set of marginal transformations was proposed by Andrews et al. (1971) in order to achieve *joint normality* for the transformed data.

Definition 6.4.6. Transformation to joint normality. Suppose $X_j^{(\lambda_j)}$, $j = 1, \cdots, k$ denote the marginal transformations, and suppose the vector $\lambda = (\lambda_1, \cdots, \lambda_k)$ denotes the set of parameters that yields joint normality of the vector $\mathbf{x}^{(\lambda)} = (X_1^{(\lambda_1)}, \cdots, X_k^{(\lambda_k)})'$. Suppose the mean and covariance of this multivariate normal distribution are μ and Σ. The joint density function of $\mathbf{x}$ is

$$f(\mathbf{x}; \mu, \Sigma, \lambda) = (2\pi)^{-k/2}|\Sigma|^{-1/2}|J| \exp\{-\frac{1}{2}(\mathbf{x}^{(\lambda)} - \mu)'\Sigma^{-1}(\mathbf{x}^{(\lambda)} - \mu)\}, \quad (6.4.9)$$

where the Jacobian of the transformation is given by

$$J = \prod_{j=1}^{k} X_j^{(\lambda_j)}.$$

Given N independent observations $\mathbf{x}_1, \cdots, \mathbf{x}_N$, the estimate of λ, along with μ and Σ is obtained by numerically maximizing the likelihood function which has the form in (6.4.9). There are some situations where nonnormality is manifest only in some directions in the k-dimensional space. Andrews et al. (1971) suggested an approach (a) to identify these directions, and (b) to then estimate a power transformation of the projections of $\mathbf{x}_1, \cdots, \mathbf{x}_N$ onto these selected directions in order to improve the normal approximation.

Exercises

6.1. Express the maximized likelihood function in (6.1.10) as a function of the generalized variance $|\mathbf{S}_N|$ of the random sample $\mathbf{x}_1, \cdots, \mathbf{x}_N$.

6.2. Prove the identities (6.1.4).

6.3. If $\mathbf{S}_N \sim W_k(\Sigma, N-1)$, and $\mathbf{a} = (a_1, \cdots, a_k)'$ is an arbitrary vector, show that $\max_{\mathbf{a}}(\mathbf{a}'\mathbf{S}_N\mathbf{a}/\mathbf{a}'\Sigma\mathbf{a})$ and $\min_{\mathbf{a}}(\mathbf{a}'\mathbf{S}_N\mathbf{a}/\mathbf{a}'\Sigma\mathbf{a})$ are respectively the largest and smallest roots of the determinantal equation $|\mathbf{S}_N - c\Sigma| = 0$.

6.4. Suppose $\mathbf{S}_{N_1} \sim W_k(\Sigma, N_1-1)$ and is independent of $\mathbf{S}_{N_2} \sim W_k(\Sigma, N_2-1)$. For any $\mathbf{a} = (a_1, \cdots, a_k)'$, find the distribution of $\mathbf{a}'\mathbf{S}_{N_1}\mathbf{a}/\mathbf{a}'\mathbf{S}_{N_2}\mathbf{a}$.

6.5. Derive the joint distribution of S_{jj}, S_{ll} and r.

6.6. The following table gives the means and the variance-covariance matrix of four variables X_0, X_1, X_2, and X_3:

	X_0	X_1	X_2	X_3	Means
X_0	60.516	0.998	3.511	21.122	18.3
X_1		15.129	23.860	1.793	14.9
X_2			54.756	3.633	30.5
X_3				18.225	7.8

(a) Compute the multiple correlation coefficient of X_0 on X_1, X_2 and X_3.

(b) Compute the partial correlation coefficient between X_0 and X_3, eliminating the effects of X_1 and X_2.

6.7. Suppose $\mathbf{S}$ is partitioned as in (6.2.9). Evaluate $\hat{\rho}_{0(1,\cdots,k)}^2$ in terms of $|\mathbf{S}|$, $|\mathbf{S}^{(1)}|$ and S_{00}.

6.8. When $\rho_{0(1,\cdots,k)} = 0$, show that the statistic $\widehat{\rho}_{0(1,\cdots,k)}^2$ follows a Beta distribution. What are the parameters of this distribution?

6.9. Find $E(d_j^2)$, where d_j^2 are the squared generalized distances.

6.10. Let $\mathbf{x} \sim N(\mu, \Sigma)$. Show that $b_{1,k}$ and $b_{2,k}$ defined in (6.3.3) and (6.3.4) are invariant under a nonsingular linear transformation $\mathbf{y} = \mathbf{Px} + \mathbf{q}$ (where $\mathbf{P}$ is nonsingular). Discuss whether these coefficients depend on μ and Σ.

Chapter 7

Inference for the General Linear Model

In this chapter, we describe classical inference for the general linear model that we introduced in Chapter 4. The least squares estimation did not require any distributional assumptions on the model errors. However, in many cases, one is interested in constructing interval estimates for the parameters of interest, as well as in testing hypotheses about these parameters or functions of these parameters. Parametric inference proceeds by assuming that the errors are generated by some probability model. The most widely used assumption is that of normality, and the multivariate normal distribution was defined in Chapter 5. We also introduced some alternate distributions that enable us to incorporate skewness and heavy tailed behavior in the distribution of the model errors. In Chapter 6, we saw how it is possible to assess the multivariate normal assumption in practice, and introduced transformations to approximate normality. This has the advantage of allowing for greater modeling flexibility, thereby enhancing the scope of these models. The properties of the multivariate normal distribution ensures that the least squares estimates of the general linear model parameters are also multivariate normal, as Result 7.1.1 shows. Using results from distributions of quadratic forms that were discussed in section 5.4, we derive tests of hypotheses.

7.1 Properties of least squares estimates

Suppose the error vector ε in the general linear model (4.1.1) follows a multivariate normal distribution, i.e., $\varepsilon \sim N(\mathbf{0}, \sigma^2 \mathbf{I}_N)$ with pdf

$$
\begin{aligned}
f(\varepsilon; \sigma^2 \mathbf{I}_N) &= \frac{1}{(2\pi\sigma^2)^{N/2}} \exp\{-\frac{1}{2\sigma^2}\varepsilon'\varepsilon\} \\
&= \frac{1}{(2\pi\sigma^2)^{N/2}} \exp\{-\frac{1}{2\sigma^2}\sum_{i=1}^{N}\varepsilon_i^2\}, \quad \varepsilon \in \mathcal{R}^N.
\end{aligned}
$$

In Chapter 4, we derived the least squares solutions β^0 and $\hat{\sigma}^2$. For the general linear model, we show that the least squares estimate of any estimable function of β has a multivariate normal distribution. We derive the mean and variance of this estimator, and discuss the full rank model as a special case. Based on the point estimates and precision estimates for estimable functions of β, we construct joint confidence region and marginal confidence intervals. We develop test procedures for various hypotheses of interest about estimable functions of β. In (4.2.12), we introduced the ANOVA decomposition of the total sum of squares (SST) into the model sum of squares (SSR) and the error sum of squares (SSE). Using results from Chapter 5, we now derive the distributions of these quadratic forms in normal random vectors. We also derive the distribution of the fitted vector and the residual vector.

Result 7.1.1. Let $\varepsilon \sim N(\mathbf{0}, \sigma^2 \mathbf{I}_N)$. Then,

1. β^0 has a singular normal distribution

$$\beta^0 \sim SN(\mathbf{H}\beta, \sigma^2 \mathbf{GX'XG'}), \tag{7.1.1}$$

where $\mathbf{H} = \mathbf{GX'X}$.

2. $\hat{\mathbf{y}} \sim SN(\mathbf{X}\beta, \sigma^2 \mathbf{P})$, and $\hat{\varepsilon} \sim SN[\mathbf{0}, \sigma^2(\mathbf{I} - \mathbf{P})]$.

3. SSE has a scaled chi-square distribution:

$$\frac{SSE}{\sigma^2} \sim \chi^2_{N-r}. \tag{7.1.2}$$

4. β^0 and SSE are distributed independently.

5. The model sum of squares has a scaled noncentral chi-square distribution:

$$\frac{SSR}{\sigma^2} \sim \chi^2(r, \lambda), \quad \text{where} \quad \lambda = \frac{1}{2\sigma^2}\beta'\mathbf{X'X}\beta. \tag{7.1.3}$$

6. SSR and SSE are independently distributed.

7.

$$\frac{SSM}{\sigma^2} \sim \chi^2(1, \frac{(\mathbf{1'X}\beta)^2}{2N\sigma^2}). \tag{7.1.4}$$

8. SSM is distributed independently of SSE.

Proof. The model function is $\mathbf{y} = \mathbf{X}\beta + \varepsilon$, and $\mathbf{y} \sim N(\mathbf{X}\beta, \sigma^2 \mathbf{I}_N)$. Since $\beta^0 = \mathbf{GX'y}$ is a linear function of $\mathbf{y}$, the proof of property 1 follows from Result 5.2.6. We prove property 2 by applying Result 5.2.6 as well. Since $SSE = \mathbf{y'(I - XGX')y}$, property 3 follows from Result 5.4.4 since $(\mathbf{I} - \mathbf{XGX'})$ is idempotent with rank $N - r$. Since $\beta^0 = \mathbf{GX'y}$, and $\mathbf{G}(\mathbf{X'} - \mathbf{X'XGX'})\sigma^2 = \mathbf{0}$

(see Exercise 3.4), property 4 follows from Result 5.4.6. Property 5 follows directly by observing that $\mathbf{XGX}'$ is an idempotent matrix of rank r, so that SSR/σ^2 has a noncentral chi-square distribution with noncentrality parameter $\lambda = \beta'\mathbf{X}'\mathbf{X}\beta/2\sigma^2$. Independence of SSR and SSE is proved by invoking Result 5.4.7 since $(\mathbf{XGX}')[\mathbf{I} - \mathbf{XGX}'] = \mathbf{0}$. From properties 2, 4 and 5, and Result 5.3.9, it follows that the ratio $(N - r)SSR/rSSE$ has a noncentral F distribution with noncentrality parameter λ. Recall that $\mathbf{\bar{J}}_N = \mathbf{11}'/N$ is symmetric and idempotent of rank 1. We can write

$$SSM/\sigma^2 = \mathbf{y}'\mathbf{11}'\mathbf{y}/\sigma^2$$

so that property 8 is a direct consequence of Result 5.4.7. Similarly, independence of SSM and SSE follows from Result 5.4.7, using the fact that

$$(\mathbf{11}'/N)(\mathbf{I} - \mathbf{XGX}') = \mathbf{0}. \quad \blacksquare$$

Ansley (1985) derived these and related distributions via the QR algorithm.

Result 7.1.2.

1. Let $\mathbf{c}'_j\beta$, $j = 1, \cdots, s$ denote s estimable functions of β (see Definition 4.3.1). Then

$$\mathbf{C}'\beta^0 \sim N(\mathbf{C}'\beta, \sigma^2\mathbf{C}'\mathbf{GC}),$$

where $\mathbf{C} = (\mathbf{c}_1, \cdots, \mathbf{c}_s)$ is a $p \times s$ dimensional matrix of known coefficients which satisfies $\mathbf{C}'\mathbf{H} = \mathbf{C}'$. Also, $\mathbf{C}'\mathbf{GC}$ is nonsingular provided $\mathbf{c}_1, \cdots, \mathbf{c}_s$ are LIN.

2. For a given s-dimensional vector of constants $\mathbf{d}$,

$$Q/\sigma^2 = (\mathbf{C}'\beta^0 - \mathbf{d})'(\mathbf{C}'\mathbf{GC})^{-1}(\mathbf{C}'\beta^0 - \mathbf{d}) \sim \chi^2(s, \lambda)$$

distribution, with $\lambda = (\mathbf{C}'\beta - \mathbf{d})'(\mathbf{C}'\mathbf{GC})^{-1}(\mathbf{C}'\beta - \mathbf{d})/2\sigma^2$.

Proof. From property 1 of Result 7.1.1 and Result 4.2.6, it follows that $\mathbf{C}'\beta^0 \sim N(\mathbf{C}'\mathbf{H}\beta, \sigma^2\mathbf{C}'\mathbf{GX}'\mathbf{XG}'\mathbf{C})$. Since $\mathbf{C}' = \mathbf{T}'\mathbf{X}$, using Exercise 3.4, we see that $\mathbf{C}'\mathbf{GX}'\mathbf{XG}'\mathbf{C} = \mathbf{C}'\mathbf{GX}'\mathbf{XG}'\mathbf{X}'\mathbf{T} = \mathbf{C}'\mathbf{GX}'\mathbf{T} = \mathbf{C}'\mathbf{GC}$, and the result follows. $\blacksquare$

We state some results for the full rank case in the following corollary. In the full rank linear model, β is estimable, as is any linear function of β. Further, the least squares estimate of β, in addition to being $BLUE$, is also the minimum variance unbiased estimate ($MVUE$).

Corollary 7.1.1. When $r(\mathbf{X}) = p$,

1. $\widehat{\beta} \sim N_p(\beta, \sigma^2(\mathbf{X}'\mathbf{X})^{-1})$.

2. For any given vector $\mathbf{a} = (a_1, \cdots, a_p)'$, $\mathbf{a}'\widehat{\beta} \sim N(\mathbf{a}'\beta, \sigma^2 \mathbf{a}'(\mathbf{X}'\mathbf{X})^{-1}\mathbf{a})$.

3. $\widehat{\beta}'\mathbf{X}'\mathbf{X}\widehat{\beta}/\sigma^2 \sim \chi^2(p, \lambda)$, where $\lambda = \beta'\mathbf{X}'\mathbf{X}\beta/2\sigma^2$.

4. $Cov(\widehat{\beta}, \widehat{\varepsilon}) = \mathbf{0}$, so that $\widehat{\beta}$ is independent of SSE.

5. $SSE/\sigma^2 = (N-p)\widehat{\sigma}^2/\sigma^2 \sim \chi^2_{N-p}$.

Proof. The proof is left as an exercise.

Example 7.1.1. We continue with Example 4.1.1. For the simple regression model, it may be shown that

$$\widehat{\beta}_1 \sim N(\beta_1, \sigma^2/\sum_{i=1}^{N}(X_i - \overline{X})^2),$$

$$\widehat{\beta}_0 \sim N(\beta_0, \sum_{i=1}^{N}X_i^2\sigma^2/N\sum_{i=1}^{N}(X_i - \overline{X})^2).$$

The distributions of $\widehat{\beta}_0$ and $\widehat{\beta}_1$ involve the unknown error variance σ^2. The estimate of σ^2 is the sample variance of the residuals, i.e.,

$$\widehat{\sigma}^2 = \sum_{i=1}^{N}\widehat{\varepsilon}_i^2/(N-2) = \sum_{i=1}^{N}(Y_i - \widehat{\beta}_0 - \widehat{\beta}_1 X_i)^2/(N-2),$$

where $\widehat{\varepsilon}_i = Y_i - \widehat{Y}_i$ is the ith residual. The residual variance $\widehat{\sigma}^2$ is often called the residual mean square and provided the model assumptions are met, it is an unbiased and consistent estimator of σ^2. The residual degree of freedom (d.f.) is the sample size N minus the number of estimated model parameters, here 2. It may be shown that $(N-2)\widehat{\sigma}^2/\sigma^2$ has a chi-square distribution with $N-2$ degrees of freedom. Substituting the value of $\widehat{\sigma}^2$ for the unknown quantity σ^2, we obtain estimated variances of $\widehat{\beta}_0$ and $\widehat{\beta}_1$ as well as their estimated covariance. Let us denote the estimated standard errors of $\widehat{\beta}_0$ and $\widehat{\beta}_1$ respectively by $s_{\widehat{\beta}_0}$ and $s_{\widehat{\beta}_1}$. The estimates of β_0 and β_1 and their associated standard errors will be used in the derivation of confidence intervals and hypotheses tests.   □

Example 7.1.2.   Suppose $\mathbf{y} = \mathbf{X}\beta + \varepsilon$, $\mathbf{X}$ is an $N \times p$ matrix with $r(\mathbf{X}) = p$, and $\varepsilon \sim N(\mathbf{0}, \sigma^2\mathbf{V})$, where $\mathbf{V}$ is a known p.d. matrix. Let $\widehat{\beta}_{GLS}$ denote the GLS estimator of β. It is easy to verify that the matrix $\mathbf{P}_{GLS} = \mathbf{X}(\mathbf{X}'\mathbf{V}^{-1}\mathbf{X})^{-1}\mathbf{X}'$ is symmetric, but not idempotent. By Result 5.2.6, $\widehat{\beta}_{GLS} \sim N(\beta, \sigma^2(\mathbf{X}'\mathbf{V}^{-1}\mathbf{X})^{-1})$. We verify that

$$Q = (\mathbf{y} - \mathbf{X}\widehat{\beta}_{GLS})'\mathbf{V}^{-1}(\mathbf{y} - \mathbf{X}\widehat{\beta}_{GLS})/\sigma^2$$

has a χ^2_{N-p} distribution, and that $Q/(N-p)$ is the MINQUE of σ^2. Now, $Q/\sigma^2 = [\mathbf{y} - \mathbf{X}(\mathbf{X}'\mathbf{V}^{-1}\mathbf{X})^{-1}\mathbf{X}'\mathbf{V}^{-1}\mathbf{y}]'[\mathbf{V}^{-1}/\sigma^2][\mathbf{y} - \mathbf{X}(\mathbf{X}'\mathbf{V}^{-1}\mathbf{X})^{-1}\mathbf{X}'\mathbf{V}^{-1}\mathbf{y}] = \mathbf{y}'[\mathbf{I} - \mathbf{X}(\mathbf{X}'\mathbf{V}^{-1}\mathbf{X})^{-1}\mathbf{X}'\mathbf{V}^{-1}]'[\mathbf{V}^{-1}/\sigma^2][\mathbf{I} - \mathbf{X}(\mathbf{X}'\mathbf{V}^{-1}\mathbf{X})^{-1}\mathbf{X}'\mathbf{V}^{-1}]\mathbf{y} = \mathbf{y}'\mathbf{A}\mathbf{y}$, say. We can verify that $\sigma^2\mathbf{A}\mathbf{V}$ is idempotent, with $r(\sigma^2\mathbf{A}\mathbf{V}) = tr(\sigma^2\mathbf{A}\mathbf{V}) =$

$tr(\mathbf{I}_N) - tr[(\mathbf{X}'\mathbf{V}^{-1}\mathbf{X})(\mathbf{X}'\mathbf{V}^{-1}\mathbf{X})^{-1}] = (N - p)$, and $\beta'\mathbf{X}'\mathbf{A}\mathbf{X}\beta = 0$, so that $Q/\sigma^2 \sim \chi^2(N - p, \lambda = 0)$, i.e., $Q/\sigma^2 \sim \chi^2_{N-p}$. Then, $E[Q/(N - p)] = \sigma^2$, and since $\mathbf{y} \sim N(\mathbf{X}\beta, \sigma^2\mathbf{V})$, $Q/(N - p)$ is the MINQUE of σ^2. Further, $\hat{\mathbf{y}}_{GLS} = \mathbf{X}(\mathbf{X}'\mathbf{V}^{-1}\mathbf{X})^{-1}\mathbf{X}'\mathbf{V}^{-1}\mathbf{y} = \mathbf{P}_{GLS}\mathbf{y}$ is the fitted response vector. $\square$

7.2 General linear hypotheses

In this section, we derive tests for hypotheses about certain parametric linear functions of β. The hypothesis

$$H : \mathbf{C}'\beta = \mathbf{d} \tag{7.2.1}$$

is called a general linear hypothesis, where $\mathbf{C}$ is a $p \times s$ matrix of rank s with known coefficients and $\mathbf{d} = (d_1, \cdots, d_s)'$ is a vector of known constants. This can also be written as

$$H : \mathbf{c}_1'\beta = d_1, \mathbf{c}_2'\beta = d_2, \cdots, \mathbf{c}_s'\beta = d_s. \tag{7.2.2}$$

We assume that $r(\mathbf{C}) = s$, since otherwise, some of the relations in H are redundant, and may be obtained from the others. In practice, we expect that such redundant hypotheses about parameters have been eliminated. Unless $r(\mathbf{X}) = p$, not all such linear hypotheses are in general, testable. A hypothesis is said to be *testable* if $\mathbf{C}'\beta$ can be written in terms of estimable functions of β; otherwise, it is a non-testable hypothesis. The matrix $\mathbf{C}$ must satisfy the condition $\mathbf{T}'\mathbf{X} = \mathbf{C}'$ or $\mathbf{C}'\mathbf{H} = \mathbf{C}'$ in order that the hypothesis H is testable (see section 4.3). To obtain a solution for β under the restriction imposed by H, we use the approach in section 4.6, and minimize the function $S(\beta)$ subject to $\mathbf{C}'\beta = \mathbf{d}$. The equations corresponding to (4.6.2) and (4.6.3) are

$$\mathbf{X}'\mathbf{X}\beta_H^0 + \mathbf{C}\lambda = \mathbf{X}'\mathbf{y}, \quad \mathbf{C}'\beta_H^0 = \mathbf{d}, \tag{7.2.3}$$

where 2λ denotes the vector of Lagrangian multipliers. Provided $\mathbf{C}'\beta = \mathbf{d}$ is estimable, the restricted (under H) least squares solution of β has the form (see (4.6.6))

$$\beta_H^0 = \beta^0 - \mathbf{G}\mathbf{C}(\mathbf{C}'\mathbf{G}\mathbf{C})^{-1}(\mathbf{C}'\beta^0 - \mathbf{d}). \tag{7.2.4}$$

7.2.1 Derivation of and motivation for the F-test

We develop a statistic based on the F-distribution to test the (testable) null hypothesis $H : \mathbf{C}'\beta = \mathbf{d}$. We first define testable hypotheses.

Definition 7.2.1. Consider the normal general linear model $\mathbf{y} = \mathbf{X}\beta + \varepsilon$, where $r(\mathbf{X}) = r < p$. A hypothesis $H : \mathbf{C}'\beta = \mathbf{d}$ is testable if the s rows of $\mathbf{C}'$ are linearly dependent on the rows of $\mathbf{X}$; i.e., $\mathbf{c}_i' = \mathbf{t}_i'\mathbf{X}$, or equivalently, if there exists an $N \times s$ matrix $\mathbf{T}$ such that $\mathbf{C}' = \mathbf{T}'\mathbf{X}$. Equivalently, a hypothesis $H : \mathbf{C}'\beta = \mathbf{d}$ is testable if and only if $\mathbf{C}'\mathbf{H} = \mathbf{C}'$.

Result 7.2.1.   Assume that (7.2.1) is a consistent system of equations. When $\mathbf{y} \sim N(\mathbf{X}\beta, \sigma^2 \mathbf{I}_N)$, the test statistic

$$F(H) = \frac{Q/s}{SSE/(N-r)} \sim F(s, N-r, \lambda), \tag{7.2.5}$$

where the terms in this expression are defined below.

Proof. When $\mathbf{y} \sim N(\mathbf{X}\beta, \sigma^2 \mathbf{I})$, $\beta^0 \sim SN(\mathbf{H}\beta, \sigma^2 \mathbf{G}\mathbf{X}'\mathbf{X}\mathbf{G}')$ (see Result 7.1.1), and further,

$$\mathbf{C}'\beta^0 - \mathbf{d} \sim N_s(\mathbf{C}'\beta - \mathbf{d}, \mathbf{C}'\mathbf{G}\mathbf{C}\sigma^2).$$

It is easy to verify that the matrix $\mathbf{C}'\mathbf{G}\mathbf{C}$ is nonsingular. Consider the quadratic form

$$Q = (\mathbf{C}'\beta^0 - \mathbf{d})'[\mathbf{C}'\mathbf{G}\mathbf{C}]^{-1}(\mathbf{C}'\beta^0 - \mathbf{d}). \tag{7.2.6}$$

By Result 5.3.3,

$$Q/\sigma^2 \sim \chi^2(s, \lambda), \quad \lambda = \frac{1}{2\sigma^2}(\mathbf{C}'\beta - \mathbf{d})'[\mathbf{C}'\mathbf{G}\mathbf{C}]^{-1}(\mathbf{C}'\beta - \mathbf{d}), \tag{7.2.7}$$

a noncentral chi-square distribution with s degrees of freedom and noncentrality parameter λ. Note that under the null hypothesis, $\lambda = 0$ since $\mathbf{C}'\beta = \mathbf{d}$, and the null distribution of Q/σ^2 is a central chi-square with s degrees of freedom. We have already seen that $SSE/\sigma^2 \sim \chi^2_{N-r}$. We will now show that Q and SSE are independently distributed. Substituting $\beta^0 = \mathbf{G}\mathbf{X}'\mathbf{y}$, using $\mathbf{C}' = \mathbf{T}'\mathbf{X}$ and simplifying, we can write

$$
\begin{aligned}
Q &= [\mathbf{y} - \mathbf{X}\mathbf{C}(\mathbf{C}'\mathbf{C})^{-1}\mathbf{d}]'\mathbf{X}\mathbf{G}'\mathbf{C}[\mathbf{C}'\mathbf{G}\mathbf{C}]^{-1}\mathbf{C}'\mathbf{G}\mathbf{X}'[\mathbf{y} - \mathbf{X}\mathbf{C}(\mathbf{C}'\mathbf{C})^{-1}\mathbf{d}] \\
&= [\mathbf{y} - \mathbf{X}\mathbf{C}(\mathbf{C}'\mathbf{C})^{-1}\mathbf{d}]'\mathbf{A}_1[\mathbf{y} - \mathbf{X}\mathbf{C}(\mathbf{C}'\mathbf{C})^{-1}\mathbf{d}], \tag{7.2.8}
\end{aligned}
$$

say. We can also write

$$
\begin{aligned}
SSE &= (\mathbf{y} - \mathbf{X}\beta^0)'(\mathbf{y} - \mathbf{X}\beta^0) \\
&= \mathbf{y}'[\mathbf{I} - \mathbf{X}\mathbf{G}\mathbf{X}']\mathbf{y} \\
&= [\mathbf{y} - \mathbf{X}\mathbf{C}(\mathbf{C}'\mathbf{C})^{-1}\mathbf{d}]'[\mathbf{I} - \mathbf{X}\mathbf{G}\mathbf{X}'][\mathbf{y} - \mathbf{X}\mathbf{C}(\mathbf{C}'\mathbf{C})^{-1}\mathbf{d}] \\
&= [\mathbf{y} - \mathbf{X}\mathbf{C}(\mathbf{C}'\mathbf{C})^{-1}\mathbf{d}]'\mathbf{A}_2[\mathbf{y} - \mathbf{X}\mathbf{C}(\mathbf{C}'\mathbf{C})^{-1}\mathbf{d}]. \tag{7.2.9}
\end{aligned}
$$

It is easily verified, either algebraically, or geometrically that $\mathbf{A}_1\mathbf{A}_2 = \mathbf{0}$, so that by Result 5.4.7, Q is distributed independently of SSE. Hence, by Result 5.3.6, the statistic

$$
\begin{aligned}
F(H) &= \{Q/s\sigma^2\}/\{SSE/(N-r)\sigma^2\} \\
&= \{Q/s\}/\{SSE/(N-r)\} \sim F(s, N-r, \lambda),
\end{aligned}
$$

i.e., a noncentral F-distribution with numerator degrees of freedom s, denominator degrees of freedom $N - r$ and noncentrality parameter λ. Since $\lambda = 0$

under the null hypothesis, the statistic $F(H)$ has a central $F_{s,N-r}$ distribution under H. ■

Let Ω_H denote the estimation space Ω reduced by the hypothesis H. Figure 7.2.1 illustrates the F-test geometrically. The F-test amounts to checking whether $\mathbf{d}$ belongs to the $100(1-\alpha)\%$ confidence ellipsoid for $\mathbf{C}'\beta$, which is centered at $\mathbf{C}'\beta^0$, i.e., the ellipsoid

$$\{\mathbf{C}'\beta : (\mathbf{C}'\beta - \mathbf{C}'\beta^0)'[\mathbf{C}'(\mathbf{X}'\mathbf{X})^-\mathbf{C}]^{-1}(\mathbf{C}'\beta - \mathbf{C}'\beta^0) \leq s\widehat{\sigma}^2 F_{s,N-r}\}. \quad (7.2.10)$$

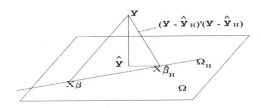

Figure 7.2.1. Geometry of the F-test.

Example 7.2.1. In the simple regression model, we have seen that the estimation space Ω is a plane spanned by $\mathbf{1}_N$ and $\mathbf{x} = (X_1, \cdots, X_N)'$. The estimation space Ω_H reduced by the null hypothesis $H : \mathbf{C}'\beta = \mathbf{d}$, i.e., $H : c_0\beta_0 + c_1\beta_1 = d$ is a straight line formed by combining the vectors $d\mathbf{x}/c_1$ (of constant length), and $\beta_0\{\mathbf{1}_N - c_0\mathbf{x}/c_1\}$ (of variable length). This straight line is parallel to $\mathbf{1}_N - c_0\mathbf{x}/c_1$, but displaced by a distance of $d\mathbf{x}/c_1$. Clearly, Ω_H is a subset of Ω, while $\Omega - \Omega_H$ is the space spanned by all vectors in Ω that are orthogonal to Ω_H. When $p = 2$, and $s = 1$, two vectors span Ω, while Ω_H and $\Omega - \Omega_H$ are each spanned by a single vector denoted respectively by $\mathbf{v} = \beta_0\mathbf{1}_N + (d - c_0\beta_0)\mathbf{x}/c_1$, and $(\mathbf{v}'\mathbf{x})\mathbf{1}_N - (\mathbf{v}'\mathbf{1}_N)\mathbf{x}$. □

Example 7.2.2. Consider the model (4.1.2). We derive the F-test for $H : \beta_j = d_j$, where d_j is a fixed constant, $1 \leq j \leq k$. We can write the hypothesis as $H : \mathbf{C}'\beta = \mathbf{d}$, where $\mathbf{C}'$ is a p-dimensional vector with 1 in the $(j+1)$th position and zero elsewhere. Straightforward calculation yields

$$Q = (\widehat{\beta}_j - d_j)^2/\{(\mathbf{X}'\mathbf{X})^{-1}\}_{jj},$$

so that under H,

$$F(H) = Q/\{SSE/(N-p)\} \sim F_{1,N-p}. \quad □$$

Example 7.2.3. Let A_1 and A_2 denote objects of unknown weights β_1 and β_2 respectively. The weights of A_1 and A_2 are measured on a balance using the following scheme, all of these actions being repeated twice:

(1) both objects on the balance, resulting in weights $Y_{1,1}$ and $Y_{1,2}$,

(2) A_1 on the balance, resulting in weights $Y_{2,1}$ and $Y_{2,2}$, and

(3) A_2 on the balance, resulting in weights $Y_{3,1}$ and $Y_{3,2}$.

We assume that $Y_{i,j}$'s are independent, normally distributed variables, with common variance σ^2. We also assume that the balance has an unknown systematic error β_0. We wish to test the hypothesis that both objects have the same weight. The model can be written as

$$
\begin{aligned}
Y_{1,1} = Y_{1,2} &= \beta_0 + \beta_1 + \beta_2 + \varepsilon_1 \\
Y_{2,1} = Y_{2,2} &= \beta_0 + \beta_1 + \varepsilon_2 \\
Y_{3,1} = Y_{3,2} &= \beta_0 + \beta_2 + \varepsilon_3,
\end{aligned}
$$

where ε_i are iid $N(0, \sigma^2)$ variables, $i = 1, 2, 3$. Let $\overline{Y}_{i.} = (Y_{i,1} + Y_{i,2})/2$. It is easy to verify that

$$
\widehat{\beta} = \begin{pmatrix} -\overline{Y}_{1.} + \overline{Y}_{2.} + \overline{Y}_{3.} \\ \overline{Y}_{1.} - \overline{Y}_{3.} \\ \overline{Y}_{1.} - \overline{Y}_{2.} \end{pmatrix}
$$

with

$$
Cov(\widehat{\beta}) = \sigma^2 \begin{pmatrix} 3/2 & -1 & -1 \\ -1 & 1 & 1/2 \\ -1 & 1/2 & 1 \end{pmatrix},
$$

and that $\widehat{\beta}$ has a normal distribution with mean β and this covariance. Also,

$$
\widehat{\sigma}^2 = \tfrac{1}{3} \sum_{i=1}^{3} \sum_{j=1}^{2} (Y_{i,j} - \overline{Y}_{i.})^2 \sim \chi_3^2.
$$

The test of $H : \beta_1 = \beta_2$ can be written as $H : \mathbf{C}'\beta = \mathbf{d}$, with $\mathbf{C} = (0, 1, -1)$, and $d = 0$. The test statistic is

$$
F(H) = (\overline{Y}_{2.} - \overline{Y}_{3.})^2 / \widehat{\sigma}^2 \sim F_{1,3}
$$

under H. $\square$

An alternative derivation of the F-statistic is shown below. The least squares solution for β in the linear model $\mathbf{y} = \mathbf{X}\beta + \varepsilon$ subject to the linear restriction $H : \mathbf{C}'\beta = \mathbf{d}$ was given in (7.2.4). We see that

$$
\begin{aligned}
SSE_H &= (\mathbf{y} - \mathbf{X}\beta_H^0)'(\mathbf{y} - \mathbf{X}\beta_H^0) \\
&= [\mathbf{y} - \mathbf{X}\beta^0 + \mathbf{X}(\beta^0 - \beta_H^0)]'[\mathbf{y} - \mathbf{X}\beta^0 + \mathbf{X}(\beta^0 - \beta_H^0)] \\
&= (\mathbf{y} - \mathbf{X}\beta^0)'(\mathbf{y} - \mathbf{X}\beta^0) + (\beta^0 - \beta_H^0)'\mathbf{X}'\mathbf{X}(\beta^0 - \beta_H^0) \\
&= SSE + (\mathbf{C}'\beta^0 - \mathbf{d})'(\mathbf{C}'\mathbf{G}\mathbf{C})^{-1}\mathbf{C}'\mathbf{G}'\mathbf{X}'\mathbf{X}\mathbf{G}\mathbf{C}(\mathbf{C}'\mathbf{G}\mathbf{C})^{-1}(\mathbf{C}'\beta^0 - \mathbf{d})
\end{aligned}
$$

$$(7.2.11)$$

since $\mathbf{X}'(\mathbf{y} - \mathbf{X}\beta^0) = 0$. Estimability of $\mathbf{C}'\beta$ implies that $\mathbf{C}' = \mathbf{T}'\mathbf{X}$, so that $\mathbf{C}'\mathbf{G}'\mathbf{X}'\mathbf{X}\mathbf{G}\mathbf{C}(\mathbf{C}'\mathbf{G}\mathbf{C})^{-1} = \mathbf{I}$. It follows that $SSE_H = SSE + Q$, where Q was defined in (7.2.6). The statistic for testing $H : \mathbf{C}'\beta = \mathbf{d}$ may be written as

$$F(H) = \frac{(SSE_H - SSE)/s}{SSE/(N - r)} \qquad (7.2.12)$$

which has an $F_{s,N-r}$ distribution when H is true. Golub and Styan (1973) have suggested a numerically efficient procedure for computing Q.

Here is a motivation for the F-test statistic. Let us consider the quantity Q/s. We have seen that Q/σ^2 has a noncentral $\chi^2(s, \lambda)$ distribution, with $\lambda = (\mathbf{C}'\beta - \mathbf{d})'[\mathbf{C}'(\mathbf{X}'\mathbf{X})^{-1}\mathbf{C}]^{-1}(\mathbf{C}'\beta - \mathbf{d})/2\sigma^2$. By Result 5.3.4, we have

$$E(Q/\sigma^2) = s + 2\lambda,$$

so that

$$E(Q/s) = \sigma^2 + (\mathbf{C}'\beta - \mathbf{d})'[\mathbf{C}'(\mathbf{X}'\mathbf{X})^{-1}\mathbf{C}]^{-1}(\mathbf{C}'\beta - \mathbf{d})/s.$$

We know that $E(\widehat{\sigma}^2) = \sigma^2$. Under $H : \mathbf{C}'\beta - \mathbf{d} = 0$, the second term in $E(Q/s)$ becomes zero, and $E(Q/s) = \sigma^2$. We therefore expect that under H, the statistic $F(H)$ is approximately equal to 1. When the null hypothesis is false, $E(Q/s) > \sigma^2 = E(\widehat{\sigma}^2)$. Now,

$$E\{F(H)\} = E(Q/s)E(1/\widehat{\sigma}^2)$$

and we know from the Markov inequality that $E(1/\widehat{\sigma}^2) > 1/E(\widehat{\sigma}^2)$. Therefore,

$$E\{F(H)\} > E(Q/s)\big/E(\widehat{\sigma}^2) > 1,$$

and H is rejected if $F(H)$ is significantly large.

Example 7.2.4. Sets of regression lines. Consider L regression lines

$$Y_{l,i} = \beta_{l,0} + \beta_{l,1}X_{l,i} + \varepsilon_{l,i}, \quad i = 1, \cdots, n_l, \ l = 1, \cdots, L, \qquad (7.2.13)$$

which can be written in the form (4.1.1) with

$$\mathbf{y} = \begin{pmatrix} Y_{1,1} \\ \vdots \\ Y_{1,n_1} \\ Y_{2,1} \\ \vdots \\ Y_{2,n_2} \\ \vdots \\ Y_{L,1} \\ \vdots \\ Y_{L,n_L} \end{pmatrix}, \quad \varepsilon = \begin{pmatrix} \varepsilon_{1,1} \\ \vdots \\ \varepsilon_{1,n_1} \\ \varepsilon_{2,1} \\ \vdots \\ \varepsilon_{2,n_2} \\ \vdots \\ \varepsilon_{L,1} \\ \vdots \\ \varepsilon_{L,n_L} \end{pmatrix}, \quad \beta = \begin{pmatrix} \beta_{1,0} \\ \vdots \\ \beta_{L,0} \\ \beta_{1,1} \\ \vdots \\ \beta_{L,1} \end{pmatrix}$$

$$\mathbf{X} = \begin{pmatrix}
1 & 0 & \cdots & 0 & X_{1,1} & 0 & \cdots & 0 \\
\vdots & \vdots & \ddots & \vdots & \vdots & \vdots & \ddots & \vdots \\
1 & 0 & \cdots & 0 & X_{1,n_1} & 0 & \cdots & 0 \\
0 & 1 & \cdots & 0 & 0 & X_{2,1} & \cdots & 0 \\
\vdots & \vdots & \ddots & \vdots & \vdots & \vdots & \ddots & \vdots \\
0 & 1 & \cdots & 0 & 0 & X_{2,n_2} & \cdots & 0 \\
\vdots & \vdots & \vdots & \ddots & \vdots & \vdots & \vdots & \vdots \\
0 & 0 & \cdots & 1 & 0 & 0 & \cdots & X_{L,1} \\
\vdots & \vdots & \ddots & \vdots & \vdots & \vdots & \vdots & \vdots \\
0 & 0 & 0 & 1 & 0 & 0 & \cdots & X_{L,n_L}
\end{pmatrix},$$

where $E(\varepsilon_{l,i}) = 0$, $Var(\varepsilon_{l,i}) = \sigma^2$, and $\varepsilon_{l,i}$'s are uncorrelated, for $i = 1, \cdots, n_l$, $l = 1, \cdots, L$. Here, $N = \sum_{l=1}^{L} n_l$, $p = 2L$, and $r(X) = 2L$. The least squares estimate of the parameter vector β is obtained by minimizing the function $S(\beta) = (\mathbf{y} - \mathbf{X}\beta)'(\mathbf{y} - \mathbf{X}\beta)$ and the coefficients are

$$\widehat{\beta}_{l,1} = \frac{\sum\limits_{i=1}^{n_l} (Y_{l,i} - \overline{Y}_{l\cdot})(X_{l,i} - \overline{X}_{l\cdot})}{\sum\limits_{i=1}^{n_l} (X_{l,i} - \overline{X}_{l\cdot})^2}, \qquad (7.2.14)$$

$$\widehat{\beta}_{l,0} = \overline{Y}_{l\cdot} - \widehat{\beta}_{l,1}\overline{X}_{l\cdot}. \qquad (7.2.15)$$

where $\overline{Y}_{l\cdot} = \sum_{i=1}^{n_l} Y_{l,i}/n_l$, and $\overline{X}_{l\cdot} = \sum_{i=1}^{n_l} X_{l,i}/n_l$, for $l = 1, \cdots, L$. Then,

$$\begin{aligned}
SSE &= \sum_{l=1}^{L} \left[\sum_{i=1}^{n_l} (Y_{l,i} - \overline{Y}_{l\cdot})^2 - \widehat{\beta}_{l,1}^2 \sum_{i=1}^{n_l} (X_{l,i} - \overline{X}_{l\cdot})^2 \right] \\
&= \sum_{l=1}^{L}\sum_{i=1}^{n_l} (Y_{l,i} - \overline{Y}_{l\cdot})^2 - \sum_{l=1}^{L} \widehat{\beta}_{l,1}^2 \sum_{i=1}^{n_l} (X_{l,i} - \overline{X}_{l\cdot})^2. \qquad (7.2.16)
\end{aligned}$$

Suppose we impose the linear restriction that the slopes of the L lines are the same, i.e., we hypothesize that

$$H : \beta_{1,1} = \beta_{2,1} = \cdots = \beta_{L,1} = \beta.$$

The least squares estimates of $\beta_{l,0}$, $l = 1, \cdots, L$ and β are obtained by minimizing the function

$$S(\beta_{1,0}, \cdots, \beta_{L,0}, \beta) = \sum_{l=1}^{L}\sum_{i=1}^{n_l} (Y_{l,i} - \beta_{l,0} - \beta X_{l,i})^2$$

with respect to $\beta_{l,0}$, $l = 1, \cdots, L$, and β. The normal equations are

$$\sum_{i=1}^{n_l} (Y_{l,i} - \widehat{\beta}_{l,0,H} - \widehat{\beta}_H X_{l,i}) = 0, \quad l = 1, \cdots, L,$$

$$\sum_{l=1}^{L}\sum_{i=1}^{n_l} (Y_{l,i} - \widehat{\beta}_{l,0,H} - \widehat{\beta}_H X_{l,i}) X_{l,i} = 0;$$

solving these simultaneously, we obtain the least squares estimates of the parameters under the reduction imposed by H as

$$\widehat{\beta}_{l,0,H} = \overline{Y}_{l\cdot} - \widehat{\beta}_H \overline{X}_{l\cdot}, \tag{7.2.17}$$

$$\widehat{\beta}_H = \frac{\sum\limits_{l=1}^{L}\sum\limits_{i=1}^{n_l} X_{l,i}(Y_{l,i} - \overline{Y}_{l\cdot})}{\sum\limits_{l=1}^{L}\sum\limits_{i=1}^{n_l} X_{l,i}(X_{l,i} - \overline{X}_{l\cdot})}. \tag{7.2.18}$$

Clearly, SSE is the error sum of squares in (7.2.16), while

$$SSE_H = \sum_{l=1}^{L}\sum_{i=1}^{n_l}\{Y_{l,i} - \overline{Y}_{l\cdot} - \widehat{\beta}_H(X_{l,i} - \overline{X}_{l\cdot})\}^2$$

$$= \sum_{l=1}^{L}\sum_{i=1}^{n_l}(Y_{l,i} - \overline{Y}_{l\cdot})^2 - \widehat{\beta}_H^2\sum_{l=1}^{L}\sum_{i=1}^{n_l}(X_{l,i} - \overline{X}_{l\cdot})^2, \tag{7.2.19}$$

so that

$$SSE_H - SSE = \sum_{l=1}^{L}\widehat{\beta}_l^2\sum_{i=1}^{n_l}(X_{l,i} - \overline{X}_{l\cdot})^2 - \widehat{\beta}_H^2\sum_{l=1}^{L}\sum_{i=1}^{n_l}(X_{l,i} - \overline{X}_{l\cdot})^2.$$

The test statistic is

$$F(H) = \frac{(SSE_H - SSE)/(L-1)}{SSE/(N-2L)} \tag{7.2.20}$$

which follows an $F_{L-1,N-2L}$ distribution under H. $\quad\square$

In Chapter 8, we will further explore inference for sets of regression lines. We next discuss the relation between the F-test statistic and the coefficient of determinant R^2 in the full-rank model.

Result 7.2.2. In the model (4.1.2) where ε_i are iid $N(0,\sigma^2)$ variables, consider the test of $H : \beta_1 = \beta_2 = \cdots = \beta_k = 0$. The F-test statistic can be written in terms of the coefficient of determination as

$$F(H) = (N - k - 1)R^2/[k(1 - R^2)] \sim F_{k,N-k-1}$$

under H. The null distribution of R^2 is $Beta(k/2, (N-k-1)/2)$.

Proof. Under H, the model is $Y_i = \beta_0 + \varepsilon_i$, with $\widehat{\beta}_H = \overline{Y}$ and $SSE_H = SST = \sum_{i=1}^{N}(Y_i - \overline{Y})^2$. From (7.2.12) and Definition 4.2.4, the form of $F(H)$ in terms of R^2 follows. Since $F(H) \sim F_{k,N-k-1}$ under H, the null distribution of R^2 follows directly from (A14). $\quad\blacksquare$

In Chapter 4, we introduced sums of squares associated with the general linear model. In particular, we distinguished two ways of writing the ANOVA decomposition, $SST = SSR + SSE$, or $SST_c = SSR_c + SSE$, where SST, and SSR denote the total and model sums of squares respectively, SSE denotes the residual sum of squares, while SST_c and SSR_c denote the mean corrected total and model sums of squares. SSM is the sum of squares due to fitting the mean. We now present the ANOVA table in special cases.

Example 7.2.5. Suppose we wish to test the hypothesis $H : \mathbf{X}\beta = \mathbf{0}$ in the general linear model (4.1.1). Since $\mathbf{X}\beta$ includes all estimable parametric functions of β, this hypothesis requires that all estimable parametric functions are null. Clearly this is a testable hypothesis. The F-statistic has the form

$$F(H) = \{SSR/r\} / \{SSE/(N-r)\} \sim F(r, N-r, \beta'\mathbf{X}'\mathbf{X}\beta/2\sigma^2);$$

under H, the noncentrality parameter is zero since $\mathbf{X}\beta = \mathbf{0}$, so that the null distribution of the test statistic $F(H)$ is an $F_{r,N-r}$ distribution. It is not surprising that the numerator degrees of freedom is r, since there are exactly r LIN estimable functions in $\mathbf{X}\beta$ (see Result 4.3.3). It is usual to represent this information via an ANOVA table as shown in Table 7.2.1.

Table 7.2.1. ANOVA table for Example 7.2.5

Source	d.f.	SS	MS
Model	r	$SSR = \beta^{0\prime}\mathbf{X}'\mathbf{y}$	$MSR = SSR/r$
Residual	$N-r$	$SSE = \mathbf{y}'\mathbf{y} - \beta^{0\prime}\mathbf{X}'\mathbf{y}$	$MSE = SSE/(N-r)$
Total	N	$SST = \mathbf{y}'\mathbf{y}$	

It is important to keep in mind that this statistic does not provide a test of $\beta = \mathbf{0}$; in fact, unless $r(\mathbf{X}) = p$, β is not even estimable, so that $\beta = \mathbf{0}$ is *not a testable hypothesis*. In the full rank case when $(\mathbf{X}'\mathbf{X})^{-1}$ exists, the hypotheses $\mathbf{X}\beta = \mathbf{0}$ and $\beta = \mathbf{0}$ are equivalent, since $\mathbf{X}\beta = \mathbf{0}$ implies that $\mathbf{X}'\mathbf{X}\beta = \mathbf{0}$. It is left as an exercise to the reader to verify that SSR, and hence the F-test is unchanged if we replace $\mathbf{X}\beta = \mathbf{0}$ by $\mathbf{L}\beta = \mathbf{0}$, where $\mathbf{L}\beta$ is a different set of r LIN estimable parametric functions of β. The ANOVA table separating out the mean fitting is shown in Table 7.2.2.

Table 7.2.2. ANOVA table separating out the mean

Source	d.f.	SS	MS
Mean	1	$SSM = N\overline{Y}^2$	$MSM = SSM/1$
Mean Corrected Model	$r-1$	$SSR_c = \beta^{0\prime}\mathbf{X}'\mathbf{y} - N\overline{Y}^2$	$MSR_c = SSR/r$
Residual	$N-r$	$SSE = \mathbf{y}'\mathbf{y} - \beta^{0\prime}\mathbf{X}'\mathbf{y}$	$MSE = SSE/(N-r)$
Total	N	$SST_c = \mathbf{y}'\mathbf{y} - N\overline{Y}^2$	

Under the null hypothesis $H : \mathbf{X}\beta = \mathbf{0}$, $F_M = MSM/MSE \sim F_{1,N-r}$, while $F_c = MSR_c/MSE \sim F_{r-1,N-r}$. While F_M tests whether $E(\overline{Y}) = 0$, F_c tests for effects apart from the mean. $\square$

Example 7.2.6. Consider the linear model

$$
\begin{aligned}
Y_1 &= \beta_1 + 3\beta_2 + \varepsilon_1 \\
Y_2 &= 2\beta_1 - \beta_2 + \varepsilon_2 \\
Y_3 &= 3\beta_1 - 4\beta_2 + \varepsilon_3,
\end{aligned}
$$

where ε_i are iid $N(0,\sigma^2)$ variables, $i = 1,2,3$. We derive the F-statistic for testing $H : \beta_1 = \beta_2$, which can be written as $\mathbf{C}'\beta = \mathbf{d}$, with $\mathbf{C}' = (1,-1)$, $\beta = (\beta_1,\beta_2)'$, and $d = 0$. We can verify that $\widehat{\beta}$ and $\mathbf{I} - \mathbf{P}$ are

$$
\widehat{\beta} = \frac{1}{243}\begin{pmatrix} 59Y_1 + 41Y_2 + 34Y_3 \\ 53Y_1 + 8Y_2 - 23Y_3 \end{pmatrix}, \quad
\mathbf{I} - \mathbf{P} = \frac{1}{243}\begin{pmatrix} 25 & -65 & 35 \\ -65 & 169 & -91 \\ 35 & -91 & 49 \end{pmatrix},
$$

$\mathbf{C}'\widehat{\beta} - d = (6Y_1 + 33Y_2 + 57Y_3)/243$, $\mathbf{C}'(\mathbf{X}'\mathbf{X})^{-1}\mathbf{C} = 2/27$. Also, $\widehat{\sigma}^2 = \mathbf{y}'(\mathbf{I} - \mathbf{P})\mathbf{y}$. The F-test statistic has the form in (7.2.5), and has an $F_{1,1}$ distribution under H. $\square$

Example 7.2.7. We continue with Example 4.1.3. In the one-way fixed-effects ANOVA model, our primary interest is in testing equality of the a treatment means, viz.,

$$
\begin{aligned}
H_0 &: \quad \mu_1 = \mu_2 = \cdots = \mu_a, \text{ versus} \\
H_1 &: \quad \mu_i \neq \mu_j \text{ for at least one pair } (i,j),
\end{aligned}
$$

or equivalently, the hypothesis that the a treatment effects are equal, viz.,

$$
\begin{aligned}
H_0 &: \quad \tau_1 = \tau_2 = \cdots = \tau_a, \text{ versus} \\
H_1 &: \quad \tau_i \neq \tau_j \text{ for at least one pair } (i,j).
\end{aligned}
$$

The ANOVA identity leads to the orthogonal partitioning of the total variability in the response variable Y into its component parts:

$$
\sum_{i=1}^{a}\sum_{j=1}^{n_i}(Y_{ij} - \overline{Y}_{..})^2 = \sum_{i=1}^{a} n_i(\overline{Y}_{i.} - \overline{Y}_{..})^2 + \sum_{i=1}^{a}\sum_{j=1}^{n_i}(Y_{ij} - \overline{Y}_{i.})^2 .
$$

The term on the left is the total corrected sum of squares SST_c. The first term on the right side is a sum of squares of the differences *between* treatment means and the grand mean and is called the treatment sum of squares, $SSTr$, while the second term on the right is the sum of squares of the differences of observations *within* a treatment from the treatment mean and is the error sum of squares, SSE. Symbolically, we can write the decomposition as

$$
SST_c = SSTr + SSE.
$$

This algebraic identity is easily verified by seeing that $N\overline{Y}.. = Y.. = \sum_{i=1}^{a} n_i \overline{Y}_{i\cdot\cdot}$. Each of these sums of squares is a quadratic form in an N-dimensional normal random vector $\mathbf{y} = (Y_{11}, Y_{12,}, \cdots, Y_{1n_1}, \cdots, Y_{a1}, Y_{a2}, \cdots, Y_{a,n_a})'$. It may be shown using standard linear model theory for normal random variables that $SST \,/\, \sigma^2$ and $SSTr \,/\, \sigma^2$ have chi-square distributions with $N-1$ and $a-1$ degrees of freedom respectively when H_0 is true, while $SSE \,/\, \sigma^2$ has a chi-square distribution with $N - a$ degrees of freedom. Moreover, $SSTr$ and SSE are independently distributed. We define the mean squares, $MSTr = SSTr/(a-1)$ and $MSE = SSE/(N - a)$; it is easily seen that $E(MSE) = \sigma^2$, while $E(MSTr) = \sigma^2 + \sum_{i=1}^{a} n_i \, \tau_i^2/(a-1)$.

The ANOVA identity provides us with two alternate estimates of σ^2, one based on the variability within treatments and the other based on the variability between treatments. Specifically, MSE is an estimate of σ^2 and $MSTr$ estimates σ^2 under H_0. If there are significant differences in the treatment means, then $E(MSTr)$ exceeds σ^2. The F-statistic for testing H_0 compares $MSTr$ with MSE. From the independent chi-square distributions of $SSTr/\sigma^2$ and SSE/σ^2 under H_0, it follows that the ratio

$$F(H_0) = \{SSTr/(a-1)\} \,/\, \{SSE/(N-a)\} = MSTr/MSE$$

is distributed as a Snedecor's F-distribution with $a - 1$ and $N - a$ degrees of freedom. $F(H_0)$ is the test statistic for testing H_0. These details are summarized in Table 7.2.3.

Table 7.2.3. ANOVA table for the one-factor model

Source	d.f.	SS	MS
Treatment	$a-1$	$SSTr = \sum\limits_{i=1}^{a} n_i(\overline{Y}_{i\cdot} - \overline{Y}..)^2$	$MSTr = SSTr/(a-1)$
Residual	$N-a$	$SSE = \sum\limits_{i=1}^{a}\sum\limits_{j=1}^{n_i}(Y_{ij} - \overline{Y}_{i\cdot})^2$	$MSE = SSE/(N-a)$
Corrected			
Total	$N-1$	$SST_c = \sum\limits_{i=1}^{a}\sum\limits_{j=1}^{n_i}(Y_{ij} - \overline{Y}..)^2$	

We saw that under H_0, both $MSTr$ and MSE are unbiased estimates of σ^2. Under the alternative hypothesis however, $E(MSTr) > \sigma^2$. Hence, if the null hypothesis were false, the expected value of the numerator would be significantly greater than the expectation of the denominator, and consequently, we would reject H_0 for a large value of the test statistic $F(H_0)$. That is, we reject H_0 at $\alpha\%$ level of significance if $F(H_0) > F_{a-1,N-a,\alpha}$, where, $F_{a-1,N-a,\alpha}$ denotes the upper $\alpha\%$ critical point from an $F_{a-1,N-a}$ distribution. Alternatively, in practice, we may compute the p-value of the test as $P\{F > F(H_0)\}$. Most statistical software give the p-value of this upper-tailed test. If the p-value is less than α, we reject H_0. $\square$

Numerical Example 7.1. Fixed-effects one-factor model. Four speci-
mens (n) of each of five brands (a) of a synthetic wood veneer material are
subjected to a friction test. A measure of wear, Y, is determined for each spec-
imen. All tests are made on the same machine in completely random order.
The five brands are ACME, CHAMP, AJAX, TUFFY, and XTRA. The brands
ACME and AJAX are produced by a U.S. company A-line while CHAMP is
produced by a U.S. company C-line. TUFFY and XTRA are produced by a
foreign company (see Littell, Freund and Spector, 1991). The ANOVA table is
shown below.

ANOVA table for Numerical Example 7.1.

Source	d.f.	SS	MS	F-value	$Pr > F$
Model	4	0.617	0.154	7.40	0.0017
Error	15	0.313	0.021		
Corrected					
Total	19	0.930			

The F-test rejects $H : \tau_i$'s are equal, $i = 1, \cdots, 5$. We will continue with this
example in section 7.3. ▲

Example 7.2.8.   We continue with Example 4.2.6. The ANOVA decomposition for the *main effects* model is

$$SST_c = SS_A + SS_B + SSE$$

where

$$SST_c = \sum_{k=1}^{n}\sum_{i=1}^{a}\sum_{j=1}^{b}(Y_{ijk} - \overline{Y}...)^2 \text{ with } N - 1 = nab - 1 \text{ d.f.}$$

$$SS_A = nb\sum_{i=1}^{a}(\overline{Y}_{i..} - \overline{Y}...)^2 \text{ with } a - 1 \text{ d.f.}$$

$$SS_B = na\sum_{j=1}^{b}(\overline{Y}_{.j.} - \overline{Y}...)^2 \text{ with } b - 1 \text{ d.f.}$$

$$SSE = \sum_{k=1}^{n}\sum_{i=1}^{a}\sum_{j=1}^{b}(Y_{ijk} - \overline{Y}_{i..} - \overline{Y}_{.j.} + \overline{Y}...)^2 \text{ with } nab - a - b + 1 \text{ d.f.}$$

The ANOVA table is shown in Table 7.2.4. The test statistic for the hypothesis
$H_A : \tau_1 = \cdots = \tau_a$, is $F_A = MS_A/MSE$, which has an $F_{a-1,nab-a-b+1}$ distribution under H_A. The test statistic for $H_B : \beta_1 = \cdots = \beta_b$ is $F_B = MS_B/MSE$,
which has an $F_{b-1,nab-a-b+1}$ distribution under H_B. For the model with no
replication, we set $n = 1$ in the above formulas. In the balanced model, it can
be shown that the τ effects and β effects are *orthogonal*, so that it is irrelevant
which effect we test first. This unfortunately does not hold in the unbalanced
case which is discussed in Chapter 9.

Table 7.2.4. ANOVA table for the two-factor main effects model

Source	d.f.	SS
Mean μ	1	$SS_M = abn\overline{Y}_{...}^2$
τ after μ	$a-1$	$SS_A = nb\sum_i(\overline{Y}_{i..} - \overline{Y}_{...})^2$
β after (μ, τ)	$b-1$	$SS_B = na\sum_j(\overline{Y}_{.j.} - \overline{Y}_{...})^2$
Error	$nab - a - b + 1$	$SSE = \sum_{ijk}(Y_{ijk} - \overline{Y}_{i..} - \overline{Y}_{.j.} + \overline{Y}_{...})^2$
Total	nab	$SST = \sum_{ijk}Y_{ijk}^2$

The ANOVA table for the *model with interaction* between Factor A and Factor B model is shown in Table 7.2.5.

Table 7.2.5. ANOVA table for two-factor model with interaction

Source	d.f.	SS
Mean μ	1	$SS_M = abn\overline{Y}_{...}^2$
τ after μ	$a-1$	$SS_A = nb\sum_i(\overline{Y}_{i..} - \overline{Y}_{...})^2$
β after (μ, τ)	$b-1$	$SS_B = na\sum_j(\overline{Y}_{.j.} - \overline{Y}_{...})^2$
$(\tau\beta)$ after (μ, τ, β)	$(a-1)(b-1)$	$SS_{AB} = n\sum_{ij}(\overline{Y}_{ij.} - \overline{Y}_{i..} - \overline{Y}_{.j.} + \overline{Y}_{...})^2$
Error	$ab(n-1)$	$SSE = \sum_{ijk}(Y_{ijk} - \overline{Y}_{ij.})^2$
Total	anb	$SST = \sum_{ijk}Y_{ijk}^2$

Let $\gamma_{i.} = \sum_{j=1}^{b}\gamma_{ij}$, $\gamma_{.j} = \sum_{i=1}^{a}\gamma_{ij}$ and $\gamma_{..} = \sum_{j=1}^{b}\sum_{i=1}^{a}\gamma_{ij}$. Although γ_{ij}'s are not estimable, $\gamma_{ij}^* = \gamma_{ij} - \gamma_{i.} - \gamma_{.j} + \gamma_{..}$, $i = 1, \cdots, a$, $j = 1, \cdots, b$ are estimable. We first test for no interaction effects, i.e., $H_{AB} : \gamma_{ij}^* = 0$ for all i, j, using the test statistic

$$F_{AB} = \{SS_{AB}/(a-1)(b-1)\}/\{SSE/ab(n-1)\} \sim F_{(a-1)(b-1),ab(n-1)}$$

under H_{AB}. We next test the hypothesis of no difference among the levels of Factor B. This does not lead to testing $\beta_1 = \cdots = \beta_b$, since this has no meaning in the model with interaction. We test that the effects due to the levels of Factor B are equal, averaged over all levels of Factor A, i.e., $H_B : \beta_j + \sum_i \gamma_{ij}/a$ equal for all j, using the test statistic

$$F_B = \{SS_B/(b-1)\}/\{SSE/ab(n-1)\} \sim F_{(b-1),ab(n-1)}$$

under H_B. Similarly, we test that effects due to the levels of Factor A are equal, averaged over all levels of Factor B; i.e., we test the hypothesis $H_A : \tau_i + \sum_j \gamma_{ij}/b$ equal for all i, using the test statistic

$$F_A = \{SS_A/(a-1)\} / \{SSE/ab(n-1)\} \sim F_{(a-1),ab(n-1)}$$

under H_A. $\square$

Numerical Example 7.2. Fixed-effects two-factor model. An engineer is designing a battery for use in a device that would be subjected to extreme variations in temperature. Three choices of the plate material are possible, and the engineer tests these at three temperature levels. Four batteries are tested at each plate material/temperature combination, all 36 tests being run in random order. We make inference based on fitting a two-factor model to lifetimes of the batteries (in hours) (Montgomery, 1991). The ANOVA table is shown below.

ANOVA table for Numerical Example 7.2.

Source	d.f.	SS	MS	F-value	$\Pr > F$
Model	8	59416.222	7427.028	11.00	0.0001
Plate	2	10683.722	5341.861	7.91	0.0020
Temp	2	39118.722	19559.361	28.97	0.0001
Plate × temp	4	9613.778	2403.444	3.56	0.0186
Error	27	18230.750	675.213		
Corrected					
Total	35	77646.972			

All the effects are significant. ▲

7.2.2 Power of the F-test

By definition, the power of the F-test for the general linear hypothesis H is

$$P(\text{Reject}\,H|H \text{ is false}) = P\left[\frac{(SSE_H - SSE)/s}{SSE/(N-r)} > F_{s,N-r,\alpha}|H \text{ is false}\right]$$

$$= \int_{F_{s,N-r,\alpha}}^{\infty} g(\xi)d\xi,$$

where the random variable

$$\xi = \{(SSE_H - SSE)/s\} / \{SSE/(N-r)\}$$
$$= \{(SSE_H - SSE)/(s\sigma^2)\} / \{SSE/(N-r)\sigma^2\}$$

has pdf $g(\xi)$, which we know has a noncentral $F(s, N-r, \lambda)$ distribution (see Chapter 5). We may derive an explicit expression for $g(\xi|s, N-r, \lambda)$ using the distribution of $(SSE_H - SSE)$ and SSE, and transforming to ξ (see Kendall and Stuart, 1963 for details). In order to evaluate the integral involved in the power calculation, we may use Tang's tables (1938), which are given in terms of a random variable $E^2 = s\xi/(N - r + s\xi)$; see Pearson and Hartley (1970) for charts of the power function.

It is clear that an evaluation of the power function requires an estimate of the noncentrality parameter λ. If $U \sim \chi^2(k, \lambda)$, it is easy to see that $(U - k)/2$ is an unbiased estimator of λ. However, since it may assume negative values, it is not a useful estimator, and we prefer to use $(U - k)^+/2$. The MLE of λ does not have a closed form and must be solved numerically (Saxena and Alam, 1982).

7.2.3   Testing independent and orthogonal contrasts

Let $\mathbf{c}_i'$ and $\mathbf{c}_j'$ denote two distinct rows of the $k \times s$ matrix $\mathbf{C}$. The quadratic forms

$$
\begin{aligned}
Q_i &= \beta^{0\prime}\mathbf{c}_i(\mathbf{c}_i'\mathbf{G}\mathbf{c}_i)^{-1}\mathbf{c}_i'\beta^0 = \mathbf{y}'\mathbf{X}\mathbf{G}'\mathbf{c}_i(\mathbf{c}_i'\mathbf{G}\mathbf{c}_i)^{-1}\mathbf{c}_i'\mathbf{G}\mathbf{X}'\mathbf{y}, \text{ and} \\
Q_j &= \beta^{0\prime}\mathbf{c}_j(\mathbf{c}_j'\mathbf{G}\mathbf{c}_j)^{-1}\mathbf{c}_j'\beta^0 = \mathbf{y}'\mathbf{X}\mathbf{G}'\mathbf{c}_j(\mathbf{c}_j'\mathbf{G}\mathbf{c}_j)^{-1}\mathbf{c}_j'\mathbf{G}\mathbf{X}'\mathbf{y}
\end{aligned}
$$

appear as the numerator sums of squares in the F-statistics for testing $H_i : \mathbf{c}_i'\beta = 0$, and $H_j : \mathbf{c}_j'\beta = 0$. That is,

$$
F(H_i) = Q_i/\{SSE/(N - r)\} \sim F_{1,N-r}
$$

under H_i, so that we reject H_i at level of significance α if $F(H_i) > F_{1,N-r,\alpha}$. It can be verified that Q_i and Q_j are independently distributed if and only if

$$
\mathbf{X}\mathbf{G}'\mathbf{c}_i(\mathbf{c}_i'\mathbf{G}\mathbf{c}_i)^{-1}\mathbf{c}_i'\mathbf{G}\mathbf{X}'\mathbf{X}\mathbf{G}'\mathbf{c}_j(\mathbf{c}_j'\mathbf{G}\mathbf{c}_j)^{-1}\mathbf{c}_j'\mathbf{G}\mathbf{X}' = \mathbf{0},
$$

which in turn is true if and only if $\mathbf{c}_i'\mathbf{G}\mathbf{X}'\mathbf{X}\mathbf{G}'\mathbf{c}_j = 0$. Since $\mathbf{c}_j' = \mathbf{t}_j'\mathbf{X}$, the condition is equivalent to $\mathbf{c}_i'\mathbf{G}\mathbf{X}'\mathbf{X}\mathbf{G}'\mathbf{X}'\mathbf{t}_j = 0$. Since $\mathbf{X}'\mathbf{X}\mathbf{G}'\mathbf{X}' = \mathbf{X}'$, this in turn is equivalent to $\mathbf{c}_i'\mathbf{G}\mathbf{X}'\mathbf{t}_j = 0$, i.e.,

$$
\mathbf{c}_i'\mathbf{G}\mathbf{c}_j = 0. \tag{7.2.21}
$$

(7.2.21) gives a necessary and sufficient condition for independence of Q_i and Q_j. If (7.2.21) holds, we refer to $\mathbf{c}_i'\beta$ and $\mathbf{c}_j'\beta$ as orthogonal contrasts. It can be verified that when $\mathbf{c}_i'\mathbf{G}\mathbf{X}'\mathbf{t}_j = 0$, for $i, j = 1, \cdots, s$, $i \neq j$, then $(\mathbf{C}'\mathbf{G}\mathbf{C})^{-1}$ reduces to a diagonal matrix. The statistic for testing the general linear hypothesis $H : \mathbf{C}'\beta = \mathbf{d}$, can then be written as

$$
\begin{aligned}
Q &= \sum_{i=1}^{s}(\mathbf{c}_i'\beta^0 - d_i)'(\mathbf{c}_i'\mathbf{G}\mathbf{c}_i)^{-1}(\mathbf{c}_i'\beta^0 - d_i) \\
&= \sum_{i=1}^{s}\frac{(\mathbf{c}_i'\beta^0 - d_i)^2}{\mathbf{c}_i'\mathbf{G}\mathbf{c}_i} = \sum_{i=1}^{s}Q_i.
\end{aligned}
$$

7.3 Confidence intervals and multiple comparisons

The least squares approach and the method of maximum likelihood (see section 7.5.1) provide point estimates for the vector β. Under the assumption of normal errors, we now construct the joint confidence region for an estimable function $\mathbf{C}'\beta$ as well as marginal confidence intervals for each estimable function $\mathbf{c}'_j\beta$, $j = 1, \cdots, s$.

7.3.1 Joint and marginal confidence intervals

Let $\mathbf{C}'\beta$ denote a vector of estimable functions of β, where $\mathbf{C}$ is a $p \times s$ matrix of known coefficients. We have seen that the least squares estimator of $\mathbf{C}'\beta$ is $\mathbf{C}'\beta^0$, with covariance $\sigma^2\mathbf{C}'\mathbf{G}\mathbf{C}$.

Result 7.3.1. The $100(1 - \alpha)\%$ joint confidence region for $\mathbf{C}'\beta$ is

$$(\mathbf{C}'\beta^0 - \mathbf{C}'\beta)'(\mathbf{C}'\mathbf{G}\mathbf{C})^{-1}(\mathbf{C}'\beta^0 - \mathbf{C}'\beta) \leq s\hat{\sigma}^2 F_{s,N-r,\alpha} \qquad (7.3.1)$$

where $F_{s,N-r,\alpha}$ denotes the upper $\alpha\%$ critical point from an $F_{s,N-r}$ distribution.

Proof. This result directly follows from inverting the F-statistic in (7.2.5). ∎

Corollary 7.3.1. In the full rank case, the $100(1 - \alpha)\%$ joint confidence region for the parameter vector β is

$$(\hat{\beta} - \beta)'(\mathbf{X}'\mathbf{X})(\hat{\beta} - \beta) \leq p\hat{\sigma}^2 F_{p,N-p,\alpha}. \qquad (7.3.2)$$

In Figure 7.3.1, for $k = 2$, the ellipsoid represents the joint confidence region for β, while the marginals intervals for β_1 and β_2 form the rectangle ABCD.

The marginal $100(1-\alpha)\%$ confidence intervals for s estimable functions $\mathbf{c}'_i\beta$, $i = 1, \cdots, s$ of β are given by

$$\mathbf{c}'_i\beta^0 \pm t_{N-r,\alpha/2}\hat{\sigma}(\mathbf{c}'_i\mathbf{G}\mathbf{c}_i)^{1/2}, \quad i = 1, \cdots, s. \qquad (7.3.3)$$

While each marginal interval contains the true parameter $\mathbf{c}'_i\beta$ with probability $(1 - \alpha)$, the probability that "simultaneously" all s functions $\mathbf{c}'_i\beta$, $i = 1, \cdots, s$ are contained in the intervals in (7.3.3) is certainly much less than $(1 - \alpha)$. We may, of course, construct simultaneous confidence intervals for estimable functions of β, as described in section 7.3.2.

Example 7.3.1. Continuing with Example 4.1.1, we construct confidence intervals for the model parameters and functions of the parameters in a simple regression model by inverting t-tests (or, equivalently, F-tests having one numerator degree of freedom). We can test the null hypothesis $H_0 : \beta_1 = \beta_{1,0}$

using the t-statistic $t = (\widehat{\beta}_1 - \beta_{1,0})/s_{\widehat{\beta}_1}$, which has a Student t-distribution with $(N-2)$ degrees of freedom under H_0. For a two-sided alternative $H_1 : \beta_1 \neq \beta_{1,0}$, the test rejects the null hypothesis at level of significance α if $|t_{obs}| > t_{N-2,\alpha/2}$, i.e., the observed test statistic is greater in absolute value than the upper $\alpha/2$ percent critical value from a t-distribution with $(N-2)$ degrees of freedom. The $100(1-\alpha)\%$ confidence interval for β_1 is given by $\widehat{\beta}_1 \pm s_{\widehat{\beta}_1} t_{N-2,\alpha/2}$. Using a similar procedure, the $100(1-\alpha)\%$ confidence interval for β_0 is given by $\widehat{\beta}_0 \pm s_{\widehat{\beta}_0} t_{N-2,\alpha/2}$. □

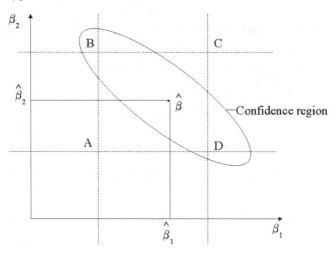

Figure 7.3.1.   Joint confidence region for β.

Example 7.3.2.   We continue with Example 4.1.2. From the distributional properties of the multiple regression model, it follows that $\widehat{\sigma}^2(\mathbf{X'X})^{-1}$ is an unbiased estimator of $Cov(\widehat{\beta})$. Since (i) $\widehat{\beta}_j - \beta_j, j = 0, \cdots, k$ has a normal distribution with mean 0 and variance $\sigma^2(\mathbf{X'X})^{-1}_{jj}$ (which is the jth diagonal element of $Cov(\widehat{\beta})$), (ii) $(N-k-1)\widehat{\sigma}^2/\sigma^2$ is distributed as a chi-square with $(N-k-1)$ degrees of freedom, and (iii) $(N-k-1)\widehat{\sigma}^2/\sigma^2$ is distributed independently of $\widehat{\beta}_j - \beta_j, j = 0, \cdots, k$, it follows that the statistic

$$t = (\widehat{\beta}_j - \beta_j)/s_{\widehat{\beta}_j} \qquad (7.3.4)$$

has a t-distribution with $(N-k-1)$ degrees of freedom. This framework enables us to carry out hypothesis tests on the components of β as well as to construct confidence intervals for β_j. To test the null hypothesis $H_0 : \beta_j = \beta_{j,0}$, we substitute $\beta_{j,0}$ for β_j in (7.3.4); if the observed value of the statistic is greater than the upper $\alpha/2$ critical value from a t-distribution with $(N-k-1)$ degrees of freedom, we reject the null hypothesis at level of significance α. The $100(1-\alpha)\%$ confidence interval for β_j is

$$\widehat{\beta}_j \pm s_{\widehat{\beta}_j} t_{N-k-1,\alpha/2}. \qquad \square$$

Example 7.3.3. We continue with Example 4.5.1, where we looked at GLS estimation of β in a model with AR(1) errors. We see that

$$\widehat{\beta}_{GLS} \sim N(\beta, \sigma^2(\mathbf{x}'\mathbf{V}^{-1}\mathbf{x})^{-1}), \quad \text{and} \quad (N-1)\widehat{\sigma}^2_{GLS} \sim \chi^2_{N-1}$$

(see Example 7.1.2). Hence,

$$(\widehat{\beta}_{GLS} - \beta)/\{\widehat{\sigma}^2_{GLS}(\mathbf{x}'\mathbf{V}^{-1}\mathbf{x})^{-1}\}^{1/2} \sim t_{N-1}.$$

The $100(1-\alpha)\%$ confidence interval for β is

$$\widehat{\beta}_{GLS} \pm t_{N-1,\alpha/2}\sqrt{\widehat{\sigma}^2_{GLS}(\mathbf{x}'\mathbf{V}^{-1}\mathbf{x})^{-1}},$$

where $t_{N-1,\alpha/2}$ denotes the upper $100\alpha/2$th percentile from a Student's t-distribution with $(N-1)$ degrees of freedom. $\square$

Example 7.3.4. Suppose

$$
\begin{aligned}
Y_1 &= \beta_1 + \varepsilon_1, \\
Y_2 &= 2\beta_1 - \beta_2 + \varepsilon_2, \\
Y_3 &= \beta_1 + 2\beta_2 + \varepsilon_3,
\end{aligned}
$$

where ε_i are iid $N(0,\sigma^2)$ variables, $i = 1,2,3$. We construct a 95% confidence interval for $\theta = \beta_1 + 3\beta_2$. By Corollary 7.1.1, the b.l.u.e. of θ is $\widehat{\theta} = \widehat{\beta}_1 + 3\widehat{\beta}_2 = (5Y_1 - 8Y_2 + 41Y_3)/30$, while $\widehat{\sigma}^2 = \sum_{i=1}^{3} Y_i^2 - \frac{1}{6}(Y_1 + 2Y_2 + Y_3)^2 + \frac{1}{5}(-Y_2 + 2Y_3)^2$. We can verify that $E(\widehat{\theta}) = \theta$ and $est.Var(\widehat{\theta}) = 59\widehat{\sigma}^2/30$. The 95% confidence interval for θ is

$$\widehat{\theta} \pm t_{1,.025}(59\widehat{\sigma}^2/30)^{1/2}. \qquad \square$$

Example 7.3.5. Consider the linear model

$$
\begin{pmatrix} Y_1 \\ Y_2 \\ Y_3 \end{pmatrix} = \begin{pmatrix} 1 & 1 & 0 \\ 1 & 0 & 1 \\ 1 & 1 & 0 \end{pmatrix} \begin{pmatrix} \beta_1 \\ \beta_2 \\ \beta_3 \end{pmatrix} + \begin{pmatrix} \varepsilon_1 \\ \varepsilon_2 \\ \varepsilon_3 \end{pmatrix},
$$

where $\varepsilon \sim N(\mathbf{0}, \sigma^2\mathbf{I})$. We construct a 95% confidence interval for $\beta_1 + \beta_2/3 + 2\beta_3/3$. First, see that since $r(\mathbf{X}) = 2$, we must verify that the linear function of β is estimable. Given $\mathbf{c}' = (c_1, c_2, c_3)$, it is easy to verify using (4.3.3) that $\mathbf{c}'\beta$ is estimable if and only if $c_1 = c_2 + c_3$ (see Example 4.3.1). Based on

$$\mathbf{G} = (\mathbf{X}'\mathbf{X})^- = \begin{pmatrix} 0 & 1/2 & 0 \\ 0 & 0 & 0 \\ 1 & -3/2 & 0 \end{pmatrix}, \text{ and } \beta^0 = \begin{pmatrix} (Y_1 + Y_3)/2 \\ 0 \\ Y_2 - (Y_1 + Y_3)/2 \end{pmatrix},$$

the least squares estimate of $\beta_1 + \beta_2/3 + 2\beta_3/3$ is $\mathbf{c}'\beta^0 = (Y_1 + 4Y_2 + Y_3)/6$. Using (7.3.3), the 95% confidence interval of $\mathbf{c}'\beta$ is

$$\mathbf{c}'\beta^0 \pm t_{2,.025}\widehat{\sigma}(\mathbf{c}'\mathbf{G}\mathbf{c})^{1/2}. \qquad \square$$

7.3.2   Simultaneous confidence intervals

The marginal $100(1-\alpha)\%$ confidence intervals for s contrasts $\mathbf{c}_i'\beta$, $i = 1, \cdots, s$ given in (7.3.3) provide coverage probability of $(1-\alpha)$ for *each* $\mathbf{c}_i'\beta$. For simultaneous inference, we wish to claim in general that $P[\mathbf{c}_i'\beta \in I_{\mathbf{c}_i}, \mathbf{c}_i \in \mathcal{S}] = 1 - \alpha$, where $\mathcal{S}$ is a finite or infinite collection of such vectors $\mathbf{c}_i$; then, $\{I_{\mathbf{c}_i}, \mathbf{c}_i \in \mathcal{S}\}$ is called a "family" of confidence intervals with confidence coefficient $(1-\alpha)$.

Let $\mathcal{F} = \{S_f\} = \{S_1, \cdots, S_{N(\mathcal{F})}\}$ denote a family of statements in a confidence interval estimation or a hypothesis testing problem, where $N(\mathcal{F})$ is the number of statements in the family. Let $N_w(\mathcal{F})$ denote the number of incorrect statements in $\mathcal{F}$.

Definition 7.3.1.   For $N(\mathcal{F}) < \infty$, the error rate

$$Er(\mathcal{F}) = N_w(\mathcal{F})/N(\mathcal{F}) \tag{7.3.5}$$

is a random variable.

The probability of a nonzero error rate is $P\{Er(\mathcal{F}) > 0\}$. The probability that at least one statement in $\mathcal{F}$ is *incorrect* is

$$P(\mathcal{F}) = P\{N_w(\mathcal{F})/N(\mathcal{F}) > 0\} = P\{N_w(\mathcal{F}) > 0\},$$

so that $1 - P(\mathcal{F})$ denotes the probability that all statements in $\mathcal{F}$ are correct, and provides a simultaneous probability statement for $\mathcal{F}$. If $N(\mathcal{F}) < \infty$, the expected error rate is

$$E(\mathcal{F}) = E\{N_w(\mathcal{F})/N(\mathcal{F})\}.$$

Let $I(S_f) = 1$ if S_f is an incorrect statement in $\mathcal{F}$, and $I(S_f) = 0$ if S_f is a correct statement. Let us denote the level of significance by $\alpha_f = P\{I(S_f) = 1\} = P(S_f$ is incorrect $) = E\{I(S_f)\}$, $f = 1, \cdots, N(\mathcal{F})$. Now, $E\{N_w(\mathcal{F})\} = E\{I(S_1)\} + \cdots + E\{I(S_{N(\mathcal{F})})\}$, and, since $N(\mathcal{F})$ is not a random variable, $E(\mathcal{F}) = \{\alpha_1 + \cdots + \alpha_{N(\mathcal{F})}\}/N(\mathcal{F})$. For the assessment and comparison of simultaneous inference procedures, including multiple comparisons of means, $P(\mathcal{F})$ or $E(\mathcal{F})$ is a useful criterion. The following result may be interpreted as a statement that the use of $P(\mathcal{F})$ is an adequate criterion.

Result 7.3.2.   If $N(\mathcal{F}) < \infty$, then $E(\mathcal{F}) \leq P(\mathcal{F}) \leq N(\mathcal{F})E(\mathcal{F})$.

Proof.   By definition, $P(\mathcal{F}) \geq \alpha_f$, $f = 1, \cdots, N(\mathcal{F})$. Clearly, $E\{I(S_f)\} = \alpha_f$, $f = 1, \cdots, N(\mathcal{F})$, so that $E\{N_w(\mathcal{F})\} = \sum_{f=1}^{N(\mathcal{F})} \alpha_f$, and

$$E(\mathcal{F}) = \sum_{f=1}^{N(\mathcal{F})} \alpha_f / N(\mathcal{F}) . \tag{7.3.6}$$

The probability that at least one statement is incorrect is

$$P(\mathcal{F}) = P(\cup_{f=1}^{N(\mathcal{F})}\{S_f \text{ is incorrect }\}) = P(N_w(\mathcal{F}) > 0)$$

$$\leq \sum_{f=1}^{N(\mathcal{F})} P(S_f \text{ is incorrect }) = \sum_{f=1}^{N(\mathcal{F})} \alpha_f,$$

by Boole's inequality. That is, $P(\mathcal{F}) \leq \sum_{f=1}^{N(\mathcal{F})} \alpha_f = E(\mathcal{F})N(\mathcal{F})$. Since by definition, $P(\mathcal{F}) \geq \alpha_f$, $f = 1, \cdots, N(\mathcal{F})$, it follows that $\sum_{f=1}^{N(\mathcal{F})} P(\mathcal{F}) \geq \sum_{f=1}^{N(\mathcal{F})} \alpha_f$, i.e., $N(\mathcal{F})P(\mathcal{F}) \geq \sum_{f=1}^{N(\mathcal{F})} \alpha_f$, i.e., $P(\mathcal{F}) \geq \sum_{f=1}^{N(\mathcal{F})} \alpha_f/N(\mathcal{F}) = E(\mathcal{F})$, which proves the result. ∎

We describe the construction of simultaneous confidence intervals for s contrasts $\mathbf{c}_i'\beta$. We first describe a procedure due to Scheffe, and then discuss Bonferroni t-intervals.

Scheffe intervals

Scheffe (1953) proposed a method for comparing *all possible contrasts* in β such that the probability of type I error is at most α for any of the possible comparisons. In other words, the probability is $1 - \alpha$ that the associated confidence intervals simultaneously contain the true values of *all* the contrasts in β. Let $\mathcal{L} = \{\mathbf{c} = (c_1, \cdots, c_p)'\} \subset \mathcal{C}(\mathbf{X})$, with $\dim(\mathcal{L}) = s$, say. That is, $\mathcal{L}$ is a fixed s-dimensional linear subspace of $\mathcal{C}(\mathbf{X})$, $s \leq r$. The objective is to construct confidence intervals for $\mathbf{c}'\beta = \sum_{i=1}^p c_i\beta_i$ for all $\mathbf{c} \in \mathcal{L}$ with simultaneous $100(1-\alpha)\%$ coverage. Here, $\mathcal{F} = \mathcal{L}$, which can denote a family of contrasts, or arbitrary estimable linear functions of β, or individual coordinates of dimension s, etc. For example, in the fixed-effects one-way ANOVA model, we are often interested in estimating contrasts. In simple linear regression, we might be interested in confidence intervals on all linear combinations $c_0\beta_0 + c_1\beta_1$. If $\dim(\mathcal{L}) = 1$, we would obtain a single confidence interval. Consider s LIN combinations with coefficients $\mathbf{c}_i = (c_{i1}, \cdots, c_{ip})'$, $i = 1, \cdots, s$. Consider the $s \times p$ matrix

$$\mathbf{L}' = \begin{pmatrix} c_{11} & \cdots & c_{1p} \\ & \vdots & \\ c_{s1} & \cdots & c_{sp} \end{pmatrix}$$

with $r(\mathbf{L}') = s$, so that the rows of $\mathbf{L}'$ form a basis of $\mathcal{L}$. From Result 5.2.6, $\mathbf{L}'\beta^0 \sim N_s(\mathbf{L}'\beta, \sigma^2\mathbf{L}'\mathbf{GL})$. A test of $H : \mathbf{L}'\beta = \mathbf{b}^*$, say, is based on

$$(\mathbf{L}'\beta^0 - \mathbf{b}^*)'(\mathbf{L}'\mathbf{GL})^{-1}(\mathbf{L}'\beta^0 - \mathbf{b}^*)/s\widehat{\sigma}^2 \sim F_{s,N-r} \qquad (7.3.7)$$

under the null hypothesis.

Result 7.3.3. The $100(1 - \alpha)\%$ simultaneous confidence intervals via the "F- projections" approach for estimable functions $\mathbf{c}'\beta$ for all $\mathbf{c} \in \mathcal{L}$ are given by

$$\mathbf{c}'\beta^0 \pm \widehat{\sigma}\{s(\mathbf{c}'\mathbf{Gc})F_{s,N-r,\alpha}\}^{1/2}. \qquad (7.3.8)$$

The simultaneous confidence interval for any $\mathbf{c}'\beta$, $\mathbf{c} \in \mathcal{L}$ is the projection of the confidence ellipsoid (7.2.10) onto the one-dimensional subspace of $\mathcal{L}$ generated by $\mathbf{c}$.

Proof.   Let $\mathbf{P} = \mathbf{C}'\mathbf{GC}$, $\gamma = s\widehat{\sigma}^2 F_{s,N-r,\alpha}$, and $\mathbf{C}'\beta^0 - \mathbf{C}'\beta = \mathbf{b}$. Using Result 2.4.6,

$$
\begin{aligned}
1 - \alpha &= P(F_{s,N-r} \leq F_{s,N-r,\alpha}) \\
&= P\{(\mathbf{C}'\beta^0 - \mathbf{C}'\beta)'(\mathbf{C}'\mathbf{GC})^{-1}(\mathbf{C}'\beta^0 - \mathbf{C}'\beta) \leq s\widehat{\sigma}^2 F_{s,N-r,\alpha}\} \\
&= P\{\mathbf{b}'\mathbf{P}^{-1}\mathbf{b} \leq \gamma\} = P\{\sup_{\mathbf{h}\neq\mathbf{0}}[\frac{(\mathbf{h}'\mathbf{b})^2}{\mathbf{h}'\mathbf{Ph}}] \leq \gamma\} \\
&= P\{\frac{(\mathbf{h}'\mathbf{b})^2}{\mathbf{h}'\mathbf{Ph}} \leq \gamma \text{ for all } \mathbf{h} \neq \mathbf{0}\} \\
&= P\left\{\frac{|\mathbf{h}'\mathbf{C}'\beta^0 - \mathbf{h}'\mathbf{C}'\beta|}{\widehat{\sigma}(\mathbf{h}'\mathbf{Ph})^{1/2}} \leq [sF_{s,N-r,\alpha}]^{1/2} \text{ for all } \mathbf{h} \neq \mathbf{0}\right\}.
\end{aligned}
$$

Setting $\mathbf{c} = \mathbf{Lh}$, gives $1 - \alpha = P\{|\mathbf{c}'\beta^0 - \mathbf{c}'\beta| \leq \{s\mathbf{c}'\mathbf{Gc}F_{s,N-r,\alpha}\}^{1/2} \text{ for all } \mathbf{c}\}$, which proves the result.   ∎

In Exercise 7.9, we ask the reader to derive the Scheffe F-intervals for the linear model with a p.d. covariance structure. For ANOVA models, Scheffe's method is generally recommended when (a) the sample sizes n_i, $i = 1, \cdots, a$ are unequal, and (b) we are interested in more complicated comparisons between treatment means than simple pairwise comparisons.

Example 7.3.6.   We apply Scheffe's simultaneous procedure to simple linear regression to construct simultaneous confidence intervals for $c_0\beta_0 + c_1\beta_1$, which are given by

$$
\{(c_0\widehat{\beta}_0 + c_1\widehat{\beta}_1) \pm [2 \text{ est. } Var(c_0\widehat{\beta}_0 + c_1\widehat{\beta}_1)F_{2,N-2,\alpha}]^{1/2}\},
$$

where, $Var(c_0\widehat{\beta}_0 + c_1\widehat{\beta}_1) = c_0^2 Var(\widehat{\beta}_0) + c_1^2 Var(\widehat{\beta}_1) + 2c_0 c_1 Cov(\widehat{\beta}_0, \widehat{\beta}_1)$ can be computed from (4.2.28). Letting $c_0 = 1$, and $c_1 = X$, we can obtain the simultaneous confidence intervals for $\beta_0 + \beta_1 X$.   □

Suppose $r(\mathbf{X}) = p$. To obtain simultaneous confidence surfaces for the entire regression, we have from Scheffe's procedure that the unknown Y corresponding to all values of $\mathbf{x}$ lies in

$$
\mathbf{x}'\widehat{\beta} \pm \widehat{\sigma}\{pF_{p,N-p,\alpha}[\mathbf{x}(\mathbf{X}'\mathbf{X})^{-1}\mathbf{x}]\}^{1/2}. \tag{7.3.9}
$$

Bonferroni t-intervals

Let us consider the problem of constructing simultaneous $100(1-\alpha)\%$ confidence intervals for L pairwise treatment differences $\tau_i - \tau_k$, $i \neq k$, $i, k = 1, \cdots, a$, such that the probability that the intervals jointly contain the true differences is at least $1 - \alpha$. This goal can be achieved by using the Bonferroni inequality. For any events $A_1, \cdots, A_L$, we have

$$P(A_1 \cap \cdots \cap A_L) = 1 - P(\bar{A}_1 \cup \cdots \cup \bar{A}_L),$$

where $\bar{A}_j$ denotes the complement of the event A_j, and

$$P(\bar{A}_1 \cup \cdots \cup \bar{A}_L) \leq \sum_{i=1}^{L} P(\bar{A}_i).$$

The first-order Bonferroni inequality gives

$$P(A_1 \cap \cdots \cap A_L) \geq 1 - \sum_{i=1}^{L} P(\bar{A}_i).$$

Suppose we denote the confidence intervals by $I_1, \cdots, I_L$, and suppose $P(\theta_i \in I_i) = 1 - \alpha_i$, $i = 1, \cdots, L$, where θ_i denotes a difference between any two treatment means. Let A_i denote the event $\{\theta_i \in I_i\}$. Then

$$P(\theta_1 \in I_1, \cdots, \theta_L \in I_L) \geq 1 - \sum_{i=1}^{L} P(\theta_i \notin I_i) = 1 - \sum_{i=1}^{L} \alpha_i.$$

If $\alpha_i = \alpha$ for all $i = 1, \cdots, L$, then the simultaneous confidence coefficient could be as small as $(1 - L\alpha) < (1 - \alpha)$ when $L > 1$. For example, if $L = 10$ and $\alpha = 0.05$, the joint confidence coefficient is 0.50! We achieve an overall confidence of $1 - \alpha$ by setting $\sum_{i=1}^{L} \alpha_i = \alpha$. One way to do this is to have each individual confidence coefficient to be $1 - (\alpha/L)$. The Bonferroni procedure can be conservative.

For constructing Bonferroni intervals, we see that

$$T_i = (\mathbf{c}_i'\beta^0 - \mathbf{c}_i'\beta) / \left\{ \hat{\sigma} (\mathbf{c}_i'\mathbf{G}\mathbf{c}_i)^{1/2} \right\}, \quad i = 1, \cdots, s$$

has a Student's t-distribution with $(N - r)$ degrees of freedom. Let $t_{\alpha/2s}$ denote upper $\alpha/2s$th percentile points from this distribution. Suppose E_i denotes the event that the interval $\mathbf{c}_i'\beta^0 \pm t_{\alpha/2}\hat{\sigma}[\mathbf{c}_i'\mathbf{G}\mathbf{c}_i]^{1/2}$ contains $\mathbf{c}_i'\beta$, for $i = 1, \cdots s$, so that $P(E_i) = 1 - \alpha/s$. Hence, the probability that $\mathbf{c}_i'\beta$ lies in the interval $\mathbf{c}_i'\beta^0 \pm t_{\alpha/2s}\hat{\sigma}[\mathbf{c}_i'\mathbf{G}\mathbf{c}_i]^{1/2}$, for all $i = 1, \cdots, s$ is at least $(1 - \alpha)$.

7.3.3 Multiple comparison procedures

We describe multiple comparison procedures which are widely used for comparing fixed-effect means in ANOVA procedures. In the one-way fixed-effects ANOVA model with a treatments, suppose the F-test rejects the null hypothesis of equal treatment effects; this does not give the user any information on how the test was rejected, i.e., which of the $\binom{a}{2}$ pairs of means were significantly different. A naive approach would be to compare all pairs of treatment means based on the usual t-tests. If we do this, we run into a problem that although each individual comparison would have a Type I error rate of α, simultaneous comparison of all pairs would have a rate which may be considerably less than α. The solution to this problem is offered by a variety of multiple comparison procedures, ranging from simple and elegant graphical techniques, to sophisticated significance tests, which were pioneered by Tukey and Scheffe (see Miller, 1981; or Hochberg and Tamhane, 1987).

The effects to be compared must be planned in advance. To illustrate, suppose we wish to test $H_0 : \mu_1 = \mu_2 = \mu_3 = \mu_4 = \mu_5$, and suppose we reject the null hypothesis. Assume that during the ANOVA analysis, we had observed that $\overline{Y}_1$. was the largest sample mean and $\overline{Y}_3$. was the smallest and *then* decided to test for the difference between μ_1 and μ_3. Since this is *not* a predetermined comparison, the level of significance of this single test will not be α. In general, comparisons must be planned *before* looking at the sample information. Otherwise, an analyst will be guilty of indulging in *data dredging* or *data snooping*. These are the alternate names given to the practice of first looking at the sample information and then choosing to analyze those comparisons that appear to be interesting. However, it is perfectly acceptable to use a multiple comparison procedure with a given confidence coefficient to cover all comparisons that could be carried out after observing the sample data. It is important that users have protection against drawing erroneous conclusions. While the error rate with a single comparison is the Type I error rate, the notion of error rate in multiple comparisons can be complicated. We give two definitions.

Definition 7.3.2.   The comparisonwise Type I error rate is defined as the ratio of the number of comparisons incorrectly declared significant to the total number of nonsignificant comparisons tested.

Definition 7.3.3.   The experimentwise Type I error rate is defined as the ratio of the number of experiments with one or more comparisons incorrectly declared significant to the total number of experiments with at least two treatment means.

The experimentwise error rate is more conservative. Although the choice of error rates is subjective, the comparisonwise error rate should be used if one incorrect inference from an experiment does not affect other inferences from that experiment. The following results describe methods for the pairwise comparison of treatment means using the LSD method, Duncan's multiple range procedure, the Newman-Keuls method, and Tukey's procedure.

Numerical Example 7.3.   We use a numerical example (Montgomery, 1991) to clarify the procedures. Consider a balanced one-way ANOVA setup with $a = 5$, $n = 5$, (so that $N = 25$), $\overline{Y}_1. = 9.8$, $\overline{Y}_2. = 15.4$, $\overline{Y}_3. = 17.6$, $\overline{Y}_4. = 21.6$, $\overline{Y}_5. = 10.8$, $\overline{Y}.. = 15.04$, and $MSE = 8.06$. The overall F-statistic is 14.76, which is significant at the 5% level of significance.   ▲

LSD procedure

Fisher's *least significance difference* (LSD) procedure is useful for making pairwise comparisons among a set of a population means. We define the least significance difference to be the observed difference between two sample means that is required in order to decide that the corresponding population means are distinct. For a given level α, the LSD for comparing μ_i and μ_j in an unbalanced one-factor fixed-effects ANOVA model is

$$LSD = t_{N-a,\alpha/2}\sqrt{\widehat{\sigma}^2\left(1/n_i + 1/n_j\right)},$$

while for a balanced model with $n_i = n, i = 1, \cdots, a$, it is

$$LSD = t_{N-a,\alpha/2}\sqrt{2\widehat{\sigma}^2/n}.$$

All pairs of sample means are compared. If $\left|\overline{Y}_{i\cdot} - \overline{Y}_{j\cdot}\right| > LSD$, we decide that μ_i is significantly different from μ_j, with a Type I error probability of α. Note that the LSD procedure is similar to a two-sample test for any two population means, the difference being that we use the estimate $\widehat{\sigma}^2$ instead of the pooled variances from the ith and jth samples. To implement this procedure, we compute the LSD for all pairs of sample means.

In general, the LSD procedure is criticized for inflating the Type I error rate. That is, the overall probability of incorrectly declaring some pair of means significantly different, when they are in fact equal, is substantially higher than the specified α value. The α level of the LSD procedure is valid for a given pairwise comparison only if the procedure is used for LIN and orthogonal contrasts or for preplanned comparisons. In practice however, the procedure is more loosely used because of its simplicity and ease of implementation. For this reason, it has been recommended that Fisher's LSD procedure be used only after the F-test for treatments is seen to be significant. This revised procedure is sometimes called Fisher's protected LSD, and some simulation studies show that the error rate for the protected LSD procedure is controlled on an experimentwise basis at a level that is approximately equal to α.

Numerical Example 7.3. (continued). To illustrate, the LSD at level of significance $\alpha = 0.05$ is

$$LSD = t_{20,0.025}\sqrt{2(8.06)/5} = 3.75.$$

The differences in the five treatment averages are $\overline{Y}_{1\cdot} - \overline{Y}_{2\cdot} = -5.6$; $\overline{Y}_{1\cdot} - \overline{Y}_{3\cdot} = -7.8$; $\overline{Y}_{1\cdot} - \overline{Y}_{4\cdot} = -11.8$; $\overline{Y}_{1\cdot} - \overline{Y}_{5\cdot} = -1.0$; $\overline{Y}_{2\cdot} - \overline{Y}_{3\cdot} = -2.2$; $\overline{Y}_{2\cdot} - \overline{Y}_{4\cdot} = -6.2$; $\overline{Y}_{2\cdot} - \overline{Y}_{5\cdot} = 4.6$; $\overline{Y}_{3\cdot} - \overline{Y}_{4\cdot} = -4.0$; $\overline{Y}_{3\cdot} - \overline{Y}_{5\cdot} = 6.8$; and $\overline{Y}_{4\cdot} - \overline{Y}_{5\cdot} = 10.8$. Treatment means whose absolute difference is bigger than 3.75 are significantly different. Thus, the only pairs that do not differ significantly are (1,5), and (2,3). ▲

Duncan's multiple range procedure

Duncan's multiple range procedure is widely used for comparing all pairs of means. We arrange the treatment means $\overline{Y}_{i\cdot}$ in ascending order. If $n_i = n$, $i = 1, \cdots, a$, the standard error of each $\overline{Y}_{i\cdot}$ is $\widehat{\sigma}/\sqrt{n}$. If not all the n_i's are equal, we compute their harmonic mean $n_H = a/\sum_{i=1}^{a}(1/n_i)$, and obtain the standard error of $\overline{Y}_{i\cdot}$ to be $s_{\overline{Y}_{i\cdot}} = \widehat{\sigma}/\sqrt{n_H}$. Duncan (1955) produced tables of significant ranges $r_\alpha(p, f)$, for $p = 2, 3, \cdots, a$, where f denotes the error degrees of freedom. We convert these significant ranges into a set of $a-1$ least significant ranges

$$R_p = r_\alpha(p, f)s_{\overline{Y}_{i\cdot}}, \quad \text{for } p = 2, 3, \cdots, a.$$

We test the observed differences between treatment means as follows. First, we compute the difference between the largest and the smallest means, which is compared to the least significant range R_a. Next, we compute the difference between the largest and the second smallest mean and compare it to R_{a-1}. We continue until we have exhausted differences between the largest mean and all other treatment means. If an observed difference is greater than the corresponding least significant range, we conclude that there is a significant difference between that pair of means. Next, we compute the difference between the second largest and the smallest mean and compare it to R_{a-1}, etc. We continue this process of comparisons until we have exhausted differences between all $\binom{a}{2}$ pairs.

Duncan's test is powerful, i.e., it is effective in detecting real differences between treatment means, and is therefore widely used. As the number of treatment means to be compared increases, this test requires a greater observed difference between the means to detect significance. When we compare two means, the critical value R_2 is exactly equal to the LSD value. To a lesser extent than the LSD procedure, Duncan's multiple range procedure may also inflate the Type I error rate.

Numerical Example 7.3. (continued).   To illustrate, we rank the treatment means in ascending order: $\overline{Y}_{1\cdot} = 9.8$; $\overline{Y}_{5\cdot} = 10.8$; $\overline{Y}_{2\cdot} = 15.4$; $\overline{Y}_{3\cdot} = 17.6$; and $\overline{Y}_{4\cdot} = 21.6$. Each has standard error $\sqrt{MSE/5} = 1.27$. From the tables of significant ranges for Duncan's test, we obtain corresponding to $\alpha = 0.05$: $r_{0.05}(2, 20) = 2.95$, $r_{0.05}(3, 20) = 3.10$, $r_{0.05}(4, 20) = 3.18$, and $r_{0.05}(5, 20) = 3.25$. The least significant ranges are computed as $R_2 = (2.95)(1.27) = 3.75$; $R_3 = (3.10)(1.27) = 3.94$; $R_4 = (3.18)(1.27) = 4.04$; and $R_5 = (3.25)(1.27) = 4.13$. These comparisons show that all pairs of treatment means except (3,2) and (5,1) are significantly different. This conclusion is identical to the one given by the LSD procedure (although in general, results from the two procedures need not coincide).   ▲

Tukey's procedure

Tukey's method is based on the distribution of the Studentized range statistic (see the appendix). Assume that $n_i = n$, $i = 1, \cdots, a$. Since ε_i are iid $N(0, \sigma^2)$ variables, it follows that $\overline{Y}_{i\cdot} - \mu_i$ are independently distributed as $N(0, \sigma^2/n)$ variables. Since all the treatment difference pairs are less than some number if and only if the largest difference is, we have $P\{|(\overline{Y}_{i_1\cdot} - \mu_{i_1}) - (\overline{Y}_{i_2\cdot} - \mu_{i_2})| \leq C_\alpha$, for all i_1 and $i_2\} = P\{\max_{i_1,i_2} |(\overline{Y}_{i_1\cdot} - \mu_{i_1}) - (\overline{Y}_{i_2\cdot} - \mu_{i_2})| \leq C_\alpha\}$. Tukey derived the distribution of the random variable

$$\max_{i_1,i_2}\{|(\overline{Y}_{i_1\cdot} - \mu_{i_1}) - (\overline{Y}_{i_2\cdot} - \mu_{i_2})|\}/\{\hat{\sigma}/\sqrt{n}\},$$

where the maximum is taken over all pairs i_1 and i_2 from 1 to a. This distribution is called the Studentized range distribution with parameters a and $a(n-1)$. Let $q_\alpha(a, N - a)$ denote the upper 100α percentage point of this distribution.

Then $100(1 - \alpha)\%$ set of confidence intervals that hold simultaneously for all pairwise treatment mean differences $\mu_{i_1} - \mu_{i_2}$ is $\left(\overline{Y}_{i_1 \cdot} - \overline{Y}_{i_2 \cdot}\right) \pm q_\alpha(a, N - a) \, s_{\overline{Y}_{i \cdot}}$. If the intervals do not include zero, we reject the null hypothesis that there is no difference between μ_{i_1} and μ_{i_2} for all i_1 and i_2 at level α. We can compute $T_\alpha = q_\alpha(a, N - a) \, s_{\overline{Y}_{i \cdot}}$, and decide that two means are significantly different if the absolute difference between them exceeds T_α. Note that, unlike the Duncan and the Newman-Keuls procedures, a single critical value is used in all comparisons. Tukey's test procedure has Type I error rate of α for all pairwise comparisons. It has a smaller Type I error rate than Duncan or Newman-Keuls procedures, and is therefore more conservative. It is less powerful than either of those procedures.

Numerical Example 7.3. (continued). From the table of the Studentized range distribution, we compute the value $q_{0.05}(5, 20) = 4.24$, and then $T_{0.05} = (4.24)(1.27) = 5.38$. The comparisons indicate that all pairs of treatment means except (4,3), (3,2) and (5,1) are significantly different (similar to the LSD procedure and Duncan's procedure). ▲

Newman-Keuls procedure

We next discuss the Newman-Keuls procedure. Newman (1939) first derived this test, which got its name due to the revival of the method by Keuls (1954). The overall nature of this test is very similar to Duncan's multiple range test, except for an alternate approach for computing differences between the treatment means. For the Newman-Keuls test, we compute a set of critical values

$$K_p = q_\alpha(p, f)s_{\overline{Y}_{i \cdot}}, \quad p = 2, 3, \cdots, a,$$

where $q_\alpha(p, f)$ denotes the upper 100α percentage point of the Studentized range for groups of means of size p and error degrees of freedom f. We now compare extreme pairs of means in groups of size p with the value of K_p, just like we did for Duncan's test. The Studentized range is defined as the random variable

$$q = \left(\overline{Y}_{\max} - \overline{Y}_{\min}\right) \Big/ \left(\sqrt{MSE/N}\right)$$

where $\overline{Y}_{\max}$ and $\overline{Y}_{\min}$ are respectively the largest and the smallest treatment means out of a group of p means.

This test is more conservative than Duncan's test, i.e., it has a smaller type I error probability, and is less powerful. It is therefore easier to decide that a pair of means are significantly different using Duncan's procedure than it is using Newman-Keuls procedure.

Numerical Example 7.3. (continued). We compute $K_2 = q_{0.05}(2, 20)(1.27) = (2.95)(1.27) = 3.75$; $K_3 = q_{0.05}(3, 20)(1.27) = (3.58)(1.27) = 4.55$; $K_4 = q_{0.05}(4, 20)(1.27) = (3.96)(1.27) = 5.03$; and $K_5 = q_{0.05}(5, 20)(1.27) = (4.24)(1.27) = 5.39$. The comparisons are similar to Duncan's procedure, and all pairs of treatment means except (3,2) and (5,1) are significantly different (similar to the LSD and Duncan's procedures). ▲

Dunnett's procedure

In many experiments, one treatment is the control, and there is interest in comparing each of the other $a - 1$ treatments with this control (using $(a - 1)$ comparisons). To apply Dunnett's (1964) procedure for this purpose, suppose that treatment a is the control, and we wish to test the hypothesis $H_0 : \tau_i = \tau_a$ versus $H_a : \tau_i \neq \tau_a$ for $i = 1, \cdots, a - 1$. For each of the $(a - 1)$ hypotheses, compute observed differences in the sample means $|\overline{Y}_{i\cdot} - \overline{Y}_{a\cdot}|$, $i = 1, \cdots, a - 1$. At the joint significance level α, H_0 is rejected if

$$|\overline{Y}_{i\cdot} - \overline{Y}_{a\cdot}| > d_\alpha(a - 1, N - a)\{\widehat{\sigma}^2(1/n_i + 1/n_a)\}^{1/2},$$

where $(N - a)$ is the error degrees of freedom, and the values of $d_\alpha(a-1, N-a)$ have been tabulated for different values of $(a - 1)$ and $N - a$. It is usually recommended that more observations be used for the control than for other treatments. A rule of thumb is to choose these numbers such that $n_a/n = \sqrt{a}$, where n_a is the number of observations for the control and n denotes the (same) number of observations for each of the other $(a - 1)$ treatments.

Numerical Example 7.3. (continued).   To illustrate, let treatment 5 be the control. The table value is $d_{0.05}(4, 20) = 2.65$, yielding a critical difference of $(2.65)\sqrt{(2)(8.06)/5} = 4.76$. Thus, any treatment mean that differs from the control by more than 4.76 is significantly different. The comparisons indicate that treatment 3 and treatment 4 are significantly different from the control treatment 5.   ▲

Choice of procedure

Which multiple comparison procedure should one use? Unfortunately, there is no precise answer to this question, and there are varied opinions about the relative merits of these procedures. There have been some simulation studies that compare these procedures for different situations. The LSD and Duncan's multiple range test appear to be most powerful for detecting true differences in treatment means. The LSD procedure can be carried out using the widely available tables of t-values, whereas the other pairwise comparison procedures require specialized tables. The Newman-Keuls test is more conservative than Duncan's test in that the Type I error rate is smaller, and the test is less powerful. Hence, it is more difficult to declare that two treatment means are significantly different using the Newman-Keuls test than it is using Duncan's test. Scheffe's procedure is used for all possible comparisons and may therefore be extremely conservative when applied to a finite set of treatment differences. Certainly, Dunnett's procedure, which is a modification of the usual t-test is useful when treatment means are compared to a control mean.

Numerical Example 7.1. (continued).   We obtained the ANOVA table and the F-test for this example in section 7.1. The means and standard errors of the treatment means are shown in the next table, while t-tests from the LSD procedure at the 5% level of significance are given in the following table. This test controls the Type I comparisonwise error rate, and not the experimentwise error rate. The critical t-value is 2.131, while the least significant difference is 0.218. In the table, means with the same letter are not significantly different.

Least squares estimates of treatment means

BRAND	N	Mean	s.e.
ACME	4	2.325	0.171
AJAX	4	2.050	0.129
CHAMP	4	2.375	0.171
TUFFY	4	2.600	0.141
XTRA	4	2.375	0.096

Comparison of effects using the LSD procedure

t grouping	Mean	N	BRAND
A	2.600	4	TUFFY
B	2.375	4	XTRA
B			
B	2.375	4	CHAMP
B			
B	2.325	4	ACME
C	2.050	4	AJAX

It is possible to test hypotheses on various contrasts of interest, as results in the next table show.

Tests of selected contrasts

Contrast	d.f.	Contrast SS	MS	F-value	$\Pr > F$
US VS FOREIGN	1	0.271	0.271	13.00	0.0026
US VS FOREIGN	1	0.271	0.271	13.00	0.0026
ALINE VS CLINE	1	0.094	0.094	4.50	0.0510
ACME VS AJAX	1	0.151	0.151	7.26	0.0166
TUFFY VS XTRA	1	0.101	0.101	4.86	0.0435
US VS FOREIGN	1	0.271	0.271	13.00	0.0026
ALINE VS CLINE	1	0.094	0.094	4.50	0.0510
ACME VS AJAX	1	0.151	0.151	7.26	0.0166
TUFFY VS XTRA	1	0.101	0.101	4.86	0.0435
US BRANDS	2	0.245	0.123	5.88	0.0130

The least squares estimate for the contrast ACME versus AJAX is 0.275, with s.e. 0.102, so that the t-value is 2.69, and the p-value is 0.017. For the contrast US AVERAGE, the estimate and s.e. are 2.250 and 0.042 respectively, while the t-value is 54.00, with p-value < 0.0001. The reader is referred to the first author's website for more details. ▲

7.4   Restricted and reduced models

In Chapter 4, we discussed estimation subject to linear restrictions on the parameters. We now describe partitioning of the sums of squares under such restrictions. We will also discuss reduced models, and restricted, reduced models in detail. These ideas are extremely useful for building a general theory of hypothesis testing in a linear model. We now describe the situation where the linear model $\mathbf{y} = \mathbf{X}\beta + \varepsilon$ is subject to the "natural" restriction $\mathbf{A}'\beta = \mathbf{b}$, and we wish to test the hypothesis $H : \mathbf{C}'\beta = \mathbf{d}$. We develop inference in the framework of a nested sequence of hypotheses.

7.4.1   Nested sequence of hypotheses

Let $\mathcal{C}(\mathbf{X})$ denote the column space of $\mathbf{X}$ in (4.1.1); since $r(\mathbf{X}) = r$, $\dim[\mathcal{C}(\mathbf{X})] = r$. Let us introduce the following notation. Let $\mathcal{S}_{H_0} \equiv \mathcal{M}(\mathbf{X})$ be the space spanned by $\mathbf{X}$ corresponding to the full model, viz., $E(\mathbf{y}) = \mathbf{X}\beta$. For $l = 1, 2, \cdots$, let $\mathcal{S}_{H_l}$ be the space spanned by $\mathbf{X}\beta$ subject to $\mathbf{C}'_j\beta = d_j$, $j = 1, \cdots, l$, and let $\mathcal{S}_{H_L}$ correspond to $\mathbf{y} = \varepsilon$. Suppose that $\mathbf{C}'_j$ is an $(s_j \times p)$ matrix with $r(\mathbf{C}'_j) = s_j$, $j = 1, \cdots, L$. Therefore, L sets of restrictions takes us from the full model down to random error. Clearly,

$$\mathcal{S}_{H_0} \supset \mathcal{S}_{H_1} = \{\mathbf{X}\beta : \mathbf{C}'_1\beta = \mathbf{d}_1\}$$
$$\supset \mathcal{S}_{H_2} = \{\mathbf{X}\beta : \mathbf{C}'_1\beta = \mathbf{d}_1, \mathbf{C}'_2\beta = \mathbf{d}_2\}$$
$$\vdots$$
$$\supset \mathcal{S}_{H_l} = \{\mathbf{X}\beta : \mathbf{C}'_j\beta = \mathbf{d}_j, \ j = 1, \cdots, l\}$$
$$\vdots$$
$$\supset \mathcal{S}_{H_L} = \{\mathbf{0}\}.$$

Note that $\dim(\mathcal{S}_{H_0}) = r > \dim(\mathcal{S}_{H_1}) = r - s_1 > \cdots > \dim(\mathcal{S}_{H_l}) = r - \sum_{i=1}^{l} s_i > \cdots > \dim(\mathcal{S}_{H_L}) = r - \sum_{i=1}^{L} s_i = 0$. We can also see this from

$$\dim(\mathcal{S}_{H_1}) = r \begin{pmatrix} \mathbf{X} \\ \mathbf{C}'_1 \end{pmatrix} - r(\mathbf{C}'_1).$$

Geometrically, $\mathbf{P}_{H_l}$ denotes the projection of $\mathbf{y}$ onto $\mathcal{S}_{H_l}$, i.e., $\mathbf{P}_{H_l} = \mathbf{X}_l\mathbf{G}_l\mathbf{X}'_l$, where $\mathbf{X}_l$ is the design matrix under the lth hypothesis, and $\mathbf{G}_l = (\mathbf{X}'_l\mathbf{X}_l)^-$. Then, $\hat{\mathbf{y}}_{H_l} = \mathbf{P}_{H_l}\mathbf{y}$, and $Q(H_l) = \mathbf{y}'\mathbf{P}_{H_l}\mathbf{y}$, $l = 0, \cdots, L$. The reduction in the model sum of squares due to $H_l, l = 0, \cdots, L$ is

$$Q(H_l) = \mathbf{y}'\mathbf{P}_{H_l}\mathbf{y} = \mathbf{y}'\mathbf{X}_l\mathbf{G}_l\mathbf{X}'_l\mathbf{y}.$$

$Q(H_0) = \mathbf{y}'\mathbf{P}_{H_0}\mathbf{y}$ corresponds to the full model sum of squares SSR, while $Q(H_L) = 0$. At the lth stage, $Q(H_l)$ corresponds to the reduced SSR due to fitting the model $\mathbf{y} = \mathbf{X}\beta + \varepsilon$ subject to $\mathbf{C}'_j\beta = \mathbf{d}_j$, $j = 1, \cdots, l$. Consider the

lth and $(l+1)$th stages of the nesting. We denote by $Q(H_l|H_{l+1})$ the reduced model sum of squares due to the fit under H_l beyond that obtained by fitting (4.1.1) under H_{l+1}. In other words, $Q(H_l|H_{l+1})$ is the sum of squares for H_l adjusted for H_{l+1}, and is defined to be

$$Q(H_l|H_{l+1}) = Q(H_l) - Q(H_{l+1}).$$

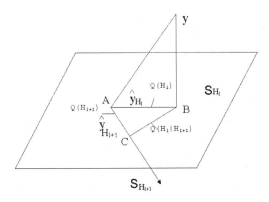

Figure 7.4.1. Nested sequence of hypotheses.

Note that the fitted model has more parameters under H_l than under H_{l+1}. In the triangle in Figure 7.4.1 with vertices A, B, C, we see that $\| AB \|$ denotes the length of the vector $\widehat{\mathbf{y}}_{H_l}$, so that

$$\| AB \| = (\widehat{\mathbf{y}}'_{H_l}\widehat{\mathbf{y}}_{H_l})^{1/2} = \mathbf{y}'\mathbf{P}_{H_l}\mathbf{y} = Q(H_l).$$

Similarly, $\| AC \|$ denotes the length of $\widehat{\mathbf{y}}_{H_{l+1}}$, which is $(\widehat{\mathbf{y}}'_{H_{l+1}}\widehat{\mathbf{y}}_{H_{l+1}})^{1/2} = \mathbf{y}'\mathbf{P}_{H_{l+1}}\mathbf{y} = Q(H_{l+1})$. Hence,

$$\| CB \| = \| AB \| - \| AC \| = Q(H_l) - Q(H_{l+1}) = Q(H_l|H_{l+1}).$$

The quantity $Q(H_l|H_{l+1})$ tests whether $\mathcal{S}_{H_{l+1}}$ is acceptable, given that we are in $\mathcal{S}_{H_l}$. Consider the following partition of SST:

$$\begin{aligned} SST &= Q(H_0) + SSE_{H_0} \\ &= Q(H_1) + Q(H_0|H_1) + SSE_{H_0} = Q(H_1) + SSE_{H_1} \end{aligned}$$

$$\vdots$$

$$= \sum_{l=0}^{L-1} Q(H_l|H_{l+1}) + SSE_{H_0} = Q(H_L) + SSE_{H_L}.$$

The statistic $Q(H_l|H_{l+1})$ has a noncentral $\chi^2(s_{l+1}, \lambda_{l+1})$ distribution, where the noncentrality parameter is $\lambda_{l+1} = \frac{1}{2\sigma^2}(\mu_{H_l} - \mu_{H_{l+1}})'(\mu_{H_l} - \mu_{H_{l+1}})$, where $\mu_{H_l} \in \mathcal{S}_{H_l}$, and $\mu_{H_{l+1}} \in \mathcal{S}_{H_{l+1}}$. When $\mathbf{C}'_{l+1}\beta = \mathbf{d}_{l+1}$, the noncentrality parameter is zero, and

$$\{Q(H_l|H_{l+1})/s_{l+1}\}/\{SSE_{H_0}/(N-r)\} \sim F_{s_{l+1}, N-r}$$

under $\mathbf{C}'_{l+1}\beta = \mathbf{d}_{l+1}$, which is the usual "partial F-test" in linear model applications. We may compute these sums of squares as follows:

$$
\begin{aligned}
Q(H_l) &= \widehat{\mathbf{y}}'_{H_l}\widehat{\mathbf{y}}_{H_l}, \\
Q(H_l|H_{l+1}) &= \widehat{\mathbf{y}}'_{H_l}\widehat{\mathbf{y}}_{H_l} - \widehat{\mathbf{y}}'_{H_{l+1}}\widehat{\mathbf{y}}_{H_{l+1}} \\
&= (\widehat{\mathbf{y}}_{H_l} - \widehat{\mathbf{y}}_{H_{l+1}})'(\widehat{\mathbf{y}}_{H_l} - \widehat{\mathbf{y}}_{H_{l+1}}).
\end{aligned}
$$

Example 7.4.1.   Consider the model $\mathbf{y} = \beta + \varepsilon$, where $\varepsilon \sim N_4(\mathbf{0}, \sigma^2\mathbf{I})$, and $\sum_{i=1}^{4}\beta_i = \mathbf{1}'\beta = 0$. We derive the test statistic for $H : \beta_1 = \beta_2$. The estimate of β subject to the restriction $\mathbf{1}'\beta = 0$ is

$$\widetilde{\beta} = \mathbf{y} - \tfrac{1}{4}\mathbf{1}'\mathbf{y}.$$

The hypothesis $H : \beta_1 = \beta_2$ can be written as $\mathbf{C}'\beta = \mathbf{d}$ with $\mathbf{C}' = (1, -1, 0, 0)$, and $d = 0$. It is a straightforward exercise to verify that $SSE = (\sum_{i=1}^{4} Y_i)^2/4$, and $Q = (Y_1 - Y_2)^2/2$, so that $F = \{2(Y_1 - Y_2)^2\}/\{(\sum Y_i)^2\} \sim F_{1,1}$ under H.
$\square$

The reduced model setup enables us to discuss consequences of model misspecification on solution vectors and predictions. Consider a partition of the general linear model $\mathbf{y} = \mathbf{X}\beta + \varepsilon$ as

$$\mathbf{y} = \mathbf{X}_1\beta_1 + \mathbf{X}_2\beta_2 + \varepsilon, \tag{7.4.1}$$

where $\mathbf{y}$ and ε are both N-dimensional vectors, $\mathbf{X}_1$ and $\mathbf{X}_2$ are respectively $N \times p_1$ and $N \times p_2$ matrices with ranks r_1 and r_2, $r(\mathbf{X}) = r = r_1 + r_2$, β_1 and β_2 are p_1 and p_2-dimensional vectors, $E(\varepsilon) = \mathbf{0}$, and $Cov(\varepsilon) = \sigma^2\mathbf{I}_N$. Let $\mathbf{P}_i = \mathbf{X}_i(\mathbf{X}'_i\mathbf{X}_i)^-\mathbf{X}'_i$, $i = 1, 2$. The least squares solutions of β_1 and β_2 under (7.4.1) are obtained by solving simultaneously the normal equations

$$
\begin{aligned}
\mathbf{X}'_1\mathbf{X}_1\beta_1^0 + \mathbf{X}'_1\mathbf{X}_2\beta_2^0 &= \mathbf{X}'_1\mathbf{y} \\
\mathbf{X}'_2\mathbf{X}_1\beta_1^0 + \mathbf{X}'_2\mathbf{X}_2\beta_2^0 &= \mathbf{X}'_2\mathbf{y}.
\end{aligned}
$$

Let $\mathbf{M}_2 = \mathbf{X}'_2(\mathbf{I} - \mathbf{P}_1)\mathbf{X}_2$. Then,

$$
\begin{aligned}
\beta_1^0 &= (\mathbf{X}'_1\mathbf{X}_1)^-\mathbf{X}'_1(\mathbf{y} - \mathbf{X}_2\beta_2^0), \quad \text{and,} \\
\beta_2^0 &= [\mathbf{X}'_2(\mathbf{I} - \mathbf{P}_1)\mathbf{X}_2]^-\mathbf{X}'_2(\mathbf{I} - \mathbf{P}_1)\mathbf{y} = \mathbf{M}_2^-\mathbf{X}'_2(\mathbf{I} - \mathbf{P}_1)\mathbf{y},
\end{aligned}
$$

while the corresponding error mean square is

$$MSE = \tfrac{1}{N-r}(\mathbf{y} - \mathbf{X}_1\beta_1^0 - \mathbf{X}_2\beta_2^0)'(\mathbf{y} - \mathbf{X}_1\beta_1^0 - \mathbf{X}_2\beta_2^0).$$

In the full rank case with $r(\mathbf{X}) = p$, $r(\mathbf{X}_i) = p_i$, $i = 1, 2$, and $p_1 + p_2 = p$, it can be shown that for testing $H : \beta_1 = \mathbf{0}$, $E(Q) = E(SSE_H - SSE) = \sigma^2 p_1 + \beta_1' \mathbf{X}_1' (\mathbf{I}_N - \mathbf{P}_2) \mathbf{X}_1 \beta_1$.

Example 7.4.2. We describe hypothesis tests in three situations that correspond to imposing a restriction on the (unrestricted) one-way ANOVA model (4.1.7). We show that if a parametric function of β is estimable under the unrestricted model, it must be estimable under the restricted model. When the natural restriction is not an estimable function, an interesting situation develops. We see that under different restrictions, the same parameter μ is estimable, whereas it is non-estimable in the unrestricted model. However, its b.l.u.e. is different under each restriction; in fact, its b.l.u.e. under a particular restriction is equal to the b.l.u.e. of that estimable function in the *unrestricted model* from which we obtain μ under the restriction. In the following result, we use the solution vector $\beta^0 = (0, \overline{Y}_{1.}, \cdots, \overline{Y}_{a.})'$, and corresponding g-inverse $\mathbf{G} = \begin{pmatrix} 0 & 0 \\ 0 & \mathbf{D} \end{pmatrix}$, where $\mathbf{D} = \mathrm{diag}(1/n_1, \cdots, 1/n_a)$.

Consider the unrestricted one-way ANOVA model in (4.1.7).

1. The test for $H : \mu = 0$ in the model (4.1.7) subject to the constraint $\sum_{i=1}^{a} n_i \tau_i = 0$ is equivalent to testing $H : \mu + \frac{1}{N} \sum_{i=1}^{a} n_i \tau_i = 0$ in the unrestricted model, and the test statistic $SSM / \hat{\sigma}^2$ follows an $F_{1,N-a}$ distribution under H.

2. The test for $H : \mu = 0$ in the model (4.1.7) subject to the constraint $\sum_{i=1}^{a} c_i \tau_i = 0$ such that $\sum_{i=1}^{a} c_i = 1$ is equivalent to testing $H : \mu + \sum_{i=1}^{a} c_i \tau_i / \sum_{i=1}^{a} c_i = 0$ in the unrestricted model, and the test statistic $\left[\sum_{i=1}^{a} \overline{Y}_{i.} \right]^2 / [\hat{\sigma}^2 \sum_{i=1}^{a} (1/n_i)]$ follows an $F_{1,N-a}$ distribution under H.

3. The test for $H : \mu = 0$ in the model (4.1.7) subject to the constraint $\sum_{i=1}^{a} \tau_i = 0$ is equivalent to testing $H : \mu + \frac{1}{a} \sum_{i=1}^{a} \tau_i = 0$ in the unrestricted model, and the test statistic $\left[\sum_{i=1}^{a} c_i \overline{Y}_{i.} \right]^2 / [\hat{\sigma}^2 \sum_{i=1}^{a} (c_i^2/n_i)]$ follows an $F_{1,N-a}$ distribution under H.

These results are easily verified. The function $\mu + \frac{1}{N} \sum_{i=1}^{a} n_i \tau_i$ is estimable under the unrestricted model, and yields μ upon imposing the restriction $\sum_{i=1}^{a} n_i \tau_i = 0$. Therefore testing $H : \mu + \frac{1}{N} \sum_{i=1}^{a} n_i \tau_i = 0$, or equivalently, $H : N\mu + \sum_{i=1}^{a} n_i \tau_i = 0$ in the unrestricted model is the same as testing $H : \mu = 0$ in the model with the constraint $\sum_{i=1}^{a} n_i \tau_i = 0$. In the notation of this section, the hypothesis $H : N\mu + \sum_{i=1}^{a} n_i \tau_i = 0$ can be written as $H : \mathbf{c}' \beta = 0$, where $\mathbf{c} = (N, n_1, \cdots, n_a)'$ is an $(a + 1)$-dimensional vector. By Result 7.4.1, $F_0 = Q/\hat{\sigma}^2 \sim F_{1,N-a}$ under H, where $Q = \beta^{0'} \mathbf{c} (\mathbf{c}' \mathbf{G} \mathbf{c})^{-1} \mathbf{c}' \beta^0 = N\overline{Y}_{..}^2 = SSM$. This proves property 1. To show property 2 and property 3, we again write the hypothesis under the unrestricted model as $H : \mathbf{c}' \beta = 0$, where $\mathbf{c}'$ is the vector $(1, 1/a, \cdots, 1/a)$ for property 2, and the vector $(1, c_1/c_., \cdots, c_a/c_.)$ for property 3, where $c_. = \sum_{i=1}^{a} c_i$. In each case, the F-test statistic follows from Result 7.4.1. □

Example 7.4.3.   Consider the fixed-effects two-way ANOVA model for the balanced case shown in (4.2.31). Writing as a sequence of nested hypotheses,

$$S_{H_0} = \{Y_{ij} = \mu + \tau_i + \beta_j + \varepsilon_{ij}, \sum_{i=1}^{a} \tau_i = 0, \sum_{j=1}^{b} \beta_j = 0\}$$

$$\supset S_{H_1} = \{Y_{ij} = \mu + \tau_i + \beta_j + \varepsilon_{ij}, \sum_{i=1}^{a} \tau_i = 0, \sum_{j=1}^{b} \beta_j = 0, \beta_j = 0 \; \forall \; j\}$$

$$= \{Y_{ij} = \mu + \tau_i + \varepsilon_{ij}, \sum_{i=1}^{a} \tau_i = 0\}$$

$$\supset S_{H_2} = \{Y_{ij} = \mu + \tau_i + \beta_j + \varepsilon_{ij}, \sum_{i=1}^{a} \tau_i = 0, \sum_{j=1}^{b} \beta_j = 0, \beta_j = 0 \; \forall \; j,$$

$$\tau_i = 0 \; \forall \; i\}$$

$$= \{Y_{ij} = \mu + \varepsilon_{ij}\}$$

$$\supset S_{H_3} = \{Y_{ij} = \mu + \tau_i + \beta_j + \varepsilon_{ij}, \sum_{i=1}^{a} \tau_i = 0, \sum_{j=1}^{b} \beta_j = 0,$$

$$\beta_j = 0 \; \forall \; j, \tau_i = 0 \; \forall \; i, \mu = 0\}$$

$$= \{Y_{ij} = \varepsilon_{ij}\}.$$

As mentioned earlier, the constraints are represented in matrix notation by $\mathbf{A}'\beta = \mathbf{0}$. In S_{H_1}, we have in addition to this constraint, the reduction imposed by the null hypothesis $H_1 : \beta_j$'s equal, $j = 1, \cdots, b$, viz., $\mathbf{C}_1'\beta = \mathbf{0}$, say, where the $(b-1) \times p$ matrix $\mathbf{C}_1'$ has the form

$$\mathbf{C}_1' = \begin{pmatrix} 1 & -1 & 0 & 0 & \cdots & 0 \\ 1 & 0 & -1 & 0 & \cdots & 0 \\ \vdots & \vdots & \vdots & \vdots & \ddots & \vdots \\ 1 & 0 & 0 & 0 & \cdots & -1 \end{pmatrix}.$$

Similarly, in S_{H_2}, we have the constraint $\mathbf{A}'\beta = \mathbf{0}$, the reduction $\mathbf{C}_1'\beta = \mathbf{0}$, and additionally, the reduction by $H_2 : \tau_i$'s equal, $i = 1, \cdots, a$, viz. $\mathbf{C}_2'\beta = \mathbf{0}$, say, where the $(a-1) \times p$ matrix $\mathbf{C}_2'$ has the form

$$\mathbf{C}_2' = \begin{pmatrix} 1 & -1 & 0 & 0 & \cdots & 0 \\ 1 & 0 & -1 & 0 & \cdots & 0 \\ \vdots & \vdots & \vdots & \vdots & \ddots & \vdots \\ 1 & 0 & 0 & 0 & \cdots & -1 \end{pmatrix}.$$

Note that $\dim[\mathcal{S}_{H_0}] = a+b+1-2 = a+b-1$, $\dim[\mathcal{S}_{H_1}] = p - r(\,\mathbf{A}'\quad\mathbf{C}_1'\,)' = a+b+1-(b+1) = a$, and $\dim[\mathcal{S}_{H_2}] = p-r\left(\mathbf{A}'\quad\mathbf{C}_1'\quad\mathbf{C}_2'\right)' = a+b+1-(a+b) = 1$. Here, $\mathcal{S}_{H_1}$ corresponds to the one-way ANOVA model, while $\mathcal{S}_{H_2}$ corresponds to the model with overall mean only. The numerator degrees of freedom in the F-test for H_1 is $\dim[\mathcal{S}_{H_0}] - \dim[\mathcal{S}_{H_1}] = b - 1$, and in the F-test for H_2 is $\dim[\mathcal{S}_{H_1}] - \dim[\mathcal{S}_{H_2}] = a - 1$. We have,

$$\hat{\mathbf{y}}_{H_0} = (\hat{Y}_{11}, \cdots, \hat{Y}_{1b}, \cdots, \hat{Y}_{a1}, \cdots, \hat{Y}_{ab})'$$

where $\hat{Y}_{ij}$ was defined under Example 4.2.6. Also,

$$\hat{\mathbf{y}}_{H_1} = (\overline{Y}_{1\cdot}, \cdots, \overline{Y}_{1\cdot}, \cdots, \overline{Y}_{a\cdot}, \cdots, \overline{Y}_{a\cdot})'$$

and $\hat{\mathbf{y}}_{H_2} = (\overline{Y}_{\cdot\cdot}, \cdots, \overline{Y}_{\cdot\cdot})'$, while $\hat{\mathbf{y}}_{H_3} = \mathbf{0}$. $\square$

In a balanced model, it does not matter in what order we test for the τ effects and the β effects. This is possible as long as the "manifolds" of the $\mathbf{X}$ columns corresponding to these effects are orthogonal. To make this more precise, let us write $\mathbf{X} = \left(\mathbf{X}_1 \quad \mathbf{X}_2 \quad \mathbf{X}_3\right)$, where $\mathbf{X}_1$ has dimension $N \times 1$, and contains the first column of $\mathbf{X}$ (corresponding to the parameter μ), $\mathbf{X}_2$ is an $N \times a$ matrix consisting of the next a columns of $\mathbf{X}$ (corresponding to $\tau_i, i = 1, \cdots, a$), and $\mathbf{X}_3$ is an $N \times b$ matrix consisting of the last b columns of $\mathbf{X}$ (corresponding to $\beta_j, j = 1, \cdots, b$). Letting $\mathcal{M}(\mathbf{X})$ denote the manifold of $\mathbf{X}$, we can see that $\mathcal{M}(\mathbf{X}) = \mathcal{M}(\mathbf{X}_1) \oplus \mathcal{M}(\mathbf{X}_2) \oplus \mathcal{M}(\mathbf{X}_3)$, and $\mathcal{M}(\mathbf{X}_i) \perp \mathcal{M}(\mathbf{X}_j)$, $i \neq j$, $i,j = 1,2,3$. The manifolds are orthogonal for the following reasons. An arbitrary member in $\mathcal{M}(\mathbf{X}_1)$ is $(c, \cdots, c)'$; an arbitrary member in the manifold $\mathcal{M}(\mathbf{X}_2)$ is $(d_1, \cdots, d_1, \cdots, d_a, \cdots, d_a)'$; and an arbitrary member in $\mathcal{M}(\mathbf{X}_3)$ is $(e_1, \cdots, e_b, \cdots, e_1, \cdots, e_b)'$. Let $\mathbf{x}_l$ be an arbitrary column in $\mathcal{M}(\mathbf{X}_l)$, $l = 1,2,3$. Then, $\mathbf{x}_1'\mathbf{x}_2 = cb\sum_{i=1}^a d_i = 0$, since in $\mathcal{M}(\mathbf{X}_2)$ $\sum_{i=1}^a \tau_i = 0$; $\mathbf{x}_1'\mathbf{x}_3 = ca\sum_{j=1}^b e_j = 0$ since in $\mathcal{M}(\mathbf{X}_3)$, $\sum_{j=1}^b \beta_j = 0$; and then, $\mathbf{x}_2'\mathbf{x}_3 = \sum_{i=1}^a d_i \sum_{j=1}^b e_j = 0$. We present this in an alternate way in the following result.

Result 7.4.1. Consider the model (4.2.31) with $n_{ij} = 1$, $i = 1, \cdots, a$, $j = 1, \cdots, b$.

1. The function $\sum_{i=1}^a c_i\tau_i$ is estimable if and only if $\sum_{i=1}^a c_i = 0$, i.e., the function is a contrast in τ_i.

2. Contrasts in $\{\tau_i\}$ are orthogonal to contrasts in $\{\beta_j\}$.

Proof. Suppose $\sum_{i=1}^a c_i\tau_i$ is estimable. We must have

$$\sum_{i=1}^a c_i\tau_i = \sum_{i=1}^a f_i(\tau_1 - \tau_i) = \tau_1\sum_{i=1}^a f_i - \sum_{i=1}^a f_i\tau_i$$

$$= (\sum_{i=1}^a f_i - f_1)\tau_1 - \sum_{i=2}^a f_i\tau_i,$$

which implies that $c_1 = \sum_{i=1}^{a} f_i - f_1 = \sum_{i=2}^{a} f_i, c_2 = -f_2, \cdots, c_a = -f_a$, so that $\sum_{i=1}^{a} c_i = 0$. Conversely, if $\sum_{i=1}^{a} c_i = 0$, then $\sum_{i=1}^{a} c_i \tau_i$ is a contrast, and contrasts in the effects are estimable. This proves property 1. To prove property 2, let $\sum_{i=1}^{a} c_i \tau_i$ be a contrast in $\{\tau_i\}$ and let $\sum_{j=1}^{b} d_j \beta_j$ be a contrast in $\{\beta_j\}$. Since $\sum_{i=1}^{a} c_i = 0$, the b.l.u.e. of $\sum_{i=1}^{a} c_i \tau_i$ is $\sum_{i=1}^{a} c_i \tau_i^0 = \sum_{i=1}^{a} c_i (\overline{Y}_{i.} - \overline{Y}_{..}) = \sum_{i=1}^{a} c_i \overline{Y}_{i.}$ with variance

$$\sum_{i=1}^{a} c_i^2 Var(\overline{Y}_{i.}) = \sum_{i=1}^{a} c_i^2 Var(\sum_{j=1}^{b} Y_{ij}/b) = \sum_{i=1}^{a} (c_i^2/b^2) b\sigma^2 = \sum_{i=1}^{a} c_i^2 \sigma^2/b.$$

Substituting $\hat{\sigma}^2 = SSE/\{(a-1)(b-1)\}$ into the above expression gives the estimated variance of the b.l.u.e. Similarly, since $\sum_{j=1}^{b} d_j = 0$, it follows that the b.l.u.e. of $\sum_{j=1}^{b} d_j \beta_j$ is $\sum_{j=1}^{b} d_j \overline{Y}_{.j}$, with estimated variance $\sum_{j=1}^{b} d_j^2 \hat{\sigma}^2/a$. Also,

$$
\begin{aligned}
Cov(\sum_{i=1}^{a} c_i \tau_i, \sum_{j=1}^{b} d_j \beta_j) &= \sum_{i=1}^{a} \sum_{j=1}^{b} Cov(\overline{Y}_{i.}, \overline{Y}_{.j}) \\
&= \sum_{i=1}^{a} \sum_{j=1}^{b} \frac{c_i d_j}{ab} \sigma^2 \\
&= \frac{\sigma^2}{ab} \sum_{i=1}^{a} c_i \sum_{j=1}^{b} d_j = 0
\end{aligned}
$$

using the formula $Cov(\overline{Y}_{i.}, \overline{Y}_{.j}) = Cov\{\sum_{j=1}^{b} Y_{ij}/b, \sum_{i=1}^{a} Y_{ij}/a\} = \sigma^2/ab$, which proves the result. ∎

One consequence of this orthogonality is that in a balanced two-way model, we have

$$R(\tau|\mu) = R(\tau|\mu, \beta) \quad \text{and} \quad R(\beta|\mu) = R(\beta|\mu, \tau).$$

In other words, it does not matter in what order we test for the τ effects and the β effects. This result does not hold for unbalanced models which we will discuss in Chapter 9.

Example 7.4.4. In the two-way fixed-effects model with interaction effects, consider a sequence of nested hypotheses,

$$\mathcal{S}_{H_0} \supset$$

$$\mathcal{S}_{H_1} = \{Y_{ijk} = \mu + \tau_i + \beta_j + \varepsilon_{ijk}, \sum_{i=1}^{a}\tau_i = 0, \sum_{j=1}^{b}\beta_j = 0\}$$

$$\supset \mathcal{S}_{H_2} = \{Y_{ijk} = \mu + \tau_i + \varepsilon_{ijk}, \sum_{i=1}^{a}\tau_i = 0\}$$

$$\supset \mathcal{S}_{H_3} = \{Y_{ijk} = \mu + \varepsilon_{ijk}\}$$

$$\supset \mathcal{S}_{H_4} = \{Y_{ijk} = \varepsilon_{ijk}\}$$

The vectors of fitted values under the models are

$$\begin{aligned}
\widehat{\mathbf{y}}_{H_0} &= \{\mu^0 + \tau_i^0 + \beta_j^0 + \gamma_{ij}^0\} = \{\overline{Y}_{ij\cdot}\}, \\
\widehat{\mathbf{y}}_{H_1} &= \{\mu^0 + \tau_i^0 + \beta_j^0\} = \{\overline{Y}_{i\cdot\cdot} + \overline{Y}_{\cdot j\cdot} - \overline{Y}_{\cdots}\}, \\
\widehat{\mathbf{y}}_{H_2} &= \{\mu^0 + \tau_i^0\} = \{\overline{Y}_{i\cdot\cdot}\}, \\
\widehat{\mathbf{y}}_{H_3} &= \{\mu^0\} = \{\overline{Y}_{\cdots}\}.
\end{aligned}$$

Also,

$$SST = \sum_{i=1}^{a}\sum_{j=1}^{b}\sum_{k=1}^{n} Y_{ijk}^2,$$

$$R(H_0) = \widehat{\mathbf{y}}_{H_0}'\widehat{\mathbf{y}}_{H_0} = \sum_{i=1}^{a}\sum_{k=1}^{n}\frac{1}{n}Y_{ij\cdot}^2, \text{ and}$$

$$SSE = SST - R(H_0) = \sum_{i=1}^{a}\sum_{j=1}^{b}\sum_{k=1}^{n}(Y_{ijk} - \overline{Y}_{ij\cdot})^2.$$

$R(H_0) \sim \chi_{ab}^2$ under H_0, while $SSE \sim \chi_{ab(n-1)}^2$. We first test the hypothesis that there are no interaction effects. Here,

$$R(H_1) = \widehat{\mathbf{y}}_{H_1}'\widehat{\mathbf{y}}_{H_1} = \sum_{i=1}^{a}\sum_{j=1}^{b}(\overline{Y}_{i\cdot\cdot} + \overline{Y}_{\cdot j\cdot} - \overline{Y}_{\cdots})^2,$$

and it follows that the *interaction sum of squares* is

$$\begin{aligned}
R(H_0|H_1) &= R(H_0) - R(H_1) \\
&= \sum_{i=1}^{a}\sum_{j=1}^{b}[\frac{1}{n}Y_{ij\cdot}^2 - (\overline{Y}_{i\cdot\cdot} + \overline{Y}_{\cdot j\cdot} - \overline{Y}_{\cdots})^2] \\
&= n\sum_{i=1}^{a}\sum_{j=1}^{b}(\overline{Y}_{ij\cdot} - \overline{Y}_{i\cdot\cdot} - \overline{Y}_{\cdot j\cdot} + \overline{Y}_{\cdots})^2,
\end{aligned}$$

which follows a $\chi^2_{(a-1)(b-1)}$ under H_1. The statistic for testing H_1 is

$$F(H_1) = \frac{R(H_0|H_1)/(a-1)(b-1)}{SSE/ab(n-1)} \sim F_{(a-1)(b-1),ab(n-1)} \text{ under } H_1. \quad (7.4.2)$$

The model $\mathcal{S}_{H_2}$ corresponds to a hypothesis of no difference among the b levels of Factor B. This does not refer to a test of $H : \beta_1 = \cdots = \beta_b$ under the full model, since the β_j's are not even estimable functions, nor are $\sum_{j=1}^{b} d_j \beta_j$. Also, in a model with interaction, it is meaningless to test whether β_j's are equal. For instance, suppose Factor A denotes operators of type i, $i = 1, \cdots, a$, and Factor B denotes machines of type j, $j = 1, \cdots, b$. If there are interaction effects γ_{ij}, it is meaningless to compare two machine effects β_j and $\beta_{j'}$ unless we consider their performance averaged over all levels of Factor A (operators), i.e., we test the hypothesis that $\beta_j + \sum_{i=1}^{a} \gamma_{ij}/a$ are equal, $j = 1, \cdots, b$. Notice that under the constraint $\sum_{i=1}^{a} \gamma_{ij} = 0$, $\beta_j + \sum_{i=1}^{a} \gamma_{ij}/a$ becomes β_j. Then,

$$F(H_2) = \frac{R(H_1|H_2)/(b-1)}{SSE/ab(n-1)} \sim F_{(b-1),ab(n-1)} \quad (7.4.3)$$

under H_2, where

$$
\begin{aligned}
R(H_1|H_2) &= (\widehat{\mathbf{y}}_{H_1} - \widehat{\mathbf{y}}_{H_2})'(\widehat{\mathbf{y}}_{H_1} - \widehat{\mathbf{y}}_{H_2}) \\
&= \sum_{i=1}^{a}\sum_{j=1}^{b}\sum_{k=1}^{n}(\overline{Y}_{\cdot j\cdot} - \overline{Y}_{\cdots})^2 \\
&= an\sum_{j=1}^{b}(\overline{Y}_{\cdot j\cdot} - \overline{Y}_{\cdots})^2 \sim \chi^2_{b-1} \text{ under } H_2.
\end{aligned}
$$

Therefore,

$$F(H_2) = \frac{an\sum_{j=1}^{b}(\overline{Y}_{\cdot j\cdot} - \overline{Y}_{\cdots})^2/(b-1)}{SSE/ab(n-1)} \sim F_{(b-1),ab(n-1)} \quad (7.4.4)$$

under H_2.

$\mathcal{S}_{H_3}$ corresponds to the hypothesis of no difference among a levels of Factor A, i.e., $H_3 : \tau_i + \sum_{j=1}^{b} \gamma_{ij}/b$ are equal for $i = 1, \cdots, a$. Here,

$$R(H_2|H_3) = (\widehat{\mathbf{y}}_{H_2} - \widehat{\mathbf{y}}_{H_3})'(\widehat{\mathbf{y}}_{H_2} - \widehat{\mathbf{y}}_{H_3})$$

where $\widehat{\mathbf{y}}_{H_2} - \widehat{\mathbf{y}}_{H_3} = (\overline{Y}_{i\cdot\cdot} - \overline{Y}_{\cdots})$, so that

$$
\begin{aligned}
F(H_3) &= \frac{R(H_2|H_3)/(a-1)}{SSE/ab(n-1)} \\
&= \frac{nb\sum_{i=1}^{a}(\overline{Y}_{i\cdot\cdot} - \overline{Y}_{\cdots})^2/(a-1)}{SSE/ab(n-1)} \sim F_{a-1,ab(n-1)}
\end{aligned}
$$

under H_3. Finally, H_4 corresponds to testing $\mu = 0$ in the restricted model. Then,

$$
\begin{aligned}
R(H_3|H_4) &= (\widehat{\mathbf{y}}_{H_3} - \widehat{\mathbf{y}}_{H_4})'(\widehat{\mathbf{y}}_{H_3} - \widehat{\mathbf{y}}_{H_4}) \\
&= \sum_{i=1}^{a}\sum_{j=1}^{b}\sum_{k=1}^{n}\overline{Y}_{...}^2 = nab\overline{Y}_{...}^2 \sim \chi_1^2 \text{ under } H_4,
\end{aligned}
$$

so that

$$
F(H_4) = nab\overline{Y}_{...}^2 / \{SSE/ab(n-1)\} \sim F_{1,ab(n-1)}
$$

under H_4. $\qquad \square$

Example 7.4.5. Two-way nested or hierarchical model. In Example 4.2.7, we derived the least squares solutions of the parameters in the balanced model. The ANOVA decomposition is

$$
SST = SS_A + SS_{B(A)} + SSE
$$

where

$$
SST = \sum_{i=1}^{a}\sum_{j=1}^{b}\sum_{k=1}^{n}(Y_{ijk} - \overline{Y}_{...})^2 \text{ with } (abn - 1) \text{ d.f.}
$$

$$
SS_A = nb\sum_{i=1}^{a}(\overline{Y}_{i..} - \overline{Y}_{...})^2 \text{ with } (a - 1) \text{ d.f.}
$$

$$
SS_{B(A)} = n\sum_{i=1}^{a}\sum_{j=1}^{b}(\overline{Y}_{ij.} - \overline{Y}_{i..})^2 \text{ with } a(b - 1) \text{ d.f.}
$$

$$
SSE = \sum_{i=1}^{a}\sum_{j=1}^{b}\sum_{k=1}^{n}(Y_{ijk} - \overline{Y}_{ij.})^2 \text{ with } ab(n - 1) \text{ d.f.}
$$

The ANOVA table is shown in Table 7.4.1.

Table 7.4.1. ANOVA table for the two-way balanced nested model

Source	SS	d.f.	MS
Factor A	SS_A	$a - 1$	MS_A
Factor B (within Factor A)	$SS_{B(A)}$	$a(b - 1)$	$MS_{B(A)}$
Error	SSE	$ab(n - 1)$	MSE
Total	SST	$abn - 1$	

The expected mean squares are

$$E(MS_A) = \sigma^2 + \frac{bn\sum_{i=1}^{a}\tau_i^2}{a-1},$$

$$E(MS_{B(A)}) = \sigma^2 + \frac{n\sum_{i=1}^{a}\sum_{j=1}^{b}\beta_{j(i)}^2}{a(b-1)},$$

$$E(MSE) = \sigma^2.$$

The hypothesis $H_0 : \tau_i$'s equal, $i = 1, \cdots, a$ is tested by

$$F = MS_A/MSE \sim F_{a-1,ab(n-1)}$$

under H_0. The test statistic for $H_0 : \beta_{j(i)}$'s equal, $j = 1, \cdots, b$, $i = 1, \cdots, a$ is

$$F = MS_{B(A)}/MSE \sim F_{a(b-1),ab(n-1)}$$

under H_0.   □

Example 7.4.6. Higher-order nested models.   We can generalize the two-stage nested model to an m-stage nested model. For instance, a three-stage completely nested model (balanced case) is given by

$$Y_{ijkl} = \mu + \tau_i + \beta_{j(i)} + \gamma_{k(ij)} + \varepsilon_{(ijk)l},$$

for $i = 1, \cdots, a$, $j = 1, \cdots, b$, $k = 1, \cdots, c$, and $l = 1, \cdots, n$. For example, consider an experiment where a factory wishes to investigate the hardness of two different formulations of a metal alloy. Three heats of each alloy formulation are made, two ingots are selected at random from each heat, and two hardness measurements are made on each ingot. Thus, heats are nested within the levels of the factor alloy formulation, while ingots are nested within the levels of the factor heats. There are two replicates in this three-stage nested model. The ANOVA table for the three-stage nested model is shown in Table 7.4.2, based on which we can develop hypotheses tests as in the two-stage case.

Table 7.4.2. ANOVA table for a three-way balanced nested model

Source	SS	d.f.	MS
Factor A	$\frac{1}{bcn}\sum_{i}Y_{i\cdots}^2 - \frac{1}{abcn}Y_{\cdots\cdots}^2$	$a-1$	MS_A
Factor B (within A)	$\frac{1}{cn}\sum_{i}\sum_{j}Y_{ij\cdots}^2 - \frac{1}{bcn}\sum_{i}Y_{i\cdots}^2$	$a(b-1)$	$MS_{B(A)}$
Factor C (within B)	$\frac{1}{n}\sum_{i}\sum_{j}\sum_{k}Y_{ijk\cdot}^2 - \frac{1}{cn}\sum_{i}\sum_{j}Y_{ij\cdots}^2$	$ab(c-1)$	$MS_{C(B)}$
Error	$\sum_{i}\sum_{j}\sum_{k}\sum_{l}Y_{ijkl}^2 - \frac{1}{n}\sum_{i}\sum_{j}\sum_{k}Y_{ijk\cdot}^2$	$abc(n-1)$	MSE
Total	$\sum_{i}\sum_{j}\sum_{k}\sum_{l}Y_{ijkl}^2 - \frac{1}{abcn}Y_{\cdots\cdots}^2$	$abcn-1$	

This may be extended to higher order models in a similar way. □

Example 7.4.7. Consider the balanced model with nested and crossed factors:

$$Y_{ijkl} = \mu + \tau_i + \beta_j + \gamma_{k(j)} + (\tau\beta)_{ij} + (\tau\gamma)_{ik(j)} + \varepsilon_{(ijk)l}, \qquad (7.4.5)$$

$i = 1, \cdots, a; \; j = 1, \cdots, b; \; k = 1, \cdots, c;$ and $l = 1, \cdots, n$. It may be verified that the ANOVA decomposition is

$$SST = SS_A + SS_B + SS_{C(B)} + SS_{AB} + SS_{AC(B)} + SSE, \qquad (7.4.6)$$

where

$$SST = \sum_{i=1}^{a}\sum_{j=1}^{b}\sum_{k=1}^{c}\sum_{l=1}^{n}(Y_{ijkl} - \overline{Y}_{....})^2 \quad \text{with } (abcn - 1) \text{ d.f.}$$

$$SS_A = \sum_{i=1}^{a}\frac{Y_{i...}^2}{bcn} - \frac{Y_{....}^2}{abcn} \quad \text{with } (a - 1) \text{ d.f.}$$

$$SS_B = \sum_{j=1}^{b}\frac{Y_{.j..}^2}{acn} - \frac{Y_{....}^2}{abcn} \quad \text{with } (b - 1) \text{ d.f.}$$

$$SS_{C(B)} = \sum_{j=1}^{b}\sum_{k=1}^{c}\frac{Y_{.jk.}^2}{an} - \frac{Y_{.j..}^2}{acn} \quad \text{with } b(c - 1) \text{ d.f.}$$

$$SS_{AB} = \sum_{i=1}^{a}\sum_{j=1}^{b}\frac{Y_{ij..}^2}{cn} - \frac{Y_{....}^2}{abcn} - SS_A - SS_B \quad \text{with } (a - 1)(b - 1) \text{ d.f.}$$

$$SS_{AC(B)} = \sum_{i=1}^{a}\sum_{j=1}^{b}\sum_{k=1}^{c}\frac{Y_{ijk.}^2}{n} - \sum_{j=1}^{b}\sum_{k=1}^{c}\frac{Y_{.jk.}^2}{an} - \sum_{i=1}^{a}\sum_{j=1}^{b}\sum_{j=1}^{b}\frac{Y_{.j..}^2}{acn}$$
$$\text{with } b(a - 1)(c - 1) \text{ d.f.},$$

completing this example. □

Example 7.4.8. Higher-order crossed models. It is possible to extend the methods of the two-factor models to deal with models involving several factors. We illustrate the ideas using three factors, Factor A, Factor B and Factor C with levels a, b, and c respectively. We only consider the balanced case. The three-way cross-classified model with all possible interactions is

$$Y_{ijkl} = \mu + \tau_i + \beta_j + \gamma_k + (\tau\beta)_{ij} + (\tau\gamma)_{ik} + (\beta\gamma)_{jk} + (\tau\beta\gamma)_{ijk} + \varepsilon_{ijkl},$$

for $i = 1, \cdots, a$, $j = 1, \cdots, b$, $k = 1, \cdots, c$, and $l = 1, \cdots, n$, with $n > 1$. We assume that $\varepsilon_{ijkl} \sim N(0, \sigma^2)$. The effects $(\tau\beta)_{ij}$, $(\tau\gamma)_{ik}$ and $(\beta\gamma)_{jk}$ are called two-factor interactions, while $(\tau\beta\gamma)_{ijk}$ is a three-factor interaction. Suppose all three factors are fixed effects. We obtain least squares solutions of the main effects, two-way and three-way interactions by imposing the following constraints on the normal equations:

$$\sum_{i=1}^{a} \tau_i = \sum_{j=1}^{b} \beta_j = \sum_{k=1}^{c} \gamma_k = 0,$$

$$\sum_{i=1}^{a} (\tau\beta)_{ij} = \sum_{j=1}^{b} (\tau\beta)_{ij} = \sum_{i=1}^{a} (\tau\gamma)_{ik} = \sum_{k=1}^{c} (\tau\gamma)_{ik} = 0,$$

$$\sum_{j=1}^{b} (\beta\gamma)_{jk} = \sum_{k=1}^{c} (\beta\gamma)_{ik} = 0,$$

$$\sum_{i=1}^{a} (\tau\beta\gamma)_{ijk} = \sum_{j=1}^{b} (\tau\beta\gamma)_{ijk} = \sum_{k=1}^{c} (\tau\beta\gamma)_{ijk} = 0.$$

For $i = 1, \cdots, a$, $j = 1, \cdots, b$, $k = 1, \cdots, c$, and $l = 1, \cdots, n$, the solutions of the parameters are

$$
\begin{aligned}
\mu^0 &= \overline{Y}_{\cdots} \\
\tau_i^0 &= \overline{Y}_{i\cdots} - \overline{Y}_{\cdots}, i = 1, \cdots, a, \\
\beta_j^0 &= \overline{Y}_{\cdot j\cdot\cdot} - \overline{Y}_{\cdots}, j = 1, \cdots, b, \\
\gamma_k^0 &= \overline{Y}_{\cdot\cdot k\cdot} - \overline{Y}_{\cdots}, k = 1, \cdots, c,
\end{aligned}
$$

$$
\begin{aligned}
(\tau\beta)_{ij}^0 &= \overline{Y}_{ij\cdot\cdot} - \overline{Y}_{i\cdots} - \overline{Y}_{\cdot j\cdot\cdot} + \overline{Y}_{\cdots}, i = 1, \cdots, a; j = 1, \cdots, b, \\
(\tau\gamma)_{ik}^0 &= \overline{Y}_{i\cdot k\cdot} - \overline{Y}_{i\cdots} - \overline{Y}_{\cdot\cdot k\cdot} + \overline{Y}_{\cdots}, i = 1, \cdots, a; k = 1, \cdots, c,
\end{aligned}
$$

$$
\begin{aligned}
(\beta\gamma)_{jk}^0 &= \overline{Y}_{\cdot jk\cdot} - \overline{Y}_{\cdot j\cdot\cdot} - \overline{Y}_{\cdot\cdot k\cdot} + \overline{Y}_{\cdots}, j = 1, \cdots, b; k = 1, \cdots, c, \\
(\tau\beta\gamma)_{ijk}^0 &= \overline{Y}_{ijk\cdot} - \overline{Y}_{ij\cdot\cdot} - \overline{Y}_{i\cdot k\cdot} - \overline{Y}_{\cdot jk\cdot} + \overline{Y}_{i\cdots} + \overline{Y}_{\cdot j\cdot\cdot} + \overline{Y}_{\cdot\cdot k\cdot} - \overline{Y}_{\cdots}.
\end{aligned}
$$

The ANOVA decomposition is

$$SST_c = SS_A + SS_B + SS_C + SS_{AB} + SS_{AC} + SS_{BC} + SS_{ABC} + SSE,$$

where

$$SST_c = \sum_{i=1}^{a}\sum_{j=1}^{b}\sum_{k=1}^{c}\sum_{l=1}^{n}(Y_{ijkl} - \overline{Y}....)^2 \text{ with } (abcn - 1) \text{ d.f.}$$

$$SS_A = \sum_{i=1}^{a}\frac{Y_{i...}^2}{bcn} - \frac{Y_{....}^2}{abcn} \text{ with } (a-1) \text{ d.f.}$$

$$SS_B = \sum_{j=1}^{b}\frac{Y_{.j..}^2}{acn} - \frac{Y_{....}^2}{abcn} \text{ with } (b-1) \text{ d.f.}$$

$$SS_C = \sum_{k=1}^{c}\frac{Y_{..k.}^2}{abn} - \frac{Y_{....}^2}{abcn} \text{ with } (c-1) \text{ d.f.}$$

$$SS_{AB} = \sum_{i=1}^{a}\sum_{j=1}^{b}\frac{Y_{ij..}^2}{cn} - \frac{Y_{....}^2}{abcn} - SS_A - SS_B \text{ with } (a-1)(b-1) \text{ d.f.}$$

$$SS_{AC} = \sum_{i=1}^{a}\sum_{k=1}^{c}\frac{Y_{i.k.}^2}{bn} - \frac{Y_{....}^2}{abcn} - SS_A - SS_C \text{ with } (a-1)(c-1) \text{ d.f.}$$

$$SS_{BC} = \sum_{j=1}^{b}\sum_{k=1}^{c}\frac{Y_{.jk.}^2}{an} - \frac{Y_{....}^2}{abcn} - SS_B - SS_C \text{ with } (b-1)(c-1) \text{ d.f.}$$

$$SS_{ABC} = \sum_{i=1}^{a}\sum_{j=1}^{b}\sum_{k=1}^{c}\frac{Y_{ijk.}^2}{n} - \frac{Y_{....}^2}{abcn} - SS_A - SS_B - SS_C - SS_{AB}$$
$$-SS_{AC} - SS_{BC} \text{ with } (a-1)(b-1)(c-1) \text{ d.f.} \,,$$

while SSE is obtained by subtracting these sums of squares from SST_c and has a χ^2 distribution with $abc(n-1)$ d.f. These may be used to construct confidence interval estimates of estimable functions of the parameter vector as well as for carrying out various tests of hypotheses.

The model simplifies considerably when there are no interactions:

$$Y_{ijkl} = \mu + \tau_i + \beta_j + \gamma_k + \varepsilon_{ijkl},$$

for $i = 1, \cdots, a$, $j = 1, \cdots, b$, $k = 1, \cdots, c$, and $l = 1, \cdots, n$. We assume that $\varepsilon_{ijkl} \sim N(0, \sigma^2)$. Suppose all three factors are fixed effects. We obtain least squares solutions of the main effects by imposing the following constraints on the normal equations:

$$\sum_{i=1}^{a}\tau_i = \sum_{j=1}^{b}\beta_j = \sum_{k=1}^{c}\gamma_k = 0.$$

The ANOVA decomposition in this case is

$$SST_c = SS_A + SS_B + SS_C + SSE,$$

where

$$SST_c = \sum_{i=1}^{a}\sum_{j=1}^{b}\sum_{k=1}^{c}\sum_{l=1}^{n}(Y_{ijkl} - \overline{Y}_{....})^2 \text{ with } (abcn - 1) \text{ d.f.}$$

$$SS_A = \sum_{i=1}^{a}\frac{Y_{i...}^2}{bcn} - \frac{Y_{....}^2}{abcn} \text{ with } (a - 1) \text{ d.f.}$$

$$SS_B = \sum_{j=1}^{b}\frac{Y_{.j..}^2}{acn} - \frac{Y_{....}^2}{abcn} \text{ with } (b - 1) \text{ d.f.}$$

$$SS_C = \sum_{k=1}^{c}\frac{Y_{..k.}^2}{abn} - \frac{Y_{....}^2}{abcn} \text{ with } (c - 1) \text{ d.f.,}$$

while SSE is obtained by subtracting these sums of squares from SST_c and has a χ^2 distribution with $abcn - a - b - c + 1$ d.f. Based on this decomposition, we can test for the significance of these main effect differences.

If all three factors have a levels each, and $n = 1$, the design corresponds to an $a \times a$ Latin Square Design (LSD):

$$Y_{ijk} = \mu + \tau_i + \beta_j + \gamma_k + \varepsilon_{ijk},$$

for $i, j, k = 1, \cdots, a$. We assume that $\varepsilon_{ijkl} \sim N(0, \sigma^2)$. This corresponds to a square with a rows (Factor A) and a columns (Factor B); each of the resulting a^2 cells contains one of the a levels of Factor C occurring once and only once in each row and each column. Note that in an LSD, $N = a^2$. The ANOVA decomposition is

$$SST_c = SS_A + SS_B + SS_C + SSE,$$

where

$$SST_c = \sum_{i=1}^{a}\sum_{j=1}^{a}\sum_{k=1}^{a}(Y_{ijk} - \frac{1}{N}Y_{...})^2 \text{ with } (a^2 - 1) \text{ d.f.}$$

$$SS_A = \sum_{i=1}^{a}\frac{Y_{i..}^2}{a} - \frac{Y_{...}^2}{N} \text{ with } (a - 1) \text{ d.f.}$$

$$SS_B = \sum_{j=1}^{a}\frac{Y_{.j.}^2}{a} - \frac{Y_{...}^2}{N} \text{ with } (a - 1) \text{ d.f. and}$$

$$SS_C = \sum_{k=1}^{a}\frac{Y_{..k}^2}{a} - \frac{Y_{...}^2}{N} \text{ with } (a - 1) \text{ d.f.}$$

To test the null hypothesis of no difference in effects due to Factor C, the test statistic is $F = MS_C/MSE$ which has an $F_{(a-1),(a-1)(a-2)}$ distribution under the null hypothesis. $\square$

Example 7.4.9.   Consider the two-phase regression model

$$\begin{cases} E(Y) = \beta_{1,0} + \beta_{1,1}X, & \text{if } X \leq \delta \\ E(Y) = \beta_{2,0} + \beta_{2,1}X, & \text{if } X > \delta, \end{cases} \tag{7.4.7}$$

with $\beta_{1,0} + \beta_{1,1}\delta = \beta_{2,0} + \beta_{2,1}\delta = \eta$, say. The parameters δ and η respectively denote the changeover point and the changeover value. Given data (Y_i, X_i), $i = 1, \cdots, N$, we derive the F-test of $H : \delta = \delta_0$, where $\delta_0 \in (X_n, X_{n+1})$. This is a test for concurrence of the two regression lines at $X = \delta_0$. The least squares estimates of $\widehat{\beta}_{l,1}$ and $\widehat{\beta}_{l,0}$, $l = 1, 2$ have the form (7.2.14) and (7.2.15), while SSE has the form (7.2.16) with $L = 2$. To compute $\widehat{\beta}_{l,1,H}$ and $\widehat{\beta}_{l,0,H}$, we must minimize the expression

$$S = \sum_{l=1}^{2} \sum_{i=1}^{n_l} (Y_{li} - \beta_{l,0} - \beta_{l,1}X_{li})^2 + 2\lambda\{\beta_{2,0} - \beta_{1,0} + \delta_0(\beta_{2,1} - \beta_{1,1})\},$$

where -2λ is the Lagrange multiplier. Let $N^* = n_1 n_2/(n_1 + n_2)$, and let

$$a_{ll} = \sum_i (X_{li} - \overline{X}_{l\cdot})^2 + N^*(\overline{X}_{l\cdot} - \delta_0)^2, \quad l = 1, 2,$$

$$a_{12} = a_{21} = -N^*(\overline{X}_{1\cdot} - \delta_0)(\overline{X}_{2\cdot} - \delta_0), \text{ and}$$

$$a_{l3} = \sum_i (Y_{li} - \overline{Y}_{l\cdot})(X_{li} - \overline{X}_{l\cdot}) + (-1)^l N^*(\overline{Y}_{2\cdot} - \overline{Y}_{1\cdot})(\overline{X}_{l\cdot} - \delta_0), \quad l = 1, 2.$$

After some algebra, we see that $\widehat{\beta}_{l,1,H}$, $l = 1, 2$ are solutions to

$$a_{11}\widehat{\beta}_{1,1,H} + a_{12}\widehat{\beta}_{2,1,H} = a_{13}$$
$$a_{21}\widehat{\beta}_{1,1,H} + a_{22}\widehat{\beta}_{2,1,H} = a_{23}.$$

We solve for λ as

$$\widehat{\lambda}_H = N^*\{\overline{Y}_{2\cdot} - \overline{Y}_{1\cdot} + \widehat{\beta}_{1,1,H}(\overline{X}_{1\cdot} - \delta_0) - \widehat{\beta}_{2,1,H}(\overline{X}_{2\cdot} - \delta_0)\},$$

while

$$\widehat{\beta}_{l,0,H} = \overline{Y}_{l\cdot} - \widehat{\beta}_{l,1,H}\overline{X}_{l\cdot} + (-1)^{l-1}\widehat{\lambda}_H n_l^{-1}, \quad l = 1, 2.$$

It may be verified that (Sprent, 1961)

$$SSE_H - SSE = \sum_{l=1}^{2}(\widehat{\beta}_{l,1} - \widehat{\beta}_{l,1,H})\sum_{i=1}^{n_l}(Y_{li} - \overline{Y}_{l\cdot})(X_{li} - \overline{X}_{l\cdot}) + \lambda(\overline{Y}_{2\cdot} - \overline{Y}_{1\cdot}),$$

and

$$F = \{SSE_H - SSE\}/\{SSE/(N - 4)\} \sim F_{1,N-4}$$

under H.   □

    The following result summarizes the consequences of underfitting, and suggests that deleting variables corresponding to small coefficients (relative to their standard errors) will lead to higher precision in the estimates of coefficients corresponding to the retained variables.

Result 7.4.2. Underfitting.   Suppose the true model is given by (7.4.1), but the model fitted to the data is

$$\mathbf{y} = \mathbf{X}_1\beta_1 + \varepsilon. \tag{7.4.8}$$

Let $\beta_{1,H}^0 = (\mathbf{X}_1'\mathbf{X}_1)^-\mathbf{X}_1'\mathbf{y}$ be the solution vector for β_1 (possibly after imposing some restriction $\mathbf{A}'\beta_1 = \mathbf{b}$), and let $\widehat{\sigma}_{1,H}^2 = \{\mathbf{y}'(\mathbf{I} - \mathbf{P}_1)\mathbf{y}\}/(N - r_1)$ denote the estimate of σ^2. Let MSE_H denote the error mean squares under (7.4.8). Then,

1. $E(\beta_{1,H}^0) = \mathbf{H}_1\beta_1 + (\mathbf{X}_1'\mathbf{X}_1)^-\mathbf{X}_1'\mathbf{X}_2\beta_2$, where $\mathbf{H}_1 = (\mathbf{X}_1'\mathbf{X}_1)^-\mathbf{X}_1'\mathbf{X}_1$. In the full rank case, $E(\widehat{\beta}_{1,H}) = \beta_1 + (\mathbf{X}_1'\mathbf{X}_1)^{-1}\mathbf{X}_1'\mathbf{X}_2\beta_2$.

2. $E(\widehat{\sigma}_{1,H}^2) = \sigma^2 + \frac{1}{N-r_1}\beta_2'\mathbf{X}_2'(\mathbf{I} - \mathbf{P}_1)\mathbf{X}_2\beta_2$.

3. Let $\widehat{Y}_{0,H} = \mathbf{X}_{1,0}\beta_1^0$ denote the prediction corresponding to $\mathbf{X}_{1,0}$. Then

$$E(\widehat{Y}_{0,H}) = \mathbf{X}_{1,0}[\beta_1 + (\mathbf{X}_1'\mathbf{X}_1)^-\mathbf{X}_1'\mathbf{X}_2\beta_2].$$

4. If the matrix $Cov(\beta_2^0) - \beta_2\beta_2'$ is p.s.d, $MSE \geq MSE_H$.

Proof.   The model (7.4.8) corresponds to imposing the reduction $H : \mathbf{X}_2\beta_2 = \mathbf{0}$ on the model (7.4.1). The solution vector under the reduced fitted model has covariance $Cov(\beta_1^0) = \sigma^2(\mathbf{X}_1'\mathbf{X}_1)^-$. Now,

$$
\begin{aligned}
E(\beta_{1,H}^0) &= (\mathbf{X}_1'\mathbf{X}_1)^-\mathbf{X}_1'E(\mathbf{y}) \\
&= (\mathbf{X}_1'\mathbf{X}_1)^-\mathbf{X}_1'(\mathbf{X}_1\beta_1 + \mathbf{X}_2\beta_2) \\
&= (\mathbf{X}_1'\mathbf{X}_1)^-\mathbf{X}_1'\mathbf{X}_1\beta_1 + (\mathbf{X}_1'\mathbf{X}_1)^-\mathbf{X}_1'\mathbf{X}_2\beta_2 \\
&= \mathbf{H}_1\beta_1 + (\mathbf{X}_1'\mathbf{X}_1)^-\mathbf{X}_1'\mathbf{X}_2\beta_2.
\end{aligned}
$$

Let $\mathbf{M}_1 = (\mathbf{X}_1'\mathbf{X}_1)^-\mathbf{X}_1'\mathbf{X}_2$. In the full rank case, $\widehat{\beta}_{1,H} = (\mathbf{X}_1'\mathbf{X}_1)^{-1}\mathbf{X}_1'\mathbf{y}$, and $E(\widehat{\beta}_{1,H}) = \beta_1 + (\mathbf{X}_1'\mathbf{X}_1)^{-1}\mathbf{X}_1'\mathbf{X}_2\beta_2$. Thus, $\widehat{\beta}_{1,H}$ is an unbiased estimate for β_1 only if either (a) $\beta_2 = \mathbf{0}$, i.e., (7.4.8) is the "correct model", or (b) $\mathbf{X}_1'\mathbf{X}_2 = \mathbf{0}$, i.e., $\mathbf{X}_1$ is orthogonal to $\mathbf{X}_2$, or both (a) and (b) hold. This proves property 1. To prove property 2, we use Result 4.2.3, setting $\mathbf{x} = \mathbf{y}$, and $\mathbf{A} = (\mathbf{I} - \mathbf{P}_1)$. Since $\mathbf{X}_1'(\mathbf{I} - \mathbf{P}_1) = \mathbf{0}$ and $tr(\mathbf{I} - \mathbf{P}_1) = N - r_1$, we see that

$$
\begin{aligned}
E(\mathbf{y}'(\mathbf{I} - \mathbf{P}_1)\mathbf{y}) &= \sigma^2 tr(\mathbf{I} - \mathbf{P}_1) + (\mathbf{X}_1\beta_1 + \mathbf{X}_2\beta_2)'(\mathbf{I} - \mathbf{P}_1)(\mathbf{X}_1\beta_1 + \mathbf{X}_2\beta_2) \\
&= (N - r_1)\sigma^2 + \beta_2'\mathbf{X}_2'(\mathbf{I} - \mathbf{P}_1)\mathbf{X}_2\beta_2,
\end{aligned}
$$

so that

$$E(\widehat{\sigma}_{1,H}^2) = \sigma^2 + \frac{1}{N-r_1}\beta_2'\mathbf{X}_2'(\mathbf{I} - \mathbf{P}_1)\mathbf{X}_2\beta_2 \neq \sigma^2$$

unless $\beta_2 = \mathbf{0}$. Property 3 follows directly since $E(\widehat{Y}_{0,H}) = E(\mathbf{X}_{1,0}\beta_{1,H}^0)$. Hence $\widehat{Y}_{0,H}$ is biased unless $\beta_2 = \mathbf{0}$, or $\mathbf{X}_1$ is orthogonal to $\mathbf{X}_2$, or both. To prove property 4, we verify that

$$
\begin{aligned}
MSE_H &= \sigma^2(\mathbf{X}_1'\mathbf{X}_1)^- + \mathbf{M}_1\beta_2\beta_2'\mathbf{M}_1', \text{ and} \\
MSE &= \sigma^2(\mathbf{X}_1'\mathbf{X}_1)^- + \mathbf{M}_1Cov(\beta_2^0)\mathbf{M}_1';
\end{aligned}
$$

hence, $MSE - MSE_H = \mathbf{M}_1\{Cov(\beta_2^0) - \beta_2\beta_2'\}\mathbf{M}_1'$, and the result follows. ∎

Example 7.4.10. While the *true* model is $E(Y) = \beta_0 + \beta_1X_1 + \beta_2X_1^2$, suppose we *fit* the model $Y_i = \beta_0 + \beta_1X_1 + \varepsilon_i$, $i = 1, 2, 3$, using data $(X_1, Y_1) = (-2, 15)$, $(X_2, Y_2) = (0, 21)$, and $(X_3, Y_3) = (2, 55)$. Using Result 7.4.2, we can verify that $\widehat{\beta}_0$ has bias $8\beta_2/3$, while $\widehat{\beta}_1$ is unbiased. □

Result 7.4.3. Overfitting. Suppose the true model is (7.4.8), but we fit the full model (7.4.1) to the data. Using the earlier notation,

1. $E(\beta_1^0) = \mathbf{H}_1\beta_1$.

2. MSE is an unbiased estimate of σ^2.

Proof. Since $(\mathbf{I} - \mathbf{P}_1)\mathbf{X}_1 = \mathbf{0}$, it follows that $E(\beta_2^0) = \mathbf{M}_2^-\mathbf{X}_2'(\mathbf{I} - \mathbf{P}_1)\mathbf{X}_1\beta_1 = \mathbf{0}$. Then, $E(\beta_1^0) = E(\beta_{1,H}^0) = E\{(\mathbf{X}_1'\mathbf{X}_1)^-\mathbf{X}_1'(\mathbf{y} - \mathbf{X}_2\beta_2^0)\} = \mathbf{H}_1\beta_1$. This proves property 1. The proof of property 2 is left as an exercise (see Exercise 7.16). ∎

7.4.2 Lack of fit test

In some data sets, we observe the response variable repeatedly at the same settings of the predictor variables. Let $Y_{i,l}$ denote the lth observation of the response variable at the ith setting for X_j, $l = 1, \cdots, n_i$, $j = 1, \cdots, k$, $i = 1, \cdots, m$. The total number of observations is $N = \sum_{i=1}^m n_i$. Suppose $r(\mathbf{X}) = p$. Unless $p \leq m$, the parameters cannot be estimated. In order to test for lack of fit, we require $p < m$. Suppose $\mathbf{X}_e$ denotes an $N \times m$ matrix whose jth column contains n_i ones (in locations $n_1 + n_2 + \cdots + n_{i-1} + 1$ up to $n_1 + \cdots + n_i$) and $N - n_i$ zeroes (in the remaining locations). An explanatory variable X_j with only one setting (no repeats) would imply that the jth column of $\mathbf{X}_e$ has a single value equal to 1. Consider the linear model

$$\mathbf{y} = \mathbf{X}_e\mu + \varepsilon \tag{7.4.9}$$

where, we can express the m-dimensional vector $\mu = (\mu_1, \cdots, \mu_m)'$ in terms of β when $p \leq m$. Let $\mathbf{P}_e = \mathbf{X}_e(\mathbf{X}_e'\mathbf{X}_e)^-\mathbf{X}_e'$; then $\mathcal{C}(\mathbf{X}) \subset \mathcal{C}(\mathbf{X}_e)$, i.e., $\mathcal{C}(\mathbf{P}) \subset \mathcal{C}(\mathbf{P}_e)$, and $\mathbf{X}_e'\mathbf{X}_e = \text{diag}(n_1, \cdots, n_m)$. Let $\widehat{\mathbf{y}}_e = \mathbf{P}_e\mathbf{y}$.

Then, $\mathbf{y} - \widehat{\mathbf{y}} = (\widehat{\mathbf{y}}_e - \widehat{\mathbf{y}}) + (\mathbf{y} - \widehat{\mathbf{y}}_e)$, i.e., $(\mathbf{I} - \mathbf{P})\mathbf{y} = (\mathbf{P}_e - \mathbf{P})\mathbf{y} + (\mathbf{I} - \mathbf{P}_e)\mathbf{y}$, which represents an orthogonal decomposition of the residual vector into the *lack of fit* vector and the *pure error* vector, since $(\mathbf{P}_e - \mathbf{P})'(\mathbf{I} - \mathbf{P}_e) = \mathbf{0}$ (see Figure 7.4.2). Note that the pure errors denote deviations of the individual observations from their own group averages (for the same setting of the explanatory variables). The corresponding breakup of the residual sum of squares is

$$\mathbf{y}'(\mathbf{I} - \mathbf{P})\mathbf{y} = \mathbf{y}'(\mathbf{P}_e - \mathbf{P})\mathbf{y} + \mathbf{y}'(\mathbf{I} - \mathbf{P}_e)\mathbf{y}, \qquad (7.4.10)$$

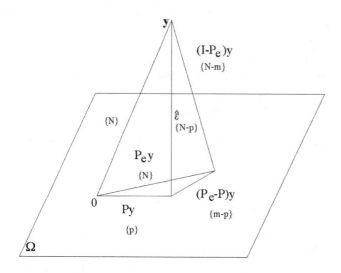

Figure 7.4.2.   Geometry of lack of fit and pure error.

while the degrees of freedom decompose correspondingly as $N - p = (m - p) + (N - m)$. Table 7.4.3 shows the ANOVA decomposition corresponding to the lack of fit and pure error.

Table 7.4.3. ANOVA table for lack of fit and pure error decomposition

Source	d.f.	SS	MS
Model	$p - 1$	SSR_c	$MSR_c = SSR_c/p$
Residual	$N - p$	$SSE = \mathbf{y}'(\mathbf{I} - \mathbf{P})\mathbf{y}$	$MSE = SSE/(N - p)$
Lack of Fit	$m - p$	$SSLF = \mathbf{y}'(\mathbf{P}_e - \mathbf{P})\mathbf{y}$	$MSLF = SSLF/(m - p)$
Pure Error	$N - m$	$SSPE = \mathbf{y}'(\mathbf{I} - \mathbf{P}_e)\mathbf{y}$	$MSPE = SSPE/(N - m)$
Corrected			
Total	$N - 1$	SST_c	

The following example provides a simple illustration.

Example 7.4.11.   Consider the data in Table 7.4.4. Suppose X refers to a level of light intensity, and Y denotes a measure of plant growth. The data are genuine repeats, i.e., observations on two *different* plants at the same light intensity were obtained, and not measurements on the same plant twice. In this example, $N = 10$, and $m = 6$.

Table 7.4.4. Illustration for lack of fit and pure error

Obs.	X_1	Y
1	2.0	1.4
2	2.0	3.1
3	3.1	1.9
4	3.1	2.5
5	3.1	3.8
6	3.5	1.6
7	4.6	1.8
8	4.6	2.2
9	5.7	3.5
10	5.9	3.1

The residual for the lth response at the ith setting of the explanatory variables is

$$\widehat{\varepsilon}_{i,l} = Y_{i,l} - \widehat{Y}_i = (Y_{i,l} - \overline{Y}_i) + (\overline{Y}_i - \widehat{Y}_i),$$

since the repeated responses at the setting X_i have the same predicted value $\widehat{Y}_i$. The residual sum of squares in this case is

$$SSE = \sum_{i=1}^{m} \sum_{l=1}^{n_i} (Y_{i,l} - \widehat{Y}_i)^2,$$

which is decomposed into the *pure error* sum of squares, and the *lack of fit* sum of squares. The overall pure error sum of squares is

$$SSPE = \sum_{i=1}^{m} \sum_{l=1}^{n_i} (Y_{i,l} - \overline{Y}_i)^2$$

with $(\sum_{i=1}^{m} n_i - m)$ degrees of freedom. The residual sum of squares is partitioned as

$$\sum_{i=1}^{m} \sum_{l=1}^{n_i} (Y_{i,l} - \widehat{Y}_i)^2 = \sum_{i=1}^{m} \sum_{l=1}^{n_i} (Y_{i,l} - \overline{Y}_i)^2 + \sum_{i=1}^{m} n_i (\widehat{Y}_i - \overline{Y}_i)^2, \text{ i.e.,}$$

$$SSE = SSPE + SSLF,$$

where $SSLF$ denotes the lack of fit sum of squares. The pure error mean square is obtained by dividing $SSPE$ by its degrees of freedom, and is an estimate of σ^2. The lack of fit mean square is obtained by dividing $SSLF$ by its degrees of freedom, viz., $m - r$. The reader is referred to Draper and Smith (1998) for more details. $\square$

7.4.3   Non-testable hypotheses

Suppose that $\mathbf{C}'\beta$ is not estimable, i.e., $\mathbf{C}' \neq \mathbf{T}'\mathbf{X}$ for any $\mathbf{T}'$ (see (4.3.2)). This in turn implies that $\mathbf{C}' \neq (\mathbf{T}'\mathbf{X}\mathbf{G})\mathbf{X}'\mathbf{X}$ for any $\mathbf{T}'$ (see Exercise 3.4 (a)), so that the rows of $\mathbf{C}'$ are LIN of the rows of $\mathbf{X}'\mathbf{X}$. Since $r(\mathbf{X}'\mathbf{X}) = r$, this requires that $\mathbf{C}$ contains no more than $(p - r)$ LIN rows. Now,

$$\beta^0 = \mathbf{G}\mathbf{X}'\mathbf{y} + (\mathbf{H} - \mathbf{I})\mathbf{z} \tag{7.4.11}$$

is a solution to the unrestricted normal equations $\mathbf{X}'\mathbf{X}\beta^0 = \mathbf{X}'\mathbf{y}$. Consider the equations

$$\mathbf{C}'(\mathbf{H} - \mathbf{I})\mathbf{z} = \mathbf{d} - \mathbf{C}'\mathbf{G}\mathbf{X}'\mathbf{y} \tag{7.4.12}$$

in $\mathbf{z}$. Since $r(\mathbf{H} - \mathbf{I}) = p - r$, for arbitrary $\mathbf{z}$, there are only $(p - r)$ arbitrary elements in $(\mathbf{H} - \mathbf{I})\mathbf{z}$, of which the remaining r elements are linear combinations. Hence, (7.4.12) represents a set of at most $(p - r)$ consistent equations in the $(p - r)$ unknowns $(\mathbf{H} - \mathbf{I})\mathbf{z}$; suppose that $\widetilde{\mathbf{z}}$ is a solution. Then, $\widetilde{\mathbf{z}}$ is a solution to (7.2.3). Substituting $\widetilde{\mathbf{z}}$ for $\mathbf{z}$ in (7.4.11), we see that

$$\beta_H^0 = \mathbf{G}\mathbf{X}'\mathbf{y} + (\mathbf{H} - \mathbf{I})\widetilde{\mathbf{z}}, \tag{7.4.13}$$

satisfies (7.2.3) in which $\lambda = \mathbf{0}$. Therefore, (7.4.13) is just a subset of the solutions β^0 to the unrestricted normal equations, so that

$$SSE_H = (\mathbf{y} - \mathbf{X}\beta_H^0)'(\mathbf{y} - \mathbf{X}\beta_H^0) = SSE, \tag{7.4.14}$$

and no test for $H : \mathbf{C}'\beta = \mathbf{d}$ can be derived. Searle (1973, sec. 5.5.d-e) has argued that if we compute Q for a non-testable hypothesis, the hypothesis being tested is actually $H : \mathbf{C}'\mathbf{H}\beta = \mathbf{d}$, and not $H : \mathbf{C}'\beta = \mathbf{d}$. Note that $\mathbf{C}'\mathbf{H}\beta$ is always estimable.

7.5   Likelihood based approaches

Least squares estimation does not require specification of a probability distribution for the errors ε. In this section, we assume that ε follows a specific probability distribution, derive the maximum likelihood estimate of β and study its properties. We describe two classes of distributions – the normal family, and the family of elliptically contoured distributions. In general, if $\mathbf{z} = (Z_1, \cdots, Z_N)$ is a random sample from a population with pdf or pmf $f(z; \theta)$, where $\theta = (\theta_1, \cdots, \theta_q)'$, the likelihood function is defined by

$$L(\theta; \mathbf{z}) = \prod_{i=1}^{N} f(z_i; \theta).$$

The maximum likelihood estimator of θ is a point estimator, denoted by $\widehat{\theta}_{ML}$, and is the value in the parameter space Θ that maximizes $L(\theta; \mathbf{z})$, i.e., the value in Θ for which the observed sample $\mathbf{z}$ is most likely. In practice, it is convenient to obtain $\widehat{\theta}_{ML}$ by maximizing $\log L(\theta; \mathbf{z})$, which is a monotonic function of $L(\theta; \mathbf{z})$. That is, we find $\widehat{\theta}_{ML}$ such that

$$\log L(\widehat{\theta}_{ML}; \mathbf{z}) = \sup_{\theta \in \Theta} \log L(\theta; \mathbf{z}).$$

There are situations where this supremum is attained at an interior point of Θ, and other situations where the supremum is attained on the boundary of Θ. In the former case, if $\log L(\theta; \mathbf{z})$ is a differentiable function of θ, $\widehat{\theta}_{ML}$ may be obtained as a solution to the equations

$$\partial \log L(\theta; \mathbf{z})/\partial \theta_i = 0, \quad i = 1, \cdots, q,$$

which satisfies $\log L(\theta; \mathbf{z}) \geq \log L(\widehat{\theta}_{ML}; \mathbf{z})$ for all $\theta \in \Theta$. The MLE of θ is unique if $f(z; \theta)$ is unimodal, which can be verified in practice by the log concavity of $f(z; \theta)$. For instance, suppose $f(z; \theta)$ corresponds to the mixture of normals distribution (see section 5.5.1), then $\widehat{\theta}_{ML}$ need not be unique. Consider a situation where we are interested in estimating some function $h(\theta)$, although $f(z; \theta)$ is itself indexed by θ. By the *invariance property* of the maximum likelihood estimator, $h(\widehat{\theta}_{ML})$ is the MLE of $h(\theta)$. This property is useful in linear model theory, as the following result shows. Let $\theta = \mathbf{C}'\beta$ denote an estimable function of β.

7.5.1 Maximum likelihood estimation under normality

Assuming that $\varepsilon \sim N(\mathbf{0}, \sigma^2 \mathbf{I}_N)$ in (4.1.1), we obtain the maximum likelihood estimates of parameters.

Result 7.5.1.   Consider the general linear model $\mathbf{y} = \mathbf{X}\beta + \varepsilon$ with normal errors. The maximum likelihood estimate of an estimable function $\theta = \mathbf{C}'\beta$ of β coincides with its least squares estimate, while $\widehat{\sigma}^2_{ML}$ is a scalar multiple of $\widehat{\sigma}^2$. In the full-rank case, by setting $\mathbf{C} = \mathbf{I}_N$ we obtain the MLE of β as $\widehat{\beta}_{ML} = (\mathbf{X}'\mathbf{X})^{-1}\mathbf{X}'\mathbf{y}$, while $\widehat{\sigma}^2_{ML} = (N-p)\widehat{\sigma}^2/N$.

Proof.   When $\mathbf{y} \sim N(\mathbf{X}\beta, \sigma^2 \mathbf{I}_N)$, the logarithm of likelihood function is (see (A1))

$$l(\mathbf{y}; \mathbf{X}, \beta, \sigma^2) = -\frac{N}{2}\log(2\pi\sigma^2) - \frac{1}{2\sigma^2}(\mathbf{y} - \mathbf{X}\beta)'(\mathbf{y} - \mathbf{X}\beta). \qquad (7.5.1)$$

We set the first partial derivatives of $l(\mathbf{y}; \mathbf{X}, \beta, \sigma^2)$ with respect to β and σ^2 equal to zero, and solve the resulting equations simultaneously. Specifically, using Result 2.7.2 and Result 2.7.3, we obtain the equations

$$\frac{\partial}{\partial \beta} l(\mathbf{y}; \mathbf{X}, \beta, \sigma^2) = \frac{1}{2\sigma^2}(2\mathbf{X}'\mathbf{y} - 2\mathbf{X}'\mathbf{X}\beta^0) \equiv \mathbf{0},$$

$$\frac{\partial}{\partial \sigma^2} l(\mathbf{y}; \mathbf{X}, \beta, \sigma^2) = -\frac{N}{2\widehat{\sigma}^2_{ML}} + \frac{1}{2\widehat{\sigma}^4_{ML}}(\mathbf{y} - \mathbf{X}\beta^0)'(\mathbf{y} - \mathbf{X}\beta^0) \equiv 0,$$

which we solve to obtain $\beta^0 = (\mathbf{X}'\mathbf{X})^-\mathbf{X}'\mathbf{y} = \mathbf{G}\mathbf{X}'\mathbf{y}$, and $\widehat{\sigma}^2_{ML} = (\mathbf{y} - \mathbf{X}\beta^0)'(\mathbf{y} - \mathbf{X}\beta^0)/N$. When $\mathbf{C}'\beta$ is estimable,

$$\mathbf{C'}\beta^0 = \mathbf{C'GX'y} = \mathbf{T'XGX'y}$$

using the definition of estimability. Since $\mathbf{XGX'}$ is invariant to the choice of $\mathbf{G}$, it follows that $\widehat{\mathbf{C'}\beta} = \mathbf{C'}\beta^0$ is unique, and is the MLE of $\mathbf{C'}\beta$. In the full-rank case, by setting $\mathbf{C} = \mathbf{I}_N$, we obtain the MLE of β as $\widehat{\beta}_{ML} = (\mathbf{X'X})^{-1}\mathbf{X'y}$, while $\widehat{\sigma}^2_{ML} = (\mathbf{y} - \mathbf{X}\widehat{\beta}_{ML})'(\mathbf{y} - \mathbf{X}\widehat{\beta}_{ML})/N$.   ∎

In the full-rank case, $\widehat{\beta}_{ML}$ is an unbiased estimate of β, with covariance $\sigma^2(\mathbf{X'X})^{-1}$ (obtained as the inverse of the Fisher information matrix). The minimal sufficient statistics for β and σ^2 are respectively $\widehat{\beta}$ and $\widehat{\sigma}^2$, and $\widehat{\beta}$ is the $MVUE$ of β (Rao, 1973a). Also, $E(\widehat{\sigma}^2_{ML}) = (N - p)\sigma^2/N$, so that $\widehat{\sigma}^2_{ML}$ is a biased estimator of σ^2, with the bias decreasing as N increases (relative to p).

Example 7.5.1.   Let $Y_i = \beta_0 + \beta_1 X_i + \beta_2 X_i^2 + \varepsilon_i$, $i = 1, \cdots, N$, $(N > 3)$, where $\sum_{i=1}^N X_i = 0$, $\sum_{i=1}^N X_i^3 = 0$, and ε_i are iid $N(0, \sigma^2)$ variables. We assume that $\beta_2 \neq 0$. We wish to find the value X^*, $(-\infty < X^* < \infty)$, for which the quadratic model function attains an extremum (maximum for a profit function, and minimum for a cost function). Setting the first derivative of the function $f(x) = \beta_0 + \beta_1 x + \beta_2 x^2$ equal to zero, and solving, we get $x^* = -\beta_1/2\beta_2$. Under normality, the maximum likelihood estimator of $\beta = (\beta_0, \beta_1, \beta_2)'$ coincides with its least squares estimator $\widehat{\beta} = (\mathbf{X'X})^{-1}\mathbf{X'y}$, with

$$\mathbf{X'X} = \begin{pmatrix} N & 0 & \sum X_i^2 \\ 0 & \sum X_i^2 & 0 \\ \sum X_i^2 & 0 & \sum X_i^4 \end{pmatrix} \text{ and } \mathbf{X'y} = \begin{pmatrix} \sum Y_i \\ \sum X_i Y_i \\ \sum X_i^2 Y_i \end{pmatrix},$$

i.e.,

$$\widehat{\beta}_0 = \{\sum_{i=1}^N Y_i - \widehat{\beta}_2 \sum_{i=1}^N X_i^2\}/N,$$

$$\widehat{\beta}_1 = \{\sum_{i=1}^N Y_i X_i\}/\{\sum_{i=1}^N X_i^2\}, \text{ and}$$

$$\widehat{\beta}_2 = \{\sum_{i=1}^N Y_i X_i^2 - \widehat{\beta}_0 \sum_{i=1}^N X_i^2\}/\sum_{i=1}^N X_i^4.$$

By the invariance property of the MLE, $\widehat{X}^*_{ML} = -\widehat{\beta}_1/2\widehat{\beta}_2$.   □

Example 7.5.2.   In model (4.5.1), suppose $\varepsilon \sim N(\mathbf{0}, \sigma^2 \mathbf{V})$, then $\mathbf{c'}\beta^0_{GLS}$ is the maximum likelihood estimator of the function $\mathbf{c'}\beta$ provided the function is estimable.   □

We can also motivate the F-test statistic based on the likelihood ratio test, as the following result shows.

Result 7.5.2. The statistic

$$F_0 = \frac{(N-p)}{s}[\Lambda^{-N/2} - 1] \tag{7.5.2}$$

is a monotonically decreasing function of the likelihood ratio test statistic Λ.

Proof. For the full rank case, the maximum likelihood estimates of β and σ^2 obtained by maximizing the likelihood function over the entire (unrestricted) parameter space $\mathcal{R}^p \times \mathcal{R}^+$ are

$$\widehat{\beta}_{ML} = (\mathbf{X}'\mathbf{X})^{-1}\mathbf{X}'\mathbf{y} \quad \text{and} \quad \widehat{\sigma}^2_{ML} = (\mathbf{y} - \mathbf{X}\widehat{\beta}_{ML})'(\mathbf{y} - \mathbf{X}\widehat{\beta}_{ML})/N.$$

The corresponding (unrestricted) maximized likelihood function is

$$L(\widehat{\beta}_{ML}, \widehat{\sigma}^2_{ML}) = (2\pi\widehat{\sigma}^2_{ML})^{-N/2} \exp\{-N/2\}.$$

The maximum likelihood estimates of β and σ^2 subject to the restriction $\mathbf{C}'\beta = \mathbf{d}$ under H are obtained by using the method of Lagrangian multipliers for maximizing the log-likelihood function subject to the linear constraint. It may be verified that $\widetilde{\beta}_{ML} = \widetilde{\beta}$, the restricted least squares estimate of β, while

$$\widetilde{\sigma}^2_{ML} = (\mathbf{y} - \mathbf{X}\widetilde{\beta}_{ML})'(\mathbf{y} - \mathbf{X}\widetilde{\beta}_{ML})/N.$$

The corresponding (restricted under H) maximized likelihood function is

$$L(\widetilde{\beta}_{ML}, \widetilde{\sigma}^2_{ML}) = (2\pi\widetilde{\sigma}^2_{ML})^{-N/2} \exp\{-N/2\}.$$

The likelihood ratio test statistic is

$$\Lambda = L(\widehat{\beta}_{ML}, \widehat{\sigma}^2_{ML})/L(\widetilde{\beta}_{ML}, \widetilde{\sigma}^2_{ML}) = (\widehat{\sigma}^2_{ML}/\widetilde{\sigma}^2_{ML})^{N/2},$$

and we reject H if Λ is too small. We can see that F_0 defined in (7.5.2) is a monotonically decreasing function of Λ, and we will reject H_0 if the statistic F_0 is too large. ∎

7.5.2 Elliptically contoured linear model

Consider the elliptical linear model

$$\mathbf{y} = \mathbf{X}\beta + \varepsilon, \quad \varepsilon \sim E_N(\mathbf{0}, \sigma^2\mathbf{I}_N, h), \tag{7.5.3}$$

and $r(\mathbf{X}) = p$. Then, $\mathbf{y} \sim E_N(\mathbf{X}\beta, \sigma^2\mathbf{I}_N, h)$, and the likelihood function is

$$\sigma^{-N}h\{\sigma^{-2}(\mathbf{y} - \mathbf{X}\beta)'(\mathbf{y} - \mathbf{X}\beta)\}. \tag{7.5.4}$$

The least squares estimator of β and SSE have the form in (4.2.4) and (4.2.17) respectively. It is easily verified that the maximum likelihood estimator of β coincides with its least squares estimator, i.e., $\widehat{\beta} = (\mathbf{X}'\mathbf{X})^{-1}\mathbf{X}'\mathbf{y}$ for any density generator $h(.)$ and the fitted vector and residual vector are the same too. In fact, the distribution of the MLE of β is the same for all $h(.)$ within the elliptical family. However, the distribution of the MLE of σ^2 is affected by departures from normality within the family of elliptical distributions.

Result 7.5.3. Under the model (7.5.3),

1. $\widehat{\beta} \sim E_p(\beta, \sigma^2(\mathbf{X}'\mathbf{X})^{-1}, h)$, and

2. $\widehat{\sigma}^2 = \mathbf{y}'\{\mathbf{I} - \mathbf{X}(\mathbf{X}'\mathbf{X})^{-1}\mathbf{X}'\}\mathbf{y}/(N-p)$ is an unbiased estimator of σ^2.

Proof.   Let $\mathbf{y} \sim E_N(\mathbf{X}\beta, \sigma^2\mathbf{I}_N, h)$, and suppose $M_{\mathbf{y}}(\mathbf{t})$ exists and has the form given in Definition 5.5.5. The mgf of $(\mathbf{X}'\mathbf{X})^{-1}\mathbf{X}'\mathbf{y}$ is

$$M_{\mathbf{y}}(\mathbf{X}(\mathbf{X}'\mathbf{X})^{-1}\mathbf{t}) = \psi(\mathbf{t}'(\mathbf{X}'\mathbf{X})^{-1}\mathbf{X}'(\sigma^2\mathbf{I}_N)\mathbf{X}(\mathbf{X}'\mathbf{X})^{-1}\mathbf{t})\exp\{\mathbf{t}'(\mathbf{X}'\mathbf{X})^{-1}\mathbf{X}'\mathbf{X}\beta\}$$

(see Exercise 7.30), from which property 1 follows. The proof of property 2 is left to the reader.   ∎

Also,

$$\{\mathbf{X}'\mathbf{X}/\widehat{\sigma}^2\}^{1/2}(\widehat{\beta} - \beta) \sim t_p(\mathbf{0}, \mathbf{I}_p, N-p), \tag{7.5.5}$$

where $t_p(\delta, \Omega, \nu)$ is a p-variate Student's t-distribution with ν degrees of freedom, location vector δ and scale matrix Ω (see (A25)), and

$$(\widehat{\beta} - \beta)'\mathbf{X}'\mathbf{X}(\widehat{\beta} - \beta)/\widehat{\sigma}^2 \sim pF_{p,N-p}. \tag{7.5.6}$$

Further,

$$(N-p)\widehat{\sigma}^2/\sigma^2 \sim R_{N-p}^2(h), \tag{7.5.7}$$

is the radial-squared distribution with $(N-p)$ degrees of freedom and density generator h (see (5.5.4)). Consider testing the hypothesis $H : \mathbf{C}'\beta = \mathbf{d}$ where $\mathbf{C}$ is a $p \times s$ matrix of rank s, and $\mathbf{d}$ is a known vector. By using the relationship between the likelihood ratio test statistic and the F-statistic, it can be shown that

$$F_0 = \frac{(N-p)}{s}\frac{(\mathbf{C}'\widehat{\beta} - \mathbf{d})'\{\mathbf{C}'(\mathbf{X}'\mathbf{X})^{-1}\mathbf{C}\}^{-1}(\mathbf{C}'\widehat{\beta} - \mathbf{d})}{(N-p)\widehat{\sigma}^2} \tag{7.5.8}$$

has an $F_{s,N-p}$ distribution under H (see Result 7.5.2). These distributional results facilitate inference in linear models with elliptical errors. For more details, the reader is referred to Fang and Anderson (1990) and references given there.

7.5.3   Model selection criteria

In this section, we describe criteria based on the likelihood function, such as the Akaike Information Criterion (AIC), and the Bayesian Information Criterion (BIC), that are widely used in model selection. In the linear model, these measures have simple forms, as we will show. Suppose the observed response $\mathbf{y} = (Y_1, \cdots, Y_N)' \sim N(\mathbf{X}\beta, \sigma^2\mathbf{I}_N)$. Let $\widehat{\beta}_{ML}$ and $\widehat{\sigma}_{ML}^2$ denote the maximum likelihood estimators of β and σ^2 respectively, and let

$$l(\mathbf{y}; \mathbf{X}, \widehat{\beta}_{ML}, \widehat{\sigma}_{ML}^2) = -\log(2\pi\widehat{\sigma}_{ML}^2)/N - SSE(\mathbf{y}, \widehat{\beta}_{ML})/2\widehat{\sigma}_{ML}^2$$

denote the maximized log-likelihood function, where $SSE(\mathbf{y}, \widehat{\beta}_{ML}) = (\mathbf{y} - \mathbf{X}\widehat{\beta}_{ML})'(\mathbf{y} - \mathbf{X}\widehat{\beta}_{ML})$ is the usual error sum of squares. Let $\mathbf{y}^* = (Y_1^*, \cdots, Y_N^*)'$ be an independent random vector, with the same distribution as $\mathbf{y}$. The definition of AIC is based on an estimate of $-2\log(\text{likelihood})$ for $\mathbf{y}^*$, which can be written as

$$
\begin{aligned}
-2l(\mathbf{y}^*; \mathbf{X}, \widehat{\beta}_{ML}, \widehat{\sigma}_{ML}^2) &= -2l(\mathbf{y}; \mathbf{X}, \widehat{\beta}_{ML}, \widehat{\sigma}_{ML}^2) + \{SSE(\mathbf{y}, \widehat{\beta}_{ML}) \\
&- SSE(\mathbf{y}^*, \widehat{\beta}_{ML})\}/2\widehat{\sigma}_{ML}^2.
\end{aligned}
\tag{7.5.9}
$$

While the first term on the right side of (7.5.9) can be computed from the observed data, we must estimate the second term. The distribution of $SSE(\mathbf{y}^*, \widehat{\beta}_{ML})$ is the same as the distribution of $SSE(\mathbf{y}, \widehat{\beta}_{ML})$, where $\widetilde{\beta}_{ML}$ is the MLE of β based on $\mathbf{y}^*$, and

$$
\begin{aligned}
E\{SSE(\mathbf{y}^*, \widehat{\beta}_{ML}) - SSE(\mathbf{y}, \widehat{\beta}_{ML})\} &= E\{SSE(\mathbf{y}^*, \widehat{\beta}_{ML}) - SSE(\mathbf{y}^*, \widetilde{\beta}_{ML})\} \\
&= \sigma^2 E\{(\widehat{\beta}_{ML} - \beta)'\mathbf{X}'\mathbf{X}(\widehat{\beta}_{ML} - \beta)\} \\
&+ \sigma^2 E\{(\beta - \widetilde{\beta}_{ML})'\mathbf{X}'\mathbf{X}(\beta - \widetilde{\beta}_{ML})\} \\
&= 2p\sigma^2,
\end{aligned}
$$

using property 3 of Corollary 7.1.1. The estimate of $-2l(\mathbf{y}^*; \mathbf{X}, \widehat{\beta}_{ML}, \widehat{\sigma}_{ML}^2)$ is then $-2l(\mathbf{y}; \mathbf{X}, \widehat{\beta}_{ML}, \widehat{\sigma}_{ML}^2) + 2p$, which leads to the following definition.

Definition 7.5.1. A criterion for model order selection, called the Akaike Information Criterion (AIC) (Akaike, 1974) is defined by

$$
\begin{aligned}
AIC(p) &= -2l(\mathbf{y}; \mathbf{X}, \widehat{\beta}_{ML}, \widehat{\sigma}_{ML}^2) + 2p \\
&= -N\log(\widehat{\sigma}_{ML}^2)/2 - N/2 + 2p.
\end{aligned}
\tag{7.5.10}
$$

The model order p must be chosen so as to minimize (7.5.10). The AIC criterion tends to overestimate p, and the following modified criteria were proposed by Akaike (1978) and Schwarz (1978).

Definition 7.5.2. The Bayesian Information Criterion (BIC) is defined by

$$
BIC = N\log(\widehat{\sigma}_{ML}^2) + 2(p + 2).
\tag{7.5.11}
$$

Definition 7.5.3. The Schwarz Bayesian Criterion (SBC) is defined by

$$
SBC = N\log(\widehat{\sigma}_{ML}^2) + p\log(N).
\tag{7.5.12}
$$

7.5.4 Other types of likelihood analyses

In section 7.5.1, we introduced the likelihood function of the parameters β and σ^2. In some problems, we may think of a subset of the parameter vector to be *nuisance* parameters. One way of handling nuisance parameters is to maximize

the *marginal likelihood*, also called the restricted likelihood. The general framework is discussed below. Applications to the random-effects and mixed-effects
models are given in Chapter 10. We also discuss the notion of quasi-likelihood,
and invoke it in Chapter 11 for analyzing longitudinal data, and for generalized
linear models. Finally, we look at likelihood based inference for incomplete data
problems due to missingness.

Restricted maximum likelihood

The method of restricted maximum likelihood (REML) was introduced as a technique for estimating variance components in a random-effects or mixed-effects
general linear model (Patterson and Thompson, 1971). Let $\mathbf{y} \sim N(\mathbf{X}\beta, \Omega)$,
where $\Omega = \Omega(\varphi)$, for some unknown parameter vector φ. Suppose φ is the
parameter of interest, and β is a nuisance parameter. The marginal likelihood
approach eliminates β from the likelihood function, and obtains the REML es-
timator of φ as the MLE based on a linear transformation, $\mathbf{y}^* = \mathbf{A}\mathbf{y}$, which has
zero expectation, and whose distribution is independent of the location para-
meter β. Let $\mathbf{P}$ be the usual projection matrix $\mathbf{X}(\mathbf{X}'\mathbf{X})^{-1}\mathbf{X}'$, when $r(\mathbf{X}) = p$.

Result 7.5.4.   The REML estimator $\widehat{\varphi}_{RM}$ maximizes the function

$$l_{RM}(\varphi) = -\frac{1}{2}\log|\Omega| - \frac{1}{2}\log|\mathbf{X}'\Omega^{-1}\mathbf{X}| - \frac{1}{2}(\mathbf{y} - \mathbf{X}\widehat{\beta}_{GLS})'\Omega^{-1}(\mathbf{y} - \mathbf{X}\widehat{\beta}_{GLS}),$$

$$(7.5.13)$$

where $\widehat{\beta}_{GLS} = (\mathbf{X}'\Omega^{-1}\mathbf{X})^{-1}\mathbf{X}'\Omega^{-1}\mathbf{y} = \Lambda\mathbf{y}$, say, is the GLS estimator of β.

Proof.   Let $\mathbf{B}$ denote the $N \times (N-p)$ matrix such that $\mathbf{B}\mathbf{B}' = \mathbf{I} - \mathbf{P}$, and
$\mathbf{B}'\mathbf{B} = \mathbf{I}_{N-p}$. Consider the transformation $\mathbf{z} = \mathbf{B}'\mathbf{y}$, and $\widehat{\beta}_{GLS} = \Lambda\mathbf{y}$, with
Jacobian $|\mathbf{X}'\mathbf{X}|^{-1/2}$. By Result 5.2.6, $\mathbf{z}$ and $\widehat{\beta}_{GLS}$ have normal distributions.
Further, they are independent (irrespective of the value of β) because

$$\begin{aligned}
Cov(\mathbf{z}, \widehat{\beta}_{GLS}) &= E\{\mathbf{z}(\widehat{\beta}_{GLS} - \beta)'\} = E\{\mathbf{B}'\mathbf{y}(\mathbf{y}'\Lambda' - \beta')\} \\
&= \mathbf{B}'\{Var(\mathbf{y}) + E(\mathbf{y})E(\mathbf{y})'\}\Lambda' - \mathbf{B}'E(\mathbf{y})\beta' \\
&= \mathbf{B}'\{\Omega + \mathbf{X}\beta\beta'\mathbf{X}'\}\Lambda' - \mathbf{B}'\mathbf{X}\beta\beta' = 0,
\end{aligned}$$

since it may be verified that $\mathbf{X}'\Lambda' = \mathbf{I}$, and $\mathbf{B}'\Omega\Lambda' = 0$. Also, $E(\mathbf{z}) = \mathbf{B}'E(\mathbf{y}) =
\mathbf{B}'\mathbf{X}\beta = \mathbf{B}'\mathbf{B}\mathbf{B}'\mathbf{X}\beta = \mathbf{B}'(\mathbf{I} - \mathbf{P})\mathbf{X}\beta = 0$, since $(\mathbf{I} - \mathbf{P}) \perp \mathcal{C}(\mathbf{X})$. The pdf of $\mathbf{z}$ is
singular normal and is proportional to

$$\frac{f(\mathbf{y})}{g(\widehat{\beta}_{GLS})} = (2\pi)^{-(N-p)/2}|\Omega|^{-1/2}|\mathbf{X}'\Omega^{-1}\mathbf{X}|^{-1/2}$$

$$\times \exp\{-\frac{1}{2}(\mathbf{y} - \mathbf{X}\widehat{\beta}_{GLS})'\Omega^{-1}(\mathbf{y} - \mathbf{X}\widehat{\beta}_{GLS})\}.$$

The REML estimator of φ then maximizes the (restricted) log likelihood in
(7.5.13) (see Harville, 1974, 1977). This estimator is invariant to $\mathbf{A}$; any choice

of $\mathbf{A}$ for which $E(\mathbf{z}) = \mathbf{0}$ and $Cov(\mathbf{z}, \widehat{\beta}_{GLS}) = \mathbf{0}$ will suffice. It is instructive to observe that the MLE of φ maximizes

$$l(\varphi; \mathbf{y}) = -\tfrac{1}{2} \log |\Omega| - \tfrac{1}{2}(\mathbf{y} - \mathbf{X}\widehat{\beta}_{GLS})'\Omega^{-1}(\mathbf{y} - \mathbf{X}\widehat{\beta}_{GLS}). \qquad \blacksquare$$

In estimating random effects, maximum likelihood estimation does not account for the degrees of freedom that are involved in estimating fixed effects. REML (sometimes called residual maximum likelihood) corrects this defect, and obtains estimates of variance components in a general mixed-effects linear model based on residuals from an OLS fit to the fixed-effects portion of the model.

Quasi-likelihood

In the linear model (4.1.1), supposed it is specified for each $i = 1, \cdots, N$ that $Var(Y_i) = \gamma V(\mu_i)$, where $\mu_i = E(Y_i) = \mathbf{x}_i'\beta$, $V(.)$ is some known function, and γ is a possibly unknown constant of proportionality. The quasi-likelihood function $K(Y_i, \mu_i)$ for the ith response is defined by the relation (Wedderburn, 1974)

$$\frac{\partial K(Y_i, \mu_i)}{\partial \mu_i} = \frac{(Y_i - \mu_i)}{V(\mu_i)}. \qquad (7.5.14)$$

The quasi-likelihood function may be used for estimation in much the same way as a likelihood function. For $i = 1, \cdots, N$, let $\mathbf{u}_i$ denote the p-dimensional vector with components $\partial K(Y_i, \mu_i)/\partial \beta_j$. The following result is central to the notion of quasi-likelihood estimation (for proof, see section 5 in Wedderburn, 1974).

Result 7.5.5.

1. $E(\mathbf{u}_i) = \mathbf{0}$, while the (j, k)th element of its variance-covariance matrix is $-E\{\partial^2 K(Y_i, \mu_i)/\partial \beta_j \partial \beta_k\}$.

2. $E(\sum_{i=1}^{N} \mathbf{u}_i) = \mathbf{0}$, while the (j, k)th element of its variance-covariance matrix is $-E\{\partial^2 \sum_{i=1}^{N} K(Y_i, \mu_i)/\partial \beta_j \partial \beta_k\}$.

The maximum quasi-likelihood estimate $\widehat{\beta}_Q$ is obtained by setting $\sum_{i=1}^{N} \mathbf{u}_i$ equal to its expectation of $\mathbf{0}$ and solving the resulting p equations simultaneously. This holds irrespective of whether $\gamma = 1$, or γ is an unknown parameter. If Y_i are independent, homoscedastic normal variables, then the maximum quasi-likelihood estimator $\widehat{\beta}_Q$ coincides with the least squares (or maximum likelihood) estimator.

Result 7.5.6. When $\gamma = 1$, the approximate covariance matrix of $\widehat{\beta}_Q$ is $\{E(\mathbf{H})\}^{-1}$, where $\mathbf{H}$ denotes the matrix of second derivatives of $\sum_{i=1}^{N} \mathbf{u}_i$.

Proof. We have, up to first order in $(\beta - \widehat{\beta}_Q)$,

$$\sum_{i=1}^{N} \mathbf{u}_i \approx \mathbf{H}(\beta - \widehat{\beta}_Q),$$

so that $\beta - \widehat{\beta}_Q \approx \mathbf{H}^{-1} \sum_{i=1}^{N} \mathbf{u}_i$, and approximating $\mathbf{H}$ by its expectation of $-\mathbf{D}$, we get $\widehat{\beta}_Q \approx \beta + \mathbf{D}^{-1} \sum_{i=1}^{N} \mathbf{u}_i$. The result follows since the covariance of $\mathbf{D}^{-1} \sum_{i=1}^{N} \mathbf{u}_i$ is $\mathbf{D}^{-1}$. ∎

When γ is unknown, the following estimate enables us to approximate the covariance matrix of $\beta - \widehat{\beta}_Q$:

$$\widehat{\gamma} = \{ \sum_{i=1}^{N} (Y_i - \widehat{\mu}_i)^2 / V(\widehat{\mu}_i) \} / (N - p).$$

When $V(\mu_i) = 1$, maximum quasi-likelihood estimation reduces to least squares. For a one-parameter exponential family, the log likelihood coincides with the quasi-likelihood. For a discussion of generalized estimating equations (GEE), a multivariate analogue of quasi-likelihood, see Liang and Zeger (1986).

Missing data analysis

In many situations, a portion of the data might be missing; these missing observations may have a significant impact on the statistical analysis of the non-missing data. Suppose $\mathbf{y} = (\mathbf{y}_{\text{obs}}, \mathbf{y}_{\text{mis}})$ denotes the *complete data*, where $\mathbf{y}_{\text{obs}}$ and $\mathbf{y}_{\text{mis}}$ respectively denote the N_1 and N_2-dimensional vectors of *observed data* and the *missing data*. The missing values are said to be *missing at random* (MAR) if the observed units are a random subsample of the sampled units; in this case, the missing data mechanism is ignorable. On the other hand, if the probability that Y_i is observed depends on the value of Y_i, then the missing values are not MAR, and the missing data mechanism is nonignorable (Little and Rubin, 1987). Suppose we partition the $N \times p$ predictor matrix as $\mathbf{X} = (\mathbf{X}_{\text{obs}}, \mathbf{X}_{\text{mis}})$, where $\mathbf{X}_{\text{obs}}$ is an $N_1 \times p$ matrix and $\mathbf{X}_{\text{mis}}$ is an $N_2 \times p$ matrix. In general, there are three approaches for handling missing data, viz., (i) complete case analysis, (ii) imputation for missing values, and (iii) model based techniques via the likelihood function. We take a brief look at (i) and (ii), before discussing (iii) in more detail.

As the name suggests, *complete case analysis* is usual statistical analyses using only the cases where all observations are available. Standard software may be used, which is attractive. The disadvantage is that if the percentage of missingness (which is $100N_2/N$) is large, and if the data is not MAR, such analyses tend to be inefficient. An alternative approach is *imputation of missing data*, usually in the $\mathbf{X}$ matrix. Standard procedures are then used to analyze the data with $\widehat{\mathbf{X}}^* = (\mathbf{X}_{\text{obs}}, \widehat{\mathbf{X}}^*_{\text{mis}})$. The following methods of imputation are commonly used in practice. Hot deck imputation consists of selecting imputed values from the sample distribution. In cold deck imputation, we replace a missing value by a constant, usually obtained extraneously. Mean imputation consists of replacing missing values by the averages of available observations. Sometimes, we may use model based imputation. For instance, regression (or correlation) imputation consists of fitting a regression model of the missing data on observed values, and substituting the resulting predicted values for the missing values. We next discuss model based techniques which use a factorization of the *complete data likelihood.*

Assume that the data are MAR. Let $f(\mathbf{y}|\theta) = f(\mathbf{y}_{\text{obs}}, \mathbf{y}_{\text{mis}}|\theta)$ denote the joint pdf of $\mathbf{y}_{\text{obs}}$ and $\mathbf{y}_{\text{mis}}$, from which we obtain the marginal pdf of $\mathbf{y}_{\text{obs}}$ as

$$f(\mathbf{y}_{\text{obs}}) = \int f(\mathbf{y}_{\text{obs}}, \mathbf{y}_{\text{mis}}|\theta)d\mathbf{y}_{\text{mis}}.$$

The likelihood of θ ignoring the missing-data mechanism, and based only on $f(\mathbf{y}_{\text{obs}}|\theta)$ is called the *incomplete data likelihood* and is

$$L(\theta|\mathbf{y}_{\text{obs}}) \propto f(\mathbf{y}_{\text{obs}}|\theta). \tag{7.5.15}$$

The objective is to maximize $L(\theta|\mathbf{y}_{\text{obs}})$ with respect to θ. If $L(\theta|\mathbf{y}_{\text{obs}})$ is unimodal and differentiable, the MLE of θ is obtained either as the closed-form solution to the ML equations

$$\partial \log L(\theta|\mathbf{y}_{\text{obs}})/\partial\theta = \mathbf{0},$$

or by using iterative methods such as the Newton-Raphson algorithm. In many cases, it is cumbersome to maximize the incomplete data likelihood $L(\theta|\mathbf{y}_{\text{obs}})$.

An alternative, widely used iterative approach is the Expectation - Maximization (EM) algorithm where the MLE of θ is related to the complete data likelihood $L(\theta|\mathbf{y})$. This algorithm has a wide range of applications, beyond incomplete data problems (Dempster, Laird and Rubin, 1977). Each iteration of the EM algorithm consists of an E step (expectation step) and an M step (maximization step). The E step computes the conditional expectation of $\mathbf{y}_{\text{mis}}$ given $\mathbf{y}_{\text{obs}}$ and the current estimate of θ and then substitutes these expectations for functions of $\mathbf{y}_{\text{mis}}$ that appear in $L(\theta|\mathbf{y})$ (or usually, the logarithm of this function). The M step maximizes the resulting expected log likelihood.

Let $\theta^{(m)}$ denote the estimate at the mth iteration. In the E step, we compute

$$Q(\theta|\theta^{(m)}) = \int l(\theta|\mathbf{y})f(\mathbf{y}_{\text{mis}}|\mathbf{y}_{\text{obs}}, \theta^{(m)})d\mathbf{y}_{\text{mis}}. \tag{7.5.16}$$

The M step obtains $\theta^{(m+1)}$ by maximizing the expected log-likelihood in (7.5.16) with respect to θ:

$$Q(\theta^{(m+1)}|\theta^{(m)}) \geq Q(\theta|\theta^{(m)}), \quad \text{for all } \theta. \tag{7.5.17}$$

A generalized EM (GEM) algorithm chooses $\theta^{(m+1)}$ such that

$$Q(\theta^{(m+1)}|\theta^{(m)}) > Q(\theta^{(m)}|\theta^{(m)}). \tag{7.5.18}$$

Result 7.5.7.

1. In an EM (or GEM) algorithm, the change from $\theta^{(m)}$ to $\theta^{(m+1)}$ cannot decrease the log-likelihood, i.e.,

$$l(\theta^{(m+1)}|\mathbf{y}_{\text{obs}}) - l(\theta^{(m)}|\mathbf{y}_{\text{obs}}) \geq 0, \tag{7.5.19}$$

with equality if and only if

$$Q(\theta^{(m+1)}|\theta^{(m)}) = Q(\theta^{(m)}|\theta^{(m)}). \tag{7.5.20}$$

2. The observed information matrix evaluated at the MLE $\widehat{\theta}$ is given by

$$\mathbf{I}(\widehat{\theta}|\mathbf{y}_{\mathrm{obs}}) = -\mathbf{D}^{20}Q(\widehat{\theta}|\widehat{\theta}) - E\{\mathbf{S}(\theta|\mathbf{y}_{\mathrm{obs}}, \mathbf{y}_{\mathrm{mis}})\mathbf{S}'(\theta|\mathbf{y}_{\mathrm{obs}}, \mathbf{y}_{\mathrm{mis}})|\mathbf{y}_{\mathrm{obs}}, \theta\}\,|_{\theta=\widehat{\theta}}$$

$$(7.5.21)$$

where $\mathbf{S}(\theta|\mathbf{y}_{\mathrm{obs}}, \mathbf{y}_{\mathrm{mis}})$ denotes the score function, and

$$\mathbf{D}^{20}Q(\widehat{\theta}|\widehat{\theta}) = (\partial^2/\partial\theta\partial\theta')Q(\theta|\widehat{\theta})\,|_{\theta=\widehat{\theta}}.$$

Proof.   Since we can write

$$f(\mathbf{y}|\theta) = f(\mathbf{y}_{\mathrm{obs}}, \mathbf{y}_{\mathrm{mis}}|\theta) = f(\mathbf{y}_{\mathrm{obs}}|\theta)f(\mathbf{y}_{\mathrm{mis}}|\mathbf{y}_{\mathrm{obs}}, \theta),$$

it follows that

$$l(\theta|\mathbf{y}) = l(\theta|\mathbf{y}_{\mathrm{obs}}) + \log f(\mathbf{y}_{\mathrm{mis}}|\mathbf{y}_{\mathrm{obs}}, \theta). \qquad (7.5.22)$$

If we define

$$H(\theta|\theta^{(m)}) = \int \{\log f(\mathbf{y}_{\mathrm{mis}}|\mathbf{y}_{\mathrm{obs}}, \theta)\} f(\mathbf{y}_{\mathrm{mis}}|\mathbf{y}_{\mathrm{obs}}, \theta^{(m)}) d\mathbf{y}_{\mathrm{mis}}, \text{ then}$$

$$H(\theta|\theta^{(m)}) \leq H(\theta^{(m)}|\theta^{(m)}), \qquad (7.5.23)$$

by Jensen's inequality. Then,

$$l(\theta|\mathbf{y}_{\mathrm{obs}}) = Q(\theta|\theta^{(m)}) - H(\theta|\theta^{(m)}), \text{ and}$$

$$l(\theta^{(m+1)}|\mathbf{y}_{\mathrm{obs}}) - l(\theta^{(m)}|\mathbf{y}_{\mathrm{obs}}) = \{Q(\theta^{(m+1)}|\theta^{(m)}) - Q(\theta^{(m)}|\theta^{(m)})\}$$
$$- \{H(\theta^{(m+1)}|\theta^{(m)}) - H(\theta^{(m)}|\theta^{(m)})\}.$$

$$(7.5.24)$$

That the left side of (7.5.24) is nonnegative follows from (7.5.18) and (7.5.23), proving property 1. The proof of property 2 is left as an exercise.   ■

   Dempster, Laird and Rubin (1977) showed that if $l(\theta|\mathbf{y}_{\mathrm{obs}})$ is bounded, then $l(\theta^{(m)}|\mathbf{y}_{\mathrm{obs}})$ converges to some value l^*, while if $f(Y|\theta)$ is a regular exponential family (see (A22)), and $l(\theta|\mathbf{y}_{\mathrm{obs}})$ is bounded, then $\theta^{(m)}$ converges to some stationary point θ^*. In general, the rate of convergence is inversely proportional to the proportion of missing information. When the distribution of the complete data $\mathbf{y}$ belongs to the exponential family, the EM algorithm is especially simple. Then, the E step consists of estimating the complete data sufficient statistics $\mathbf{T}(\mathbf{y})$ by

$$\mathbf{T}^{(m+1)} = E\{\mathbf{T}(\mathbf{y})|\mathbf{y}_{\mathrm{obs}}, \theta^{(m)}\},$$

while the M step obtains the new iterate $\theta^{(m+1)}$ as the solution to the likelihood equations

$$E\{\mathbf{T}(\mathbf{y})|\theta\} = \mathbf{T}^{(m+1)}.$$

Exercises

7.1. Prove Corollary 7.1.1.

7.2. Consider the model in Example 7.5.1.

    (a) How will you test $H : \beta_0 = 0$?

    (b) Derive an F-statistic to test $H : \beta_1 = \beta_2$.

    (c) For $N = 12$, how would you test $H_0 : X^* = 0$ versus $H_1 : X^* \neq 0$ at the 5% level of significance?

7.3. Let $Y_i = \beta_0 + \beta_1 X_{i1} + \cdots + \beta_5 X_{i5} + \varepsilon_i$, $i = 1, \cdots, N$, $\varepsilon_i \sim N(0, \sigma^2)$. Derive the F-statistic for testing $H : \beta_3 = \beta_4 = \beta_5 = 0$. By what amount is this test statistic changed if mean subtracted responses $Y_i - \overline{Y}$ are used instead of the original responses?

7.4. Consider the measurement error model in Exercise 4.3. Assuming that ε_i are iid $N(0, \sigma^2)$ variables, derive the distribution of the least squares estimator of the unknown force θ, and the level $(1 - \alpha)$ confidence interval for θ.

7.5. In the model (4.1.7) with $a = 3$, assume that ε_{ij} are iid $N(0, \sigma^2)$ variables. Derive a suitable test for $H : \mu + \tau_1 = \mu + \tau_2 = \mu + \tau_3$. Characterize the power function of this test.

7.6. In an experiment where several treatments are compared with a control, it may be desirable to replicate the control more than the experimental treatments, since the control enters into every difference investigated. Suppose each of m experimental treatments is replicated t times while the control is replicated c times. Let Y_{ij} denote the jth observation on the ith experimental treatment, $j = 1, \cdots, t$, $i = 1, \cdots, m$, and let Y_{0j} denote the jth observation on the control, $j = 1, \cdots, c$. Assume that $Y_{ij} = \tau_i + \varepsilon_{ij}$, $i = 0, \cdots, m$, where ε_{ij} are iid $N(0, \sigma^2)$ variables. Find the distribution of the least squares estimates of $\theta_i = \tau_i - \tau_0$, $i = 1, \cdots, m$.

7.7. Suppose $\varepsilon_1, \cdots, \varepsilon_N$ are iid random variables following a normal distribution with mean 0 and variance 1. Suppose $Y_0 = 0$, and $Y_i = \theta Y_{i-1} + \varepsilon_i$, $i = 1, \cdots, N$, and $|\theta| < 1$. Find the maximum likelihood estimate of θ.

7.8. In Exercise 4.5, assume that the errors have a normal distribution. Construct 95% confidence intervals for β_1, β_2, β_3, $\beta_1 - \beta_2$, and $\beta_1 + \beta_3$.

7.9. Consider the regression model $\mathbf{y} = \mathbf{X}\beta + \varepsilon$, $\varepsilon \sim N(\mathbf{0}, \sigma^2 \mathbf{V})$, where $\mathbf{V}$ is a known p.d. matrix. Obtain a simultaneous confidence set for $\mathbf{c}'\beta$ for all $\mathbf{c}$ in $\mathcal{L}$, using Scheffe's projection method.

7.10. Derive the F-statistic to test the hypothesis that two straight lines $Y_{l,i} = \beta_{l,0} + \beta_{l,1} X_{l,i} + \varepsilon_{l,i}$, $i = 1, \cdots, n_l$, $l = 1, 2$, $\varepsilon_{l,i} \sim N(0, \sigma^2)$ intersect at a point (x_0, y_0).

7.11. Consider two parallel regression lines $Y_{l,i} = \beta_{l,0} + \beta X_{l,i} + \varepsilon_{l,i}$, $i = 1, \cdots, n_l$, $l = 1, 2$, $\varepsilon_{l,i} \sim N(0, \sigma^2)$. Obtain a point estimate and an interval estimate for the horizontal distance $\delta = (\beta_{2,0} - \beta_{1,0})/\beta$ between the two lines.

7.12. In the less than full rank linear model, suppose we wish to test $H : \mathbf{C}'\beta = \mathbf{d}$. Let $\mathbf{G} = (\mathbf{X}'\mathbf{X})^-$. Show that $\mathbf{C}'\mathbf{G}\mathbf{C}$ is nonsingular whenever H is a testable hypothesis.

7.13. Obtain $E(R^2)$ in the multiple regression model with normal errors when $\beta_1 = \cdots = \beta_k = 0$.

7.14. [Wu, Hosking and Ravishanker, 1993]. For $i = 1, \cdots, N$, let

$$
\begin{aligned}
Y_i &= \varepsilon_i, \quad i \neq k, k+1, k+2 \\
Y_k &= \lambda_1 + \varepsilon_k \\
Y_{k+1} &= -c\lambda_1 + \lambda_2 + \varepsilon_{k+1} \\
Y_{k+2} &= -c\lambda_2 + \varepsilon_{k+2},
\end{aligned}
$$

where k is a fixed integer, $1 \leq k \leq N - 2$, $|c| < 1$ is a known constant, and ε_i's are iid $N(0, \sigma^2)$ variables. Let $\beta = (\lambda_1, \lambda_2)'$, and suppose σ^2 is known.

(a) Derive the least squares estimate of β, and the variance of the estimate.

(b) Derive the least squares estimate of β subject to the restriction $\lambda_1 + \lambda_2 = 0$. What is the variance of this estimate ?

(c) Derive a statistic for testing $H : \lambda_1 + \lambda_2 = 0$ versus the alternative hypothesis that λ_1 and λ_2 are unrestricted.

7.15. Consider the model $\mathbf{y} = \beta + \varepsilon$, where $\varepsilon \sim N_4(\mathbf{0}, \sigma^2\mathbf{I})$, and $\sum_{i=1}^{4} \beta_i = 0$. Derive the F-statistic for testing $H : \beta_1 = \beta_3$.

7.16. Prove property 2 in Result 7.4.3.

7.17. In Exercise 4.3, derive the distribution of the maximum likelihood estimator of θ, and use it to construct a $100(1 - \alpha)\%$ confidence interval for θ, assuming normal errors.

7.18. Based on N observations (Y_i, X_{ij}), $j = 1, \cdots, p$, $i = 1, \cdots, N$ following the model (4.1.1) with $\varepsilon_i \sim N(0, \sigma^2)$, suppose we wish to predict the value of a future observation, Y_0, say. Let $\widehat{\beta}$ and $\widehat{\sigma}^2$ denote the least squares estimates of β and σ^2 respectively.

(a) Show that the mean of Y_0 and $Var(Y_0 - \widehat{Y}_0)$ are respectively $\mathbf{x}_0'\beta$ and $\sigma_{Y_0}^2 = \widehat{\sigma}^2\{1 + \mathbf{x}_0'(\mathbf{X}'\mathbf{X})^{-1}\mathbf{x}_0\}$. Find the distribution of $(Y_0 - \mathbf{x}_0'\widehat{\beta})/\widehat{\sigma}\{1 + \mathbf{x}_0'(\mathbf{X}'\mathbf{X})^{-1}\mathbf{x}_0\}^{1/2}$.

(b) Find the 95% symmetric two-sided prediction interval for Y_0.

(c) Let $\eta \in (0, 0.5]$, and suppose the 100ηth percentile of the distribution of Y_0 is $\gamma(\eta) = \mathbf{x}_0'\beta + z_\eta \sigma_{Y_0}$. Find a $100(1 - \alpha)\%$ lower confidence bound for $\gamma(\eta)$.

7.19. In Example 7.5.1, test $H_0 : X^* = 0$ versus $H_1 : X^* \neq 0$ at the 5% level of significance when $N = 40$.

7.20. Consider the balanced incomplete block design (BIBD) with a levels of treatment, each replicated r times, b blocks, and k treatments per block. The total number of observations is $N = ar = bk$. Let $\lambda = r(k-1)/(a-1)$ denote the number of times each pair of treatments appears in the same block. Test the equality of treatment effects τ_i, $i = 1, \cdots, a$.

7.21. Let $Y_{ij} = \mu + \tau_i + \varepsilon_{ij}$, and $\varepsilon_{ij} \sim N(0, \sigma^2)$, $j = 1, \cdots, n$, $i = 1, \cdots, a$. Let $\beta = (\mu, \tau_1, \cdots, \tau_a)'$. For $l = 1, \cdots, (a-1)$, define

$$\mathbf{c}_l'\beta = (\textstyle\sum_{i=1}^{l} \tau_i - l\tau_{l+1})/[l(l+1)]^{1/2}.$$

Verify that $\mathbf{c}_l'\beta$ is estimable. Construct marginal and Tukey simultaneous confidence intervals for these functions of β.

7.22. In the regression model

$$Y_i = \beta_0 + \beta_1 X_i + \beta_2(3X_i^2 - 2) + \varepsilon_i, \quad i = 1, 2, 3,$$

with $X_1 = -1$, $X_2 = 0$, and $X_3 = 1$, what happens to the least squares estimates of β_0 and β_1 when $\beta_2 = 0$? Why?

7.23. Consider a two-way ANOVA model with no interaction and $n > 1$ replications per cell:

$$Y_{ijk} = \mu + \tau_i + \beta_j + \varepsilon_{ijk},$$

$i = 1, \cdots, a$, $j = 1, \cdots, b$, and $k = 1, \cdots, n$, where ε_{ijk} are iid $N(0, \sigma^2)$ random variables.

(a) Show that the MVUE of σ^2 is

$$\hat{\sigma}^2 = (T_1 + T_2)/N^*,$$

where

$$T_1 = \sum_{i=1}^{a}\sum_{j=1}^{b} n(\overline{Y}_{ij\cdot} - \overline{Y}_{i\cdot\cdot} - \overline{Y}_{\cdot j\cdot} + \overline{Y}_{\cdots})^2,$$

$$T_2 = \sum_{i=1}^{a}\sum_{j=1}^{b}\sum_{k=1}^{n} (Y_{ijk} - \overline{Y}_{ij\cdot})^2,$$

and $N^* = nab - a - b + 1$.

(b) Let $Z_1 = \sum_{i=1}^{a} c_i \tau_i^0$, and $Z_2 = \sum_{j=1}^{b} d_j \beta_j^0$. Show that Z_1, Z_2, and $U = N^* \hat{\sigma}^2 / \sigma^2$ are jointly independent.

7.24. Let $Y_1, \cdots, Y_N$ be independent normal random variables with $E(Y_i) = \beta_1 X_{i1} + \beta_2 X_{i2}$, and $Var(Y_i) = \sigma^2 X_{i1} X_{i2}$. Assume that X_{ij}'s are positive and the regression matrix $\mathbf{X}$ has full rank. Obtain the MVUE's $\widetilde{\beta}_1$ and $\widetilde{\beta}_2$ of β_1 and β_2. If $\widehat{\beta}_1$ and $\widehat{\beta}_2$ denote the OLS estimates of these parameters, obtain the efficiency of $\widehat{\beta}_1$ relative to $\widetilde{\beta}_1$, i.e., obtain $Var(\widetilde{\beta}_1)/Var(\widehat{\beta}_1)$.

7.25 Consider the model

$$
\begin{aligned}
E(Y_i) &= \beta_{1,0} + \beta_{1,1} X_i, \quad i = 1, \cdots, n \\
E(Y_i) &= \beta_{2,0} + \beta_{2,1} X_i, \quad i = n+1, \cdots, n+m,
\end{aligned}
$$

which corresponds to a two-phase regression in which the straight line changes phase between X_n and X_{n+1}. Suppose Y_i's are independent normal random variables with variance σ^2, $i = 1, \cdots, n+m$. Let γ denote the value of X at which the lines intersect.

(a) Find the MLE's of $\beta_{1,0}$, $\beta_{1,1}$, $\beta_{2,0}$, $\beta_{2,1}$, σ^2 and γ.

(b) Construct a $100(1-\alpha)\%$ confidence interval for γ. Does such an interval always exist?

7.26. In the model $Y_{ij} = \mu + \tau_i + \varepsilon_{ij}$, $j = 1, \cdots, n_i$, $i = 1, \cdots, 3$, $\varepsilon_{ij} \sim N(0, \sigma^2)$, derive a test statistic for $H : (\mu + \tau_1)/5 = (\mu + \tau_2)/10 = (\mu + \tau_3)/15$. How will you obtain the power of this test ?

7.27. In the one-way ANOVA model $Y_{ij} = \mu + \tau_i + \varepsilon_{ij}$, $j = 1, \cdots, n$, $i = 1, \cdots, a$, with $N(0, \sigma^2)$ errors, derive a test of $H : \mu + \tau_1 = 2(\mu + \tau_2) = \cdots = a(\mu + \tau_a)$.

7.28. Let $Y_{ij} = \mu + \tau_i + \varepsilon_{ij}$, $j = 1, \cdots, n$, $i = 1, \cdots, 3$, and $\varepsilon_{ij} \sim N(0, \sigma^2)$. Derive a test for $H : \tau_2 = (\tau_1 + \tau_3)/2$.

7.29. Consider the three factor model with normal errors, viz., $Y_{ijk} = \mu + \tau_i + \beta_j + (\tau\beta)_{ij} + \gamma_k + (\beta\gamma)_{jk} + \varepsilon_{ijk}$, $i = 1, \cdots, a$, $j = 1, \cdots, b$, $k = 1, \cdots, c$, with the constraints $\sum_i \tau_i = 0$, $\sum_j \beta_j = 0$, $\sum_k \gamma_k = 0$, $\sum_j (\tau\beta)_{ij} = 0$, $\sum_i (\tau\beta)_{ij} = 0$, $\sum_j (\beta\gamma)_{jk} = 0$, and $\sum_k (\beta\gamma)_{jk} = 0$. Develop a suitable sequence of nested hypotheses, giving the relevant sums of squares. Complete the ANOVA table.

7.30. Let $\mathbf{y} \sim E_k(\mu, \mathbf{V}, h)$, and let $\mathbf{B}$ be a $q \times k$ matrix of constants, with $r(\mathbf{B}) = q \leq k$. Show that the distribution of $\mathbf{By} \sim E_q(\mathbf{B}\mu, \mathbf{BVB}')$. Hint: Derive the mgf of $\mathbf{By}$.

7.31. Prove property 2 of Result 7.5.3.

7.32. Prove property 2 of Result 7.5.7.

Chapter 8

Multiple Regression Models

A regression model is a mechanism that enables us to describe the relationship between a response variable and explanatory variables via a functional form that involves some unknown parameters called the regression coefficients. We introduced these models in Chapter 4, and discussed inference in Chapter 7. Regression analysis consists of fitting the model to a set of observed data on the response and explanatory variables, that is, estimation of the regression coefficients in order to obtain a fitted regression model and then, assessing the goodness of the fit. The fitted model is then usually used for predicting the response at "new" values of the explanatory variables (see Draper and Smith, 1998).

The general regression model has the form (4.1.1), i.e., $\mathbf{y} = \mathbf{X}\beta + \varepsilon$, subject to the assumptions (4.1.4) on the errors, i.e., $E(\varepsilon) = \mathbf{0}$ and $Cov(\varepsilon) = \sigma^2 \mathbf{I}_N$. The $N \times p$ matrix $\mathbf{X}$ of predictors usually includes the vector $\mathbf{1}_N$ as the first column, and we may write $\mathbf{X} = (\mathbf{1}_N : \widetilde{\mathbf{X}})$. We have seen in Chapter 4 that the least squares estimate of β is $\widehat{\beta} = (\mathbf{X}'\mathbf{X})^{-1}\mathbf{X}'\mathbf{y}$, with $Cov(\widehat{\beta}) = \sigma^2(\mathbf{X}'\mathbf{X})^{-1}$. The symmetric and idempotent projection matrix $\mathbf{P} = \{p_{ij}\} = \mathbf{X}(\mathbf{X}'\mathbf{X})^{-1}\mathbf{X}'$ orthogonally projects the response $\mathbf{y}$ onto the p-dimensional subspace spanned by the columns of $\mathbf{X}$. Let $\mathbf{x}_i$ denote the ith row of $\mathbf{X}$. Then, $p_{ii} = \mathbf{x}_i'(\mathbf{X}'\mathbf{X})^{-1}\mathbf{x}_i$, and $p_{ij} = \mathbf{x}_i'(\mathbf{X}'\mathbf{X})^{-1}\mathbf{x}_j$. The matrix $(\mathbf{I} - \mathbf{P})$ is the projection onto the $(N-p)$-dimensional orthogonal subspace of $\mathcal{R}^N$.

8.1 Departures from model assumptions

Residual analysis is a crucial step in assessing the adequacy of a fitted regression model. The ordinary least squares residuals, defined by $\widehat{\varepsilon}_i = Y_i - \widehat{Y}_i$, $i = 1, \cdots, N$, represent the difference between the observed responses and the corresponding predictions from the fitted model. If the fitted model is accurate, the behavior of the residuals, which may be viewed as "estimates" of the errors, should be similar to the underlying errors. A careful perusal of the residuals should therefore enable us to conclude either that the fitting procedure has not violated any assumptions, or that some or all of the assumptions have indeed been violated and there is merit in revising the model fit. Recall from Chapter 4 that the assumptions include (a) normality of the residuals, (b) homoscedasticity, (c) independence and (d) linearity of the model. Regression residuals provide graphical and nongraphical summaries that enable us to verify departures from the usual assumptions. In the first subsection, we describe graphical procedures, while a few significance tests based on the F-distribution are described in the following subsection. Subsequent sections discuss heteroscedasticity and serial correlation in regression.

8.1.1   Graphical procedures

Three basic residual plots that enable verification of the regression assumptions are included routinely in almost all statistical software packages. These are described in the next subsection and include (i) a plot of residuals versus each predictor, (ii) a plot of residuals versus fitted values $\widehat{Y}_i$, and (iii) a normal probability plot of residuals. The following subsections describe more enhanced plots such as added-variable plots and partial residual plots.

Basic residual plots

In any model including an intercept, we must have $\sum_{i=1}^{N} \widehat{\varepsilon}_i = 0$, so that an ideal plot of residuals versus a predictor variable, or residuals versus fitted values should contain a random scatter of points in an approximate horizontal band centered at zero. The residuals are always correlated with the actual responses even when the model gives a perfect fit; therefore, a plot of residuals versus observed responses would be useless! On the contrary, when the model fits perfectly, the residuals are expected to be uncorrelated with the fitted values, so that presence of some correlation would indicate inadequate model fit. Departures from the "ideal" plot can occur in several ways, and correspond to violation of specific assumptions. A funnel shaped plot, which widens (becomes narrow) to the right indicates that the error variance increases (decreases) with increasing values of the predictor (or fit). This is a departure from the assumption of homoscedasticity of the errors and may be corrected by an appropriate (variance stabilizing) transformation or by using weighted (instead of ordinary) least squares for model fitting (see section 4.5). A departure from the linearity assumption will be indicated by a tendency of the scatter to exhibit curvature. In such cases, a remedy could be to include polynomial powers of the X_j's of suitable orders as additional predictors in the multiple regression model. In some cases, especially when the data is observed over time, the independence assumption on the errors is violated. A plot of residuals versus order (or time) would indicate this by a pattern of runs, i.e., high (low) values followed by high (low) values.

The normality assumption is checked via a histogram, or a stem-and-leaf plot, or a normal probability plot of the residuals. If the histogram or the stem-and-leaf plot exhibit skewness, heavy-tailed behavior, or multimodality, then the normality assumption is suspect. These plots also indicate the presence of outlying residuals, i.e., large discrepancies between the actual and fitted response values. The normal probability plot is a plot of the empirical residual quantiles versus quantiles from a standard normal distribution; departure from a straight line would indicate violation of the normality assumption. All these basic plots are now routinely available with many statistical software.

If normality is suspect, a possible remedy is a transformation of the data (see section 6.4). In general, the parameter of the transformation λ is unknown and must be estimated from the data. We give a brief description of the maximum likelihood approach for estimating λ (Box and Cox, 1964). Suppose we fit the model (4.1.2) to the data $(\mathbf{x}_i, Y_i)$, $i = 1, \cdots, N$. The estimation procedure consists of the following steps. We first choose a set of λ values in a preselected real interval, such as $(-5, 5)$. For each chosen λ, we compute the vector of transformed variables $\mathbf{y}^{(\lambda)} = (Y_1^{(\lambda)}, \cdots, Y_N^{(\lambda)})$ using (6.4.3), say. We then fit the normal linear model (4.1.2) to $(\mathbf{x}_i, Y_i^{(\lambda)})$, and compute $SSE(\lambda)$ based on the maximum likelihood estimates (which coincide with the OLS estimates under normality). In the plot of $SSE(\lambda)$ versus λ, we locate the value of λ which corresponds to the minimum value of $SSE(\lambda)$. This is the MLE of λ.

Added-variable plots

Added-variable plots, which are also called *partial regression plots* are useful for understanding the role of a single predictor variable in a multiple regression model (Cook and Weisberg, 1982). Suppose we partition $\mathbf{X} = (\mathbf{X}_1, \mathbf{x}_2)$ where $\mathbf{X}_1$ is an $N \times k$ matrix which usually includes the constant vector $\mathbf{1}_N$, with corresponding projection matrix $\mathbf{P}_1$, and $\mathbf{x}_2$ corresponds to a single predictor, i.e., X_2 corresponds to one of the predictor variables X_j, $j = 1, \cdots, k$. An added-variable plot shows the contribution made by X_2 to the variability in Y in the model

$$\mathbf{y} = \mathbf{X}_1\beta_1 + \mathbf{x}_2\beta_2 + \varepsilon, \qquad (8.1.1)$$

over and beyond the portion explained by $\mathbf{X}_1$ alone. Let $\widehat{\varepsilon}$ denote the vector of residuals from fitting the model (8.1.1).

Result 8.1.1. Let $\widehat{\varepsilon}(Y|\mathbf{X}_1) = (\mathbf{I} - \mathbf{P}_1)\mathbf{y}$ and $\widehat{\varepsilon}(\mathbf{x}_2|\mathbf{X}_1) = (\mathbf{I} - \mathbf{P}_1)\mathbf{x}_2$ respectively denote the ordinary residuals from a fit of Y on $\mathbf{X}_1$ and that of X_2 on $\mathbf{X}_1$. Then,

$$E[\widehat{\varepsilon}(\mathbf{y}|\mathbf{X}_1)] = \beta_2\widehat{\varepsilon}(\mathbf{x}_2|\mathbf{X}_1). \qquad (8.1.2)$$

Further, the OLS estimate of β_2 in the model (8.1.1) is

$$\widehat{\beta}_2 = \frac{\widehat{\varepsilon}'(\mathbf{x}_2|\mathbf{X}_1)\widehat{\varepsilon}(\mathbf{y}|\mathbf{X}_1)}{\widehat{\varepsilon}'(\mathbf{x}_2|\mathbf{X}_1)\widehat{\varepsilon}(\mathbf{x}_2|\mathbf{X}_1)}. \qquad (8.1.3)$$

Proof.   Since $\mathbf{P}_1 = \mathbf{X}_1(\mathbf{X}_1'\mathbf{X}_1)^{-1}\mathbf{X}_1'$, premultiplying both sides of (8.1.1) by $\mathbf{I} - \mathbf{P}_1$, we see that

$$(\mathbf{I} - \mathbf{P}_1)\mathbf{y} = (\mathbf{I} - \mathbf{P}_1)\mathbf{X}_1\beta_1 + \beta_2(\mathbf{I} - \mathbf{P}_1)\mathbf{x}_2 + (\mathbf{I} - \mathbf{P}_1)\varepsilon. \qquad (8.1.4)$$

The first term on the right side of (8.1.4) is zero; taking expectations on both sides of (8.1.4),

$$E[\widehat{\varepsilon}(\mathbf{y}|\mathbf{X}_1)] = \beta_2(\mathbf{I} - \mathbf{P}_1)\mathbf{x}_2 = \beta_2\widehat{\varepsilon}(\mathbf{x}_2|\mathbf{X}_1),$$

proving (8.1.2). Using results on partitioned matrices from section 2.1, and the idempotency of the matrix $(\mathbf{I} - \mathbf{P}_1)$, it is easily verified that the OLS estimate of β_2 in the model (8.1.1) is

$$\widehat{\beta}_2 = \{\mathbf{x}_2'(\mathbf{I} - \mathbf{P}_1)\mathbf{y}\}/\{\mathbf{x}_2'(\mathbf{I} - \mathbf{P}_1)\mathbf{x}_2\},$$

which leads directly to (8.1.3).   ■

   This result implies that a plot of $\widehat{\varepsilon}(\mathbf{y}|\mathbf{X}_1)$ versus $\widehat{\varepsilon}(\mathbf{x}_2|\mathbf{X}_1)$ is expected to be a straight line through the origin, with estimated slope $\widehat{\beta}_2$, which incidentally, is also the *GLS* estimate in (8.1.1), and the correct estimate to use (see Kruskal, 1968). This is the added-variable plot, which is a visual summary of the t-statistic (or extra sum of squares F-statistic) for testing $H_0 : \beta_2 = 0$. If all the points in the added-variable plot lie exactly on a straight line with slope β_2, $0 < \beta_2 < \infty$, i.e., the residuals from the fit of $\widehat{\varepsilon}(\mathbf{y}|\mathbf{X}_1)$ versus $\widehat{\varepsilon}(\mathbf{x}_2|\mathbf{X}_1)$ are all zero, then X_2 is a useful addition to the model. If, on the other hand, the points lie exactly on a horizontal line, the regression $\widehat{\mathbf{y}} = \mathbf{X}_1\widehat{\beta}_1$ explains all the variation in $\mathbf{y}$, and there is no need to include X_2 as a predictor. If the points in the added-variable plot lie on a vertical line, then $\widehat{\varepsilon}(\mathbf{x}_2|\mathbf{X}_1) = 0$, i.e., X_2 is an exact linear combination of the components of $\mathbf{X}_1$, and is therefore superfluous to the model. This is a situation that we recognize as collinearity and discuss in detail in section 8.3.

Partial residual plots

Partial residual plots, also called residual plus component plots (Larsen and McCleary, 1972 and Wood, 1973), are widely used in practice, because they are computationally more convenient than added-variable plots. Let $\mathbf{X} = (\mathbf{X}_1, \mathbf{x}_2)$ as before. The vector of *partial residuals* corresponding to X_2 is defined by

$$\varepsilon_2^* = \mathbf{y} - \mathbf{X}_1\widehat{\beta}_1 = \widehat{\varepsilon} + \mathbf{x}_2\widehat{\beta}_2.$$

In other words, these partial residuals are residuals that have not been adjusted for the predictor variable X_2.

   A plot of ε_2^* versus X_2 has estimated slope $\widehat{\beta}_2$ and is called a *partial residual plot*. In general, X_2 could correspond to any predictor variable X_j, $j = 1, \cdots, k$; the corresponding partial residuals, which we denote by ε_j^* are residuals from a regression that includes all other variables except X_j in the model. Thus, partial residuals contain the remnant variability in the response Y, after accounting for relationships between Y and X_l, $l \neq j$, $l = 1, \cdots, k$, and therefore constitute the portion of the data used for estimating β_j. A plot of these partial residuals versus X_j will show the partial relationship between Y and X_j. Although they look very different, it may be verified that the partial residual plot and the added-variable plot for X_j have the same slope and the same residuals. Cook and Weisberg (1994) have devoted an entire text to the area of regression graphics.

8.1.2 Sequential and partial F-tests

The ANOVA identity was introduced in section 4.2. In the full-rank regression case, the identity represents a partition of the total variation in Y into two orthogonal components, one due to the fitted regression, and the other due to unexplained error. It is written as $\mathbf{y'y} = \widehat{\beta}'\mathbf{X'y} + \widehat{\varepsilon}'\widehat{\varepsilon}$, or, by subtracting out the effect due to the intercept from the total and regression sum of squares, as $\mathbf{y'y} - N\overline{Y}^2 = (\widehat{\beta}'\mathbf{X'y} - N\overline{Y}^2) + \widehat{\varepsilon}'\widehat{\varepsilon}$. The ANOVA table corresponding to each of these forms is shown below. In each case, the mean squares in column 4 are obtained by dividing the sums of squares (in column 3) by the corresponding degrees of freedom (in column 2).

Table 8.1.1. ANOVA table for the multiple regression model

Source	d.f.	SS	MS
Regression	p	$SSR = \widehat{\beta}'\mathbf{X'y}$	MSR
Residual	$N - p$	$SSE = \widehat{\varepsilon}'\widehat{\varepsilon} = \mathbf{y'y} - \widehat{\beta}'\mathbf{X'y}$	MSE
Total	N	$SST = \mathbf{y'y}$	

The F-statistic for the joint hypothesis $H_0 : \beta_j = 0$, $j = 0, \cdots, k$ is given by

$$F_0 = \frac{SSR\ /p}{SSE\ /(N-p)} = \frac{MSR}{MSE} = \frac{(N-p)R^2}{p(1-R^2)}, \tag{8.1.5}$$

which has an $F_{p,N-p}$ distribution under H_0. We reject the null hypothesis at level of significance α if $F_0 > F_{p,N-p,\alpha}$.

The ANOVA table corresponding to separating the intercept from the remaining k predictor variables is shown in Table 8.1.2, where SSM denotes the sum of squares due to the intercept term (or mean) and $SSR_c = SSR - SSM$ denotes the corrected sum of squares due to regression. The ANOVA decomposition in Table 8.1.3 commonly appears in many standard statistical software. The F-statistic for the joint hypothesis $H_0 : \beta_j = 0$, $j = 1, \cdots, k$ is given by

$$F_0 = \frac{SSR_c\ /k}{SSE\ /(N-k-1)} = \frac{MSR_c}{MSE} = \frac{(N-k-1)R^2}{k(1-R^2)}, \tag{8.1.6}$$

which has an $F_{k,N-k-1}$ distribution under this null hypothesis. We reject the null hypothesis at level of significance α if $F_0 > F_{k,N-k-1,\alpha}$.

Table 8.1.2. ANOVA table for multiple regression with intercept separated

Source	d.f.	SS	MS
Intercept β_0	1	$SSM = N\overline{Y}^2$	MSM
Regression $|\beta_0$	k	$SSR_c = \widehat{\beta}'\mathbf{X}'\mathbf{y} - N\overline{Y}^2$	MSR_c
Residual	$N-k-1$	$SSE = \widehat{\varepsilon}'\widehat{\varepsilon} = \mathbf{y}'\mathbf{y} - \widehat{\beta}'\mathbf{X}'\mathbf{y}$	MSE
Total	N	$SST = \mathbf{y}'\mathbf{y}$	

Table 8.1.3. Mean corrected ANOVA table for multiple regression

Source	d.f.	SS	MS
Regression $|\beta_0$	k	$SSR_c = \widehat{\beta}'\mathbf{X}'\mathbf{y} - N\overline{Y}^2$	MSR_c
Residual	$N-k-1$	$SSE = \widehat{\varepsilon}'\widehat{\varepsilon} = \mathbf{y}'\mathbf{y} - \widehat{\beta}'\mathbf{X}'\mathbf{y}$	MSE
Total	$N-1$	$SST_c = \mathbf{y}'\mathbf{y} - N\overline{Y}^2$	

The regression sum of squares SSR or SSR_c can be partitioned into meaningful components that enable us to assess the effect of a *single* explanatory variable. The partition of $SSR_c = R(\beta_1, \cdots, \beta_k | \beta_0)$ into *sequential* regression sums of squares is given by

$$SSR_c = R(\beta_1|\beta_0) + R(\beta_2|\beta_1, \beta_0) + \cdots + R(\beta_k|\beta_{k-1}, \cdots, \beta_1, \beta_0) \qquad (8.1.7)$$

where $R(\theta|\nu)$ refers to the "regression explained by θ in the presence of ν". For example, $R(\beta_3|\beta_2, \beta_1, \beta_0)$ denotes the increase in the regression sum of squares when X_3 is included in a model that has the intercept, X_1 and X_2. Equation (8.1.7) represents a partition of SSR_c into single degree of freedom contributions from explanatory variables that are added sequentially one at a time to a model with just an intercept. Each component represents the incremental increase in the variability in Y explained by a particular explanatory variable included into the model. Alternately, we can view $R(\beta_3|\beta_2, \beta_1, \beta_0)$ as the reduction in the residual sum of squares by the inclusion of X_3 into a model that had the intercept, X_1 and X_2. This sequential sum of squares partitioning enables us to assess the contribution of each explanatory variable individually.

We can also implement a *subset* partitioning of SSR_c. Suppose we subdivide $\mathbf{X} = (\mathbf{1}_N, \mathbf{X}_1, \mathbf{X}_2)$, where $\mathbf{X}_1$ is $N \times k_1$, $\mathbf{X}_2$ is $N \times k_2$, such that $k = k_1 + k_2$; and we correspondingly subdivide $\beta = (\beta_0, \beta_1', \beta_2')'$. The linear regression model in (4.1.2) can be written as

$$\mathbf{y} = \beta_0 + \mathbf{X}_1\beta_1 + \mathbf{X}_2\beta_2 + \epsilon,$$

and $SSR_c = R(\beta_1, \beta_2 \mid \beta_0)$. We partition

$$SSR_c = R(\beta_1|\beta_0) + R(\beta_2|\beta_1, \beta_0),$$

where $R(\beta_2|\beta_1, \beta_0)$ is the *extra sum of squares* due to regression and represents the increase in the regression sum of squares by adding $\mathbf{X}_2$ to a model that already has the intercept and $\mathbf{X}_1$. This partition enables us to test whether any subset of regression coefficients is zero. Suppose we wish to test $H_0 : \beta_2 = \mathbf{0}$ versus $H_1 : \beta_2 \neq \mathbf{0}$. Under H_0, $R(\beta_2 \mid \beta_1, \beta_0) / \sigma^2 \sim \chi_{k_2}^2$, so that the partial F-statistic

$$F^* = \frac{R(\beta_2 \mid \beta_1, \beta_0)/k_2}{MSE} \qquad (8.1.8)$$

has an $F_{k_2, N-k-1}$ distribution under H_0. If $F^* > F_{k_2, N-k-1, \alpha}$, we reject the null hypothesis at level of significance α, since the extra variation explained by including $\mathbf{X}_2$ in the model in the presence of an intercept and $\mathbf{X}_1$ is greater than what we would attribute to chance. Some authors refer to F^* as a partial F-statistic only when a single regression coefficient is tested, i.e., when $k_2 = 1$ and the resulting statistic has an $F_{1, N-k-1}$ distribution under H_0. In general, the quantities $R(\beta_1|\beta_0, \beta_2, \beta_3, \cdots, \beta_k)$, $R(\beta_2|\beta_0, \beta_1, \beta_3, \cdots, \beta_k)$, $\cdots$, $R(\beta_k|\beta_0, \beta_1, \beta_2, \cdots, \beta_{k-1})$ are partial regression sums of squares. However, these sums of squares need not add up to SSR_c. Hence, these sums of squares and the resulting test statistics are not independent.

Note however that (8.1.7) corresponds to a complete partitioning of SSR_c and the sums of squares on the right side are independent. The resulting F-test statistics are called *sequential F-statistics*. Sequential F-test statistics enable us to test the significance of the contribution of an explanatory variable in a model containing the preceeding variables. Clearly, the order of entry of the variables into the model will affect the results. For example, $R(\beta_3|\beta_0, \beta_1, \beta_2) \neq R(\beta_3|\beta_0, \beta_1)$ and the contribution of X_3 to SSR_c will depend on which other variables were included in the model previously. Therefore, an objective and complete variable screening cannot be accomplished using only sequential F-tests, unless the selection is implemented in several stages. Many software packages contain both sequential and partial F-tests.

8.1.3 Heteroscedasticity

A linear regression model is heteroscedastic if $Var(\varepsilon) = \text{diag}(\sigma_1^2, \cdots, \sigma_N^2)$, where not all the σ_i^2 are necessarily the same. That is, the errors are uncorrelated, but do not have identical distributions. Heteroscedasticity is common in many applications. For example, in a cross-sectional study of firms within an industry, revenues of large firms might be more variable than revenues of smaller firms.

Example 8.1.1. Consider the simple regression model

$$Y_i = \beta_1 X_i + \varepsilon_i, \quad i = 1, \cdots, N,$$

where $\varepsilon_i \sim N(0, \sigma^2 X_i^2)$, $X_i \neq 0$. Using (4.5.5) and (4.5.6), the WLS estimates of β_1 and σ^2 are

$$\widehat{\beta}_{1,WLS} = \frac{1}{N}\sum_{i=1}^{N}\frac{Y_i}{X_i}, \text{ and}$$

$$\widehat{\sigma}^2_{WLS} = \frac{1}{N-1}\sum_{i=1}^{N}\frac{(Y_i - \widehat{\beta}_1 X_i)^2}{X_i^2}.$$

Recall that under heteroscedasticity, the OLS estimates of the regression parameters are unbiased, but no longer efficient. The estimated variances of the regression estimates are also biased estimates of the corresponding true variances, possibly resulting in misleading conclusions from hypothesis tests about regression parameters. □

Example 8.1.2. Consider the simple regression model

$$Y_i = \beta_1 X_i + \varepsilon_i, \quad i = 1, \cdots, N,$$

where $Y_i = \sum_{j=1}^{n_i} U_j/n_i$, and $X_i = \sum_{j=1}^{n_i} V_j/n_i$ are aggregated variables, and $\varepsilon_i \sim N(0, \sigma^2/n_i)$, $i = 1, \cdots, N$. The WLS estimate of β_1 in this case is

$$\widehat{\beta}_{1,WLS} = \{\textstyle\sum_{i=1}^{N} n_i X_i Y_i\} \big/ \{\textstyle\sum_{i=1}^{N} n_i X_i^2\},$$

with $Var(\widehat{\beta}_{1,WLS}) = \sigma^2/(\sum_{i=1}^{N} n_i X_i^2)$. □

The graphical methods of section 8.1.1 help us to diagnose heteroscedasticity. We can also carry out formal tests for departures from homoscedasticity, viz., a test of the null hypothesis

$$H_0 : \sigma_1^2 = \sigma_2^2 = \cdots = \sigma_N^2 = \sigma^2, \tag{8.1.9}$$

versus specific alternatives for the nature of nonconstant variance, such as the ones in the previous examples (see Judge et al., 1985, section 11.2). A detailed discussion of modeling and diagnostics under heterogeneity is given in Carroll and Ruppert (1988). The following results describe, without proof, some tests for heteroscedasticity without actually specifying its functional form. Each test procedure requires a (subjective) grouping of the data based on the heterogeneous errors. The first test is based on Bartlett's (1937) likelihood ratio test for the equality of a variances from normal populations.

Result 8.1.2. Consider the model

$$\mathbf{y}_i = \mathbf{X}_i \beta + \varepsilon_i, \quad i = 1, \cdots, a, \tag{8.1.10}$$

where for $i = 1, \cdots, a$, $\mathbf{y}_i$ and ε_i are n_i-dimensional vectors, $\mathbf{X}_i$ is an $n_i \times k$ matrix, $E(\varepsilon_i \varepsilon_i') = \sigma_i^2 \mathbf{I}$, and $E(\varepsilon_i \varepsilon_j') = \mathbf{0}$, $i \neq j$. The likelihood ratio test statistic of the null hypothesis $H_0 : \sigma_1^2 = \sigma_2^2 = \cdots = \sigma_N^2 = \sigma^2$ versus the alternative that the error variance is constant within a subgroups of the observations, but varies between the groups, is

$$\Lambda = \sum_{i=1}^{a} (\widehat{\sigma}_i^2 / \widehat{\sigma}^2)^{n_i/2} \qquad (8.1.11)$$

where $\widehat{\sigma}_i^2$ denotes the MSE from the fitted regression in the ith group, $i = 1, \cdots, a$, and $\widehat{\sigma}^2$ is the MSE from fitting the same model to all $N = \sum_{i=1}^{a} n_i$ observations. The statistic $-2 \ln \Lambda$ has an approximate χ_{a-1}^2 distribution. ∎

To improve the χ^2 approximation to this test statistic, Bartlett (1937) suggested the following statistic which consists of replacing n_i by $n_i - 1$, and dividing by a scaling constant c:

$$B = \frac{1}{c} \left\{ (N - a) \ln \widehat{\sigma}^2 - \sum_{i=1}^{a} (n_i - 1) \ln \widehat{\sigma}_i^2 \right\},$$

where $(n_i - 1)\widehat{\sigma}_i^2 = \sum_{j=1}^{n_i} (Y_{ij} - \overline{Y}_i)^2$, $(N - a)\widehat{\sigma}^2 = \sum_{i=1}^{a} (n_i - 1)\widehat{\sigma}_i^2$, and

$$c = 1 + \left(\frac{a-1}{3} \right) \left(\sum_{i=1}^{a} \frac{1}{(n_i - 1)} - \frac{1}{N - a} \right).$$

The statistic B has an approximate χ_{a-1}^2 distribution under H_0. Dyer and Keating (1980) provided exact critical values for Bartlett's test statistic for the balanced case, i.e., $n_i = n$, $i = 1, \cdots, a$. It is possible that the grouping occurs in one of the following ways. First, replications are available at each level of **X** and constitute natural grouping. Second, observations may be grouped together according to geographic region, size, or, as in the case of time series data, according to whether they correspond to a period before or after a fixed time t_0. Note that when the number of subgroups a is equal to 2, we may carry out the usual F-test for comparing two variances from normal populations. The usefulness of this test is limited to situations where the grouping of data into subgroups with approximately equal variances is possible. The test also requires an assumption of normal populations.

Another test procedure is the Goldfeld-Quandt test (Goldfeld and Quandt, 1965) which is useful in situations where the alternative hypothesis states that the error variance is an increasing function of the magnitude of the predictor variable, i.e., $H_1 : \sigma_i^2 = CX_i^2$, $i = 1, \cdots, N$. The test procedure consists of (subjectively) calculating two least squares regressions, one using data associated with the low variance errors and the other based on data corresponding to the high variance errors. A significant disparity in the residual variances from these two regressions would lead us to reject the null hypothesis. The following steps facilitate the testing procedure. We first order the data by the magnitude of one of the explanatory variables X_j. We omit the middle m observations (with m approximately equal to $N/5$). Next, we fit two regressions, one associated with $(N - m)/2$ observations corresponding to smaller X_j values, with residual sum of squares SSE_S and the other with the same number of observations corresponding to the larger X_j values and with residual sum of squares SSE_L.

Result 8.1.3.   Let $MSE_S = 2SSE_S/(N - m)$ and $MSE_L = 2SSE_L/(N - m)$ be the residual mean squares corresponding to the two groups. Under the assumption that the errors are independent and have normal distributions,

$$MSE_L/MSE_S \sim F_{(N-m-2p)/2,(N-m-2p)/2}$$

distribution under H_0.   ∎

Dropping the central observations with approximately equal error variances is known to improve the power of the test. This test is applicable only in situations where the alternative hypothesis states that the error variance is an increasing function of the magnitude of the predictor variable. When such an assumption is untenable, the Breusch-Pagan test may be used. In a normal linear regression model, suppose the heteroscedasticity is specified by

$$\sigma_i^2 = f(\gamma + \delta \mathbf{Z}_i) \tag{8.1.12}$$

where $f(.)$ is a general function which accommodates linear and logarithmic forms, while $\mathbf{Z}$ could either be a specific explanatory variable X, or a subset of other predictor variables. The Breusch-Pagan test procedure (Breusch and Pagan, 1979) consists of the following steps. First, we obtain the OLS residuals of the simple linear regression of Y on X, and compute $\widehat{\sigma}^2 = MSE$. We next fit the regression

$$\widehat{\varepsilon}_i^2/\widehat{\sigma}^2 = \gamma + \delta \mathbf{Z}_i + u_i.$$

Under the null hypothesis of homoscedasticity, the test statistic $SSR/2$ has a chi-square distribution with q degrees of freedom, where q denotes the number of variables represented by $\mathbf{Z}$. A large value of the test statistic implies a high correlation between the error variance and $\mathbf{Z}$, which leads us to reject the null hypothesis. Alternatively, we can construct a likelihood ratio test. The log-likelihood function for a normal regression model with multiplicative heteroscedasticity

$$\log(\sigma_i^2) = \gamma + \delta \log(Z_i) \tag{8.1.13}$$

has the form

$$\log(L) = -\tfrac{n}{2}\log(2\pi) - \tfrac{1}{2}\sum_{i=1}^{n}\log(\sigma_i^2) - \tfrac{1}{2}\sum_{i=1}^{n}(Y_i - \beta_0 - \beta_1 X_i)^2/\sigma_i^2.$$

Substituting (8.1.13) into the log-likelihood function and maximizing with respect to the regression and heteroscedasticity parameters yields estimates for β_0, β_1, γ and δ, based on which the test may be constructed. The assumption of normal errors is critical for this test. The test proposed by White (1980) is closely related to the Bruesch-Pagan test, but does not depend critically on normality of errors.

To implement White's test, we use the OLS residuals from the regression of Y on X to fit the regression

$$\widehat{\varepsilon}_i^2 = \gamma + \delta \mathbf{Z}_i + u_i$$

and calculate the coefficient of determination R^2. The statistic for White's test is NR^2, which has a chi-square distribution with q degrees of freedom under the null hypothesis of homoscedasticity, where once again, q denotes the number of Z variables.

8.1.4 Serial correlation

When data is observed over time, the assumption of independent errors is often suspect, as indicated by a plot of residuals versus order (time). The linear regression model with serially correlated errors has the form

$$Y_t = \beta_0 + \beta_1 X_{t1} + \cdots + \beta_k X_{tk} + \varepsilon_t, \quad t = 1, \cdots, N, \tag{8.1.14}$$

where the subscript t is used to indicate time, and error terms from different time periods are correlated. This model can be expressed in the form (4.5.1) with $E(\varepsilon\varepsilon') = \sigma^2 \mathbf{V}$, where $\mathbf{V}$ is an $N \times N$ p.d. matrix whose form is specified under an assumption that $\{\varepsilon_t\}$ is a stationary stochastic process. This assumption implies that the first two moments of the distribution of ε does not depend on t, and we can write

$$\mathbf{V} = \begin{pmatrix} 1 & \rho_1 & \rho_2 & \cdots & \rho_{N-1} \\ \rho_1 & 1 & \rho_1 & \cdots & \rho_{N-2} \\ \rho_2 & \rho_1 & 1 & \cdots & \rho_{N-3} \\ \vdots & \vdots & \vdots & \ddots & \vdots \\ \rho_{N-1} & \rho_{N-2} & \rho_{N-3} & \cdots & 1 \end{pmatrix}$$

where $\rho_j = E(\varepsilon_t \varepsilon_{t-j})/\sigma^2 = E(\varepsilon_t \varepsilon_{t+j})/\sigma^2$, $j = 1, 2, \cdots$, is the autocorrelation between two random errors j time periods apart. This specification is still rather general, and the most commonly assumed specification for the stationary stochastic process is the first-order autoregressive ($AR(1)$) process, which we introduced in Example 4.5.1.

Example 8.1.3. Consider the multiple regression model with serially correlated errors in (8.1.14), with $E(\varepsilon_t) = 0$, and $Cov(\varepsilon_t, \varepsilon_s) = \sigma^2 \rho^{|t-s|}$, $s, t = 1, \cdots, N$, with $|\rho| < 1$. Let $\widehat{\beta}$ denote the OLS estimate of the vector of regression coefficients, and let $\widehat{\varepsilon}$ denote the vector of OLS residuals. We estimate the serial correlation ρ by

$$\widehat{\rho} = (\sum_{t=2}^{N} \widehat{\varepsilon}_t \widehat{\varepsilon}_{t-1})/(\sum_{t=1}^{N} \widehat{\varepsilon}_t^2). \tag{8.1.15}$$

In addition to the residual versus time plot to detect serial correlation, we may use significance tests and enhanced graphical procedures to diagnose correlation in errors. The most popular test for serial correlation is the Durbin-Watson test (Durbin and Watson, 1950, 1951). The null hypothesis is $H_0 : \rho = 0$ while the alternative hypothesis is either $H_1 : \rho \neq 0$, or $H_1 : \rho > 0$, or $H_1 : \rho < 0$.

Result 8.1.4.   The exact distribution of the Durbin-Watson test statistic

$$DW = \{\sum_{t=2}^{N} (\widehat{\varepsilon}_t - \widehat{\varepsilon}_{t-1})^2\} \bigg/ \{\sum_{t=1}^{N} \widehat{\varepsilon}_t^2\} \qquad (8.1.16)$$

depends on $\mathbf{X}$. For a given level of significance α, the *bounds test* has the following decision rules based on lower and upper critical values (at level α) $d_{L,N,p}$ and $d_{U,N,p}$.

1. If H_1 is $\rho > 0$, reject H_0 at level of significance α if $DW < d_{L,N,p}$; do not reject H_0 if $DW > d_{U,N,p}$; and the test is inconclusive if $d_{L,N,p} \leq DW \leq d_{U,N,p}$.

2. If H_1 is $\rho < 0$, the decision rule has the form of the rule for $H_1 : \rho > 0$, replacing DW by $(4 - DW)$.

3. If H_1 is $\rho \neq 0$, reject H_0 at level of significance 2α if $DW < d_{L,N,p}$ or $4 - DW < d_{L,N,p}$; do not reject H_0 if $DW > d_{U,N,p}$ or $4 - DW > d_{U,N,p}$; and the test is inconclusive otherwise.

Proof.   The Durbin-Watson statistic can be written as

$$DW = \widehat{\varepsilon}' \mathbf{A} \widehat{\varepsilon} / \widehat{\varepsilon}' \widehat{\varepsilon}$$

where

$$\mathbf{A} = \begin{pmatrix} 1 & -1 & 0 & \cdots & 0 & 0 \\ -1 & 2 & -1 & \cdots & 0 & 0 \\ \vdots & \vdots & \vdots & \ddots & \vdots & \vdots \\ 0 & 0 & 0 & \cdots & 2 & -1 \\ 0 & 0 & 0 & \cdots & -1 & 1 \end{pmatrix}$$

is a symmetric matrix with eigenvalues $\lambda_1 \leq \lambda_2 \leq \cdots \leq \lambda_N$, $\widehat{\varepsilon} = (\mathbf{I} - \mathbf{P})\varepsilon$, and $\widehat{\varepsilon} \sim SN(\mathbf{0}, \sigma^2(\mathbf{I} - \mathbf{P}))$ (see property 2 of Result 7.1.1). Under H_0, the ratio DW can be reduced to a canonical form by simultaneous diagonalization of the numerator and denominator quadratic forms (see section 2.5). Since $\mathbf{A}$ is symmetric, there exists an orthogonal transformation $\varepsilon = \mathbf{B}\xi$ such that

$$\varepsilon' \mathbf{A} \varepsilon / \varepsilon' \varepsilon = \sum_{i=1}^{N-p} \nu_i \xi_i^2 \bigg/ \sum_{i=1}^{N-p} \xi_i^2 ,$$

ξ_i being iid $N(0, \sigma^2)$ variables, and where ν_i are the $N - p$ nonzero eigenvalues of $(\mathbf{I} - \mathbf{P})\mathbf{A}(\mathbf{I} - \mathbf{P})$. Correspondingly,

$$DW = \sum_{i=1}^{N-p} \lambda_i \xi_i^2 \Big/ \sum_{i=1}^{N-p} \xi_i^2 .$$

The exact distribution of DW depends on the eigenvalues of $\mathbf{A}$ and $(\mathbf{I} - \mathbf{P})$. Under the assumption of normality and independence of the errors, Durbin and Watson obtained upper and lower bounds for the distribution of DW and tabulated percentage points of these bounding distributions. Since

$$\lambda_i \le \nu_i \le \lambda_{i+k}, \quad i = 1, \cdots, N - p,$$

it follows that

$$d_L \le DW \le d_U,$$

where,

$$d_L = \sum_{i=1}^{N-p} \nu_i \xi_i^2 \Big/ \sum_{i=1}^{N-p} \xi_i^2 , \text{ and}$$

$$d_U = \sum_{i=1}^{N-p} \nu_{i+p} \xi_i^2 \Big/ \sum_{i=1}^{N-p} \xi_i^2 . \tag{8.1.17}$$

These bounds do not depend on the particular predictor matrix $\mathbf{X}$, and lead to the Durbin-Watson test. Since the values of DW lie between 0 and 4, and are symmetric about 2, property 2 follows. The decision for the two-sided alternative is immediate. ∎

Note that the summation in the numerator of the DW statistic runs from $t = 2$ to N since $\widehat{\varepsilon}_0$ is not available; this is referred to as an "end effect". The statistic DW lies in the range of 0 to 4, with a value of 2 indicating the absence of first-order serial correlation. When successive values of $\widehat{\varepsilon}_t$ are close together, DW is small, indicating the presence of positive serial correlation. For a relation between DW and $\widehat{\rho}$, see Exercise 8.4. It is important to realize that not rejecting the null hypothesis does not necessarily mean that the errors are uncorrelated; it simply means that there is no significant first-order autocorrelation. More complex linear stationary time series models may be employed in order to model autocorrelation in regression errors. An example is the autoregressive moving-average process of order (p, q) defined as

$$\varepsilon_t = \phi_1 \varepsilon_{t-1} + \phi_2 \varepsilon_{t-2} + \cdots + \phi_p \varepsilon_{t-p} + u_t + \theta_1 u_{t-1} + \theta_2 u_{t-2} + \cdots \theta_q u_{t-q}$$

where u_t's are iid $N(0, \sigma^2)$ variables, and the $(p + q)$ parameters $(\phi_1, \cdots, \phi_p)$, and $(\theta_1, \cdots, \theta_q)$ must satisfy certain restrictions (for details, see Brockwell and Davis, 1998). Plots of the sample autocorrelation function and partial autocorrelation function enable us to identify the model order in these cases.

If the errors in a regression model are serially correlated, an iterative estimation procedure called the Cochrane-Orcutt procedure is useful. Let $\widehat{\beta}$ denote the OLS estimate of β, and let $\widehat{\varepsilon}$ be the OLS residual vector. In this initial step, the first-order serial correlation is estimated by (8.1.15). Denote these quantities by $\widehat{\beta}^{(0)}$, $\widehat{\varepsilon}^{(0)}$ and $\widehat{\rho}^{(0)}$ respectively. Using $\widehat{\rho}^{(0)}$, we transform the original model and obtain OLS estimates from the transformed regression

$$Y_t^* = \beta_0(1 - \widehat{\rho}^{(0)}) + \beta_1 X_{t1}^* + \cdots + \beta_k X_{tk}^* + u_t, \ t = 1, \cdots, N,$$

where $Y_t^* = Y_t - \widehat{\rho}^{(0)} Y_{t-1}$, and $X_{tj}^* = X_{tj} - \widehat{\rho}^{(0)} X_{t-1,j}$, $j = 1, \cdots, k$. Let $\widehat{\beta}^{(1)}$ and $\widehat{\varepsilon}^{(1)}$ respectively denote the vector of regression estimates, and residual vector from this first iteration. We repeat this procedure several times until convergence. This procedure works well in practice, although there is always the danger that the procedure may tend to a local rather than a global maximum.

Numerical Example 8.1.   Consider data from the first quarter of 1952 to the fourth quarter of 1956 on consumer expenditure in the U.S. in billions of dollars (Y), and money stock in billions of dollars (X). Let t denote the time period (Chatterjee and Price, 1991). The regression estimates and the ANOVA table are shown below.

Least squares estimates for Numerical Example 8.1.

Parameter	d.f.	Estimate	s.e.	t-value	$\Pr > t$
Intercept	1	-154.954	19.883	-7.79	$< .0001$
X	1	2.302	0.115	20.06	$< .0001$

ANOVA table

Source	d.f.	SS	MS	F-value	$\Pr > F$
Model	1	6395.170	6395.170	402.34	$< .0001$
Error	18	286.107	15.895		
Corrected Total	19	6681.278			

Also, $\widehat{\sigma} = 3.987$, $R^2 = 957$, $R_{adj.}^2 = 955$, and the estimate of the first-order serial correlation $\widehat{\rho} = 0.752$, with s.e. 0.160. The Durbin-Watson statistic is $DW = 0.326$; comparing it to the lower and upper critical values $d_L = 1.201$ and $d_U = 1.411$, we reject $H_0 : \rho = 0$ at the 5% level of significance. One way to fit a regression model with $AR(1)$ errors to the data is via a two-step least squares procedure. The results from this fit are shown below.

Simultaneous estimates of β and ρ

Parameter	d.f.	Estimate	s.e.	t-value	$\Pr > t$
Intercept	1	-158.280	32.127	-4.93	.0001
X	1	2.327	0.186	12.54	$< .0001$

The estimate of the $AR(1)$ parameter is $\widehat{\rho} = 0.752$, with standard error 0.160.   ▲

8.1.5   Stochastic X matrix

In (4.1.1), suppose the $N \times p$ matrix $\mathbf{X}$ is stochastic. In practice, this is the case when some or all of the explanatory variables either cannot be measured accurately, or can only be measured indirectly.

Result 8.1.5.   Suppose the stochastic predictor $\mathbf{X}$ has rank p, and is independent of ε. The least squares estimator $\widehat{\beta}$ is an unbiased estimator of β with covariance matrix $\sigma^2 E\{(\mathbf{X}'\mathbf{X})^{-1}\}$. Also, $\widehat{\sigma}^2$ is an unbiased estimator of σ^2.

Proof.   The independence of $\mathbf{X}$ and ε implies that

$$E(\varepsilon|\mathbf{X}) = E(\varepsilon) = \mathbf{0}, \quad \text{and}$$
$$Cov(\varepsilon|\mathbf{X}) = Cov(\varepsilon) = \sigma^2 \mathbf{I}_N.$$

It follows that

$$E(\widehat{\beta}) = \beta + E\{(\mathbf{X}'\mathbf{X})^{-1}\mathbf{X}'\}E(\varepsilon) = \beta, \quad \text{and}$$

$$
\begin{aligned}
Cov(\widehat{\beta}) &= E\{(\mathbf{X}'\mathbf{X})^{-1}\mathbf{X}'\varepsilon\varepsilon'\mathbf{X}(\mathbf{X}'\mathbf{X})^{-1}\} \\
&= E\{E[(\mathbf{X}'\mathbf{X})^{-1}\mathbf{X}'\varepsilon\varepsilon'\mathbf{X}(\mathbf{X}'\mathbf{X})^{-1}]|\mathbf{X}\} \\
&= \sigma^2 E\{(\mathbf{X}'\mathbf{X})^{-1}\}.
\end{aligned}
$$

Also,

$$
\begin{aligned}
E(\widehat{\sigma}^2) = E\{E(\widehat{\sigma}^2)|\mathbf{X}\} &= E\{E[(N-p)^{-1}\widehat{\varepsilon}'\widehat{\varepsilon}|\mathbf{X}]\} \\
&= E\{(N-p)^{-1}E(\widehat{\varepsilon}'\widehat{\varepsilon}|\mathbf{X})\} \\
&= E\{(N-p)^{-1}(N-p)\sigma^2\} = \sigma^2. \quad \blacksquare
\end{aligned}
$$

Although $\widehat{\beta}$ is a stochastic function of $\mathbf{y}$, and is no longer considered the b.l.u.e. of β, it is still efficient if we consider its covariance conditional on a given $\mathbf{X}$. If ε has a $N(\mathbf{0}, \sigma^2\mathbf{I}_N)$ distribution, and the distribution of $\mathbf{X}$ does not involve β or σ^2, then the pdf of ε coincides with the conditional pdf of ε given $\mathbf{X}$, and the MLE of β coincides with its least squares estimator.

In some situations, the independence of $\mathbf{X}$ and ε is untenable. For example, consider the model

$$Y_t = \beta_1 X_t + \beta_2 Y_{t-1} + \varepsilon_t, \quad t = 1, \cdots, N,$$

where X_t is a deterministic predictor. By repeated substitution, we can verify that the distribution of Y_{t-1} depends on $\varepsilon_{t-1}, \varepsilon_{t-2}, \cdots$. The following result summarizes some asymptotic properties of the least squares estimator in the situation where $\mathbf{X}$ is partially independent of ε.

If the sequence of estimators $\widehat{\theta}_N$ based on N observations converges in probability to a constant θ, we say that θ is the probability limit of the sequence $\widehat{\theta}_N$, and write plim $\widehat{\theta}_N = \theta$.

Result 8.1.6.   In the model (4.1.1), suppose $\mathbf{X}$ and ε are partially independent, and assume that plim $\varepsilon'\varepsilon/N = \sigma^2$, plim $\mathbf{X}'\mathbf{X}/N = \Sigma_{xx}$ is nonsingular,
and plim $\mathbf{X}'\varepsilon/N = \mathbf{0}$. Then plim $\widehat{\beta} = \beta$, and $N^{1/2}(\widehat{\beta} - \beta)$ has a $N(\mathbf{0}, \sigma^2\Sigma_{xx}^{-1})$
distribution.

Proof.   The least squares estimator $\widehat{\beta}$ is consistent since

$$
\begin{aligned}
\text{plim } \widehat{\beta} &= \beta + \text{plim}(\mathbf{X}'\mathbf{X}/N)^{-1}(\mathbf{X}'\varepsilon/N) \\
&= \beta + \text{plim}(\mathbf{X}'\mathbf{X}/N)^{-1}\text{plim}(\mathbf{X}'\varepsilon/N) = \beta,
\end{aligned}
$$

using Slutsky's theorem (Casella and Berger, 1990). The limiting distribu-
tion of $\widehat{\beta}$ follows directly from the limiting distribution of $N^{1/2}(\widehat{\beta} - \beta) =$
$(\mathbf{X}'\mathbf{X}/N)^{-1}(\mathbf{X}'\varepsilon/N^{1/2})$.   ∎

The reader is referred to Judge et al., (1988) for more details on this topic,
particularly on measurement errors in the predictors, and instrumental variable
estimators.

8.2   Model selection in regression

We discuss procedures in regression useful for selecting variables from a set of
possible regressors $X_1, \cdots, X_k$. In particular, we describe selection of the best
regression equation via (a) all possible regressions, using criteria such as R^2,
adjusted R^2, $\widehat{\sigma}^2$, Mallows C_p statistic and the $PRESS$ statistic; (b) best subset
regression using these criteria; (c) forward selection; (d) backward elimination;
and (e) stepwise regression. We begin with a description of the selection criteria.
    Although the coefficient of determination R^2 is a traditional criterion for
regression model selection, it is not prediction performance oriented, and hence
should always be used in conjunction with other criteria for choosing the best
prediction model from a set of candidate models. Since the inclusion of a new
explanatory variable into a model can never decrease SSR, and consequently
the value of R^2, there might be a tendency to overparametrize in order to
achieve a large R^2 value. The adjusted R^2 ensures parsimony by imposing a
penalty for including marginally important explanatory variables at the cost
of error degrees of freedom. The use of $\widehat{\sigma}^2$ as a model comparison criterion
would entail choosing the model which has the smallest $\widehat{\sigma}^2$ value. Let $\widehat{\sigma}^2(k_1)$
and $\widehat{\sigma}^2(k_2)$ denote the residual mean squares from two fitted regression models
with k_1 and k_2 regressors respectively, where $k_1 < k_2$. It could happen that
$\widehat{\sigma}^2(k_1) > \widehat{\sigma}^2(k_2)$, which would perhaps imply that the reduction in residual mean
squares by fitting the model with k_1 parameters did not counterbalance the loss
in residual degrees of freedom. We define another criterion for model selection
which compares the standardized total mean squared error of prediction for the
observed data (Mallows, 1973, 1995).

Definition 8.2.1.   Mallows C_p.   Let $\mathbf{y} = \mathbf{X}\beta + \varepsilon$ denote the "true" regression model, where β is a q-dimensional vector. Let $\mathbf{y} = \mathbf{X}_1\beta_1 + \varepsilon$ denote the

fitted model, where the dimension of β_1 is p. Let $\widehat{\mathbf{y}}_1 = \mathbf{X}_1\widehat{\beta}_1$ denote the fitted vector. Then,

$$E(\widehat{\mathbf{y}}_1) = \mathbf{X}_1(\mathbf{X}_1'\mathbf{X}_1)^{-1}\mathbf{X}_1'E(\mathbf{X}\beta + \varepsilon) = \mathbf{X}_1(\mathbf{X}_1'\mathbf{X}_1)^{-1}\mathbf{X}_1'\mathbf{X}\beta = \eta_p, \text{ say.}$$

The C_p statistic which is useful for comparing various fitted models with p parameters to the full q parameter model is

$$C_p = \frac{SSE_p}{\widehat{\sigma}^2} - (N - 2p) = \frac{\mathbf{y}'(\mathbf{I} - \mathbf{P}_1)\mathbf{y}}{\widehat{\sigma}^2} - (N - 2p) \qquad (8.2.1)$$

where SSE_p is the residual sum of squares from a model with p regression coefficients (including the intercept), and $\widehat{\sigma}^2$ is the residual mean square from the "full-model" containing all the regressors and is presumed to be a reliable estimator of σ^2.

Note that C_q is a fixed quantity given by

$$\begin{aligned} C_q &= SSE_q/\widehat{\sigma}^2 - (N - 2q) \\ &= (N - q)\widehat{\sigma}^2/\widehat{\sigma}^2 - (N - 2q) = q. \end{aligned}$$

Otherwise, C_p is a random variable, which is an approximately unbiased estimator of the expected standardized total mean square of the predicted values as the following result shows.

Result 8.2.1. Let

$$J_p^* = E(\widehat{\mathbf{y}}_1 - \mathbf{X}\beta)'(\widehat{\mathbf{y}}_1 - \mathbf{X}\beta)/\sigma^2.$$

Then, $E(C_p) \approx J_p^*$.

Proof. Since $\mathbf{I} - \mathbf{P}_1$ is symmetric and idempotent,

$$\begin{aligned} E\{\mathbf{y}'(\mathbf{I} - \mathbf{P}_1)\mathbf{y}\} &= tr[(\mathbf{I} - \mathbf{P}_1)\sigma^2\mathbf{I}_N] + \beta'\mathbf{X}'(\mathbf{I} - \mathbf{P}_1)\mathbf{X}\beta \\ &= \sigma^2(N - p) + \beta'\mathbf{X}'(\mathbf{I} - \mathbf{P}_1)(\mathbf{I} - \mathbf{P}_1)\mathbf{X}\beta \\ &= \sigma^2(N - p) + (\mathbf{X}\beta - \mathbf{P}_1\mathbf{X}\beta)'(\mathbf{X}\beta - \mathbf{P}_1\mathbf{X}\beta) \\ &= \sigma^2(N - p) + (\mathbf{X}\beta - \eta_p)'(\mathbf{X}\beta - \eta_p). \qquad (8.2.2) \end{aligned}$$

Also,

$$\begin{aligned} E(\widehat{\mathbf{y}}_1 - \mathbf{X}\beta)'(\widehat{\mathbf{y}}_1 - \mathbf{X}\beta) &= E(\widehat{\mathbf{y}}_1 - \eta_p)'(\widehat{\mathbf{y}}_1 - \eta_p) + (\mathbf{X}\beta - \eta_p)'(\mathbf{X}\beta - \eta_p) \\ &= tr\{Cov(\widehat{\mathbf{y}}_1)\} + (\mathbf{X}\beta - \eta_p)'(\mathbf{X}\beta - \eta_p) \\ &= p\sigma^2 + (\mathbf{X}\beta - \eta_p)'(\mathbf{X}\beta - \eta_p). \qquad (8.2.3) \end{aligned}$$

Subtracting (8.2.3) from (8.2.2), we get

$$E(\widehat{\mathbf{y}}_1 - \mathbf{X}\beta)'(\widehat{\mathbf{y}}_1 - \mathbf{X}\beta) - E\{\mathbf{y}'(\mathbf{I} - \mathbf{P}_1)\mathbf{y}\} = (2p - N)\sigma^2. \qquad (8.2.4)$$

The proof follows by dividing both sides of (8.2.4) by $\widehat{\sigma}^2$. ■

Computed values of C_p for fitted models with different subsets of variables are useful for model selection. If the fitted model is unbiased, we have $\eta_p = \mathbf{X}\beta$, so that $E(C_p) = p$. Adequate models with C_p values close to p will be indicated in a plot of C_p versus p. Biased models with considerable lack of fit will be indicated by points that are substantially above the line $C_p = p$, although because of randomness, adequate models may sometimes fall below the line. Since the actual value of C_p is an estimate of the expected standardized total mean square of the predicted values J_p^*, the height of each plotted point is also important. As regressors are included in the model, SSE_p decreases, and C_p usually increases. The "best" regression model is one that gives the lowest possible value of C_p for which $C_p \approx p$. Note that there are multiple C_p values corresponding to a given p, i.e., corresponding to different subsets of p (out of q) regressor variables. In many cases, when the choice of model is not obvious from the C_p plot, personal judgment may be employed, or alternative approaches may be used.

We next define the *PRESS* or Prediction Sum of Squares criterion. Let $\widehat{Y}_{i,(i)} = \mathbf{x}_i'\widehat{\beta}_{(i)}$ denote the prediction for the ith response from fitting the regression model (4.1.2) with the ith case excluded. That is, we fit a regression model to observations $(Y_l, \mathbf{x}_l')$, $l \neq i$, $l = 1, \cdots, N$. Then, the estimated β vector with the ith case excluded is

$$
\begin{aligned}
\widehat{\beta}_{(i)} &= (\mathbf{X}_{(i)}'\mathbf{X}_{(i)})^{-1}\mathbf{X}_{(i)}'\mathbf{y}_{(i)} \\
&= \left((\mathbf{X}'\mathbf{X})^{-1} + \frac{(\mathbf{X}'\mathbf{X})^{-1}\mathbf{x}_i\mathbf{x}_i'(\mathbf{X}'\mathbf{X})^{-1}}{1 - p_{ii}} \right) \mathbf{X}_{(i)}'\mathbf{y}_{(i)}. \quad (8.2.5)
\end{aligned}
$$

The last equation on the right follows from observing that $(\mathbf{X}_{(i)}'\mathbf{X}_{(i)})^{-1} = (\mathbf{X}'\mathbf{X} - \mathbf{x}_i\mathbf{x}_i')^{-1}$ and property 5 of Result 1.2.10. Let

$$
\widehat{\varepsilon}_{i(i)} = Y_i - \widehat{Y}_{i(i)}, \quad i = 1, \cdots, N \quad (8.2.6)
$$

denote the corresponding prediction residuals or *PRESS* residuals. Corresponding to each candidate model that we fit, there will be N *PRESS* residuals based on which we define the *PRESS* statistic.

Definition 8.2.2.   The *PRESS* statistic is defined as

$$
PRESS = \sum_{i=1}^{N}(Y_i - \widehat{Y}_{i(i)})^2 = \sum_{i=1}^{N}\widehat{\varepsilon}_{i(i)}^2. \quad (8.2.7)
$$

This statistic condenses information in the form of N validations, each with a fitting sample of size $(N - 1)$. The model which has the smallest computed *PRESS* statistic value is preferred. Although it seems that in order to construct the *PRESS* statistic, we must run N separate regressions, this cumbersome computation is not necessary since the *PRESS* residuals are related to the ordinary residuals as the next result shows.

Result 8.2.2. The predicted residual is related to the ordinary residual by

$$\widehat{\varepsilon}_{i(i)} = \frac{\widehat{\varepsilon}_i}{1 - p_{ii}}. \tag{8.2.8}$$

Proof. It is left as an exercise for the reader to verify that $\widehat{\beta}_{(i)}$ may be written as

$$\widehat{\beta}_{(i)} = \widehat{\beta} - \frac{\widehat{\varepsilon}_i(\mathbf{X}'\mathbf{X})^{-1}\mathbf{x}_i}{1 - p_{ii}}. \tag{8.2.9}$$

Substituting (8.2.9) into (8.2.6), the result follows. If the regression errors are normally distributed, $\widehat{\varepsilon}_{i(i)}$ have the same correlation structure as the $\widehat{\varepsilon}_i$, have 0 means and variances equal to $\sigma^2/(1 - p_{ii})$. Use of $\widehat{\varepsilon}_{i(i)}$ will tend to emphasize cases with large p_{ii}, while use of $\widehat{\varepsilon}_i$ will emphasize cases with smaller p_{ii}. ∎

Using this result, the *PRESS* statistic is easily computed as

$$PRESS = \sum_{i=1}^{N} \left(\frac{\widehat{\varepsilon}_i}{1 - p_{ii}}\right)^2. \tag{8.2.10}$$

A related statistic based on *PRESS* residuals is

$$R^2_{pred} = 1 - \frac{PRESS}{\sum_{i=1}^{N}(Y_i - \overline{Y})^2}. \tag{8.2.11}$$

We next give a brief description of some widely used selection procedures that use these criteria in addition to t-tests and F-tests. *All Possible Regressions* is a cumbersome procedure that requires the fitting of every possible regression equation that always includes an intercept and may include any of the variables $X_1, \cdots, X_k$. Since each of the k explanatory variables can either be included or not in the regression model, we must fit 2^k possible regressions; even when $k = 10$, this requires 1024 regression fits. Each fitted regression is generally assessed on the basis of three criteria, viz., R^2, $\widehat{\sigma}^2$, and Mallows C_p statistic. In general, when there are several regressors, an analysis of all possible regressions is quite unwarranted in terms of effort and computer time. With some initial thought, a majority of the models that are considered in such an analysis could be avoided and a suitable selection procedure that compares only a subset of all possible regressions, such as *best subset regression* is usually preferred.

Stepwise regression is the most widely used approach for variable selection and is available in most standard regression packages. The procedure uses t-statistics (or corresponding p-values) to determine the significance of the predictor variables. At the outset, we choose values of α_{enter}, and α_{stay}, each of which may be equal to 0.05. Here, α_{enter} is the probability of a Type I error related to including a predictor variable into the existing regression model, while α_{stay} is the probability of a Type I error related to retaining in the model a predictor variable that was previously entered. In the first step, we consider k regression models of the form

$$Y = \beta_0 + \beta_1 X_j + \varepsilon,$$

which includes only the jth predictor, $j = 1, \cdots, k$. For each model, we compute the t-statistic (and p-value) for testing $H_0 : \beta_1 = 0$ versus $H_1 : \beta_1 \neq 0$. Let $X_{[1]}$ denote the variable corresponding to the largest absolute value of the t-statistic (i.e., the smallest p-value) and suppose the corresponding regression model is

$$Y = \beta_0 + \beta_1 X_{[1]} + \varepsilon.$$

If H_0 is not rejected (because the absolute value of the t-statistic is smaller than the $t_{N-2,\alpha/2}$ critical value, with $\alpha = \alpha_{\text{enter}}$, i.e., if the p-value is greater than α_{enter}), then the stepwise procedure terminates and the chosen model is

$$Y = \beta_0 + \varepsilon.$$

If, however the absolute value of the t-statistic is greater than $t_{N-2,\alpha/2}$, then $X_{[1]}$ is retained, since we see it as being significant at the α_{enter} level. In the second step, we then consider $k-1$ possible regressions, each with two predictor variables

$$Y = \beta_0 + \beta_1 X_{[1]} + \beta_2 X_j + \varepsilon,$$

which includes the predictor $X_{[1]}$ chosen in Step 1, and one of the other $k-1$ predictors. For each model, the t-statistic (and p-value) associated with testing $H_0 : \beta_2 = 0$ versus $H_1 : \beta_2 \neq 0$ is computed. Let $X_{[2]}$ denote the variable corresponding to the largest absolute value of the t-statistic (i.e., the smallest p-value) and suppose the corresponding regression model is

$$Y = \beta_0 + \beta_1 X_{[1]} + \beta_2 X_{[2]} + \varepsilon.$$

The variable $X_{[2]}$ is retained if the t-statistic indicates that it is significant at the α_{enter} level, and the stepwise procedure also checks to see whether or not $X_{[1]}$ should continue to remain in the model. If the p-value corresponding to $H_0 : \beta_1 = 0$ versus $H_1 : \beta_1 \neq 0$ is smaller than α_{stay}, then $X_{[1]}$ is significant and is retained; otherwise, it is dropped from the model. If $X_{[1]}$ is retained in the model, we have a two-variable model and we proceed to the next step. If, on the other hand, $X_{[1]}$ is dropped, the current one-variable model is

$$Y = \beta_0 + \beta_2 X_{[2]} + \varepsilon.$$

We now are back to the position at the start of the second step, and must search for another predictor variable that is significant and will be included in the model.

We continue with this procedure of adding predictor variables into the model, one at a time. At each step, a variable is included in the model only if it has the largest t-statistic among all variables not in the model, and further, it is significant at the α_{enter} level. After including a variable, the procedure checks all the variables in the model and excludes any variable that is not significant at the α_{stay} level. All necessary exclusions are made before the procedure attempts to include a "new" variable. The procedure terminates when all the predictor variables that are excluded are insignificant at the α_{enter} level, or when the variable to be included in the model is the one that was just removed. The choice of values for α_{enter} and α_{stay} is arbitrary and has been discussed in the literature. In general, it is recommended that α_{stay} is greater than α_{enter}, since this will preclude the subsequent "easy" inclusion of the same variable which was previously excluded. Draper and Smith (1998) suggest that α_{enter} and α_{stay} are equal, and each is either .05 or .10. If α_{enter} and α_{stay} are set higher than 0.10, more independent variables are likely to be included in the model. In general, it is likely that some important variables (such as higher order terms or interaction terms) may be omitted, while some unimportant variables may be included in the model.

The *forward selection* procedure is a sequential variable selection procedure that systematiclly adds explanatory variables to the existing regression model on the basis of partial F-tests (see section 8.1.2). The idea behind the procedure is similar to that of stepwise regression, the difference being that once a predictor variable is included in the model, it is never removed. The initial model contains only the intercept term. In the next step, the explanatory variable which corresponds to the largest partial F-value enters the model, provided it is significant at the α_{enter} level. Let us denote this variable by $X_{[1]}$. In the next step, $X_{[2]}$, the regressor which has the largest partial F-value among the predictors outside the model is included, provided it is significant at the α_{enter} level. This process is continued until we have included all significant predictors into the model. Forward selection is usually considered to be less effective than stepwise regression.

The *backward elimination* procedure is a sequential procedure that systematically removes a predictor from an existing model based on partial F-test statistics. We first consider a model which includes all k potential predictor variables and an intercept. We pick the independent variable having the smallest partial F-statistic. If this statistic is significant at the α_{stay} level, then the final model contains all k variables, and the procedure is terminated. If, however, this varaible is not significant at the α_{stay} level, it is excluded from the model. At the next step, we run a regression with the remaining $(k-1)$ predictors, and repeat the first step. The backward elimination procedure continues by excluding, if possible, one variable at a time from the regression, and terminates when no predictor variable in the model can be removed. If a modeler prefers to start the model fitting by including all possible variables, then the backward elimination procedure is a reasonable approach. Quite often, it results in the same final model that is given by the stepwise regression procedure.

Another procedure known as the *MAXR* procedure selects variables for inclusion into a regression model based on R^2 values (see 4.2.20). Unlike the other methods discussed until now, the *MAXR* method looks for the "best" j-variable model, for $j = 1, \cdots, k$. We first select the one-variable model which gives the highest R^2 value. We then consider two-variable models, by including, one at a time, the remaining $(k-1)$ predictor variables, and choose the best two-variable model yielding the largest R^2 value. Each variable in this selected two-variable model is now compared to each of the $(k-2)$ variables not in the model. In each comparison, the $MAXR$ procedure determines whether substituting one of these $(k-2)$ variables for a variable currently in the model will increase the R^2 value. This process continues until we decide that no further substitutions which increases R^2 can be made, and we have chosen the "best" two-variable model. Another variable is included in the model, and the process is continued to find the "best" three-variable model, and so on. This procedure therefore gives us k "best" models.

Numerical Example 8.2. Variable selection. The following data relates to an engineering application that was concerned with the effect of the composition of cement on heat evolved during hardening (Woods, Steinour and Starke, 1932). The data consists of 4 predictor variables, X_1, the amount of tricalcium aluminate, X_2, the amount of tricalcium silicate, X_3, the amount of tetracalcium alumino ferrite, and X_4, the amount of dicalcium silicate. The response variable is Y, the heat evolved per gram of cement (in calories). Results from the different selection procedures are summarized below. All variables left in the model are significant at the 0.10 level.

R^2 selection method

No. in model	R^2	C_p	Vars. in model
1	0.674	138.731	X_4
1	0.666	142.486	X_2
2	0.979	2.678	X_1, X_2
2	0.973	5.496	X_1, X_4
3	0.982	3.018	X_1, X_2, X_4
3	0.982	3.041	X_1, X_2, X_3
4	0.982	5.000	X_1, X_2, X_3, X_4

Summary of forward selection

Step	Var. in	No. of vars. in	Partial R^2	Model R^2	C_p	F-value	Pr > F
1	X_4	1	0.675	0.675	138.731	22.80	0.0006
2	X_1	2	0.299	0.973	5.496	108.22	< .0001
3	X_2	3	0.010	0.982	3.018	5.03	0.052

Final parameter estimates under forward selection

Var.	Estimate	s.e.	F-value	Pr $> F$
Intercept	71.648	14.142	25.67	0.0007
X_1	1.452	0.117	154.01	$< .0001$
X_2	0.416	0.186	5.03	0.052
X_4	-0.237	0.173	1.86	0.205

Summary of backward elimination

Step	Var. removed	No. vars. in	Partial R^2	Model R^2	C_p	F-value	Pr $> F$
1	X_3	3	0.000	0.982	3.018	0.02	0.896
2	X_4	2	0.004	0.979	2.678	1.86	0.205

Final parameter estimates under backward elimination

Var.	Estimate	s.e.	F-value	Pr $> F$
Intercept	52.577	2.286	528.91	$< .0001$
X_1	1.468	0.121	146.52	$< .0001$
X_2	0.662	0.046	208.58	$< .0001$

Summary of stepwise selection

Step	Var. entered	Var. removed	No. vars.	Partial R^2	Model R^2	C_p	F-value	Pr $> F$
1	X_4		1	0.675	0.675	138.731	22.80	.0006
2	X_1		2	0.298	0.973	5.496	108.22	$< .0001$
3	X_2		3	0.010	0.982	3.018	5.03	.0517
4		X_4	2	0.004	0.979	2.678	1.86	.2054

Final parameter estimates under stepwise selection

Var.	Estimate	s.e.	F-value	Pr $> F$
Intercept	52.577	2.286	528.91	$< .0001$
X_1	1.468	0.121	146.52	$< .0001$
X_2	0.662	0.046	208.58	$< .0001$

For more details, see the first author's website. ▲

8.3   Orthogonal and collinear predictors

Suppose that in the model $\mathbf{y} = \mathbf{X}\beta + \varepsilon$ we can partition the $N \times p$ matrix $\mathbf{X}$ into $(r + 1)$ sets of columns denoted in matrix form by

$$\mathbf{X} = (\mathbf{X}_0, \mathbf{X}_1, \cdots, \mathbf{X}_r),$$

and that the p-dimensional vector β is partitioned conformably so that

$$\beta' = (\beta_0, \beta_1, \cdots, \beta_r).$$

The linear regression model can be written as

$$\mathbf{y} = \mathbf{X}_0\beta_0 + \mathbf{X}_1\beta_1 + \cdots + \mathbf{X}_r\beta_r.$$

8.3.1   Orthogonality in regression

Orthogonality among the predictors comes up occasionally in regression problems. We take a brief look in this section. In Figure 8.3.1, $\mathbf{1}_N$ and $\mathbf{x}$ are orthogonal vectors. It follows that $\mathrm{OC}^2 = \mathrm{OA}^2 + \mathrm{OB}^2$.

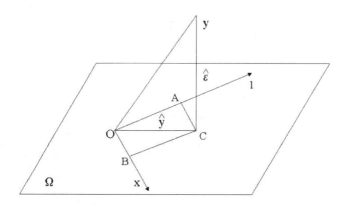

Figure 8.3.1.   Orthogonal predictors, $p = 2$.

Result 8.3.1.   Suppose that the columns of $\mathbf{X}_h$ are orthogonal to the columns of $\mathbf{X}_j$ for all $h \neq j$, i.e., $\mathbf{X}_h'\mathbf{X}_j = \mathbf{0}$. The least squares estimate of β_j in the full model $\mathbf{y} = \mathbf{X}\beta + \varepsilon$ is unchanged if any of the other β_h's are set equal to zero, i.e., if the corresponding sets of regressors $\mathbf{X}_h$'s are omitted from the model.

Proof.   The matrix $\mathbf{X}'\mathbf{X}$ in its partitioned form has a block-diagonal structure, i.e.,

$$\mathbf{X'X} = \begin{pmatrix} \mathbf{X'_0 X_0} & 0 & \cdots & 0 \\ 0 & \mathbf{X'_1 X_1} & \cdots & 0 \\ \vdots & \vdots & \vdots & \vdots \\ 0 & 0 & \cdots & \mathbf{X'_r X_r} \end{pmatrix},$$

and $\mathbf{X'y} = \begin{pmatrix} \mathbf{X'_0 y} & \mathbf{X'_1 y} & \cdots & \mathbf{X'_r y} \end{pmatrix}'$. The least squares estimator of β is then $\widehat{\beta}' = (\widehat{\beta}_0, \widehat{\beta}_1, \cdots \widehat{\beta}_r)$, where $\widehat{\beta}_j = (\mathbf{X'_j X_j})^{-1}\mathbf{X'_j y}$, $j = 0, \cdots, r$ has the form of the least squares estimate of β_j in the model $\mathbf{y} = \mathbf{X}_j \beta_j + \varepsilon$. Due to the block-diagonal structure of $(\mathbf{X'X})^{-1}$, the least squares estimate of β_j in the full model $\mathbf{y} = \mathbf{X}\beta + \varepsilon$ is unchanged if any of the other β_h's are set equal to zero, i.e., if the corresponding sets of regressors $\mathbf{X}_h$'s are omitted from the regression. This is a special property unique to orthogonal regressors. In this case the regression sum of squares is

$$\widehat{\beta}'\mathbf{X'y} = \sum_{j=0}^{r} \widehat{\beta}'_j \mathbf{X'_j y},$$

so that if we omit the regressor $\mathbf{X}_h$ from the model, the residual sum of squares is increased by $\widehat{\beta}'_h \mathbf{X'_h y}$. ■

Use of the Gram-Schmidt orthogonalization permits the full-rank model in (4.1.2) to be reparametrized and expressed as $Y_i = \gamma_0 + \gamma_1 Z_{i1} + \cdots + \gamma_k Z_{ik} + \varepsilon_i$, $i = 1, \cdots, N$, where the matrix $\mathbf{Z}$ has orthogonal columns, and for $r = 0, \cdots, k$, $\gamma_r = \gamma_{r+1} = \cdots = \gamma_k = 0$ if and only if $\beta_r = \beta_{r+1} = \cdots = \beta_k = 0$ (Seber, 1977, p. 60). Orthogonal polynomials have been used for overcoming problems, such as ill-conditioning, that are encountered in fitting polynomial regression models (Hayes, 1974), as the following examples describe.

Example 8.3.1. Orthogonal polynomials in curvilinear regression.
In the simple linear regression model (4.1.6), $E(Y|X)$ is a linear function of a predictor X. In some examples, however, there might be a curvilinear relation between the response and predictor variables, which may be adequately modeled by a polynomial model of degree m:

$$Y_i = \beta_0 + \beta_1 X_i + \beta_2 X_i^2 + \cdots + \beta_m X_i^m + \varepsilon_i, \quad i = 1, \cdots, N. \tag{8.3.1}$$

Written in the form $\mathbf{y} = \mathbf{X}\beta + \varepsilon$, with $\{\mathbf{X}\}_{i1} = 1$, and $\{\mathbf{X}\}_{ij} = X_i^j$, $j = 1, \cdots, m$, $i = 1, \cdots, N$, the properties of Corollary 7.1.1 hold for this mth order polynomial model. In practice, the degree m is unknown, and is determined using suitable tests of hypotheses (see section 7.4), which could be computationally intensive. Prior to the extensive availability of powerful computing, orthogonal polynomials in X were used.

Let $\phi_r(X_i)$ be an rth degree polynomial in X_i, $r = 0, 1, \cdots, m$, and suppose the polynomials are orthogonal over a set, i.e.,

$$\sum_{i=1}^{N} \phi_r(X_i)\phi_s(X_i) = 0, \tag{8.3.2}$$

for $r \neq s = 1, \cdots, m$. The orthogonal polynomial regression model

$$Y_i = \sum_{r=0}^{m} \beta_r \phi_r(X_i) + \varepsilon_i \qquad (8.3.3)$$

can be written in the form (4.1.1) with

$$\mathbf{X}^* = \begin{pmatrix} \phi_0(X_1) & \phi_1(X_1) & \cdots & \phi_m(X_1) \\ \phi_0(X_2) & \phi_1(X_2) & \cdots & \phi_m(X_2) \\ \vdots & \vdots & \vdots & \vdots \\ \phi_0(X_N) & \phi_1(X_N) & \cdots & \phi_m(X_N) \end{pmatrix},$$

having mutually orthogonal columns, so that $\mathbf{X}'\mathbf{X}$ is a diagonal matrix with rth diagonal element $\sum_{i=1}^{N} \phi_r^2(X_i)$, $r = 0, \cdots, m$. From (4.2.4), the least squares estimate of β is $\hat{\beta} = (\hat{\beta}_0, \cdots, \hat{\beta}_m)'$, where, for all m,

$$\hat{\beta}_r = \left\{ \sum_{i=1}^{N} \phi_r(X_i)Y_i \right\} \Big/ \left\{ \sum_{i=1}^{N} \phi_r^2(X_i) \right\}, \quad r = 0, 1, \cdots, m.$$

Due to the orthogonal structure of $\mathbf{X}$, $\hat{\beta}_r$, $r \leq m$ is independent of the polynomial degree m. If we set $\phi_0(X_i) = 1$, we get $\hat{\beta}_0 = \overline{Y}$, and

$$\begin{aligned} SSE &= \mathbf{y}'\mathbf{y} - \hat{\beta}'\mathbf{X}'\mathbf{X}\hat{\beta} \\ &= \sum_{i=1}^{N} Y_i^2 - \sum_{r=0}^{m} \hat{\beta}_r^2 \sum_{i=1}^{N} \phi_r^2(X_i) \\ &= \sum_{i=1}^{N} (Y_i - \overline{Y})^2 - \sum_{r=1}^{m} \hat{\beta}_r \sum_{i=1}^{N} \phi_r^2(X_i). \end{aligned}$$

Suppose we wish to test $H : \beta_m = 0$. By orthogonality,

$$\begin{aligned} SSE_H &= \sum_{i=1}^{N} (Y_i - \overline{Y})^2 - \sum_{r=1}^{m-1} \hat{\beta}_r^2 \sum_{i=1}^{N} \phi_r^2(X_i) \\ &= SSE + \hat{\beta}_m^2 \sum_{i=1}^{N} \phi_m^2(X_i), \end{aligned}$$

and it follows from (7.2.12) that the test statistic

$$F(H) = \left\{ \sum_{i=1}^{N} \phi_m^2(X_i)\hat{\beta}_m^2 \right\} \Big/ \{ SSE/(N - m - 1) \} \sim F_{1,N-m-1}$$

under H. $\square$

     The advantage of this approach is that the model of polynomial degree m may be easily enlarged to a model of polynomial degree $m + 1$ by simply adding one more term $\beta_{m+1}\phi_{m+1}(X_i)$ to (8.3.3), with $\phi_{m+1}(X_i)$ satisfying (8.3.2). It may be verified that the resulting computations are simplified by the assumption of orthogonality.

Example 8.3.2. Response surfaces. Consider the model

$$Y_i = \phi(X_{i1}, \cdots, X_{ik}) + \varepsilon_i, \quad i = 1, \cdots, N, \tag{8.3.4}$$

where $\phi(X_{i1}, X_{i2}, \cdots, X_{ik})$ is a polynomial of degree m in $X_1, \cdots, X_k$ (usually, $m = 2$, or $m = 3$). When $m = 2$, we can write for $i = 1, \cdots, N$,

$$Y_i = \beta_0 + \sum_{j=1}^{k} \beta_j X_{ij} + \sum_{j=1}^{k} \beta_{jj} X_{ij}^2 + \sum_{j=1}^{k} \sum_{l=1}^{k} \beta_{jl} X_{ij} X_{il} + \varepsilon_i. \tag{8.3.5}$$

The function $\phi(X_1, \cdots, X_k)$ is the *response surface*, and the model (8.3.5) can be written in the form (4.1.1) with $\mathbf{X} = (\mathbf{1}_N, \mathbf{X}_1, \mathbf{X}_2)$, where for $i = 1, \cdots, N$, $\{\mathbf{X}_1\}_{i,j} = X_{i,j}$, and $\{\mathbf{X}_2\}_{i,j}$ corresponds to values of X_{ij}^2, and $X_{ij}X_{il}$, $j, l = 1, \cdots, k$, $j \neq l$. Note that $\mathbf{X}_2$ is automatically determined once the variables in $\mathbf{X}_1$ are chosen. For details on optimum choice of $\mathbf{X}_1$ to achieve an optimum response Y, see Myers (1971). The results of Chapter 7 are useful in order to obtain the b.l.u.e.'s of the parameters and to carry out inference. □

8.3.2 Multicollinearity

A multiple regression model fit is useful if the response variable is highly correlated with the set of explanatory variables. However, it is necessary that the explanatory variables are not highly correlated among themselves. A situation where this occurs is referred to as multicollinearity. In this section, we assume that the regressors are scaled to unit length (by dividing X_{ij} by $\sqrt{\sum_{i=1}^{N} X_{ij}^2}$), but are not centered (Belsley, 1984). The resulting column-equilabrated predictor matrix $\mathbf{X}_E$ (see Example 4.1.2) is used for detecting multicollinearity. Collinearity (or multicollinearity) exists when there is "near-dependency" between the columns of $\mathbf{X}_E$, i.e., when $\mathbf{X}'_E \mathbf{X}_E$ is nearly singular. In such cases, the data/model pair is said to be ill-conditioned, and the resulting least squares estimates tend to be unstable with large variances and covariances. The presence of a high degree of multicollinearity tends to cause the following problems. First, the standard errors of the regression coefficients will be very large, resulting in small associated t-statistics, thereby leading to the conclusion that truly useful explanatory variables are insignificant in explaining the regression. Second, the sign of regression coefficients may be the opposite of what a mechanistic understanding of the problem would suggest. Third, deleting a column of the predictor matrix will cause large changes in the coefficient estimates corresponding to the other variables in a model based on the remaining data. Multicollinearity does not however, greatly affect the predicted values.

Several approaches have been suggested in the literature for the detection of multicollinearity. Detection consists of two aspects: (a) is multicollinearity

present? and (b) if it is, how severe is it? The following measures usually indicate severity of multicollinearity. The simple correlation between a pair of
predictors exceeds 0.9, or exceeds R^2. The multiple correlation coefficient between the explanatory variables is large, and some of the partial correlations
are high too, which helps in identifying problem variables. The value of the
overall F-statistic is large, but values of (some) t-statistics for individual regression coefficients are small. For $j = 1, \cdots, k$, let R_j^2 denote the coefficient of
determination of a regression of the explanatory variable X_j on the remaining
$(k-1)$ explanatory variables. A large value of R_j^2 also indicates multicollinearity.
Variance inflation factors formalize this notion.

Definition 8.3.1. Variance inflation factor.   For $j = 1, \cdots, k$, the quantity

$$VIF_j = 1/(1 - R_j^2)$$

denotes the variance inflation factor for X_j (the name is due to Marquardt).

In the ideal case when X_j is orthogonal to the other predictors, $R_j^2 = 0$, so
that $VIF_j = 1$. As R_j^2 increases from zero, VIF_j increases as well. For example,
if $R_j^2 = 0.8$, $VIF_j = 5.0$, while if $R_j^2 = 0.99$, $VIF_j = 100$. It has been suggested
in the literature that any VIF_j greater than 10 indicates multicollinearity. Alternatively, we may compute the average of the variance inflation factors, i.e.,
$\overline{VIF} = \sum_{j=1}^{k} VIF_j/k$. If $\overline{VIF}$ substantially exceeds 1, multicollinearity is indicated.

The column-equilibrated matrix $\mathbf{X}_E$ is useful in detecting multicollinearity
(Belsley, 1991). We find the singular value decomposition of $\mathbf{X}_E$ (see Result
2.2.6), i.e., $\mathbf{X}_E = \mathbf{UDV}'$, where $\mathbf{U}$ is $N \times p$, $\mathbf{D}$ is $p \times p$, $\mathbf{V}$ is $p \times p$, and
$\mathbf{U}'\mathbf{U} = \mathbf{V}'\mathbf{V} = \mathbf{VV}' = \mathbf{I}_p$. Let $\mathbf{D} = \text{diag}(d_1, \cdots, d_p)$, where the nonnegative
d_j's are the singular values of $\mathbf{X}_E$. Now

$$\mathbf{X}_E'\mathbf{X}_E = \mathbf{VDU}'\mathbf{UDV}' = \mathbf{VD}^2\mathbf{V}'$$

gives the spectral decomposition of the symmetric matrix $\mathbf{X}_E'\mathbf{X}_E$, so that $\mathbf{D}^2 =
\text{diag}(c_1, \cdots, c_p)$, where $c_j = d_j^2$ are the eigenvalues of $\mathbf{X}_E'\mathbf{X}_E$, while $\mathbf{V} = \{v_{ij}\}$
is the corresponding orthogonal eigenvector matrix. We obtain the p condition
indices in terms of d_j's and $d_{\max} = \max_{1 \leq j \leq p} d_j$.

Definition 8.3.2. Condition index.   The jth condition index is defined
by

$$\eta_j = d_{\max}/d_j, \quad j = 1, \cdots, p.$$

A value of d_j which is relatively close to zero will be associated with a
large condition index. If d_j is exactly equal to zero, there is an exact linear
relationship among the columns of $\mathbf{X}$. The quantity

$$C = d_{\max} / d_{\min},$$

where $d_{\min} = \min_{1 \leq j \leq p} d_j$, is called the condition number. The condition number C always exceeds 1. A large condition number (say, $C > 15$) indicates evidence of strong multicollinearity, and empirical evidence suggests the need for corrective action when $C > 30$. Since

$$Cov(\widehat{\beta})/\sigma^2 = (\mathbf{X}'_E \mathbf{X}_E)^{-1} = \mathbf{V}\mathbf{D}^{-2}\mathbf{V}'$$

where $\mathbf{D}^{-2} = \text{diag}(1/d_1^2, 1/d_2^2, \cdots, 1/d_p^2)$, we see that

$$Var(\widehat{\beta}_j)/\sigma^2 = \sum_{h=1}^{p} v_{jh}^2/d_h^2 = \left(\sum_{h=1}^{p} q_{jh}\right)\sum_{h=1}^{p} v_{jh}^2/d_h^2$$

is a decomposition of the variance structure of $\widehat{\beta}_j$, the q's being proportions (adding to 1) of $Var(\widehat{\beta}_j)/\sigma^2$. Large values of q_{jh} again indicate serious dependencies.

Once multicollinearity is detected, an obvious remedy is to drop from the model variables that are highly correlated with others. The disadvantage of this is that if the dropped variable is potentially valuable in an understanding of the response, we get absolutely no information about it, and moreover, it may not always be clear as to how the omission of a variable will affect the estimates of the remaining model parameters. Other statistical procedures for dealing with the problem of multicollinearity include ridge regression and principal components regression, which we discuss next.

8.3.3 Ridge regression

Hoerl (1962) first introduced the ridge trace procedure as a solution to certain multicollinearity problems in regression (see also Hoerl and Kennard, 1970a, b).

Result 8.3.2.   Consider the centered and scaled multiple regression model (see Example 4.1.2). Let $\overline{X}_j = \sum_{i=1}^{N} X_{ij}/N$, $S_{jh} = \sum_{i=1}^{N}(X_{ij} - \overline{X}_j)(X_{ih} - \overline{X}_h)$, $j, h = 1, \cdots, k$, and $S_{yy} = \sum_{i=1}^{N}(Y_i - \overline{Y})^2$. Let λ_i, $i = 1, \cdots, p$ be the eigenvalues of $\mathbf{X}^{*\prime}\mathbf{X}^*$.

1. The ridge regression estimates of the coefficients β_j^*, $j = 1, \cdots, k$ are given by

$$\widehat{\beta}^*(\theta) = (\mathbf{X}^{*\prime}\mathbf{X}^* + \theta \mathbf{I}_k)^{-1}\mathbf{X}^{*\prime}\mathbf{y}, \tag{8.3.6}$$

where θ is a positive number, usually assuming values between 0 and 1. Further, the corresponding least squares estimates of the coefficients in the model (4.1.2) are

$$\widehat{\beta}_j(\theta) = \widehat{\beta}_j^*(\theta)\sqrt{S_{yy}}/\sqrt{S_{jj}}, \quad j = 1, \cdots, k, \text{ and}$$

$$\widehat{\beta}_0(\theta) = \overline{Y} - \sum_{j=1}^{k}\widehat{\beta}_j(\theta)\overline{X}_j.$$

2. The expectation and covariance of $\widehat{\beta}^*(\theta)$ are

$$
\begin{aligned}
E\{\widehat{\beta}^*(\theta)\} &= (\mathbf{X}'\mathbf{X} + \theta\mathbf{I})^{-1}\mathbf{X}'\mathbf{X}\beta, \quad \text{and} \\
Cov\{\widehat{\beta}^*(\theta)\} &= (\mathbf{X}'\mathbf{X} + \theta\mathbf{I})^{-1}\mathbf{X}'\mathbf{X}(\mathbf{X}'\mathbf{X} + \theta\mathbf{I})^{-1}\sigma^2.
\end{aligned}
$$

3. The total mean square error of the ridge regression estimator is

$$
\begin{aligned}
E\{(\widehat{\beta}^*(\theta) - \beta)'(\widehat{\beta}^*(\theta) - \beta)\} &= \sigma^2 \sum_{j=1}^{p} \lambda_j(\lambda_j + \theta)^{-2} \\
&+ \theta^2 \beta'(\mathbf{X}'\mathbf{X} + \theta\mathbf{I})^{-2}\beta,
\end{aligned}
$$

where λ_j, $j = 1, \cdots, p$ are the eigenvalues of $\mathbf{X}'\mathbf{X}$.

Proof.   The form of $\widehat{\beta}^* = (\mathbf{X}'\mathbf{X} + \theta\mathbf{I})^{-1}\mathbf{X}'\mathbf{y}$ follows from the method of Lagrangian multipliers (see section 4.6.1). The transformation to the estimates in terms of the original coefficient vector β follows directly from the reasoning in Example 4.1.2. Since $\widehat{\beta}^*(\theta)$ is a linear function of $\mathbf{y}$, property 2 follows directly. To prove property 3, we see that by Result 2.3.4, $\mathbf{X}'\mathbf{X} = \mathbf{Q}\Delta\mathbf{Q}'$ for orthogonal $\mathbf{Q}$, so that the total variance of $\widehat{\beta}^*(\theta)$ is

$$
\begin{aligned}
tr[Var(\widehat{\beta}^*(\theta))] &= \sigma^2 tr[(\mathbf{X}'\mathbf{X} + \theta\mathbf{I})^{-1}\mathbf{X}'\mathbf{X}(\mathbf{X}'\mathbf{X} + \theta\mathbf{I})^{-1}] \\
&= \sigma^2 tr[(\mathbf{Q}\Delta\mathbf{Q}' + \theta\mathbf{I})^{-1}(\mathbf{Q}\Delta\mathbf{Q}')(\mathbf{Q}\Delta\mathbf{Q}' + \theta\mathbf{I})^{-1}] \\
&= \sigma^2 tr[(\Delta + \theta\mathbf{I})^{-1}\Delta(\Delta + \theta\mathbf{I})^{-1}] \\
&= \sigma^2 \sum_{j=1}^{p} \lambda_j(\lambda_j + \theta)^{-2},
\end{aligned}
$$

where $\Delta = \text{diag}(\lambda_1, \cdots, \lambda_p)$. Since the total mean square error of $\widehat{\beta}^*(\theta)$ is the sum of the total variance and the square of the bias, property 3 follows. Note that the total variance of the OLS estimator of β is $\sigma^2 \sum_{j=1}^{p} \lambda_j^{-1}$. When $\mathbf{X}'\mathbf{X}$ is nearly singular, some of the λ_j's may be very small, and the total variance of the OLS estimator of β is highly inflated in comparison to the total variance of the ridge estimator. ∎

When $\theta = 0$, the ridge regression estimates reduce to the usual least squares estimates. A plot of $\widehat{\beta}_j^*(\theta)$ versus θ or of $\widehat{\beta}_j(\theta)$ versus θ for $j = 1, \cdots, k$, is known as a ridge trace and is used to select a suitable value θ^* of θ using the following suggestions by Hoerl and Kennard (1970a, p. 65):

1. The estimates stabilize at a value of θ, with the general characteristics of an orthogonal system.

2. Estimated coefficients do not have unreasonable values.

3. Estimated values that had apparently incorrect signs at $\theta = 0$ have changed to the proper signs.

4. The SSE does not have an unreasonable value.

Alternatively, there is suggestion in the literature for an automatic choice of θ^* as the value

$$\theta^* = k\widehat{\sigma}^2 \Big/ \widehat{\beta}^*(0)'\widehat{\beta}^*(0)$$

where $\widehat{\sigma}^2$ is the MSE from the usual least squares fit and

$$\widehat{\beta}^*(0) = (\widehat{\beta}_1^*(0), \cdots, \widehat{\beta}_k^*(0))' = (\sqrt{S_{11}}\widehat{\beta}_1(0)/\sqrt{S_{yy}}, \cdots, \sqrt{S_{11}}\widehat{\beta}_k(0)/\sqrt{S_{yy}})'.$$

The corresponding values $\widehat{\beta}^*(\theta^*)$ are taken to be the final estimated coefficients, and can be used for prediction.

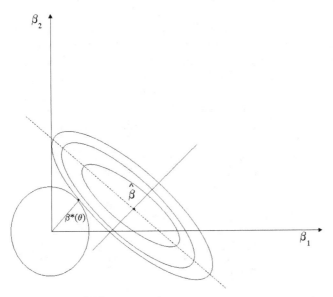

Figure 8.3.2.   Ridge regression.

We can characterize ridge regression as a restricted least squares problem. Consider least squares in the centered and scaled multiple regression model $\mathbf{y}^* = \mathbf{X}^*\beta^* + \varepsilon$ subject to the spherical restriction

$$\beta^{*\prime}\beta^* \le d^2, \tag{8.3.7}$$

for a given value d^2. Using the method of Lagrangian multipliers (see section 4.6.1) to minimize

$$S^* = (\mathbf{y}^* - \mathbf{X}^*\beta^*)'(\mathbf{y}^* - \mathbf{X}^*\beta^*) + \theta(\beta^{*\prime}\beta^* - d^2),$$

yields the equations

$$\begin{aligned}
(\mathbf{X}^{*\prime}\mathbf{X}^* + \theta\mathbf{I})\widehat{\beta}^* &= \mathbf{X}^{*\prime}\mathbf{y}^*, \text{ and}\\
\beta^{*\prime}\beta^* &= d^2,
\end{aligned}$$

whose solution leads to the ridge estimate of β^* in (8.3.6), and a solution for θ in terms of d. See Figure 8.3.2 for a geometric illustration for the case $k = 2$. While $\widehat{\beta}$ lies at the center of the innermost elliptical contour, the restricted solution lies on the innermost elliptical contour just touching the spherical restriction. As we reduce the radius from where the circle would pass through $\widehat{\beta}$ to $d = 0$, we obtain the entire sequence of ridge solutions; the *ridge* is the path traced by the solution point as the radius of the circle is increased from zero.

Note that use of an ellipsoidal restriction $\beta^{*\prime} \mathbf{A} \beta^* \leq d^2$ leads to a solution of the form

$$\widehat{\beta}^*_{\mathbf{A}}(\theta) = (\mathbf{X}^{*\prime} \mathbf{X}^* + \theta \mathbf{A})^{-1} \mathbf{X}^{*\prime} \mathbf{y}. \qquad (8.3.8)$$

The choice of the restriction can be viewed as a model selection problem.

Numerical Example 8.3. Multicollinearity.   The following data describes the manpower needs for operating a U.S. Navy bachelor officers' quarters, consisting of 25 establishments (Freund and Littell, 1991). The response variable Y is the monthly man hours needed to operate an establishment. The predictor variables are X_1, the average daily occupancy, X_2, the monthly average number of check-ins, X_3, the weekly hours of service desk operation, X_4, common use area (in sq. ft.), X_5, number of building wings, X_6, operational berthing capacity, and X_7, the number of rooms. Before we show diagnostics for multicollinearity, we give the basic results from OLS estimation. The last column in the table of least squares estimates shows the variance inflation factor for each variable.

ANOVA table for Numerical Example 8.3.

Source	d.f.	SS	MS	F-value	$\Pr > F$
Model	7	87382503	12483215	60.17	$< .0001$
Error	17	3526698	207453		
Corrected					
Total	24	90909201			

Least squares estimates

Parameter	d.f.	Estimate	s.e.	t-value	$\Pr > |t|$	VIF
Intercept	1	148.221	221.627	0.67	0.513	0
X1	1	-1.287	0.806	-1.60	0.129	2.166
X2	1	1.810	0.515	3.51	0.003	4.500
X3	1	0.590	1.800	0.33	0.747	1.406
X4	1	-21.482	10.223	-2.10	0.051	2.353
X5	1	5.619	14.756	0.38	0.708	3.653
X6	1	-14.515	4.226	-3.43	0.003	37.185
X7	1	29.360	6.370	4.61	0.0003	63.713

Condition Index

No.	Eigenvalue	Condition Index
1	6.476	1.000
2	0.594	3.302
3	0.356	4.263
4	0.268	4.914
5	0.142	6.748
6	0.083	8.840
7	0.076	9.216
8	0.005	37.448

Proportion of Variation by predictors

No.	Int.	X_1	X_2	X_3	X_4	X_5	X_6	X_7
1	.003	.005	.002	.002	.004	.003	.0003	.0002
2	.106	.111	.021	.041	.011	.001	.001	.0004
3	.052	.231	.006	.024	.113	.123	.0001	.0002
4	.0002	.464	.132	.001	.047	.048	.006	.001
5	.029	.010	.006	.002	.688	.434	$< .0001$	$< .0001$
6	.480	.0002	.187	.584	.001	.042	.025	.005
7	.328	.0001	.556	.344	.028	.045	.034	.006
8	.002	.179	.089	.001	.107	.305	.934	.987

One can also compute intercept adjusted collinearity diagnostics; see the first author's website for more details. ▲

8.3.4 Principal components regression

This is a more unified way to handle multicollinearity, but requires computations beyond standard regression computations. The procedure is based on the observation that every linear regression model can be restated in terms of a set of orthogonal predictor variables, which are constructed as linear combinations of the original variables. The new orthogonal variables are called the principal components (Johnson and Wichern, 1988) of the original variables. Principal components regression is an approach that inspects the sample data $(\mathbf{y}, \mathbf{X})$ for directions of variability and uses this information to reduce the dimensionality of the estimation problem. Let $\mathbf{X}'\mathbf{X} = \mathbf{Q}\Delta\mathbf{Q}'$ denote the spectral decomposition of $\mathbf{X}'\mathbf{X}$, where $\Delta = \mathrm{diag}(\lambda_1, \cdots, \lambda_p)$ is a diagonal matrix consisting of the (real) eigenvalues of $\mathbf{X}'\mathbf{X}$, with $\lambda_1 \geq \cdots \geq \lambda_p$ and $\mathbf{Q} = (\mathbf{q}_1, \cdots, \mathbf{q}_p)$ denotes the matrix whose columns are the orthogonal eigenvectors of $\mathbf{X}'\mathbf{X}$ corresponding to the ordered eigenvalues.

Consider the transformation

$$\mathbf{y} = \mathbf{X}\mathbf{Q}\mathbf{Q}'\beta + \varepsilon = \mathbf{Z}\theta + \varepsilon,$$

where $\mathbf{Z} = \mathbf{X}\mathbf{Q}$, and $\theta = \mathbf{Q}'\beta$. The elements of θ are known as the regression parameters of the principal components. Using this spectral decomposition, every regression model can be expressed in terms of orthogonal predictors, which are linear combinations of $X_1, \cdots, X_k$. The matrix $\mathbf{Z} = (\mathbf{z}_1, \cdots, \mathbf{z}_p)$ is called the matrix of principal components of $\mathbf{X}'\mathbf{X}$, while $\mathbf{z}_j = \mathbf{X}\mathbf{q}_j$ is the jth principal component of $\mathbf{X}'\mathbf{X}$. Note that $\mathbf{z}_j'\mathbf{z}_j = \lambda_j$, the jth largest eigenvalue of $\mathbf{X}'\mathbf{X}$. The principal components enable us to assess the presence of multicollinearity in a regression problem, and provides an alternate estimation approach. Notice however that the principal components lack a simple interpretation, each being some linear combination of the original predictors.

Principal components regression consists of deleting one or more of the variables $\mathbf{z}_j$ (which correspond to small values of λ_j), and using OLS estimation on the resulting reduced regression model. Suppose we partition $\mathbf{Z} = (\mathbf{Z}_1, \mathbf{Z}_2)$ and the other matrices and vectors conformably, so that we can write the regression model as

$$\mathbf{y} = \mathbf{Z}_1\theta_1 + \mathbf{Z}_2\theta_2 + \varepsilon.$$

Note that $\beta = \mathbf{Q}\theta = \mathbf{Q}_1\theta_1 + \mathbf{Q}_1\theta_2$. Assume that $\mathbf{Z}_1$ corresponds to the transformed predictor variables that will be retained in the model (they correspond to larger values of λ_j), while $\mathbf{Z}_2\theta_2$ will be discarded from the model. Let $\widehat{\theta}_1 = (\mathbf{Z}_1'\mathbf{Z}_1)^{-1}\mathbf{Z}_1'\mathbf{y}$ be the OLS estimator of θ_1 in the reduced model. Clearly, $E(\widehat{\theta}_1) = \theta_1$, and $Var(\widehat{\theta}_1) = \sigma^2(\mathbf{Z}_1'\mathbf{Z}_1)^{-1}$. The principal components estimator of β is

$$\widehat{\beta}_P = \mathbf{Q}_1\widehat{\theta}_1 = \mathbf{Q}(\widehat{\theta}_1', \mathbf{0}')'.$$

The principal components regression estimator $\widehat{\beta}_P$ is biased, but in general has smaller variance than $\widehat{\beta}$.

8.4   Prediction intervals and calibration

We first discuss *prediction intervals*. Example 8.4.1 illustrates this for a simple linear regression model.

Example 8.4.1.   Suppose $X_{0,1}$ is a specified value of X in a simple regression model. The predicted mean response corresponding to this value of the explanatory variable is

$$\widehat{Y}_0 = \widehat{\beta}_0 + \widehat{\beta}_1 X_{0,1} = \overline{Y} + \widehat{\beta}_1(X_{0,1} - \overline{X}_1). \tag{8.4.1}$$

Let $\mathbf{X}_0' = (1, X_{0,1})$. Then we can write $\widehat{Y}_0$ as a linear combination of $\widehat{\beta} = (\widehat{\beta}_0, \widehat{\beta}_1)'$:

$$\widehat{Y}_0 = (1, X_{0,1})\begin{pmatrix} \widehat{\beta}_0 \\ \widehat{\beta}_1 \end{pmatrix} = \mathbf{X}_0'\widehat{\beta}.$$

Therefore, $\widehat{Y}_0$ has a (singular) normal distribution with mean $E(\widehat{Y}_0) = \beta_0 + \beta_1 X_{0,1}$ and variance

$$
\begin{aligned}
Var(\widehat{Y}_0) &= Var(\overline{Y}) + (X_{0,1} - \overline{X}_1)^2 Var(\widehat{\beta}_1) \\
&= \frac{\sigma^2}{N} + \frac{(X_{0,1} - \overline{X}_1)^2 \sigma^2}{\sum_{i=1}^{N}(X_{i,1} - \overline{X}_1)^2}.
\end{aligned}
$$

Alternately, we can compute this variance using

$$
Var(\widehat{Y}_0) = Var(\widehat{\beta}_0) + X_{0,1}^2 Var(\widehat{\beta}_1) + 2X_{0,1}Cov(\widehat{\beta}_0, \widehat{\beta}_1).
$$

The estimated standard deviation of $\widehat{Y}_0$ is then

$$
est.s.e.(\widehat{Y}_0) = \widehat{\sigma}\left\{1/N + (X_{0,1} - \overline{X}_1)^2 / \sum_{i=1}^{N}(X_{i,1} - \overline{X}_1)^2\right\}^{1/2},
$$

which attains a minimum value when $X_{0,1}$ coincides with $\overline{X}_1$, and increases as the distance between the two values increases. Intuitively, this tells us that we expect inaccurate predictions for $X_{0,1}$ values that are outside the observed range of X values. We may now construct a $100(1 - \alpha)\%$ prediction interval for the mean value of the distribution of Y corresponding to a given $X_{0,1}$ value:

$$
\widehat{Y}_0 \pm t_{N-2,\alpha/2}\{est.s.e.(\widehat{Y}_0)\}
$$

where $t_{N-2,\alpha/2}$ corresponds to the upper $\alpha/2$th critical point from a t-distribution with $N - 2$ degrees of freedom. The actual (unobserved) value of Y varies about this true mean value with variance σ^2; the predicted value of an individual response corresponding to $X_{0,1}$ is still $\widehat{Y}_0$, with estimated variance

$$
est.\ Var(\widehat{Y}_0) = \widehat{\sigma}^2\left(1 + 1/N + (X_{0,1} - \overline{X}_1)^2 / \sum_{i=1}^{N}(X_{i,1} - \overline{X}_1)^2\right).
$$

Then

$$
\widehat{Y}_0 \pm t_{N-2,\alpha/2}\widehat{\sigma}\left(1 + 1/N + (X_{0,1} - \overline{X}_1)^2 / \sum_{i=1}^{N}(X_{i,1} - \overline{X}_1)^2\right)^{1/2}
$$

is the $100(1 - \alpha)\%$ prediction interval for an individual unknown response.

An extension of the marginal prediction intervals approach enables us to predict the average of L unknown future observations at $X_{0,1}$, which we denote by $\overline{Y}_0$ (when $L = 1$, we get the case we discussed above). We can verify that $\overline{Y}_0$ has a normal distribution with mean $\beta_0 + \beta_1 X_{0,1}$, and variance σ^2/L, which is independent of the distribution of $\widehat{Y}_0$. Hence,

$$
\overline{Y}_0 - \widehat{Y}_0 \sim N(0, \sigma^2/L + Var(\widehat{Y}_0));
$$

replacing σ^2 by its estimate $\widehat{\sigma}^2$, we derive the $100(1 - \alpha)\%$ confidence interval for $\overline{Y}_0$ as

$$
\widehat{Y}_0 \pm t_{N-2,\alpha/2}\,\widehat{\sigma}\left(1/L + 1/N + (X_{0,1} - \overline{X}_1)^2 / \sum_{i=1}^{N}(X_{i,1} - \overline{X}_1)^2\right)^{1/2}.
$$

These limits are wider than those for the mean response of Y corresponding to $X_{0,1}$, which is to be expected. $\square$

This procedure is useful for constructing point predictions and corresponding confidence intervals for unknown true mean responses or unknown individual responses corresponding to a set of different X values, say, $X_{0,1}, \cdots, X_{0,L}$. The confidence intervals for the responses $Y_{0,1}, \cdots, Y_{0,L}$ are called *marginal* intervals; the jth interval contains $Y_{0,j}$ with probability $1 - \alpha$. However, the joint probability that all the intervals simultaneously contain $Y_{0,j}$, $j = 1, \cdots, L$ is usually less than $1 - \alpha$. We can alternatively construct simultaneous prediction intervals, as well as simultaneous confidence curves for the whole regression function over its entire range. The latter are *confidence bands* which involve a critical value from the F-distribution.

Example 8.4.2.   We now show some results for the multiple regression models. Given a specified value of the predictors, viz., $\mathbf{x}_0' = (1, X_{1,0}, \cdots, X_{k,0})$, the predicted response is

$$\widehat{Y}_0 = \mathbf{x}_0'\widehat{\beta} = \widehat{\beta}_0 + \widehat{\beta}_1 X_{1,0} + \cdots + \widehat{\beta}_k X_{k,0} \qquad (8.4.2)$$

with mean $E(\widehat{Y}_0) = \beta_0 + \beta_1 X_{1,0} + \cdots + \beta_k X_{k,0}$ and variance

$$
\begin{aligned}
Var(\widehat{Y}_0) &= \sum_{j=1}^{k} X_{j,0}^2 Var(\widehat{\beta}_j) + \sum_{j=1}^{k}\sum_{\substack{l=1 \\ j \neq l}}^{k} X_{j,0} X_{l,0} Cov(\widehat{\beta}_j, \widehat{\beta}_l) \qquad (8.4.3) \\
&= \sigma^2 \mathbf{x}_0'(\mathbf{X}'\mathbf{X})^{-1}\mathbf{x}_0.
\end{aligned}
$$

Apart from σ^2, the prediction variance depends on the term $\mathbf{x}_0'(\mathbf{X}'\mathbf{X})^{-1}\mathbf{x}_0$, which we may denote by p_{00}. Clearly, if we let $\widehat{Y}_i$ denote $\mathbf{x}_i'\widehat{\beta}$, then $Var(\widehat{Y}_i) = p_{ii}$, the ith diagonal element of $\mathbf{P}$. The property $1/N \leq p_{ii} \leq 1$ implies that $1/N \leq Var(\widehat{Y}_i)/\sigma^2 \leq 1$. Apart from σ^2, the sum of the prediction variances over the N data locations is equal to the number of regression parameters, i.e., $\sum_{i=1}^{N} Var(\widehat{Y}_i)/\sigma^2 = tr(\mathbf{P}) = k+1$. This suggests the advantage of parsimonious models from the point of view of reducing the overall prediction variance. The $100(1 - \alpha)\%$ confidence interval for the true mean value of Y at $\mathbf{x}_0'$ is given by

$$\widehat{Y}_0 \pm t_{N-k-1,\alpha/2}\, \widehat{\sigma}\sqrt{\mathbf{x}_0'(\mathbf{X}'\mathbf{X})^{-1}\mathbf{x}_0}. \qquad (8.4.4)$$

On the other hand, if we wish to construct a prediction estimate of an individual Y response given $\mathbf{x}_0'$, the point estimate is still $\widehat{Y}_0$, while the $100(1 - \alpha)\%$ confidence interval is

$$\widehat{Y}_0 \pm t_{N-k-1,\alpha/2}\, \widehat{\sigma}\sqrt{1 + \mathbf{x}_0'(\mathbf{X}'\mathbf{X})^{-1}\mathbf{x}_0}. \quad \square \qquad (8.4.5)$$

Calibration is the problem of constructing confidence intervals for an unknown X_0 given Y_0. Consider fitting a straight line regression model to the pairs of observations $(X_i, Y_i), i = 1, \cdots, N$, for which the fitted line is $\widehat{Y} = \widehat{\beta}_0 + \widehat{\beta}_1 X$. Our interest is in obtaining point and interval estimates of the predictor variable X_0 corresponding to an observed Y_0. From the fitted least squares model, we may write $Y_0 = \widehat{\beta}_0 + \widehat{\beta}_1 \widehat{X}_0$, so that $\widehat{X}_0 = (Y_0 - \widehat{\beta}_0)/\widehat{\beta}_1$. This estimator $\widehat{X}_0$, which is also the MLE of X_0, is in general, biased. We consider two situations under which the confidence interval for X_0 is determined. First, let Y_0 denote the true mean value of the underlying response distribution. We solve for X_L and X_U as points of intersection of the line

$$Y = Y_0 = \widehat{\beta}_0 + \widehat{\beta}_1 \widehat{X}_0$$

and the curves (see Figure 8.4.1)

$$Y = Y_L - t_{N-2, \alpha/2} \left\{ \frac{\widehat{\sigma}^2}{N} + \frac{\widehat{\sigma}^2 (X_L - \overline{X})^2}{s_{XX}} \right\}^{1/2},$$

$$Y = Y_U + t_{N-2, \alpha/2} \left\{ \frac{\widehat{\sigma}^2}{N} + \frac{\widehat{\sigma}^2 (X_U - \overline{X})^2}{s_{XX}} \right\}^{1/2},$$

where $s_{XX} = \sum_{i=1}^{N} (X_i - \overline{X})^2$, $Y_L = \widehat{\beta}_0 + \widehat{\beta}_1 X_L$ and $Y_U = \widehat{\beta}_0 + \widehat{\beta}_1 X_U$. That is, we draw a horizontal line parallel to the x-axis at a height Y_0. From the point of intersection of the fitted line and this horizontal line, we drop a perpendicular to the x-axis, which gives the inverse point estimate $\widehat{X}_0$.

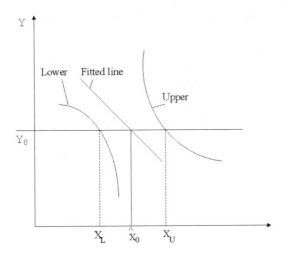

Figure 8.4.1. Calibration.

From the points where this line cuts the confidence interval curves, we drop perpendiculars onto the x-axis to give the lower and upper $100(1 - \alpha)\%$ inverse confidence limits X_L and X_U. Williams (1959) referred to these as "fiducial limits". Algebraically, we set

$$\widehat{\beta}_0 + \widehat{\beta}_1 \widehat{X}_0 = \widehat{\beta}_0 + \widehat{\beta}_1 X^* \pm t \left\{ \widehat{\sigma}^2/N + \widehat{\sigma}^2 (X_L - \overline{X})^2 / s_{XX} \right\}^{1/2},$$

where X^* represents X_L or X_U and we denote $t_{N-2,\alpha/2}$ simply by t. This simplifies to a quadratic expression in X^*:

$$\left(\widehat{\beta}_1^2 - t^2 \widehat{\sigma}^2 s_{XX} \right) X^{*2} + 2 \left(\overline{X} t^2 \widehat{\sigma}^2 / s_{XX} - \widehat{X}_0 \widehat{\beta}_1^2 \right) X^* +$$
$$\left(\widehat{\beta}_1^2 \widehat{X}_0^2 - t^2 \widehat{\sigma}^2 / N - \overline{X}^2 t^2 \widehat{\sigma}^2 / s_{XX} \right).$$

Setting this equal to zero and solving, we obtain

$$X_L = \overline{X} + \frac{\widehat{\beta}_1 (Y_0 - \overline{Y}) - t\widehat{\sigma} \left\{ (Y_0 - \overline{Y})^2 / s_{XX} + \widehat{\beta}_1^2 / N - t^2 \widehat{\sigma}^2 / N s_{XX} \right\}^{1/2}}{\widehat{\beta}_1^2 - t^2 \widehat{\sigma}^2 / s_{XX}},$$

$$X_U = \overline{X} + \frac{\widehat{\beta}_1 (Y_0 - \overline{Y}) + t\widehat{\sigma} \left\{ (Y_0 - \overline{Y})^2 / s_{XX} + \widehat{\beta}_1^2 / N - t^2 \widehat{\sigma}^2 / N s_{XX} \right\}^{1/2}}{\widehat{\beta}_1^2 - t^2 \widehat{\sigma}^2 / s_{XX}}.$$

In general, inverse estimation is not very informative unless the regression of Y on X is significant, i.e., β_1 is significantly different from zero. In such cases, it might happen that (a) the two roots of the quadratic equation in X^* are complex, or (b) the roots X_L and X_U are real-valued, but the interval (X_L, X_U) does not contain $\widehat{X}_0$ because the endpoints lie on the same side of the regression line.

We next assume that Y_0 denotes an individual value from the response distribution. In this case, we solve for X_L and X_U as points of intersection of the line $Y = Y_0 = \widehat{\beta}_0 + \widehat{\beta}_1 \widehat{X}_0$ and the curves

$$Y = Y_L - t_{N-2,\alpha/2} \left\{ \widehat{\sigma}^2 + \frac{\widehat{\sigma}^2}{N} + \frac{\widehat{\sigma}^2 (X_L - \overline{X})^2}{s_{XX}} \right\}^{1/2},$$

$$Y = Y_U + t_{N-2,\alpha/2} \left\{ \widehat{\sigma}^2 + \frac{\widehat{\sigma}^2}{N} + \frac{\widehat{\sigma}^2 (X_U - \overline{X})^2}{s_{XX}} \right\}^{1/2}.$$

Setting

$$\widehat{\beta}_1^2 (\widehat{X}_0 - X^*)^2 / t^2 \widehat{\sigma}^2 = \left(1 + 1/N + (X^* - \overline{X})^2 / s_{XX} \right),$$

we solve the resulting quadratic equation in X^* for X_L and X_U:

$$\left(\widehat{\beta}_1^2 - \frac{t^2 \widehat{\sigma}^2}{s_{XX}} \right) X^{*2} + 2 \left(\frac{\overline{X} t^2 \widehat{\sigma}^2}{s_{XX}} - \widehat{X}_0 \widehat{\beta}_1^2 \right) X^* +$$
$$\left(\widehat{\beta}_1^2 \widehat{X}_0^2 - t^2 \widehat{\sigma}^2 - \frac{t^2 \widehat{\sigma}^2}{N} - \frac{\overline{X}^2 t^2 \widehat{\sigma}^2}{s_{XX}} \right) = 0.$$

Numerical Example 8.4. Inverse simple linear regression. The data consists of observations taken at intervals from a steam plant which is part of a large industry. The data is a portion of a larger data set used to fit a multiple regression model (Draper and Smith, 1998). The response and predictor variables are respectively Y, the monthly use of steam (pounds), and X, the average atmospheric pressure (degrees F). Given a true mean response value of $Y_0 = 10$, we construct a point estimate and an interval estimate of the predictor X_0 corresponding to Y_0. The least squares estimates and ANOVA table for the regression of Y on X are shown below.

Least squares estimates for Numerical Example 8.4.

Variable	d.f.	Estimate	s.e.	t-value	$\Pr > |t|$
Intercept	1	13.623	0.581	23.43	$< .0001$
X	1	-0.080	0.011	-7.59	$< .0001$

ANOVA table

Source	d.f.	SS	MS	F-value	$\Pr > F$
Model	1	45.592	45.592	57.54	$< .0001$
Error	23	18.223	0.792		
Corrected Total	24	63.816			

Also, $\widehat{\sigma} = 0.89$, $R^2 = 0.714$, $\overline{X} = 52.6$, $s_{xx} = 7063.4$, and $t_{22,.025} = 2.069$. When $Y_0 = 10$ is the true mean response, we compute $\widehat{X}_0 = 45.4$, and also solve for $(X_L, X_U) = (40.576, 48.881)$. If on the other hand, Y_0 is an *individual* value, the value of $\widehat{X}_0$ remains the same, while $(X_L, X_U) = (20.356, 69.102)$. ▲

8.5 Regression diagnostics

In this section, we continue to explore aspects of regression model fitting. In particular, we look more closely at properties of the residuals and the projection matrix that enable us to diagnose abnormal features in the regression model. *Diagnostic measures* are statistical measures used for detecting problems with regression models and/or observations or variables in the data set, including problems of model misspecification, outliers, influential observations, and collinearity. Belsley, Kuh and Welsch (1980) give an extensive description of these topics, while a more theoretical discussion is found in Chatterjee and Hadi (1988).

8.5.1   Further properties of the projection matrix

As seen earlier, the symmetric and idempotent *hat matrix* or *projection matrix* $\mathbf{P} = \{p_{ij}\} = \mathbf{X}(\mathbf{X'X})^{-1}\mathbf{X'}$ plays an important role in regression analysis. We write $p_{ii} = \mathbf{x}_i'(\mathbf{X'X})^{-1}\mathbf{x}_i$, $i = 1, \cdots, N$, and $p_{ij} = \mathbf{x}_i'(\mathbf{X'X})^{-1}\mathbf{x}_j$, $i, j = 1, \cdots, N$. The matrix $(\mathbf{I} - \mathbf{P})$ is also symmetric and idempotent and is often called the *residuals matrix*. We have seen in section 4.2 that $\mathbf{PX} = \mathbf{X}$, $(\mathbf{I} - \mathbf{P})\mathbf{X} = \mathbf{0}$, $\widehat{\mathbf{Y}} = \mathbf{PY}$, and $\widehat{\varepsilon} = (\mathbf{I} - \mathbf{P})\mathbf{Y} = (\mathbf{I} - \mathbf{P})\varepsilon$. That is, $\widehat{\varepsilon}_i = \varepsilon_i - \sum_{j=1}^{N} p_{ij}\varepsilon_j$, and the relation between the ith error and the ith residual only depends on $\mathbf{P}$. If p_{ij}'s are sufficiently small, then $\widehat{\varepsilon}$ is a reasonable substitute for ε. Further, $Var(\widehat{Y}_i) = \sigma^2 p_{ii}$, $Var(\widehat{\varepsilon}_i) = \sigma^2(1 - p_{ii})$, and $Cov(\widehat{\varepsilon}_i, \widehat{\varepsilon}_j) = -\sigma^2 p_{ij}$, $i, j = 1, \cdots, N$. The ith predicted response can be written as

$$\widehat{Y}_i = \sum_{i=1}^{N} p_{ij}Y_j = p_{ii}Y_i + \sum_{i \neq j} p_{ij}Y_j, \ i = 1, \cdots, N, \qquad (8.5.1)$$

from which we see that

$$\partial \widehat{Y}_i / \partial Y_i = p_{ii}, \ i = 1, \cdots, N \quad \text{and} \quad \partial \widehat{Y}_i / \partial Y_j = p_{ij}, \ i, j = 1, \cdots, N. \quad (8.5.2)$$

Suppose $\mathbf{X} = \begin{pmatrix} \mathbf{X}_1 & \mathbf{X}_2 \end{pmatrix}$, where $\mathbf{X}_1$ is an $N \times q$ matrix of rank q, and $\mathbf{X}_2$ is an $N \times (p - q)$ matrix of rank $(p - q)$. Let $\mathbf{P}_j = \mathbf{X}_j(\mathbf{X}_j'\mathbf{X}_j)^{-1}\mathbf{X}_j'$ denote the projection matrix for $\mathbf{X}_j$, $j = 1, 2$. Let $\mathbf{X}_2^*$ denote the projection of $\mathbf{X}_2$ onto $\mathcal{C}^\perp(\mathbf{X}_1)$, i.e., $\mathbf{X}_2^* = (\mathbf{I} - \mathbf{P}_1)\mathbf{X}_2$. Let $\mathbf{P}_2^* = \mathbf{X}_2^*(\mathbf{X}_2^{*'}\mathbf{X}_2^*)^{-1}\mathbf{X}_2^{*'} = (\mathbf{I} - \mathbf{P}_1)\mathbf{X}_2(\mathbf{X}_2'(\mathbf{I} - \mathbf{P}_1)\mathbf{X}_2)^{-1}\mathbf{X}_2'(\mathbf{I} - \mathbf{P}_1)$. The projection of $\mathbf{y}$ onto $\mathcal{C}(\mathbf{X})$ can be partitioned into the sum of two projections, i.e., $\mathbf{P} = \mathbf{P}_1 + \mathbf{P}_2^*$ (see Example 2.1.2).

Result 8.5.1.   Let $\mathbf{P} = \{p_{ij}\}$ denote the $N \times N$ projection matrix. Then,

1. $\sum_{i=1}^{N} \sum_{j=1}^{N} p_{ij}^2 = p.$

2. $0 \le p_{ii} \le 1$, $i = 1, \cdots, N$.

3. $-0.5 \le p_{ij} \le 0.5$, $i, j = 1, \cdots, N$, $i \neq j$.

4. In the regression model with intercept, $p_{ii} \ge 1/N$, $i = 1, \cdots, N$.

Proof.   Since $\mathbf{P}$ is symmetric and idempotent, $\sum_{i=1}^{N} \sum_{j=1}^{N} p_{ij}^2 = tr(\mathbf{P}^2) = r(\mathbf{P}) = p$, proving property 1. Also, since $p_{ii} = \sum_{j=1}^{N} p_{ij}^2 = p_{ii}^2 + \sum_{j \neq i} p_{ij}^2$, property 2 follows directly. To prove property 3, we write $p_{ii} = p_{ii}^2 + p_{ij}^2 + \sum_{l \neq i,j} p_{il}^2$, so that $p_{ij}^2 \le p_{ii}(1 - p_{ii})$, i.e., $-0.5 \le p_{ij} \le 0.5$, using property 2. We next prove property 4. Let $\mathbf{X} = (\mathbf{1}_N, \mathbf{X}_2)$. Here $\mathbf{P}_1 = \mathbf{1}_N(\mathbf{1}_N'\mathbf{1}_N)^{-1}\mathbf{1}_N' = \mathbf{1}_N\mathbf{1}_N'/N$, $\mathbf{X}_2^* = (\mathbf{I} - \mathbf{P}_1)\mathbf{X}_2 = (\mathbf{I} - \mathbf{1}_N\mathbf{1}_N'/N)\mathbf{X}_2 = (\mathbf{I} - \overline{\mathbf{J}}_N)\mathbf{X}_2$, and $\mathbf{P}_2^* = \mathbf{X}_2^*(\mathbf{X}_2^{*'}\mathbf{X}_2^*)^{-1}\mathbf{X}_2^{*'}$. Then, $\mathbf{P} = \mathbf{P}_1 + \mathbf{P}_2^*$ (see Example 2.1.2); $(\mathbf{P}_1)_{ii} = 1/N$,

$i = 1, \cdots, N$, and $(\mathbf{P}_2^*)_{ii} \geq 0$, $i = 1, \cdots, N$ (since $\mathbf{P}_2^*$ is a projection matrix), from which it follows that $p_{ii} \geq 1/N$, $i = 1, \cdots, N$. ∎

The relationship between the elements of $\mathbf{P}$ and the residuals $\widehat{\varepsilon}_i$ is stated below and will be useful for a later discussion on the relative usefulness of different transformed residuals for diagnostic purposes. Notice that if p_{ii} is large (i.e., near 1), or small (i.e., near 0), then p_{ij}, $j \neq i$ will be small. Also, $p_{ii} + \widehat{\varepsilon}_i^2/\widehat{\varepsilon}'\widehat{\varepsilon} \leq 1$, where $\widehat{\varepsilon}'\widehat{\varepsilon} = \sum_{i=1}^N \widehat{\varepsilon}_i^2$, so that observations with larger p_{ii} will tend to have smaller residuals $\widehat{\varepsilon}_i$, and the usual residual plots will not identify these observations as anomalies.

8.5.2 Types of residuals

In Chapter 4, we defined ordinary least squares residuals $\widehat{\varepsilon}_i$, $i = 1, \cdots, N$. We have seen that the vector $\widehat{\varepsilon} = (\widehat{\varepsilon}_1, \cdots, \widehat{\varepsilon}_N)$ has mean $\mathbf{0}$, while $E(\widehat{\varepsilon}\widehat{\varepsilon}') = \sigma^2(\mathbf{I}-\mathbf{P})$. We now introduce four transformations of the ordinary residuals, viz., normalized residuals, standardized residuals, internally Studentized residuals and externally Studentized residuals. In general, the ith transformed residual is defined by

$$\widehat{\varepsilon}_i^* = \widehat{\varepsilon}_i/\sigma_i, \quad i = 1, \cdots, N, \tag{8.5.3}$$

where σ_i is the standard deviation of the ith residual $\widehat{\varepsilon}_i$ (the square-root of the ith diagonal element of $\sigma^2(\mathbf{I}-\mathbf{P})$). By using different estimates for the unknown parameter σ_i in (8.5.3), we obtain the four definitions shown below.

Definition 8.5.1. The ith *normalized residual* is defined by

$$a_i = \frac{\widehat{\varepsilon}_i}{(\widehat{\varepsilon}'\widehat{\varepsilon})^{1/2}}, \quad i = 1, \cdots, N. \tag{8.5.4}$$

Definition 8.5.2. The ith *standardized residual* is defined by

$$b_i = \frac{\widehat{\varepsilon}_i}{\widehat{\sigma}}, \quad i = 1, \cdots, N, \tag{8.5.5}$$

where $\widehat{\sigma} = \{\widehat{\varepsilon}'\widehat{\varepsilon}/(N-p)\}^{1/2}$.

Definition 8.5.3. The ith *internally Studentized residual* is

$$r_i = \frac{\widehat{\varepsilon}_i}{\widehat{\sigma}(1-p_{ii})^{1/2}}, \quad i = 1, \cdots, N. \tag{8.5.6}$$

Definition 8.5.4. The ith *externally Studentized residual* is

$$r_i^* = \frac{\widehat{\varepsilon}_i}{\widehat{\sigma}_{(i)}(1-p_{ii})^{1/2}}, \quad i = 1, \cdots, N, \tag{8.5.7}$$

where

$$\widehat{\sigma}^2_{(i)} = SSE_{(i)}/(N-p-1) = \mathbf{y}'_{(i)}(\mathbf{I} - \mathbf{P}_{(i)})\mathbf{y}_{(i)}/(N-p-1), \quad i = 1, \cdots, N$$

is the residual mean square estimate when the ith observation is omitted from the fit, and

$$\mathbf{P}_{(i)} = \mathbf{X}_{(i)}[\mathbf{X}'_{(i)}\mathbf{X}_{(i)}]^{-1}\mathbf{X}'_{(i)}, \quad i = 1, \cdots, N$$

is the projection matrix for $\mathbf{X}_{(i)}$, the matrix of explanatory variables when the ith observation is omitted.

Result 8.5.2.   The following relationships between the residuals hold:

1. $b_i = a_i(N-p)^{1/2}$.

2. $r_i = b_i/(1-p_{ii})^{1/2} = a_i(N-p)^{1/2}/(1-p_{ii})^{1/2}$.

3. $r_i^* = a_i(N-p-1)^{1/2}/(1-p_{ii}-a_i^2)^{1/2} = r_i(N-p-1)^{1/2}/(N-p-r_i^2)^{1/2}$.

Proof.   The proof of the first two relations follows directly from their definitions. To prove property 3, observe that omission of the ith observation is equivalent to fitting the *mean-shift outlier model*

$$E(Y) = \mathbf{X}\beta + \mathbf{u}_i\theta = (\mathbf{X}, \mathbf{u}_i)(\beta', \theta)',$$

where $\mathbf{u}_i$ is an N-dimensional vector with 1 in the ith position, and zero elsewhere, and θ is the corresponding regression coefficient. Using results from section 2.1, we can show that

$$
\begin{aligned}
SSE_{(i)} &= \mathbf{y}'_{(i)}(\mathbf{I} - \mathbf{P}_{(i)})\mathbf{y}_{(i)} \\
&= \mathbf{y}'[(\mathbf{I} - \mathbf{P}) - \frac{(\mathbf{I}-\mathbf{P})\mathbf{u}_i\mathbf{u}'_i(\mathbf{I}-\mathbf{P})}{\mathbf{u}'_i(\mathbf{I}-\mathbf{P})\mathbf{u}_i}]\mathbf{y} \\
&= SSE - \frac{\widehat{\varepsilon}_i^2}{1-p_{ii}},
\end{aligned}
$$

so that, dividing throughout by $(N-p-1)$, and using $r_i^2 = \widehat{\varepsilon}_i^2/\widehat{\sigma}^2(1-p_{ii})$,

$$
\begin{aligned}
\widehat{\sigma}^2_{(i)} &= \frac{(N-p)}{(N-p-1)}\widehat{\sigma}^2 - \frac{\widehat{\varepsilon}_i^2}{(N-p-1)(1-p_{ii})} \\
&= \frac{(N-p-r_i^2)}{(N-p-1)}\widehat{\sigma}^2.
\end{aligned}
$$

Substituting this result into the definition of r_i^*, we get

$$
\begin{aligned}
r_i^* &= \frac{\widehat{\varepsilon}_i}{\widehat{\sigma}_{(i)}(1-p_{ii})^{1/2}} \\
&= \frac{\widehat{\varepsilon}_i(N-p-1)^{1/2}}{\widehat{\sigma}(1-p_{ii})^{1/2}(N-p-r_i^2)^{1/2}},
\end{aligned}
$$

from which property 3 follows.   ∎

Thus, r_i^* is a monotonic transformation of r_i, which itself is a monotonic transformation of a_i. As $r_i^2 \to (N - p)$, $r_i^{*2} \to \infty$, and therefore the latter reflects large deviations more dramatically. Both being constant multiples of $\widehat{\varepsilon}_i$, the normalized residuals a_i and the standardized residuals b_i are equivalent as diagnostic measures. A disadvantage may be that neither residual takes into account $Var(\widehat{\varepsilon}_i)$, i.e., the diagonal elements of the projection matrix. Although this might not be critically important in some situations, it would be preferable to use the r_i when the p_{ii} vary substantially. We state two distributional properties (for proof, see Chatterjee and Hadi, 1988, section 4.2). Result 8.5.3, which is due to Ellenberg (1973), implies that $|r_i|$ cannot exceed $(N - p)^{1/2}$, while Result 8.5.4, which was proved by Beckman and Trussel (1974), shows that the square of the externally Studentized residual follows an F-distribution.

Result 8.5.3. If $r(\mathbf{X}_{(i)}) = p$, then $r_i^2 / (N - p)$, $i = 1, \cdots, N$ are identically distributed as $Beta(1/2, (N - p - 1)/2)$ variables, and the covariance between r_i and r_j is $Cov(r_i, r_j) = -(1 - p_{ii})^{-1/2}(1 - p_{jj})^{-1/2}p_{ij}$. ∎

Result 8.5.4. Provided $r(\mathbf{X}_{(i)}) = p$, r_i^*, $i = 1, \cdots, N$ are identically distributed as Student t-variables with $(N - p - 1)$ degrees of freedom. ∎

The externally Studentized residuals r_i^* are usually preferred since $\widehat{\sigma}_{(i)}$ is robust to gross errors in the ith observation and the r_i^* itself has a t-distribution for which critical values are easily available. Note that the Studentized residuals stabilize the variance in the ordinary residuals $\widehat{\varepsilon}_i$, but leave the correlation pattern unchanged. We now define other residuals that also play a useful role in regression analysis. Let $\mathbf{X} = (\mathbf{X}_1, \mathbf{x}_i)$.

Definition 8.5.5. The vector of *partial residuals* corresponding to the predictor X_j is defined by

$$\varepsilon_j^* = \mathbf{y} - \mathbf{X}_1\widehat{\beta}_1 = \widehat{\varepsilon} + \mathbf{x}_j\widehat{\beta}_j.$$

These partial residuals are residuals that have not been adjusted for the predictor variable X_j. In section 8.1.1, we saw that the *partial residual plot* or *residual plus component plot* of ε_j^* versus X_j has estimated slope $\widehat{\beta}_j$.

Definition 8.5.6. The ith *predicted residual* is defined by

$$\widehat{\varepsilon}_{i(i)} = Y_i - \mathbf{x}_i'\widehat{\beta}_{(i)}, \quad i = 1, \cdots, N$$

where $\widehat{\beta}_{(i)}$ denotes the least squares estimate of β with the ith case excluded.

Unlike the ordinary and Studentized residuals, the ith predicted residual vector $\widehat{\varepsilon}_{(i)}$ is based on a fit to the data with the ith case excluded. We may think of $\widehat{\varepsilon}_{i(i)}$ as a prediction error, since we exclude the ith case while obtaining the fit. From Result 8.2.2, it is clear that if the errors are normally distributed, $\widehat{\varepsilon}_{i(i)}$ will have the same correlation structure as the $\widehat{\varepsilon}_i$, with zero means and variances equal to $\sigma^2/(1 - p_{ii})$. It is preferable to use Studentized versions of $\widehat{\varepsilon}_{i(i)}$, which gives back the internally and externally Studentized residuals r_i and r_i^*, as the reader may verify.

Definition 8.5.7.   We define a vector of $BLUS$ (best linear unbiased and possessing a scalar covariance matrix) residuals to be a vector of uncorrelated residuals $\widehat{\mathbf{u}} = (\widehat{u}_1, \cdots, \widehat{u}_N)$ which is a linear function of $\mathbf{y}$, say $\mathbf{By}$, such that $E(\widehat{\mathbf{u}}) = \mathbf{0}$, and $E(\widehat{\mathbf{u}}\widehat{\mathbf{u}}') = \sigma^2\mathbf{I}$.

In order to choose a matrix $\mathbf{B}$ that defines the $BLUS$ residuals $\widehat{\mathbf{u}}$, we look at properties of the projection matrix $\mathbf{P}$. Recall that $\mathbf{I} - \mathbf{P}$ has $N - p$ eigenvalues equal to unity while the remaining p eigenvalues are zero. Let $\mathbf{B}$ be an $(N-p)\times p$ matrix containing the eigenvectors of $\mathbf{I} - \mathbf{P}$ corresponding to the nonzero eigenvalues. Using properties of the linear regression model and the spectral decomposition of symmetric matrices it can be shown that $\mathbf{BX} = \mathbf{0}$, $\mathbf{BB}' = \mathbf{I}, \mathbf{B}'\mathbf{B} = \mathbf{I} - \mathbf{P}$, $\widehat{\mathbf{u}} = \mathbf{BY} = \mathbf{B}\varepsilon = \mathbf{B}\widehat{\varepsilon}$, and $E(\widehat{\mathbf{u}}\widehat{\mathbf{u}}') = \sigma^2\mathbf{B}(\mathbf{I} - \mathbf{P})\mathbf{B}' = \sigma^2\mathbf{I}_{N-p}$. Note that the order of $\widehat{\mathbf{u}}$ is at most $N - p$, and further, $\widehat{\mathbf{u}}$ is not unique. This is a serious disadvantage in terms of using $\widehat{u}_i$ as case statistics for regression diagnostics, since identification of these $N - p$ residuals based on the N cases is messy and lacks interpretation. Also, the independence of the $BLUS$ residuals holds only if the regression errors are normally distributed and are homoscedastic. Hence, $\widehat{\mathbf{u}}$ is not very useful for testing the normality assumption, although it has been used to construct a test for serial correlation (see Theil, 1965) and a test for heteroscedasticity (Heyadat et al., 1977).

Recursive residuals (Brown, Durbin, and Evans, 1975) are another example of $BLUS$ residuals, but lacking the minimum variance property of the $BLUS$ residuals. Let $\mathbf{X}_j$ be a $j \times p$ matrix consisting of the first j rows of the matrix $\mathbf{X}$, where $j \geq p$, and let $\mathbf{x}'_{j+1}$ be the $(j+1)$th row of $\mathbf{X}$. Let $\mathbf{X}_{j+1} = (\mathbf{X}'_j, \mathbf{x}'_{j+1})'$, $\mathbf{y}_j = (Y_1, \cdots, Y_j)'$, and $\mathbf{W}_j = (\mathbf{X}'_j\mathbf{X}_j)^{-1}$, while $\widehat{\beta}_j = \mathbf{W}_j\mathbf{X}'_j\mathbf{y}_j$ denotes the least squares estimate of β based on the first j observations.

Definition 8.5.8.   The $(N - p)$-dimensional vector of *recursive residuals* is defined by

$$\widehat{\varepsilon}_j^R = \frac{Y_j - \mathbf{x}'_j\widehat{\beta}_{j-1}}{(1 + \mathbf{x}'_j\mathbf{W}_{j-1}\mathbf{x}_j)^{1/2}}, \quad j = p+1, \cdots, N$$

$$\widehat{\varepsilon}_j^R = 0, \quad j = 1, \cdots, p.$$

Result 8.5.5.   The following relationships are useful for the computation of recursive residuals:

$$\widehat{\beta}_j = \widehat{\beta}_{j-1} + \frac{\mathbf{W}_{j-1}\mathbf{x}_j(Y_j - \mathbf{x}'_j\widehat{\beta}_{j-1})}{1 + \mathbf{x}'_j\mathbf{W}_{j-1}\mathbf{x}_j}, \text{ and}$$

$$\mathbf{W}_j = \mathbf{W}_{j-1} - \frac{\mathbf{W}_{j-1}\mathbf{x}_j\mathbf{x}'_j\mathbf{W}_{j-1}}{1 + \mathbf{x}'_j\mathbf{W}_{j-1}\mathbf{x}_j}. \quad \blacksquare$$

For the normal linear regression model with homoscedastic errors, $\widehat{\varepsilon}_j^R$, $j > p$ are independent $N(0, \sigma^2)$ variables. Heyadat and Robson (1970) and Harvey and Phillips (1974) constructed tests for heteroscedasticity using recursive residuals, while Phillips and Harvey (1974) used them in order to develop a test for serial correlation.

8.5.3 Outliers and high leverage observations

Violations in the regression model assumptions can occur in a variety of ways. Frequently, the data may contain outliers, i.e., anomalous observations that do not reasonably fit the assumed model. In general, an observation may be influential in the regression fit either because it is an outlying response, or it is a high-leverage point, or both. In the framework of linear regression, we classify the ith observation as an outlier if the magnitude of r_i or r_i^* is large by comparison with the rest of the observations in the data set. The presence of outliers may seriously bias parameter estimation and inference. The traditional tool for detecting outliers is an analysis of the residuals $\widehat{\varepsilon}_i$, $i = 1, \cdots, N$. There are two approaches for outlier detection, viz., use of formal test procedures, and informal graphical displays. We describe both approaches.

From (8.5.1) and (8.5.2), it follows that we may interpret p_{ij} as the amount of *leverage* each Y_j has on determining $\widehat{Y}_i$, irrespective of its actual value (Hoaglin and Welsch, 1978). The leverage of the ith case is p_{ii}, which is the ith diagonal element of the projection matrix $\mathbf{P}$, while the reciprocal $1/p_{ii}$ is the effective or equivalent number of observations that determine $\widehat{Y}_i$ (Huber, 1981). When $p_{ii} = 1/2$, an equivalent of two observations determine the fitted value $\widehat{Y}_i$; when $p_{ii} = 1$, Y_i solely determines $\widehat{Y}_i$; while if $p_{ii} = 0$, Y_i has no influence on $\widehat{Y}_i$. Huber suggested that if $p_{ii} > 0.2$, then the ith case is a high-leverage point. Since $\sum_{i=1}^{N} p_{ii} = p$, Hoaglin and Welsch suggested that cases with $p_{ii} > 2p/N$ may be classified as high-leverage points. A wide variation in the values of p_{ii} indicate nonhomogeneous spacing of the rows of $\mathbf{P}$.

Geometrically, suppose $\mathbf{X}$ contains a constant column $\mathbf{1}_N$, or suppose that the columns of $\mathbf{X}$ are centered at their respective averages. For a p-dimensional vector $\mathbf{u}$, and a constant c, the quadratic form $\mathbf{u}'(\mathbf{X}'\mathbf{X})^{-1}\mathbf{u} = c$ determines p-dimensional elliptical contours centered at $\overline{\mathbf{x}}$. The smallest convex set which contains the scatter of N sample values of $\mathbf{X}$ lies within ellipsoids of radius c, where $c \leq \max(p_{ii})$. The implication is that a large value of p_{ii} indicates that $\mathbf{x}_i$ is far removed from the center $\overline{\mathbf{x}}$, i.e., it is an outlier in the X space. We define the following quantities that enable us to measure the distance of $\mathbf{x}_i$ from the rest of the cases. Assume that we have a regression model with intercept, and recall that $\mathbf{X} = (\mathbf{1}_N, \widetilde{\mathbf{X}})$.

Definition 8.5.9.   The *Mahalanobis distance* is defined by (see section 6.3)

$$M_i = (N-2)(\widetilde{\mathbf{x}}_i - \overline{\widetilde{\mathbf{X}}}_{(i)})'\{\widetilde{\mathbf{X}}'_{(i)}(\mathbf{I} - (N-1)^{-1}\mathbf{1}\mathbf{1}')\widetilde{\mathbf{X}}_{(i)}\}^{-1}(\widetilde{\mathbf{x}}_i - \overline{\widetilde{\mathbf{X}}}_{(i)}), \quad (8.5.8)$$

for $i = 1, \cdots, N$, where, $\overline{\widetilde{\mathbf{X}}}_{(i)}$ is the average of $\widetilde{\mathbf{X}}_{(i)}$. It is easily shown that

$$M_i = N(N-2)(p_{ii} - 1/N)/(N-1)(1 - p_{ii}), \quad i = 1, \cdots, N.$$

Definition 8.5.10.   The *weighted squared standardized distance* (WSSD) is defined as the weighted sum of squared distances of X_{ij} from the mean of X_j, the weights being $\widehat{\beta}_j$ (Daniel and Wood, 1971):

$$W_i^* = \sum_{j=1}^{p} c_{ij}^2 / S_Y^2, \quad i = 1, \cdots, N, \quad (8.5.9)$$

where $c_{ij} = \widehat{\beta}_j(X_{ij} - \overline{X}_j)$, $i = 1, \cdots, N$, $j = 1, \cdots, p$ denotes the effect of X_j on $\widehat{Y}_i$, and $\sum_{j=1}^{p} c_{ij} = \widehat{Y}_i - \overline{Y}$. If X_{ij} is far removed from $\overline{X}$, or if $\widehat{\beta}_j$ is large, or both, then W_i^* will be large, and the ith case is influential on the distance between $\widehat{Y}_i$ and $\overline{Y}$.

An $L-R$ plot combines information about leverages and residuals into a single graphical display, and enables us to distinguish between high-leverage points and outliers. It is a scatterplot of leverages p_{ii} versus the squared normalized residuals a_i^2. The scatter of points must lie within the triangle defined by these conditions: (i) $0 \leq p_{ii} \leq 1$, (ii) $0 \leq a_i^2 \leq 1$, and (iii) $p_{ii} + a_i^2 \leq 1$. Points that lie in the lower right corner of the $L-R$ plot are outliers, while points that lie in the upper left corner have high leverage. Neither outliers nor high-leverage points are necessarily influential. We discuss measures based on the influence function in the next section.

8.5.4   Diagnostic measures based on influence functions

The study of *influence* is the study of the dependence of conclusions and inferences on various aspects of a statistical problem formulation. This is implemented via a perturbation scheme in which data are modified by deletion of cases, either singly, or in groups (Hampel, 1974). Suppose $(z_1, \cdots, z_N)$ denotes a large random sample from a population with cdf F. Let $\widehat{F}_N = F_N(z_1, \cdots, z_N)$ denote the empirical cdf and let $T_N = T(z_1, \cdots, z_N)$ be a (scalar or vector-valued) statistic of interest. The study of influence consists of assessing the change in T_N when some specific aspect of the problem is slightly changed. The first step is to find a statistical functional T which maps (a subset of) the set of all cdf's onto $\mathcal{R}^p$, so that $T(\widehat{F}_N) = T_N$. We assume that F_N converges to F

and that T_N converges to T. For example, when $T_N = \overline{Z}$, the corresponding functional is $T(F) = \int z\,dF(z)$, and $T(\widehat{F}_N) = \int z\,d\widehat{F}_N = \overline{Z}$. The influence of an estimator T_N is said to be unbounded if it is sensitive to extreme observations, in which case, T_N is said to be nonrobust. To assess this, one more observation z is added to the *large* sample, and we monitor the change in T_N, and the conclusions based on T_N. In this section, we present results describing the influence of the ith case on the least squares regression estimates, $\widehat{\beta}$, $\widehat{\sigma}^2$, as well as on $Cov(\widehat{\beta})$, $\widehat{\mathbf{y}}$, and $Cov(\widehat{\mathbf{y}})$. We use measures based on the theoretical influence function (Hampel, 1974 and Huber, 1981).

Definition 8.5.11.   Let z denote one observation that is added to the large sample $(z_1, \cdots, z_N)$ drawn from a population with cdf F, and let T denote a functional of interest. The influence function is defined by

$$\psi(z, F, T) = \lim_{\varepsilon \to 0} \frac{1}{\varepsilon}[T\{(1 - \varepsilon)F + \varepsilon\delta_z\} - T\{F\}], \qquad (8.5.10)$$

provided the limit exists for every $z \in \mathcal{R}$, and where $\delta_z = 1$ at z and zero otherwise. The influence curve is the ordinary right-hand derivative, evaluated at $\varepsilon = 0$, of the function $T[(1 - \varepsilon)F + \varepsilon\delta_z]$ with respect to ε.

The influence curve is useful for studying asymptotic properties of an estimator as well as for comparing estimators. For example, if $T = \mu = \int z\,dF$, then

$$\psi[z, F, T] = \lim_{\varepsilon \to 0}\{[(1 - \varepsilon)\mu + \varepsilon z] - \mu\}/\varepsilon = z - \mu,$$

which is "unbounded", so that $T_N = \overline{Z}$ is nonrobust. To use the influence function in the regression context, we must first construct appropriate functionals corresponding to β and σ^2.

Result 8.5.7.   The functionals for β and σ^2 are

$$\begin{aligned}
\beta(F) &= \Sigma_{\mathbf{xx}}^{-1}(F)\Sigma_{\mathbf{x}Y}(F), \\
\sigma^2(F) &= \sigma_{YY}(F) - \Sigma_{\mathbf{x}Y}'(F)\Sigma_{\mathbf{xx}}^{-1}(F)\Sigma_{\mathbf{x}Y}(F) \\
&= \sigma_{YY}(F) - \Sigma_{\mathbf{x}Y}'(F)\beta(F), \qquad (8.5.11)
\end{aligned}$$

where $(\mathbf{x}', Y)$ has cdf F, and

$$E[(\mathbf{x}', Y)'(\mathbf{x}', Y)] = \left(\begin{array}{cc} \Sigma_{\mathbf{xx}}(F) & \Sigma_{\mathbf{x}Y}(F) \\ \Sigma_{\mathbf{x}Y}'(F) & \sigma_{YY}(F) \end{array} \right).$$

Proof.   Recall that the least squares regression estimates $\widehat{\beta}$ and $\widehat{\sigma}^2$ are obtained by simultaneously solving the equations

$$\frac{1}{N}\sum_{i=1}^{N}\mathbf{x}_i(Y_i - \mathbf{x}_i'\widehat{\beta}) = \mathbf{0},$$

$$\frac{1}{N - p}\sum_{i=1}^{N}(Y_i - \mathbf{x}_i'\widehat{\beta})^2 = \widehat{\sigma}^2. \qquad (8.5.12)$$

Corresponding to (8.5.12), we can write

$$\int\limits_{(\mathbf{x}',Y)} \mathbf{x}(Y - \mathbf{x}'\beta)d\widehat{F}_N(\mathbf{x}',Y) = \mathbf{0},$$

$$\int\limits_{(\mathbf{x}',Y)} (Y - \mathbf{x}'\beta)^2 d\widehat{F}_N(\mathbf{x}',Y) = \sigma^2, \tag{8.5.13}$$

the solution of which gives the required functionals for β and σ^2.   ■

Result 8.5.8. The influence curves for $\widehat{\beta}$ and $\widehat{\sigma}^2$ are respectively

$$
\begin{aligned}
IC_{\beta,F}(\mathbf{x}',Y) &= \Sigma_{\mathbf{xx}}^{-1}(F)\mathbf{x}[y - \mathbf{x}'\beta(F)], &(8.5.14)\\
IC_{\sigma^2,F}(\mathbf{x}',Y) &= [Y - \mathbf{x}'\beta(F)]^2 - \sigma_{YY}(F) + \Sigma_{\mathbf{x}Y}'(F)\beta(F). &(8.5.15)
\end{aligned}
$$

Proof.   Substitute $(\mathbf{x}',Y)$ for z, and $\beta(F)$ from (8.5.11) for the functional T into (8.5.10) to get

$$\psi\{(\mathbf{x}',Y),F,\beta(F)\} = \lim_{\varepsilon \to 0}\frac{1}{\varepsilon}[\beta\{(1-\varepsilon)F + \varepsilon\delta_{(\mathbf{x}',Y)}\} - \beta\{F\}]. \tag{8.5.16}$$

Using property 8 of Result 1.2.10, we can write $\frac{1}{\varepsilon}[\beta\{(1-\varepsilon)F + \varepsilon\delta_{(\mathbf{x}',Y)}\} - \beta\{F\}]$ as

$$
\begin{aligned}
&\frac{1}{\varepsilon}[\Sigma_{\mathbf{xx}}^{-1}\{(1-\varepsilon)F + \varepsilon\delta_{(\mathbf{x}',Y)}\}\Sigma_{\mathbf{x}Y}\{(1-\varepsilon)F + \varepsilon\delta_{(\mathbf{x}',Y)}\} - \Sigma_{\mathbf{xx}}^{-1}(F)\Sigma_{\mathbf{x}Y}(F)]\\
=\ &\frac{1}{\varepsilon}[\{(1-\varepsilon)\Sigma_{\mathbf{xx}}(F) + \varepsilon\mathbf{xx}'\}^{-1}\{(1-\varepsilon)\Sigma_{\mathbf{x}Y}(F) + \varepsilon\mathbf{x}Y\} - \Sigma_{\mathbf{xx}}^{-1}(F)\Sigma_{\mathbf{x}Y}(F)]\\
=\ &\frac{1}{\varepsilon}[\{\Sigma_{\mathbf{xx}}(F) + \varepsilon(\mathbf{xx}' - \Sigma_{\mathbf{xx}}(F))\}^{-1}\{\Sigma_{\mathbf{x}Y}(F) + \varepsilon(\mathbf{x}Y - \Sigma_{\mathbf{x}Y}(F))\}\\
&-\Sigma_{\mathbf{xx}}^{-1}(F)\Sigma_{\mathbf{x}Y}(F)]\\
=\ &\frac{1}{\varepsilon}[\{\mathbf{I} + \varepsilon\Sigma_{\mathbf{xx}}^{-1}(F)(\mathbf{xx}' - \Sigma_{\mathbf{xx}}(F))\}^{-1}\Sigma_{\mathbf{xx}}^{-1}(F)\{\Sigma_{\mathbf{x}Y}(F) + \varepsilon(\mathbf{x}Y\\
&-\Sigma_{\mathbf{x}Y}(F))\} - \Sigma_{\mathbf{xx}}^{-1}(F)\Sigma_{\mathbf{x}Y}(F)]\\
=\ &\frac{1}{\varepsilon}[\{\mathbf{I} - \varepsilon\Sigma_{\mathbf{xx}}^{-1}(F)(\mathbf{xx}' - \Sigma_{\mathbf{xx}}(F)) + o(\varepsilon^2)\}\{\beta(F) + \varepsilon\Sigma_{\mathbf{xx}}^{-1}(F)(\mathbf{x}Y\\
&-\Sigma_{\mathbf{x}Y}(F))\} - \Sigma_{\mathbf{xx}}^{-1}(F)\Sigma_{\mathbf{x}Y}(F)].
\end{aligned}
$$

In the limit as $\varepsilon \to 0$, this expression yields $IC_{\beta,F}(\mathbf{x}',Y)$. Since $(Y - \mathbf{x}'\beta(F))$ is unbounded, $IC_{\beta,F}(\mathbf{x}',Y)$ is unbounded, i.e., the least squares estimate $\widehat{\beta}$ is a nonrobust estimator.

Similarly, substituting the form of the functional $\sigma^2(F)$ from (8.5.11) into (8.5.10), we see that $\sigma^2\{(1-\varepsilon)F + \varepsilon\delta_{(\mathbf{x}',Y)}\} - \sigma^2\{F\} = \sigma_{YY}(F) + \varepsilon Y^2 - \varepsilon\sigma_{YY}(F) - \Sigma_{\mathbf{x}Y}'(F)\beta(F) - \varepsilon\beta'(F)\mathbf{x}(Y - \mathbf{x}'\beta(F)) - \varepsilon(Y\mathbf{x}' - \Sigma_{\mathbf{x}Y}(F))\beta(F) - \varepsilon^2(Y\mathbf{x}' - \beta'(F)\mathbf{x}(Y - \mathbf{x}'\beta(F)) - \sigma_{YY}(F) + \Sigma_{\mathbf{x}Y}'(F)\beta(F) = Y^2 - \sigma_{YY}(F) - 2Y\mathbf{x}'\beta(F) + (\mathbf{x}'\beta(F))^2 + \Sigma_{\mathbf{x}Y}'(F)\beta(F)$, which after some simplification yields

$IC_{\sigma^2,F}(\mathbf{x}',Y)$. Once again, $IC_{\sigma^2,F}(\mathbf{x}',Y)$ is unbounded, so that $\widehat{\sigma}^2$ is not a robust estimate of σ^2. ■

The theoretical functions are intended to measure the influence on $\widehat{\beta}$ and $\widehat{\sigma}^2$ due to adding one observation $(\mathbf{x}',Y)$ to a very large sample. We do not, however, always have very large samples in practice, and therefore need finite sample approximations of these influence functions. Four approximations to $IC_{\beta,F}(\mathbf{x}',Y)$ are shown below. For more details, see Cook and Weisberg (1982), or Chatterjee and Hadi (1988).

Result 8.5.9. Four approximations to the theoretical influence function $IC_{\beta,F}(\mathbf{x}',Y)$ are given below.

1. The *empirical influence function (EIC)* based on N observations is

$$EIC_i = N(\mathbf{X}'\mathbf{X})^{-1}\mathbf{x}_i\widehat{\varepsilon}_i, \quad i=1,\cdots,N. \qquad (8.5.17)$$

2. The *empirical influence function based on* $(N-1)$ *observations,* $(EIC_{(i)})$ has the form

$$EIC_{(i)} = (N-1)(\mathbf{X}'\mathbf{X})^{-1}\mathbf{x}_i\frac{\widehat{\varepsilon}_i}{(1-p_{ii})^2}, \quad i=1,\cdots,N. \qquad (8.5.18)$$

3. The *sample influence function (SIC)* based on N observations is

$$SIC_i = (N-1)(\mathbf{X}'\mathbf{X})^{-1}\mathbf{x}_i\frac{\widehat{\varepsilon}_i}{1-p_{ii}}, \quad i=1,\cdots,N. \qquad (8.5.19)$$

4. The *sensitivity curve* (SC_i) based on N observations is

$$SC_i = N(\mathbf{X}'\mathbf{X})^{-1}\mathbf{x}_i\frac{\widehat{\varepsilon}_i}{(1-p_{ii})}, \quad i=1,\cdots,N. \qquad (8.5.20)$$

Proof. The function EIC_i is obtained by setting $(\mathbf{x}',Y) = (\mathbf{x}_i',Y_i)$, $F = \widehat{F}_N$, $\beta(F) = \widehat{\beta}$ and $\Sigma_{\mathbf{xx}}^{-1}(F) = N(\mathbf{X}'\mathbf{X})^{-1}$ in (8.5.14). The function $EIC_{(i)}$ is obtained by setting $(\mathbf{x}',Y) = (\mathbf{x}_i',Y_i)$, $F = \widehat{F}_{N(i)}$, $\beta(F) = \widehat{\beta}_{(i)}$ and $\Sigma_{\mathbf{xx}}^{-1}(F) = (N-1)(\mathbf{X}_{(i)}'\mathbf{X}_{(i)})^{-1}$ in (8.5.14), which gives, for $i = 1,\cdots,N$,

$$EIC_{(i)} = (N-1)(\mathbf{X}_{(i)}'\mathbf{X}_{(i)})^{-1}\mathbf{x}_i(Y_i - \mathbf{x}_i'\widehat{\beta}_{(i)}).$$

Using (2.1.22) and (8.2.8), property 2 follows. The sample influence curve SIC_i is obtained by setting $(\mathbf{x}',Y) = (\mathbf{x}_i',Y_i)$, $F = \widehat{F}_N$, and $\varepsilon = -1/(N-1)$ in (8.5.16), omitting the limit and simplifying. The proof is left as an exercise (Exercise 8.10). To obtain SC_i, set $(\mathbf{x}',Y) = (\mathbf{x}_i',Y_i)$, $F = \widehat{F}_{N(i)}$, and $\varepsilon = 1/N$ in (8.5.16), omit the limit and simplify. ■

The main difference between these approximate influence functions is in the power of $(1-p_{ii})$. We see that EIC_i is least sensitive to high leverage points, while $EIC_{(i)}$ is the most sensitive. Note that SIC_i and SC_i are equivalent and are proportional to the distance $(\widehat{\beta} - \widehat{\beta}_{(i)})$. Note that each of these approximate influence curves for $\widehat{\beta}$ is a p-dimensional vector, which is unwieldy. In practice, it would be useful to obtain an ordering of the N observations based on a scalar summary measure of influence. The quantity

$$D_i(\mathbf{M}, c) = [\psi'\{\mathbf{x}_i', Y_i, F, \beta(F)\}\mathbf{M}\psi\{\mathbf{x}_i', Y_i, F, \beta(F)\}]/c$$

for appropriate choices of $\mathbf{M}$ and c is useful. If $D_i(\mathbf{M}, c)$ is large, then the ith observation has strong influence on $\widehat{\beta}$ relative to $\mathbf{M}$ and c. Four different choices of $\mathbf{M}$ and c leads to the following measures that are popular regression diagnostics measures – (a) Cook's distance (C_i), (b) Modified Cook's distance (MC_i), (c) $DFFITS$ or Welsch-Kuh's distance (WK_i), and (d) Welsch's distance (W_i). The essential difference between these is in the choice of scale. Further, C_i only measures the influence of the ith observation on $\widehat{\beta}$, whereas the other three statistics measure the influence on both $\widehat{\beta}$ and $\widehat{\sigma}^2$.

Definition 8.5.12.   *Cook's distance* is defined by (Cook and Weisberg, 1982 and Atkinson, 1985) as

$$
\begin{aligned}
C_i &= D_i(\mathbf{X}'\mathbf{X}, \frac{p\widehat{\sigma}^2}{(N-1)^2}) \\
&= \frac{(\widehat{\beta} - \widehat{\beta}_{(i)})'(\mathbf{X}'\mathbf{X})(\widehat{\beta} - \widehat{\beta}_{(i)})}{p\widehat{\sigma}^2}, \quad i = 1, \cdots, N. \quad (8.5.21)
\end{aligned}
$$

The $100(1 - \alpha)\%$ joint ellipsoidal confidence region for β given in (7.3.2) is centered at $\widehat{\beta}$. The quantity C_i measures the change in the center of this ellipsoid when the ith observation is omitted, and thereby assesses its influence. C_i may be interpreted as the scaled distance between $\widehat{\beta}$ and $\widehat{\beta}_{(i)}$, or alternately, as the scaled distance between $\widehat{\mathbf{y}}$ and $\widehat{\mathbf{y}}_{(i)}$. The following result summarizes alternate forms for Cook's distance.

Result 8.5.10.   For $i = 1, \cdots, N$,

$$C_i = \frac{(\widehat{\mathbf{y}} - \widehat{\mathbf{y}}_{(i)})'(\widehat{\mathbf{y}} - \widehat{\mathbf{y}}_{(i)})}{p\widehat{\sigma}^2}, \quad \text{or} \quad (8.5.22)$$

$$C_i = \frac{\mathbf{x}_i'(\mathbf{X}'\mathbf{X})^{-1}\mathbf{x}_i}{p(1 - p_{ii})}\frac{\widehat{\varepsilon}_i^2}{\widehat{\sigma}^2(1 - p_{ii})} = \frac{1}{p}\frac{p_{ii}}{(1 - p_{ii})}r_i^2. \quad (8.5.23)$$

Proof.   By partitioning $\mathbf{X} = (\mathbf{X}_{(i)}, \mathbf{x}_i)$ and $\mathbf{y} = (\mathbf{y}_{(i)}, Y_i)$, we can write

$$\widehat{\beta} = (\mathbf{X}'\mathbf{X})^{-1}\mathbf{X}_{(i)}'\mathbf{y}_{(i)} + (\mathbf{X}'\mathbf{X})^{-1}\mathbf{x}_i'Y_i. \quad (8.5.24)$$

Using the form for $\widehat{\beta}_{(i)}$ in (8.2.5) and simplifying, it follows that

$$\widehat{\beta} - \widehat{\beta}_{(i)} = (\mathbf{X}'\mathbf{X})^{-1}\mathbf{x}_i \frac{\widehat{\varepsilon}_i}{1 - p_{ii}}. \tag{8.5.25}$$

Substituting (8.5.25) into (8.5.21), we prove (8.5.23). ∎

It is clear from the previous result that we certainly need not run $(N+1)$ regressions (one with all N observations, and N regressions successively omitting observations one at a time). The quantity C_i will be large if p_{ii} is large, or if r_i^2 is large, or both. Although it has been suggested that each C_i be compared to percentiles of the $F_{p,N-p}$ distribution to see if it is large, we can also use a Boxplot or stem-and-leaf plot or index plot of C_i to answer the question "how large is large?" An *index plot* is a plot of Cook's distance against observation number. Points that are above some threshold value such as the 50th percentile of an $F_{p,N-p}$ distribution are regarded as influential observations. Several modifications of Cook's distance are available for normal regression models (Chatterjee and Hadi, 1988, section 4.2, and section 5.4), while Pregibon (1981) used a one-step approximation to extend this statistic to binary response models as well (see section 11.4). Atkinson (1981) suggested a modification of C_i in order to (a) give more emphasis to extreme points, and (b) be more suitable for graphical displays such as the normal probability plots. The modification consists of replacing $\widehat{\sigma}^2$ by $\widehat{\sigma}_{(i)}^2$, taking the square root of C_i, and adjusting C_i for sample size.

Definition 8.5.13. We define the modified Cook's distance by

$$MC_i = |r_i^*| \left[\frac{p_{ii}}{(1 - p_{ii})} \frac{(N - p)}{p} \right]^{1/2}. \tag{8.5.26}$$

In the case where $p_{ii} = p/N$, $i = 1, \cdots, N$, the plot of MC_i versus i is identical to the plot of $|r_i^*|$.

Figures 8.5.1 (a) and (b) give graphical interpretations of Cook's distance and the modified Cook's distance for a 2-dimensional vector β. In (a), the ellipsoid is centered at $\widehat{\beta}$. Cases i and l are equally influential on $\widehat{\beta}$ in (a), while case m is more influential since $\widehat{\beta}_{(m)}$ lies on an outer contour corresponding to a larger value of Cook's distance. The modified Cook's distance in (b) measures the distance from $\widehat{\beta}_{(i)}$ to $\widehat{\beta}$ relative to the ellipsoids constructed using all the observations, but with a scale $\widehat{\sigma}_{(i)}^2$ specific to the ith case. Since MC_i does not compare cases relative to a fixed metric, the ellipsoids in (b) can have different shapes. Two other measures are related to the ellipsoidal confidence region for β and are defined next.

Definition 8.5.14. The Andrews-Pregibon statistic is defined as (Andrews and Pregibon, 1978)

$$AP_i = 1 - \frac{SSE_{(i)}|\mathbf{X}_{(i)}'\mathbf{X}_{(i)}|}{SSE|\mathbf{X}'\mathbf{X}|}, \quad i = 1, \cdots, N, \tag{8.5.27}$$

which measures the influence of the ith observation on the volume of the confidence ellipsoids for β, with and without the ith observation.

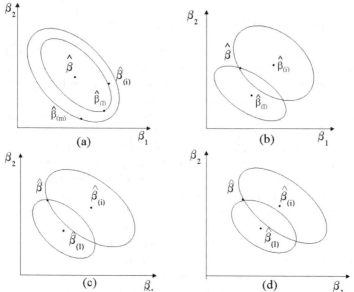

Figure 8.5.1.   Graphical interpretation of distance measures.

We leave it to the reader to verify the relationships between AP_i and the values of p_{ii} and r_i (Exercise 8.15). In particular, since $1 - AP_i = (1 - p_{ii})\{1 - r_i^2/(N-p)\}$, AP_i combines information about high-leverage and outliers, and is therefore potentially less informative than p_{ii} and r_i (Draper and John, 1981).

Definition 8.5.15.   The Cook-Weisberg statistic (Cook and Weisberg, 1980) is defined by

$$CW_i = \log\left\{\left(\frac{|\mathbf{X}'_{(i)}\mathbf{X}_{(i)}|}{|\mathbf{X}'\mathbf{X}|}\right)^{1/2}\frac{\widehat{\sigma}^p}{\widehat{\sigma}^p_{(i)}}\left(\frac{F_{p,N-p,\alpha}}{F_{p,N-p-1,\alpha}}\right)^{p/2}\right\} \qquad (8.5.28)$$

Definition 8.5.16.   The *Welsch-Kuh distance* or $DFFITS_i$ measures the influence of the ith observation on $\widehat{Y}_i$ by the change in the prediction at $\mathbf{x}_i$ by omitting the ith observation relative to $s.e.(\widehat{Y}_i)$ as

$$
\begin{aligned}
DFFITS_i = WK_i &= \frac{|\mathbf{x}'_i(\widehat{\beta} - \widehat{\beta}_{(i)})|}{\widehat{\sigma}_{(i)}\sqrt{p_{ii}}} \\
&= \frac{|[\widehat{\varepsilon}_i/(1-p_{ii})]\mathbf{x}'_i(\mathbf{X}'\mathbf{X})^{-1}\mathbf{x}_i|}{\widehat{\sigma}_{(i)}\sqrt{p_{ii}}} \\
&= |r_i^*|\sqrt{\frac{p_{ii}}{1-p_{ii}}}. \qquad (8.5.29)
\end{aligned}
$$

Definition 8.5.17.   Weslch's distance is defined by

$$W_i = \left[(N-1)r_i^{*2} \frac{p_{ii}}{(1-p_{ii})^2} \right]^{1/2} \tag{8.5.30}$$

$$= WK_i \sqrt{\frac{N-1}{1-p_{ii}}}, \tag{8.5.31}$$

and clearly gives more emphasis to high leverage points than does WK_i.

Note that the relation between MC_i and WK_i is

$$MC_i = WK_i \sqrt{(N-p)/p}.$$

WK_i is also called $DFFITS_i$ (Belsley et al., 1980) because it is the scaled difference between $\widehat{Y}_i$ and $\widehat{Y}_{i(i)}$. It provides a measure of the influence of the ith observation on the prediction at $\mathbf{x}_i$. Large values of $DFFITS_i$ indicate that the ith observation is influential on the fitted regression. Again, "how large is large? " Velleman and Welsch (1981) recommended that "values greater than 1 or 2 seem reasonable to nominate for special attention". Based on the t_{N-p-1} distribution for r_i^*, a cut-off point for WK_i of $t_{N-p-1,\alpha/2}[p/(N-p)]^{1/2}$ could be used. Alternately, we could replace $t_{N-p-1,\alpha/2}$ by 2 to get a cut-off point. Similarly, the influence of the ith observation on the prediction at $\mathbf{x}_h, h \neq i$ is given by $|\mathbf{x}_h'(\widehat{\beta} - \widehat{\beta}_{(i)})|/(\sigma\sqrt{p_{hh}})$, which can be shown to be at most equal to WK_i. The implication is that if the ith observation is not seen to be influential on the prediction at $\mathbf{x}_i$, as indicated by a small WK_i value, then the ith observation cannot be influential on the prediction at any other $\mathbf{x}_h, h \neq i$.

Figures 8.5.1 (c) and (d) give graphical representations of the Welsch distance and the Welsch-Kuh distance. While W_i measures the distance from $\widehat{\beta}_{(i)}$ to $\widehat{\beta}$ relative to the ellipsoid centered at $\widehat{\beta}_{(i)}$, W_j measures the distance from $\widehat{\beta}_{(j)}$ to $\widehat{\beta}$ relative to the ellipsoid centered at $\widehat{\beta}_{(j)}$. Similar to the modified Cook's distance, the Welsch-Kuh distance measures the distance from $\widehat{\beta}_{(i)}$ to $\widehat{\beta}$ using the entire data, but with a different scale for each case.

Until now, we looked at measures that study the influence of the ith observation on the entire regression coefficient vector. In some cases, we may be especially interested in certain components of β. It might happen that an observation is influential only on one dimension (predictor variable). Further, an observation which has moderate influence on all the β_j's may be judged to be more influential than an observation which has large influence on just one regression coefficient, and negligible influence on the other coefficients. The following result describes the influence of an observation on a single β_j. Suppose that without loss of generality, we partition $\mathbf{X} = (\mathbf{X}_{(j)}, \mathbf{x}_j)$, and

$$\mathbf{y} = \mathbf{X}_{(j)}\beta_{(j)} + \mathbf{x}_j\beta_j + \varepsilon.$$

Let $\mathbf{P} = \mathbf{P}_{(j)} + \mathbf{w}_j\mathbf{w}_j'/\mathbf{w}_j'\mathbf{w}_j$, where $\mathbf{w}_j = (\mathbf{I} - \mathbf{P}_{(j)})\mathbf{x}_j$ is the residual vector when regressing X_j on $\mathbf{X}_{(j)}$.

Result 8.5.11.   Then

$$\widehat{\beta}_j - \widehat{\beta}_{j(i)} = \frac{\widehat{\varepsilon}_i}{(1 - p_{ii})}\frac{w_{ij}}{\mathbf{w}_j'\mathbf{w}_j}. \tag{8.5.32}$$

Proof.   Using (2.1.22), we can write

$$\widehat{\beta}_{(i)} = \{(\mathbf{X}'\mathbf{X})^{-1} + [(\mathbf{X}'\mathbf{X})^{-1}\mathbf{x}_i\mathbf{x}_i'(\mathbf{X}'\mathbf{X})^{-1}]/(1 - p_{ii})\}\mathbf{X}_{(i)}'\mathbf{y}_{(i)}.$$

We can also write

$$\widehat{\beta} = (\mathbf{X}'\mathbf{X})^{-1}\mathbf{X}_{(i)}'\mathbf{y}_{(i)} + (\mathbf{X}'\mathbf{X})^{-1}\mathbf{x}_iY_i,$$

which implies that

$$\widehat{\beta} = \widehat{\beta}_{(i)} - (\mathbf{X}'\mathbf{X})^{-1}\mathbf{x}_iY_i.$$

These equations yield the required result after some simplification.   ∎

In addition to the four measures which quantify the influence of the ith observation on the entire vector $\widehat{\beta}$, it is possible to measure its influence on a single regression coefficient $\widehat{\beta}_j$ using statistics called $DFBETAS_{ij}$ which are defined as follows.

Definition 8.5.18.

$$DFBETAS_{ij} = r_i\frac{w_{ij}}{\sqrt{\mathbf{W}_j'\mathbf{W}_j}}\frac{1}{\sqrt{1 - p_{ii}}}, \quad \text{using estimate } \widehat{\sigma}, \text{ or}$$

$$= r_i^*\frac{w_{ij}}{\sqrt{\mathbf{W}_j'\mathbf{W}_j}}\frac{1}{\sqrt{1 - p_{ii}}}, \quad \text{using estimate } \widehat{\sigma}_{(i)}$$

$$\tag{8.5.33}$$

where $\mathbf{X} = (\mathbf{X}_{(j)}, \mathbf{x}_j)$, the linear model is $\mathbf{y} = \mathbf{X}_{(j)}\beta_{(j)} + \mathbf{x}_j\beta_j + \varepsilon$, $\mathbf{P}_{(j)} = \mathbf{X}_{(j)}[\mathbf{X}_{(j)}'\mathbf{X}_{(j)}]^{-1}\mathbf{X}_{(j)}'$, $\mathbf{W}_j = [\mathbf{I} - \mathbf{P}_{(j)}]\mathbf{x}_j$, and

$$\mathbf{P} = \mathbf{P}_{(j)} + \frac{(\mathbf{I}-\mathbf{P}_{(j)})\mathbf{x}_j\mathbf{x}_j'(\mathbf{I}-\mathbf{P}_{(j)})}{\mathbf{x}_j'(\mathbf{I}-\mathbf{P}_{(j)})\mathbf{x}_j} = \mathbf{P}_{(j)} + \frac{\mathbf{W}_j\mathbf{W}_j'}{\mathbf{W}_j'\mathbf{W}_j}.$$

Note that $\mathbf{P}_{(j)}$ denotes the projection matrix for $\mathbf{X}_{(j)}$, while $\mathbf{W}_j$ denotes the residual vector when $\mathbf{x}_j$ is regressed on $\mathbf{X}_{(j)}$; w_{ij} denotes the ith element of $\mathbf{W}_j$. Belsley et al. (1980) suggested that values of $|DFBETAS_{ij}|$ exceeding $2/N$ are influential on $\widehat{\beta}_j$.

Definition 8.5.19. A diagnostic measure (Belsley et al., 1980) which assesses the influence of the ith observation by comparing the estimated variance of $\widehat{\beta}$ and $\widehat{\beta}_{(i)}$ is called the Covratio, and has the form

$$CR_i = \frac{|\widehat{\sigma}^2_{(i)}(\mathbf{X}'_{(i)}\mathbf{X}_{(i)})^{-1}|}{|\widehat{\sigma}^2(\mathbf{X}'\mathbf{X})^{-1}|}, \quad i = 1, \cdots, N. \tag{8.5.34}$$

Now, CR_i will be approximately equal to one when all the N observations have equal influence on $Cov(\widehat{\beta})$, so that deviation of CR_i from unity suggests that the ith observation is influential. Exercise 8.14 shows a relationship between CR_i and the values of p_{ii} and r_i, and the resulting calibration points for CR_i. The Cook-Weisberg statistic is equivalent to CR_i since

$$CW_i = -\log(CR_i)/2 + p\log(F_{p,N-p,\alpha}/F_{p,N-p-1,\alpha})/2.$$

Numerical Example 8.5. Influence diagnostics in regression. The following analysis pertains to a study of production waste and land use. There are $N = 40$ observations on a response variable Y and five regressor variables. The response Y is solid waste (in millions of tons), while X_1 is industrial land (acres), X_2 is fabricated metals (acres), X_3 denotes trucking and wholesale trade (acres), X_4 denotes retail trade (acres), and X_5 is number of restaurants and hotels. The data is taken from Golueke and McGauhey (1970), and is discussed in Chatterjee and Hadi (1988). Graphical summaries of the Studentized residuals and some influence diagnostics, as well as a summary of least squares fit are shown below. $R^2 = 0.85$, the F-statistic is 38.39 and $\widehat{\sigma}^2 = 0.023$.

Residuals and influence diagnostics for Numerical Example 8.5.

Obs.	r_i	p_{ii}	C_i	Dffits	Obs.	r_i	p_{ii}	C_i	Dffits
1	−1.17	0.07	0.02	−0.31	21	−0.99	0.04	0.01	−0.20
2	4.41	0.73	5.62	7.21	22	−0.34	0.04	< 0.01	−0.07
3	0.03	0.04	< 0.01	0.01	23	−1.21	0.13	0.04	−0.47
4	0.74	0.36	0.05	0.56	24	−0.57	0.04	< 0.01	−0.12
5	0.16	0.04	< 0.01	0.04	25	−0.32	0.05	< 0.01	−0.07
6	0.10	0.04	< 0.01	0.02	26	0.06	0.03	< 0.01	0.011
7	−0.63	0.13	0.01	−0.24	27	−0.47	0.04	< 0.01	−0.01
8	−2.55	0.23	0.28	−1.40	28	−1.37	0.20	0.08	−0.68
9	1.50	0.04	0.02	0.32	29	0.40	0.03	< 0.01	0.07
10	1.45	0.04	0.02	0.31	30	0.28	0.08	< 0.01	0.08
11	0.51	0.03	< 0.01	0.09	31	3.15	0.92	14.68	10.54
12	0.36	0.03	< 0.01	0.06	32	0.14	0.03	< 0.01	0.03
13	−0.19	0.03	< 0.01	−0.04	33	−1.14	0.05	0.01	−0.25
14	0.56	0.04	< 0.01	0.11	34	−1.14	0.08	0.02	−0.34
15	2.68	0.61	1.59	3.36	35	1.24	0.47	0.22	1.15
16	1.85	0.09	0.05	0.58	36	−0.19	0.05	< 0.01	−0.04
17	−0.52	0.04	< 0.01	−0.10	37	1.89	0.04	0.02	0.38
18	−0.41	0.04	< 0.01	−0.08	38	−0.39	0.03	< 0.01	−0.07
19	0.12	0.04	< 0.01	0.03	39	−0.60	0.03	< 0.01	−0.11
20	−0.29	0.06	< 0.01	−0.07	40	−4.51	0.89	17.24	−12.74

Least squares results for Numerical Example 8.5.

Parameter	d.f.	Estimate	s.e.	t-value	$\Pr > |t|$
Intercept	1	0.122	0.032	3.85	0.0005
X_1	1	-0.00005	0.00002	-2.96	0.0056
X_2	1	0.00004	0.0002	0.30	0.7691
X_3	1	0.0002	0.0001	2.83	0.0079
X_4	1	-0.0009	0.0004	-2.30	0.0275
X_5	1	0.0134	0.0022	5.87	$< .0001$

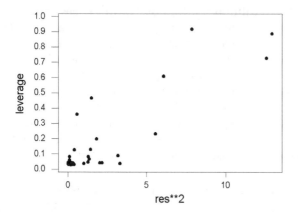

$L - R$ plot for Numerical Example 8.5

These results indicate that cases 2, 15, 31 and 40 are influential. The $L - R$ plot enables us to distinguish outliers from high leverage points.   ▲

8.6   Dummy variables in regression

The explanatory variables in a regression model may be quantitative variables or qualitative variables. Quantitative variables assume continuous values over some interval on the real line. The explanatory variables are qualitative or categorical, when they assume one of a few discrete values. A dummy variable, or indicator variable is any variable in a regression equation that assumes one of a finite number of discrete values and identifies different categories of a nominal variable. The values assumed by such variables do not represent any meaningful measurement; they are values such as 0, 1, or -1, and indicate the category into which the subject falls. If the nominal regressor has L categories, we can create L dummy variables to index these categories. We must include exactly $L - 1$

of these indicator variables in a regression model which includes an intercept term, whereas if the regression model does not include an intercept, then we may include all L indicator variables. An example of a dummy variable is gender, i.e., $W_1 = 1$ if the subject is a female, and $W_1 = 0$ if the subject is a male. Suppose a qualitative variable represents the location of a factory in one of three geographic regions of the U.S., South, West, or Midwest. Two dummy variables suffice: let $W_1 = 1$ if the factory is in the South, and zero otherwise; let $W_2 = 1$ if the factory is in the West, and zero otherwise. In practice, a response variable Y may be explained by L dummy variables and k quantitative predictors. This situation leads to a set of L parallel planes, each representing a regression equation between Y and the k quantitative predictors for a particular level of the dummy variable predictor. When $k = 1$, the model corresponds to sets of L regression lines.

In Example 7.2.4, we discussed sets of L regression lines, which can be represented by

$$S_{H_0} = \{Y_{l,i} = \beta_{l,0} + \beta_{l,1}X_{l,i} + \varepsilon_{l,i}, \quad i = 1, \cdots, n_l, l = 1, \cdots, L\}.$$

We derived the least squares estimates both under the assumption of different slopes, and the assumption of the same slope. We also derived a test for parallelism. We continue with inference for sets of regression lines, and derive tests that enable us to compare these lines. Although the notation gets cumbersome, this approach can be easily extended to compare L regression planes as well. In each case, the number of model parameters when there is no restriction is $p = 2L$, while the total number of observations is $N = \sum_{l=1}^{L} n_l$.

Result 8.6.1. Test for concurrence. The null hypothesis of concurrence of L regression lines at a point on the y-axis, (i.e., when $X = 0$) is $H_1 : \beta_{1,0} = \beta_{2,0} = \cdots = \beta_{L,0} = \beta_0$, say. The test statistic has an $F_{L-1,N-2L}$ distribution under the null hypothesis.

Proof. We can write

$$S_{H_1} = \{Y_{l,i} = \beta_0 + \beta_{l,1}X_{l,i} + \varepsilon_{l,i}, \quad i = 1, \cdots, n_l, l = 1, \cdots, L\}.$$

The least squares estimates of the common intercept and L slopes under H_1 may be derived using (4.6.6) as

$$\tilde{\beta}_0 = \frac{Y_{..} - \{\sum_{l=1}^{L} X_{l\cdot} \sum_{i=1}^{n_l} Y_{l,i}X_{l,i} / \sum_{i=1}^{n_l} X_{l,i}^2\}}{N - \{\sum_{l=1}^{L} X_{l\cdot}^2 / \sum_{i=1}^{n_l} X_{l,i}^2\}}, \tag{8.6.1}$$

$$\tilde{\beta}_{l,1} = \frac{\sum_{i=1}^{n_l} (Y_{l,i} - \tilde{\beta}_0)X_{l,i}}{\sum_{i=1}^{n_l} X_{l,i}}, \quad l = 1, \cdots, L. \tag{8.6.2}$$

It follows that

$$SSE_{H_1} = \sum_{l=1}^{L}\sum_{i=1}^{n_l}(Y_{l,i} - \widetilde{\beta}_0 - \widetilde{\beta}_{l,1}X_{l,i})^2, \text{ and}$$

$$R(H_0|H_1) = SSE_{H_1} - SSE_{H_0},$$

so that

$$F(H_0|H_1) = \{R(H_0|H_1)/(L-1)\}/\{SSE/(N-2L)\} \sim F_{L-1,N-2L}$$

distribution under H_1. ∎

Result 8.6.2. Test for coincidence.   The hypothesis of coincidence of L regression lines is given by $H_1 : \beta_{1,0} = \beta_{2,0} = \cdots = \beta_{L,0} = \beta_0$ and $\beta_{1,1} = \beta_{2,1} = \cdots, \beta_{L,1} = \beta_1$. The test statistic has an $F_{2(L-1),N-2L}$ distribution under the null hypothesis.

Proof. The least squares estimates of the common intercept and common slope under H_1 may be derived using (4.6.6) as

$$\widetilde{\beta}_0 = \overline{Y}.., \text{ and}$$

$$\widetilde{\beta}_{l,1} = \frac{\sum_{l=1}^{L}\sum_{i=1}^{n_l}(Y_{l,i} - \overline{Y}..)(X_{l,i} - \overline{X}..)}{\sum_{l=1}^{L}\sum_{i=1}^{n_l}(X_{l,i} - \overline{X}..)^2}. \tag{8.6.3}$$

We can show that

$$SSE_{H_1} = \sum_{l=1}^{L}\sum_{i=1}^{n_l}(Y_{l,i} - \overline{Y}..)^2 - \widetilde{\beta}^2\sum_{l=1}^{L}\sum_{i=1}^{n_l}(X_{l,i} - \overline{X}..)^2 \text{ and}$$

$$F(H_0|H_1) = \frac{(SSE_{H_1} - SSE_{H_0})/(2L-2)}{SSE/(N-2L)} \sim F_{2(L-1),N-2L}$$

under H_1. ∎

Numerical Example 8.6. Dummy variables in regression.   The data consists of weights (in lbs.) and the ages (in weeks) of 13 Thanksgiving turkeys. Of these 13 birds, four were reared in Georgia (G), four in Virginia (V) and five in Wisconsin (W). Let Y denote the weight, X denote the age, and O denote the origin of these turkey (Draper and Smith, 1998). The least squares estimates and ANOVA for a regression between Y and X, ignoring the grouping by origin are shown below.

Least squares estimates of Y versus X, ignoring O

Variable	d.f.	Estimate	s.e.	t-value	Pr > $|t|$	SS
Intercept	1	1.983	2.332	0.85	0.413	2124.803
X	1	0.417	0.089	4.67	0.0007	26.202

Analysis of variance for Y versus X, ignoring O

Source	d.f.	SS	MS	F-value	Pr > F
Model	1	26.202	26.202	21.81	0.0007
Error	11	13.215	1.201		
Corrected					
Total	12	39.417			

We have $\widehat{\sigma} = \sqrt{MSE} = 1.096$, $R^2 = 0.665$, and $R^2_{adj.} = 0.634$. We next seek to verify a linear relationship between weights and ages, incorporating the effect of different origins into the model, and compare whether the effect of age on weight is the same for each origin in the context of sets of regression lines (testing for parallelism).

Least squares estimates of Y versus X, G, and V

Variable	d.f.	Estimate	s.e.	t-value	Pr > |t|	SS
Intercept	1	1.431	0.657	2.18	0.0575	2124.803
X	1	0.487	0.026	18.91	< .0001	26.202
G	1	−1.918	0.202	−9.51	< .0001	2.717
V	1	−2.192	0.211	−10.37	< .0001	9.687

Analysis of variance for Y versus X, G, and V

Source	d.f.	SS	MS	F-value	Pr > F
Model	3	38.606	12.869	142.78	< .0001
Error	9	0.811	0.090		
Corrected					
Total	12	39.417			

In this model, $\widehat{\sigma} = 0.3$, $R^2 = 0.979$ and $R^2_{adj.} = 0.973$. The estimated variance-covariance matrix of the estimates is

$$\begin{pmatrix} 0.432 & -0.017 & -0.010 & 0.023 \\ -0.017 & 0.001 & -0.0003 & -0.002 \\ -0.010 & -0.0003 & 0.041 & 0.019 \\ 0.023 & -0.002 & 0.019 & 0.045 \end{pmatrix}. \quad \blacktriangle$$

8.7 Robust regression

Least squares estimates have several optimality properties within the class of normal linear models, which in addition to their computational simplicity, have made this procedure popular. However, the method of least squares can be extremely sensitive to (a) a departure of the error distribution from normality, and (b) the presence of outliers, even under normality. In general, the class of L_d-estimators are obtained by minimizing the L_d-norm $\{\sum_{i=1}^{N} |\varepsilon_i|^d\}^{1/d}$, $d \geq 1$. When $d = 2$, we have the Euclidean metric, or L_2-norm, and leads to the least squares estimator. The case $d = 1$ corresponds to the *absolute* metric or L_1-norm, and yields the L_1-estimator or LAD estimator, which we discuss below. Note that $d = \infty$ leads to the minimax method (Berger, 1980).

Many robust and resistant methods have been developed since the 1960's with the purpose of obtaining statistical procedures that are less sensitive to outliers or anomalous data values, and are reasonably efficient with data from the ideal Gaussian distribution or a range of alternative distributions. Robust methods are designed to have high efficiency in a neighborhood of an assumed model (Huber, 1964). In the following sections, we describe LAD or L_1-regression and M-regression (see Birkes and Dodge, 1993).

8.7.1   Least absolute deviations (LAD) regression

Least Absolute Deviation(LAD) regression or L_1-regression is a natural generalization of the median to a regression problem and consists of finding the estimator $\widehat{\beta}_{LAD}$ as any solution to the minimization problem

$$\min_b \sum_{i=1}^{N} |Y_i - \mathbf{x}_i'\beta| = \min_b \sum_{i=1}^{N} |\varepsilon_i|, \qquad (8.7.1)$$

where ε_i are iid having a continuous distribution with location 0, scale σ^2 and cdf $F(.)$.

Example 8.7.1.   Suppose the errors ε_i are random samples from a double exponential distribution,

$$f(\varepsilon_i) = (2\sigma)^{-1} \exp(-|\varepsilon_i|/\sigma), \quad -\infty < \varepsilon_i < \infty$$

(see (A16)). Assuming that σ is fixed, it is clear that maximum likelihood estimation of β involves minimization of the expression in (8.7.1).   □

In the literature, LAD regression has alternately been referred to as MAD (Minimum Absolute Deviations) regression, or MAE (Minimum Absolute Errors) regression, or LAR (Least Absolute Residuals) regression, or LAV (Least Absolute Values) regression, or simply L_1-regression. The L_1-regression is a special case of L_p-regression where we minimize $\sum_{i=1}^{N} |Y_i - \mathbf{x}_i'\beta|^p$. Although there is a solution that fits (8.7.1) exactly at p observations, this solution is not necessarily unique. The computation of the solution may be carried out by reducing the problem to one of linear programming (Charnes, Cooper and Ferguson, 1955). The argument is that the minimum of the criterion $\sum_{i=1}^{N} |\varepsilon_i|$ occurs at one of the finite set of points on a piecewise convex surface. Therefore, any minimum of the L_1-norm must lie at one of the vertices of a finite set of

$\binom{N}{p}$ points in $\mathcal{R}^p$. This enables the linear programming algorithm to search among the finite number of vertices for a solution.

The problem is to minimize $\sum_{i=1}^{N} |\varepsilon_i|$, where ε and β are unrestricted in sign. Define nonnegative variables ε_i^+ and ε_i^- by

$$\varepsilon_i^+ = \begin{cases} \varepsilon_i, & \text{if } \varepsilon_i > 0 \\ 0, & \text{if } \varepsilon_i \leq 0, \text{ and} \end{cases}$$

$$\varepsilon_i^- = \begin{cases} 0, & \text{if } \varepsilon_i > 0 \\ -\varepsilon_i, & \text{if } \varepsilon_i \leq 0; \end{cases}$$

either ε_i^+ or ε_i^- will be zero, $|\varepsilon_i| = \varepsilon_i^+ + \varepsilon_i^-$, and $\varepsilon_i = \varepsilon_i^+ - \varepsilon_i^-$. Geometrically, ε_i^+ and ε_i^- can be interpreted respectively as the vertical deviations above and below the fitted hyperplane corresponding to the estimated parameters. We then minimize the function $(\sum_{i=1}^{N} \varepsilon_i^+ + \sum_{i=1}^{N} \varepsilon_i^-)$ subject to $\varepsilon_i^+ \geq 0$, $\varepsilon_i^- \geq 0$, and the equation $e_i^+ - e_i^- = e_i = Y_i - \mathbf{x}_i'\beta$, while β is unrestricted. Since we are minimizing a continuous function which is bounded below over a convex set, the problem always has an optimal solution, although this solution need not be unique, even when $r(\mathbf{X}) = p$. The solution is $\widehat{\beta}_{LAD}$. In some cases (Dodge and Jureckova, 2000), LAD regression is faster than OLS for sufficiently large N and moderate p. Provided the cdf of ε_i has a continuous and positive derivative in a neighborhood of the population median, it is true that as $N \to \infty$, $\widehat{\beta}_{LAD} \sim N(\beta, \sigma^2(\mathbf{X}'\mathbf{X})^{-1})$. In practice, σ^2 is unknown, and is estimated as follows based on the LAD residuals $\widehat{\varepsilon}_{i,LAD} = Y_i - \mathbf{x}_i'\widehat{\beta}_{LAD}$, $i = 1, \cdots, N$. Arrange the $M = (N - p - 1)$ nonzero residuals in ascending order, and denote these by $\widehat{\varepsilon}_{(1),LAD} \leq \cdots \leq \widehat{\varepsilon}_{(M),LAD}$. Let $K_1 = [(M+1)/2 - \sqrt{M}]$ and $K_2 = [(M+1)/2 + \sqrt{M}]$. Then

$$\widehat{\sigma}_{LAD}^2 = \frac{\sqrt{M}\{\widehat{\varepsilon}_{(K_2),LAD} - \widehat{\varepsilon}_{(K_1),LAD}\}}{2z_{\alpha/2}}, \qquad (8.7.2)$$

where $z_{\alpha/2}$ is the upper $\alpha/2$th critical value from a standard normal distribution.

Example 8.7.2. Consider the simple linear regression model $Y_i = \beta_0 + \beta_1 X_i + \varepsilon_i$. The LAD estimates of β_0 and β_1, as well as σ^2 are obtained as described above. It is clear that the p-value of the test $H_0 : \beta_1 = 0$ is $P(|T| > |t|)$, where

$$|t| = \{|\widehat{\beta}_{1,LAD}|[\sum_{i=1}^{N}(X_i - \overline{X})^2]^{1/2}\}/\widehat{\sigma}_{LAD},$$

and $T \sim t_{N-2}$. It has been proved that $\sqrt{N}(\widehat{\beta}_{LAD} - \beta)$ converges in distribution (as $N \to \infty$) to a $N(\mathbf{0}, \{2f(0)\}^{-2}\mathbf{Q}^{-1})$ distribution, where $f(0)$ is the pdf at the median, and $\mathbf{Q} = \lim \mathbf{X}'\mathbf{X}/N$. $\square$

A more general formulation given by Bassett and Koenker (1978) is useful. Suppose as before that the errors ε_i in the linear model are iid with cdf $F(.)$, which is symmetric about 0. The θth regression quantile ($0 < \theta < 1$) is defined as any solution to the minimization problem

$$\min_{\beta} \left[\sum_{\{i:Y_i \geq \mathbf{x}_i'\beta\}} \theta \, |Y_i - \mathbf{x}_i'\beta| + \sum_{\{i:Y_i < \mathbf{x}_i'\beta\}} (1-\theta)\,|Y_i - \mathbf{x}_i'\beta| \right]. \tag{8.7.3}$$

When $\theta = 1/2$, this is equivalent to minimizing $\sum_{i=1}^{N} |Y_i - \mathbf{x}_i'\beta|$, and the resulting estimator coincides with $\widehat{\beta}_{LAD}$. Let $\widehat{\beta}^*(\theta)$ denote the solution to (8.7.3). For a general discussion of asymptotic properties of this estimator, and for a discussion of the trimmed least squares estimator, see Bassett and Koenker (1978) and Ruppert and Carroll (1980).

Example 8.7.3. Censored Regression. We describe a *limited dependent variable* model in which the response variable, which is observed over time, is censored. The tobit model is, for $t = 1, \cdots, N$,

$$Y_t^* = \begin{cases} Y_t = \mathbf{x}_t'\beta + \varepsilon_t, & \text{if } Y_t > 0 \\ 0, & \text{if } Y_t < 0, \end{cases} \tag{8.7.4}$$

where we assume that ε_t, $t = 1, \cdots, N$ are iid, whose cdf $F(.)$ has positive derivative $f(0)$ at zero, and has median zero. We also assume that the true regression parameter belongs to a bounded open set of $\mathcal{R}^p$. Let I denote the indicator function of a set of values; i.e., $I(u) = 1$ if u belongs to that set, otherwise $I(u) = 0$. The tobit model can also be written as

$$Y_t^+ = (\mathbf{x}_t'\beta + \varepsilon_t)^+, \quad t = 1, \cdots, N, \tag{8.7.5}$$

where the function q_t^+ denotes $q_t I(q_t > 0)$. Powell (1984) studied the properties of the LAD estimator of β which is obtained by minimizing

$$\sum_{i=1}^{N} |Y_t^+ - (\mathbf{x}_t'\widehat{\beta}_{LAD})^+|. \tag{8.7.6}$$

Under some regularity conditions, Powell (1984), and Rao and Zhao (1993) proved the asymptotic normality of this estimator.

Suppose we wish to test $H_0 : \mathbf{C}'\beta = \mathbf{d}$ versus the alternative $H_1 : \mathbf{C}'\beta \neq \mathbf{d}$, where as before, $\mathbf{C}$ is a $p \times s$ matrix of rank s, and $\mathbf{d}$ is a constant vector. Let $\widehat{\beta}_{LAD,H_0}$ denote the solution to (8.7.6) subject to H_0. The likelihood ratio test statistic is

$$LRT = \sum_{i=1}^{N} |Y_t^+ - (\mathbf{x}_t'\widehat{\beta}_{LAD,H_0})^+| - \sum_{i=1}^{N} |Y_t^+ - (\mathbf{x}_t'\widehat{\beta}_{LAD})^+|. \tag{8.7.7}$$

In practice, $f(0)$ is unknown and is estimated by

$$
\begin{aligned}
\widehat{f}_N(0) &= h[\sum_{i=1}^{N} I(\mathbf{x}_t'\widehat{\beta}_{LAD} > 0)^{-1}] \\
&\times [\sum_{i=1}^{N} I(\mathbf{x}_t'\widehat{\beta}_{LAD} > 0)I(\mathbf{x}_t'\widehat{\beta}_{LAD} < Y_t^+ \le \mathbf{x}_t'\widehat{\beta}_{LAD} + h)]. \quad (8.7.8)
\end{aligned}
$$

Under certain conditions (see Rao and Zhao, 1993), $4\widehat{f}(0)LRT$ has a limiting χ_s^2 distribution under H_0. $\square$

8.7.2 *M*-regression

The *M*-estimator, which was introduced by Huber (1964), is a robust alternative to the least squares estimator in the linear model. It is attractive because it is relatively simple to compute, and offers good performance and flexibility. In the model (4.1.2), we assume that ε_i are iid random variables with cdf $F(.)$, which is symmetric about 0. The distribution of ε_i can be fairly general; in fact we need not assume existence of the mean and variance of the distribution. Recall from section 7.5.1 that the MLE of β is obtained as a solution to the likelihood equations

$$
\sum_{i=1}^{N} \mathbf{x}_i\{f'(Y_i - \mathbf{x}_i'\beta)/f(Y_i - \mathbf{x}_i'\beta)\} = \mathbf{0}, \quad (8.7.9)
$$

where $f(.)$ denotes the pdf of ε_i, and $f'(.)$ denotes its first derivative. Suppose (8.7.9) cannot be solved explicitly; by replacing $f'(.)/f(.)$ by a suitable function $\psi(.)$, we obtain a "pseudo maximum likelihood" estimator of β, which is called its *M*-estimator. The function $\psi(.)$ is generally chosen such that it leads to an estimator $\widehat{\beta}_M$ which is robust to alternative specifications of $f(.)$. Suppose $\rho(.)$ is a convex, continuously differentiable function on $\mathcal{R}$, and suppose $\psi(.)$ denotes the first derivative of $\rho(.)$, i.e., $\psi(t) = (d/dt)\rho(t)$. The *M*-estimator $\widehat{\beta}_M$ of β in the model (4.1.2) is obtained by minimizing, over β, the objective function

$$
\sum_{i=1}^{N} \rho(Y_i - \mathbf{x}_i'\beta), \quad (8.7.10)
$$

or, equivalently, by solving the set of p equations

$$
\sum_{i=1}^{N} \mathbf{x}_i\psi(Y_i - \mathbf{x}_i'\beta) = \mathbf{0}. \quad (8.7.11)
$$

When (a) the function $\rho(.)$ is not convex, or (b) the first derivative of $\rho(.)$ is not continuous, or (c) the first derivative exists everywhere except at a finite or countably infinite number of points, we consider $\widehat{\beta}_M$ to be a solution of (8.7.10), since (8.7.11) might not have a solution, or might lead to an incorrect solution. By a suitable choice of $\rho(.)$ and $\psi(.)$, we can obtain an estimator which is robust to possible heavy-tailed behavior in $f(.)$.

To ensure that $\widehat{\beta}_M$ is scale-invariant, we generalize (8.7.10) and (8.7.11) respectively to

$$\sum_{i=1}^{N} \rho\{(Y_i - \mathbf{x}_i'\beta)/\sigma\}, \text{ and} \qquad (8.7.12)$$

$$\sum_{i=1}^{N} \mathbf{x}_i \psi\{(Y_i - \mathbf{x}_i'\beta)/\sigma\} = \mathbf{0}. \qquad (8.7.13)$$

In practice, σ is unknown, and is replaced by a robust estimate. One such estimate is the median of the absolute residuals from an LAD regression.

As we have seen, M-regression generalizes least-squares estimation by allowing a choice of objective functions. Least squares regression corresponds to $\rho(t) = t^2$. In general, we have considerable flexibility in choosing the function $\rho(t)$, and this choice in turn determines the properties of $\widehat{\beta}_M$. The choice involves a balance between efficiency and robustness.

Example 8.7.3. Median regression.   Suppose the true regression function is the conditional median of $\mathbf{y}$ given $\mathbf{X}$. The choice of $\rho(t)$ is $|t|$, and the corresponding problem is called median regression.   □

Example 8.7.4. W-regression is an alternative form of M-regression; $\widehat{\beta}_W$ is a solution to the p simultaneous equations

$$\sum_{i=1}^{N} \left(\frac{Y_i - \mathbf{x}_i'\beta}{\sigma}\right) w_i \mathbf{x}_i' = \mathbf{0}, \qquad (8.7.14)$$

where $w_i = w\{(Y_i - \mathbf{x}_i'\beta)/\sigma\}$. The equations in (8.7.14) are obtained by replacing $\psi(t)$ by $tw(t)$ in (8.7.10); $w(t)$ is called a weight function.   □

8.8   Nonparametric regression methods

The parametric approach to linear model inference assumes that the functional form of the relationship between the response and predictors is linear and known, so that the problem reduces to that of estimation and inference pertaining to the parameters (under some distributional assumption on the errors). On the other hand, nonparametric methods only make a few general assumptions about the regression surface. For instance, in smoothing techniques with kernel, nearest-neighbor, or spline methods (Hastie and Tibsirani, 1990; Thisted, 1988), the estimate of the regression surface at a point $\mathbf{x}_0$ is the average of the responses of those observations with predictors in the neighborhood of $\mathbf{x}_0$. In this section, we give a brief introduction to computer-intensive regression methods that are useful for nonparametric fitting, when the set of explanatory vectors is high-dimensional, or when a parametric linear model does not satisfactorily explain the relationship between Y and $\mathbf{X}$. Although these methods do not involve non-linear parameterizations, the procedures do allow for the possibility of choosing a nonlinear function of the explanatory variables.

Additive models and projection pursuit regression are described in the next two subsections. The additive model is a generalization of the linear regression model, where the usual linear function of observed covariates is replaced by a sum of unspecified smooth functions of these covariates. Projection pursuit (Friedman and Tukey, 1974) is an exploratory procedure which seeks to unravel structure within a high-dimensional predictor set by finding interesting orthogonal linear projections of the data onto a low-dimensional linear subspace, such as a line or a plane.

8.8.1 Additive models

An additive model is defined by

$$Y_i = \tau + \sum_{j=1}^{p} g_j(X_{ij}) + \varepsilon_i, \quad E(\varepsilon_i) = 0, Var(\varepsilon_i) = \sigma^2, \tag{8.8.1}$$

where the g_j's are arbitrarily defined functions, one for each predictor. A simple assumption may be that each of these component functions is univariate and smooth; however, the smoothness assumption may be relaxed, and it is possible to have a function that is continuous and multi-dimensional, or even categorical. One attractive feature of the additive model is that the variation of the response surface obtained by holding all other predictors but one fixed does not depend on the values of these predictors. Hence, after fitting the additive model to data, it is possible to plot the p coordinate functions separately in order to assess their usefulness in modeling Y.

In an additive model, no parametric form is imposed on the functions and they are estimated nonparametrically in an iterative way using *smoothers*. A smoother is a nonparametric tool for estimating the trend of a response Y as a function of predictors $X_1, \cdots, X_k$. The estimated trend is less variable than Y itself, which leads to the name "smoother". The *scatterplot smoother* is a special case when there is a single predictor. Given data $\mathbf{y} = (Y_1, \cdots, Y_n)'$ and $\mathbf{x} = (X_1, \cdots, X_n)'$, a scatterplot smoother is a function of $\mathbf{x}$ and $\mathbf{y}$. When there are several predictors, we have multiple predictor smoothers. The primary functions of smoothers are (a) as graphical descriptions of the data by enhancing the scatterplot of Y versus $\mathbf{X}$, and (b) as vehicles for estimation of the dependence of Y on $\mathbf{X}$ in the context of additive models. If there is a single categorical predictor, the smoother is very simple and consists of averaging the Y values in each category corresponding to the predictor. For continuous predictors, we may use the notion of local averaging, i.e., averaging Y values in the neighborhood of a target predictor value. Two questions to be resolved are

(a) the size of these neighborhoods, and (b) the nature of the averaging within the chosen neighborhoods, i.e., the type of smoother to use. A large neighborhood produces an estimate with low variance but high bias, with the converse for small neighborhoods. There is thus a tradeoff between bias and variance of estimation. The size of the neighborhood is expressed in terms of an adjustable smoothing parameter.

The estimated model consists of a function for each covariate. Apart from their use in predicting the response variable, additive models enable us to explore the appropriate shape of each covariate effect on the response. The idea behind the scatterplot smoother is to explore and delineate the functional dependence in multivariate data without a rigid parametric assumption about that dependence, such as linearity, or an exponential form, etc. Hastie and Tibsirani (1990) present a detailed description of this procedure for data analysis.

The most general approach for fitting additive models to data consists of estimating each component function by an arbitrary smoother, such as cubic smoothing splines, locally-weighted running lines, or kernel smoothers. The fitting then proceeds *iteratively*, possibly by minimizing the appropriate penalized least squares criterion; the back fitting algorithm is a general algorithm that enables us to fit an additive model to data. The algorithm consists of the following steps.

(i) Initialization: Set $\tau = ave(Y_i)$, where *ave* could be the mean, median, etc., and set $g_j = g_j^0$, $j = 1, \cdots, p$.

(ii) Update: For $j = 1, \cdots, p$, set $g_j = S_j(\mathbf{Y} - \tau - \sum_{j \neq k} g_j(X_j) \,|\mathbf{X}_k)$, where S_j denotes the jth scatterplot smoother.

(iii) Continue (ii) until the individual functions do not change.

The backfitting algorithm is motivated by the fact that, if the additive model is correct, then for any k,

$$E\{Y - \tau - \sum_{j \neq k} g_j(X_j)|\mathbf{X}_k\} = g_k(X_k). \qquad (8.8.2)$$

The usual linear regression estimates may be used for the initialization. By design, the algorithm is only given as a modular skeleton; details for a particular user would depend on the choice of smoother and the data analytic context in which the model is employed. It has been pointed out that when the smoothers are linear operators, the back fitting algorithm is a Gauss-Seidel algorithm for solving a certain set of estimating equations, and convergence in many practical situations has been proven. When all the smoothers S_j are projection operators, the whole back fitting algorithm may be replaced by a global projection that involves no iteration and whose convergence is guaranteed. Although smoothers such as smoothing splines are not projections, they do possess properties of projections that guarantee that the solution converges.

Generalized additive models (GAMs) are an extension to the class of generalized linear models (GLIMs), where the linear form $\tau + \sum_{j=1}^p X_{ij}\beta_j$ is replaced by the sum of component functions, $\tau + \sum_{j=1}^{p} g_j(X_{ij})$. A suitable link function between the predictors and the response which has a general probability distribution is chosen similar to the GLIM setup (see section 11.4).

8.8.2 Projection pursuit regression

In the linear regression model (4.1.2), we assumed that the response surface has a fixed linear form. In projection pursuit regression, the regression surface is approximated by a sum of smooth functions of linear combinations $\mathbf{c}'\mathbf{X}$ of the predictors, viz.,

$$PPR(\mathbf{X}) = c_0 + \sum_{j=1}^{J} S_{\mathbf{c}_j}(\mathbf{c}_j'\mathbf{X}), \qquad (8.8.3)$$

and $\mathbf{y} = PPR(\mathbf{X}) + \varepsilon$. In other words, projection pursuit regression employs an additive model on predictor variables which are obtained as projections of $\mathbf{X}$ in J chosen directions. The terms in (8.8.3) are constant in all directions except one, and are called ridge functions. As shown by Diaconis and Shahshahani (1984), these models can approximate arbitrary continuous functions of $\mathbf{X}$ when J is sufficiently large.

Definition 8.8.1. Consider a set of observations (Y_i, Z_i), $i = 1, \cdots, N$. Based on the notion of local averaging, we define a *smooth representation* of Y as ordered in ascending value of Z by

$$S(Z_i) = \underset{i-k \le j \le i+k}{AVE}(Y_j),$$

where AVE can denote any average, such as the mean, median, etc.

Definition 8.8.2. We define a criterion of fit $I(\mathbf{a}, \mathbf{v}, \mathbf{U})$ by

$$I(\mathbf{a}, \mathbf{v}, \mathbf{U}) = 1 - \sum_{i=1}^{N}\{V_i - S_{\mathbf{a}}(\mathbf{a}'\mathbf{u_i})\}^2 / \sum_{i=1}^{N} V_i^2,$$

where $\mathbf{v}' = (V_1, \cdots, V_N)$, $\mathbf{U} = (\mathbf{u}_1, \cdots, \mathbf{u}_p)$, $\mathbf{u}_j$ is an N-dimensional vector, and $S_{\mathbf{a}}(\mathbf{a}'\mathbf{u_i})$ follows from Definition 8.8.1.

Given data $(Y_i, \mathbf{x}_i')$, $i = 1, \cdots, N$, the iterative algorithm (Friedman and Stuetzle, 1981) applies an additive model to projected variables and consists of the following steps. Let δ denote a user-supplied threshold value (lower bound) for smoothness.

(i) Set the iteration counter $J = 0$, and initialize residuals to the centered responses, $\widehat{\varepsilon}_i^{(0)} = Y_i - \overline{Y}$, $i = 1, \cdots, N$.

(ii) Search for the next term in the model. For a chosen vector $\mathbf{c}$, obtain the one-dimensional projection $Z_i = \mathbf{c}'\mathbf{x}_i$, $i = 1, \cdots, N$. Construct a smooth representation of the current residuals sequenced in ascending order of Z. Find the vector $\mathbf{c}_{J+1}$ that maximizes $I(\mathbf{c}, \widehat{\varepsilon}, \mathbf{X})$. Let $S_{\mathbf{c}_{J+1}}$ denote the corresponding smooth.

(iii) If the criterion of fit is smaller than δ, we terminate the procedure. If not, we increment the iteration counter to $J + 1$, and update the residuals to

$$\widehat{\varepsilon}_i^{(J+1)} = \widehat{\varepsilon}_i^{(J)} - S_{\mathbf{c}_{J+1}}(\mathbf{c}_{J+1}'\mathbf{x}_i), \quad i = 1, \cdots, N,$$

and repeat from Step (ii).

Notice that the models at the jth step are sums of j smooth functions of arbitrary linear combinations of $X_1, \cdots, X_p$.

Unlike additive models, projection pursuit regression models can include interactions between the X_j's in the model function, and are therefore useful for representing general regression surfaces.

8.8.3   Neural networks regression

Neural networks are mathematical objects representing a system of interconnected computational units (Cheng and Titterington, 1994; Hertz, Krogh and Palmer, 1991). That is, they constitute a collection of a possibly large number of simple computational units which are interlinked by a system of possibly intricate connections. In the neural networks framework, specification of the general linear model and associated parametric inference are handled by constructing a network of nodes and links from which the linear model can be written down. The most common neural-networks approach to linear models is multilayer perceptrons and generalizations of single-layer perceptrons. This approach is extremely valuable when the problem involves very high-dimensional vectors and matrices which impose a limitation on the usual matrix methods that we discussed in earlier chapters. In most applications of neural networks, there is no explicit assumption of randomness or an ensuing probabilistic structure in the underlying variables. Instead, the aim is function approximation, and optimality criteria that enable the choice of the approximant, such as the least squares criterion, can no longer be interpreted as a log-likelihood function (under a normality assumption, say). A flexible approach to generalize linear regression functions uses feed-forward neural networks.

The simplest feed-forward network is the single-unit perceptron, which consists of K input units (covariates) $X_1, \cdots, X_k$, and one output (response) Y. The mean response is related to the covariates via the function

$$E(Y) = g(\mathbf{x}, \mathbf{w}) = w_0 + \sum_{j=1}^{N} w_j X_j, \tag{8.8.4}$$

where w_j is the weight corresponding to X_j, $j = 1, \cdots, K$, and $g(.)$ is a known activation function. Given N sets of observations $(\mathbf{x}_i, Y_i)$, $i = 1, \cdots, N$ in a *training sample*, we must determine the vector of weights such that the *energy function* or *learning function*

$$E(\mathbf{w}) = \sum_{i=1}^{N} \{Y_i - g(\mathbf{x}_i, \mathbf{w})\}^2 \tag{8.8.5}$$

is minimized with respect to $\mathbf{w}$. Using the least squares approach, we must solve the system of estimation equations

$$\frac{\partial E(\mathbf{w})}{\partial w_k} = \sum_{i=1}^{N}[Y_i - g(\mathbf{x}_i, \mathbf{w}]\frac{\partial g(\mathbf{x}_i, \mathbf{w})}{\partial w_k} = 0, \quad k = 0, 1, \cdots, K \qquad (8.8.6)$$

using numerical techniques such as the generalized delta rule or error back-propagation (Rumelhart et al., 1986), or gradient methods (Thisted, 1988).

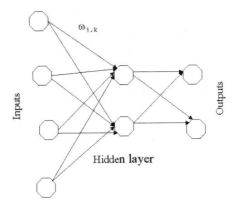

Figure 8.8.1.   A feed-forward neural network with one hidden layer.

A neural network with one hidden layer is shown in Figure 8.8.1. The input units distribute the inputs to the *hidden* units in the second layer. The hidden units cumulate their inputs, together with a constant term (the bias). An activation function ϕ_k is applied to this sum. The output units have the same form, except with output function ϕ_0. This gives

$$Y_i = \phi_0\{\tau_i + \sum_k \omega_{k,i}\phi_k(\tau_k + \sum_j \omega_{j,k}X_j)\}. \qquad (8.8.7)$$

The usual choice for the activation function of the hidden layer is the logistic function

$$\phi_k(u) = \exp(u)/\{1 + \exp(u)\}.$$

In practice, the weights must be chosen to minimize some fitting criterion, such as the least squares criterion which minimizes the L_2-norm between the output and the target, or in other words, minimizes $S = \sum_l \| T^l - Y^l \|^2$, where T^l is the target, and Y^l is the output for the lth pattern. Alternatively, we can minimize the function $S + \lambda D(f)$, where, for L patterns, the penalty function on the second derivatives of $g(.)$ has the form

$$D(g) = \int \sum_{i,j}(\partial^2 Y_i/\partial X_j^2)dx \approx \{\sum_{i,j,l} \partial^2 Y_i/\partial X_j^2\}/L.$$

The reader is referred to Warner and Misra (1996) for a accesible summary of this technique.

8.8.4   Curve estimation based on wavelet methods

Wavelet methods, which incorporate *wavelet bases*, are becoming increasingly useful in several branches of statistical modeling, including regression analysis. Consider the simple nonparametric regression model

$$Y_i = g(X_i) + \sigma\varepsilon_i, \quad i = 1, \cdots, N, \tag{8.8.8}$$

where the X_i's are equally spaced points, the ε_i's are iid $N(0,1)$ variables, and the regression function $g(.)$ is unknown. We can write (8.8.8) in vector notation as

$$\mathbf{y} = \mathbf{g} + \sigma\varepsilon, \tag{8.8.9}$$

where $\mathbf{g} = (g_1, \cdots, g_N)$. In the literature, two versions of this model are discussed (Antoniadis, Gregoire and McKeague, 1994). In the *fixed design model*, the X_i's are nonrandom design points, usually denoted by t_i, and ordered, i.e., $0 \leq t_1 \leq \cdots \leq t_N \leq 1$; the ε_i are iid with zero mean and variance σ^2. The *random design model* assumes that the (X_i, Y_i)'s are independently distributed, $g(x) = E(Y|X = x)$, and $\varepsilon_i = Y_i - g(X_i)$. Under both versions, the objective is to estimate $\mathbf{g}$ based on (Y_i, X_i), $i = 1, \cdots, N$ using functions of wavelets. To be more specific, our goal is to estimate the regression function $g(u)$, $0 < u < 1$ based on wavelet kernels (which are defined later).

In order to estimate $g(.)$ based on available discrete data, we must process the discrete wavelet transform, which maps the N-dimensional response vector $\mathbf{y}$ to an N-dimensional vector $\mathbf{d} = (d_1, \cdots, d_N)'$ in the wavelet domain.

Definition 8.8.3.   The discrete wavelet transformation is a linear transformation defined by

$$\mathbf{d} = \mathbf{Wy}, \tag{8.8.10}$$

where $\mathbf{W}$ is an orthogonal $N \times N$ matrix.

Let $\theta = (\theta_1, \cdots, \theta_N)' = \mathbf{Wg}$, and let $\varepsilon^* = (\varepsilon_1^*, \cdots, \varepsilon_N^*)' = \mathbf{W}\varepsilon$. By Exercise 5.9, $\varepsilon^* \sim N(\mathbf{0}, \mathbf{I}_N)$. The *wavelet image* of (8.8.8) under this orthogonal wavelet transformation is

$$d_i = \theta_i + \sigma\varepsilon_i^*, \quad i = 1, \cdots, N, \tag{8.8.11}$$

or, in vector notation,

$$\mathbf{d} = \theta + \sigma\varepsilon^*. \tag{8.8.12}$$

Since ε^* and ε have the same distribution, we can write the model in the wavelet domain as $\mathbf{d} = \theta + \sigma\varepsilon$.

The discrete wavelet estimator $\widehat{\mathbf{g}}$ which is based on thresholding in the wavelet domain was discussed by Donoho and Johnstone (1994). The procedure of constructing this estimator consists of three steps.

(i) Transform the observations Y_i, $i = 1, \cdots, N$ to the wavelet domain by applying a discrete wavelet transformation, yielding a sequence of wavelet coefficients d_i, $i = 1, \cdots, N$.

(ii) Using an estimate of σ, threshold (or shrink) the wavelet coefficients.

(iii) Invert the shrunk coefficients, obtaining $\widehat{g}_i$, $i = 1, \cdots, N$.

In the rest of this section, we describe linear wavelet regression estimators (see Vidakovic, 1999). We first give a few definitions on the set of complex numbers $\mathcal{C}$. Note that if a is a complex number, we denote its complex conjugate by $\bar{a}$.

Definition 8.8.4. Inner-product space. A complex vector space $\mathcal{H}$ is called an inner-product space if for each pair of elements x and y in $\mathcal{H}$, there exists a complex number $< x, y >$, called the inner product of x and y, such that

1. $< x, y >= \overline{< y, x >}$

2. $< x + y, z >=< x, z > + < y, z >$ for all $x, y, z \in \mathcal{H}$

3. $< \alpha x, y >= \alpha < x, y >$ for all $x, y \in \mathcal{H}$ and $\alpha \in \mathcal{C}$

4. $< x, x > \; \geq 0$ for all $x \in \mathcal{H}$

5. $< x, x > \; = 0$ if and only if $x = 0$.

Definition 8.8.5. Cauchy sequence. A sequence $\{x_n, n = 1, 2, \cdots\}$ of elements of an inner-product space is called a Cauchy sequence if

$$\| x_n - x_m \| \to 0 \text{ as } m, n \to \infty,$$

i.e., if for every $\epsilon > 0$, there exists a positive integer $N(\epsilon)$ such that

$$\| x_n - x_m \| < \epsilon \text{ for all } m, n > N(\epsilon).$$

Definition 8.8.6. Hilbert space. A Hilbert space $\mathcal{H}$ is an inner-product space which is complete, i.e., an inner-product space in which every Cauchy sequence $\{x_n\}$ converges in norm to some element $x \in \mathcal{H}$. The norm of an element $x \in \mathcal{H}$ is defined as $\| x \| = \sqrt{< x, x >}$.

A linear subspace $\mathcal{V}$ of a Hilbert space $\mathcal{H}$ is said to be a closed subspace of $\mathcal{H}$ if $\mathcal{V}$ contains all its limiting points, i.e., if $x_n \in \mathcal{V}$ and $\| x_n - x \| \to 0$ as $n \to \infty$, then $x \in \mathcal{V}$. The space $\mathcal{L}_2$ is the space of all square-integrable functions, i.e., if $f, g \in \mathcal{L}_2$, $<f, g>= \int f\overline{g}$ and $\| f \| = \sqrt{\int f\overline{f}}$. Let $\mathcal{V}$ be a subspace of $\mathcal{L}_2$ and let $\{e_1, e_2, \cdots\}$ be a complete orthonormal basis of $\mathcal{V}$.

Definition 8.8.7.   The scaling function $\varphi(x)$ is the solution of a two-scale difference equation:

$$\varphi(x) \;=\; \sum_{k \in \mathcal{Z}} c_k \varphi(2x - k), \text{ with}$$

$$\int_{\mathcal{R}} \varphi(x)dx \;=\; 1;$$

the coefficients c_k are called filter coefficients, and their choice enables the construction of wavelet functions with desirable properties.

Definition 8.8.8.   The primary wavelet function $\psi(x)$ is defined by

$$\psi(x) = \sum_{k \in \mathcal{Z}} (-1)^k c_{k+1} \varphi(2x + k),$$

where $\mathcal{Z}$ is the set of integers.

   As we said earlier, our goal is to estimate the regression function using wavelet kernels, viz., integral operators $\mathcal{K}_j(x, y)$ that project onto closed subspaces $\mathcal{V}_j$ of $\mathcal{L}_2(\mathcal{R})$, which is the space of all square-integrable functions. The increasing sequence of subspaces $\mathcal{V}_j$ form a *multiresolution analysis* of $\mathcal{L}_2(\mathcal{R})$. A multiresolution analysis (MRA) is a sequence of closed subspaces $\mathcal{V}_n$, $n \in \mathcal{Z}$ in $\mathcal{L}_2(\mathcal{R})$ such that

$$\cdots \subset \mathcal{V}_{-2} \subset \mathcal{V}_{-1} \subset \mathcal{V}_0 \subset \mathcal{V}_1 \subset \mathcal{V}_2 \subset \cdots,$$

$\cap_j \mathcal{V}_j = \{0\}$, and $\overline{\cup_j \mathcal{V}_j} = \mathcal{L}_2(\mathcal{R})$ ($\overline{A}$ denotes the closure of the set A). Further,

$$g(2^j x) \in \mathcal{V}_j \text{ if and only if } g(x) \in \mathcal{V}_0,$$

and there exists a scaling function $\phi \in \mathcal{V}_0$ such that

$$\mathcal{V}_0 = \{g \in \mathcal{L}_2(\mathcal{R}) | g(x) = \textstyle\sum_k c_k \phi(x - k)\}.$$

   For the fixed-design model, Antoniadis et al. (1994) suggest the waveletized Gasser-Mueller kernel estimator

$$\widehat{g}(x) = \sum_{i=1}^{N} Y_i \int_{A_i} \mathcal{K}_j(x, y)dy, \tag{8.8.13}$$

where

$$\mathcal{K}_j(x, y) \;=\; 2^j K(2^j x, 2^j y), \text{ with} \tag{8.8.14}$$

$$\mathcal{K}(u, v) \;=\; \sum_k \phi(u - k)\phi(v - k), \tag{8.8.15}$$

and $\mathcal{K}(u, v)$ and $\mathcal{K}_j(x, y)$ are respectively reproducing kernels of $\mathcal{V}_0$ and $\mathcal{V}_j$. The $A_i = [s_{i-1}, s_i)$ are intervals that partition $[0, 1]$ so that $x_i \in A_i$. For example, we can set $s_0 = 0$, $s_N = 1$, and $S_i = (x_i + x_{i+1})/2$, $i = 1, \cdots, N - 1$. Since the sum of the weights $\int \mathcal{K}(x, y) dy$ is equal to one, no normalizing constant is needed.

For the random design model, the proposed estimator is a wavelet version of the Nadaraya-Watson estimator (Nadaraya, 1964; Watson, 1964):

$$\hat{g}(x) = \{\sum_{i=1}^{N} Y_i \mathcal{K}_j(x, X_i)\} \Big/ \{\sum_{i=1}^{N} \mathcal{K}_j(x, X_i)\} . \qquad (8.8.16)$$

The resolution j is an integer-valued tuning parameter, and an optimal value must be selected; see Vidakovic (1999) for details on this as well as on more efficient non-linear estimators of $g(.)$. Wang(1995) discussed analysis of change-points via wavelets.

Exercises

8.1. Suppose $Y_i = \beta_0 + \beta_1(X_{i1} - \overline{X}_1) + \beta_2(X_{i2} - \overline{X}_2) + \varepsilon_i$, $i = 1, \cdots, N$, where $\overline{X}_j = \sum_{i=1}^{N} X_{ij}/N$, $j = 1, 2$, and ε_i are iid normal random variables with mean 0 and variance σ^2. Quantify the width of the marginal 95% confidence interval for β_1 in terms of r_{12}, the sample correlation between X_1 and X_2.

8.2. In the normal linear regression model $Y_i = \beta_0 + \beta_1 X_{i,1} + \cdots + \beta_k X_{i,k} + \varepsilon_i$, $i = 1, \cdots, N$, obtain a test statistic for $H : \beta_j = d$ where $0 \leq j \leq k$ and d is a constant.

8.3. In the full-rank regression model $\mathbf{y} = \mathbf{X}\beta + \varepsilon$, with $r(\mathbf{X}) = p$ and $\varepsilon \sim N(\mathbf{0}, \sigma^2 \mathbf{I})$, show that as an estimator of σ^2, $\mathbf{y}'\mathbf{A}_1\mathbf{y}$, with $\mathbf{A}_1 = (\mathbf{I}_N - \mathbf{P})/(N - p + 2)$, has smaller MSE than the least squares estimator of σ^2.

8.4. (a) Ignoring end effects, show that $DW \simeq 2(1 - \hat{\rho})$.

(b) Show that

$$
\begin{aligned}
E(DW) &= \mathbf{Q}/(N - p), \text{ and} \\
Var(DW) &= 2\{\mathbf{R} - \mathbf{Q}E(DW)\}/\{(N - p)(N - p + 2)\},
\end{aligned}
$$

where

$$
\begin{aligned}
\mathbf{Q} &= tr(\mathbf{A}) - tr[\mathbf{X}'\mathbf{A}\mathbf{X}(\mathbf{X}'\mathbf{X})^{-1}]), \text{ and} \\
\mathbf{R} &= tr(\mathbf{A}^2) - 2tr[\mathbf{X}'\mathbf{A}^2\mathbf{X}(\mathbf{X}'\mathbf{X})^{-1}] + tr[\{\mathbf{X}'\mathbf{A}\mathbf{X}(\mathbf{X}'\mathbf{X})^{-1}\}^2].
\end{aligned}
$$

8.5. Consider the regression lines $Y_{l,i} = \beta_{l,0} + \beta_{l,1} X_{l,i} + \varepsilon_{l,i}$, $l = 1, 2$, $\varepsilon_{l,i}$ being iid $N(0, \sigma^2)$ variables. Given observations $(X_{l,i}, Y_{l,i})$, $i = 1, \cdots, n_l$, $l = 1, 2$, $N = n_1 + n_2$, carry out the following tests:

(a) $H : \beta_{1,1} = \beta_{2,1}$; i.e., a test for parallelism.

(b) $H : \beta_{1,0} = \beta_{2,0}$; i.e., a test for concurrence.

(c) $H : \beta_{1,0} = \beta_{2,0}$, and $\beta_{1,1} = \beta_{2,1}$; i.e., a test for coincidence.

8.6. Consider the independent regressions

$$Y_{k,i} = \alpha_k + \beta(X_{k,i} - \overline{X}_k) + \varepsilon_{k,i}, \quad i = 1, \cdots, n_k, k = 1, 2,$$

where $\varepsilon_{k,i}$ are iid $N(0, \sigma^2)$ variables, and $\overline{X}_k = \sum_{i=1}^{n_k} X_{k,i}/n_k$.

(a) Estimate α_1, α_2 and β, and thus the vertical distance between the two lines, measured parallel to the y-axis.

(b) Construct a 95% C.I. for this distance.

8.7. Show that $\| \widehat{\beta}^*(\theta) \| < \| \widehat{\beta} \|$.

8.8. In the regression model (4.1.2), show that the MSE after deleting the ith case is given by

$$MSE_{(i)} = (N - p)MSE/(N - p - 1 - r_i^{*2}).$$

8.9. [Chatterjee and Hadi, 1988.] Let p_{zii} to be the diagonal elements of the matrix $P_Z = \mathbf{Z}(\mathbf{Z}'\mathbf{Z})^{-1}\mathbf{Z}'$ where $\mathbf{Z} = (\mathbf{X}, \mathbf{y})$. Show that

$$p_{zii} = p_{ii} + \widehat{\varepsilon}_i^2/\widehat{\varepsilon}'\widehat{\varepsilon}.$$

8.10. Derive the form of the sample influence function (SIC_i) in (8.5.19).

8.11. For the simple regression model $Y_i = \beta_0 + \beta_1 X_i + \varepsilon_i$, $i = 1, \cdots, N$, show that the weighted squared standardized distance in (8.5.9) is $W_i = \frac{(N-1)}{N}(Np_{ii} - 1)\rho_{X,Y}^2$, where $\rho_{X,Y}$ is the simple correlation between X and Y.

8.12. Show that

(a) $a_i^2 \leq (1 - p_{ii})$.

(b) As $a_i^2 \to 1 - p_{ii}$, show that $r_i^2 \to N - p$, and $r_i^{*2} \to \infty$.

8.13. Show that Cook's distance can be expressed as

$$C_i = \{\widehat{\varepsilon}_i^2/(1 - p_{ii})^2\}\{p_{ii}/p\widehat{\sigma}^2\}.$$

8.14. Show that

$$CR_i = \{(N - p - r_i^2)/(N - p - 1)\}^p/(1 - p_{ii}).$$

Show that when $|r_i| \geq 2$, and $p_{ii} = 1/N$, then $CR_i \leq 1 - \{3p/(N-p)\}$ approximately. Also show that when $r_i = 0$, and $p_{ii} \geq 2p/N$, $CR_i \geq 1 + \{3p/(N-p)\}$ approximately. Use these to arrive at the approximate calibration bounds $|CR_i - 1| \geq 3p/N$ (Belsley et al., 1980).

8.15. Show that

$$
\begin{aligned}
AP_i &= p_{ii} + \frac{\widehat{\varepsilon}_i^2}{\widehat{\varepsilon}'\widehat{\varepsilon}} \\
&= p_{ii} + (1 - p_{ii})\frac{r_i^2}{N-p}.
\end{aligned}
$$

8.16. Show that for inference on the location parameter, the influence curve for the median functional is

$$
IC_{T,F}(x) = sgn[x - T(F)]/2f[T(F)],
$$

where $f(.)$ is the pdf corresponding to the cdf $F(.)$.

Chapter 9

Fixed Effects Linear Models

Consider an experiment involving a single factor, Factor A, with a levels. In fixed-effects models, estimation and inference is required for these particular a treatment levels. By contrast, in random-effects models, the a treatments are regarded as a random sample from a large population of treatments (see Example 4.1.4). Inference for these models will be described in Chapter 10. In Chapter 4, we introduced the least squares approach for balanced fixed-effects models, and discussed the ANOVA decomposition and F-test under normality in Chapter 7. We begin this chapter with a discussion of procedures for assessing assumptions in fixed-effects ANOVA models. In the next subsection, we describe inference for unbalanced higher-order models, including cross-classified models and nested models. The final sections deal with analysis of covariance and nonparametric procedures.

9.1   Checking model assumptions

In section 8.1, we described graphical and numerical tests for normality of errors. Another assumption is that of equality of error variances. Fortunately, the assumption of equality of variances is less critical with nearly balanced data, i.e., when the sample sizes are nearly equal. When approximately equal samples are available from each population, the p-values in the ANOVA test for equality of means is only slightly distorted when the population variances are unequal. In situations where the heterogeneity of variances is a problem, a data transformation may help to stabilize the variance, after which the usual ANOVA procedure may be implemented. In this section, we present three tests for the homogeneity of variances.

Recall the two sample F-test of $H_0 : \sigma_1^2 = \sigma_2^2$ versus $H_1 : \sigma_1^2 > \sigma_2^2$, based on normal random samples of sizes n_1 and n_2. If the observed test statistic $F_0 = S_1^2/S_2^2$ is greater than the critical $F_{n_1-1,n_2-1,\alpha}$, we reject the null hypothesis at level α. We extend this approach for testing the assumption of homogeneity of variances in a populations.

Result 9.1.1. Bartlett's test of homogeneity of variances.   Consider
a test of the equality of a population variances, i.e.,

$$H_0 : \sigma_i^2 = \sigma^2, \quad i = 1, \cdots, a, \tag{9.1.1}$$

against the alternative that not all the population variances are the same. Let

$$S_i^2 = \sum_{j=1}^{n_i}(Y_{ij} - \overline{Y}_{i\cdot})^2/\nu_i, \quad i = 1, \cdots, a,$$

where $\nu_i = n_i - 1$, and

$$\overline{S}^2 = \sum_{i=1}^{a}\nu_i S_i^2 / \sum_{i=1}^{a}\nu_i.$$

Define

$$M = \sum_{i=1}^{a}\nu_i \log \overline{S}^2 - \sum_{i=1}^{a}\nu_i \log S_i^2, \text{ and}$$

$$C = 1 + \{\sum_{i=1}^{a}1/\nu_i - 1/\sum_{i=1}^{a}\nu_i\}/\{3(a-1)\}.$$

Under H_0, the quantity M/C is approximately distributed as a χ_{a-1}^2 variable.

Proof.   Clearly, each S_i^2 has a chi-square distribution with ν_i degrees of freedom. The approximate null distribution of the statistic M/C is a consequence
of the Satterthwaite approximation. In the balanced model, we have $n_i = n$, for
$i = 1, \cdots, a$. Define $\overline{S}^2 = \sum_{i=1}^{a}S_i^2/a$, and $M = (n-1)\{a\ln\overline{S}^2 - \sum_{i=1}^{a}\ln S_i^2\}$.
Let $C = 1 + (a+1)/\{3a(n-1)\}$. Under H_0, the quantity $M/C \sim \chi_{a-1}^2$.   ∎

We looked at this test in the context of heterogeneity in section 8.1.3. The
chi-square approximation is less satisfactory if most of the associated degrees of
freedom ν_i are less than 5. For such cases, special tables of critical values due
to Pearson and Hartley (1970) are useful. In many cases, an approximate quick
check of the homogeneous variances assumption is possible using Hartley's test
(for balanced data) which is described below. Bartlett's test is very sensitive to
the normality assumption. If observations come from a heavy-tailed distribution, the test would reject H_0 too often. We state the next two results without
proof.

Result 9.1.2. Hartley's test.   Consider a balanced one-factor model. Let
S_i^2 denote the variance of the ith sample, and let $S_{\max}^2$ and $S_{\min}^2$ denote the
maximum and the minimum of these sample variances. The statistic for testing
(9.1.1) is

$$HT = S_{\max}^2/S_{\min}^2,$$

which has an $F_{a,n-1}$ distribution under the null hypothesis. ■

For a specified level of significance α, Hartley's test rejects H_0 if $HT > F_{a,n-1,\alpha}$. If the model is unbalanced, we can run Hartley's test with the largest n_i as the denominator degree of freedom for the F-distribution; a consequence is that the probability of Type I error will slightly exceed the nominal level α. Hartley's test is simpler than Bartlett's test. Like the latter, it too is extremely sensitive to departures from normality, and for this reason it is not very widely used to test for homogeneity of variances. Levene's test (Levene, 1960) is an approximate test for the homogeneity of variances from a populations, and is somewhat less sensitive to departures from normality than the other two tests. This is because Levene's test uses the average of the absolute deviations instead of mean square deviations as a measure of variation within a group. As a consequence of the absence of "squaring" terms, this test is less sensitive to heavy-tailed distributions.

Result 9.1.3. Levene's test. Define the quantity

$$W_i^2 = |Y_{ij} - \overline{Y}_{i\cdot}|/n_i;$$

compute

$$\overline{W}^2 = \sum_{i=1}^a W_i^2/a$$

in the balanced case, and

$$\overline{W}^2 = \sum_{i=1}^a \nu_i W_i^2 / \sum_{i=1}^a \nu_i$$

in the unbalanced case. The statistic for Levene's test is then derived based on these expressions in a manner similar to Bartlett's test. ■

9.2 Inference for unbalanced ANOVA models

The fixed-effects one-way analysis of variance model that we discussed in Chapter 4 and Chapter 7 has the form

$$Y_{ij} = \mu + \tau_i + \varepsilon_{ij}, \quad j = 1, \cdots, n_i, \ i = 1, \cdots, a,$$

where Y_{ij} is the jth observation from the ith level of treatment, μ is the overall mean, τ_i is the ith treatment effect, and the random error components ε_{ij} are iid $N(0, \sigma^2)$ variables. If $n_i = n, i = 1, \cdots, a$, we have a balanced model; otherwise, the model is said to be unbalanced. For a detailed study of unbalanced ANOVA models, see Searle (1971, 1987). Searle (1971) describes "overparametrized" models, of which Example 4.1.3 was a special case. The *cell means model* is the primary subject of Searle (1987). In this section, a concise discussion of both these approaches is given, with slightly more emphasis on the overparametrized model, which seems to be the approach taken in most statistical software.

Unbalanced data can result either due to a planned design, or due to un-planned missingness. We focus on the former. *All-cells-filled* data refers to the situation where there is at least one observation in each cell. By contrast, *some-cells-empty* data correspond to some possibly empty cells. This distinction is of importance in determining whether inference on certain interaction effects is possible. Further, with some-cells-empty data, the extent and nature of sparsity determines which effects are estimable.

Definition 9.2.1. Connectedness.   For every main effects factor in the model, if all differences between levels of a factor are estimable, the data is said to be connected. Otherwise, the data is disconnected.

Example 9.2.1.   Consider the two-factor additive model (with no interac-tion)

$$Y_{ijk} = \mu + \tau_i + \beta_j + \varepsilon_{ijk}, \quad k = 1, \cdots, n_{ij}, i = 1, \cdots, a, j = 1, \cdots, b,$$

where the effects μ, τ_i and β_j have been defined earlier, and ε_{ijk} are iid $N(0, \sigma^2)$ variables. Table 9.2.1 shows two sets of data configurations for $a = 3$, and $b = 4$, so that there are $ab = 12$ cells. A symbol "x" in a cell indicates the presence of data while an empty cell indicates no data.

Table 9.2.1. Connected data (left) and disconnected data (right)

$$\begin{pmatrix} x & x & & \\ & x & x & x \\ & & x & x \end{pmatrix} \qquad \begin{pmatrix} x & x & & \\ & & x & x \\ & & x & x \end{pmatrix}$$

If the data are disconnected, some differences of the form $\tau_i - \tau_{i'}$, $i \neq i'$, or $\beta_j - \beta_{j'}$, $j \neq j'$ are not estimable. If every such difference can be estimated, then the cell means $\mu_{ij} = \mu + \tau_i + \beta_j$ are estimable for all i, j, irrespective of whether the cell is filled or empty. We leave it to the reader to verify that in Table 9.2.1, the data on the left is connected, while the data on the right is not connected.   □

Definition 9.2.2. *g*-connectedness.   In a two-way crossed classification, data are said to be geometrically connected, or *g*-connected when the filled cells in the $a \times b$ grid can be joined by a continuous line consisting only of horizontal and vertical segments, and which only changes direction in filled cells. All-cells-filled data are trivially *g*-connected. The data on the left in Table 9.2.1 are *g*-connected, while the data on the right are not.

Sometimes, reordering rows or columns of the $a \times b$ grid enables us to show *g*-connectedness. Weeks and Williams (1964) gave an algebraic characterization to verify connectedness in an *m*-factor model; when $m = 2$, the method reduces to *g*-connectedness. This gives a sufficient (though not necessary) condition for estimability of differences in the levels of main effects of the factors. Suppose the model has L main effects. Let the array of L subscripts on the sub-most cell mean be $[i_1, i_2, \cdots, i_L]$ (for details, see Weeks and Williams, 1964). Two such i-arrays are called "nearly identical" if they differ in only a single element. Connected data are defined as data for which the i-array of every filled sub-most cell is nearly identical to that of at least one other filled sub-most cell. If data is disconnected, separate analyses are recommended for each of the separate sets of data which are connected within themselves.

In the following subsections, we describe inference for one-factor and two-factor unbalanced models. As stressed by Searle (1987), the cell means models are a natural way for carrying out inference on fixed-effects unbalanced ANOVA models. A discussion of this approach for the one-way model is given in section 9.2.1. In the rest of this section, we describe higher-order *overparametrized* models, and defer the reader to Searle (1987) for a study of the cell means models for these situations.

9.2.1 One-way cell means model

In Chapter 4 and Chapter 7, we have described modeling and inference for a one-factor experiment with unequal replication corresponding to the factor levels. The model that we used there is often referred to as the *overparametrized model* because there are $(a + 1)$ parameters, but only a cell means $\overline{Y}_{i\cdot}$. Searle (1987) described an alternative model called the cell means model for the one-way fixed-effects classification as

$$Y_{ij} = \mu_i + \varepsilon_{ij}, \quad j = 1, \cdots, n_i, i = 1, \cdots, a, \qquad (9.2.1)$$

where μ_i is the population mean of the ith class, i.e., $E(Y_{ij}) = \mu_i$, and ε_{ij} are assumed to be iid $N(0, \sigma^2)$ variables. The least squares estimates of the unknown cell means are obtained by minimizing with respect to μ_i's the function

$$S = \sum_{i=1}^{a} \sum_{j=1}^{n_i} (Y_{ij} - \mu_i)^2.$$

Solving the resulting set of a equations

$$\sum_{j=1}^{n_i} \widehat{\mu}_i = \sum_{j=1}^{n_i} Y_{ij},$$

we obtain $\widehat{\mu}_i = \overline{Y}_{i\cdot}$, with $Var(\widehat{\mu}_i) = \sigma^2/n_i$, $i = 1, \cdots, a$. It follows that the fitted values and the residuals are respectively $\widehat{Y}_{ij} = \widehat{\mu}_i = \overline{Y}_{i\cdot}$, and $\widehat{\varepsilon}_{ij} = Y_{ij} - \overline{Y}_{i\cdot}$, $j = 1, \cdots, n_i, i = 1, \cdots, a$, while the forms of SSE and $\widehat{\sigma}^2$ coincide with (4.2.30) and (4.2.29). The ANOVA table coincides with Table 7.2.3 and is useful for testing the hypothesis $H_0 : \mu_1 = \cdots = \mu_a$.

Result 9.2.1. Let $\omega = \sum_{i=1}^{a} c_i \mu_i$ denote a linear function of the cell means, where c_i's are constants, and let d be a constant.

1. The b.l.u.e. of ω is $\widehat{\omega} = \sum_{i=1}^{a} c_i \overline{Y}_{i\cdot}$ with $Var(\widehat{\omega}) = \sigma^2 \sum_{i=1}^{a} c_i^2/n_i$.

2. A symmetric $100(1-\alpha)\%$ confidence interval for ω is

$$\widehat{\omega} \pm t_{N-a,\alpha/2}[est.Var(\widehat{\omega})]^{1/2}. \tag{9.2.2}$$

3. The statistic for testing $H : \sum_{i=1}^{a} c_i \mu_i = d$ is

$$F = \frac{(\sum_{i=1}^{a} c_i \overline{Y}_{i\cdot} - d)^2}{\widehat{\sigma}^2 \sum_{i=1}^{a} c_i^2/n_i}, \tag{9.2.3}$$

which has an $F_{1,N-a}$ distribution under H.

4. The statistic for testing $H : \sum_{i=1}^{a} c_{1,i} \mu_i = d_1$, $\sum_{i=1}^{a} c_{2,i} \mu_i = d_2$ is

$$F = \frac{(g_2 f_1^2 + g_1 f_2^2 - 2g f_1 f_2)}{2\widehat{\sigma}^2(g_1 g_2 - g^2)}, \tag{9.2.4}$$

and has an $F_{2,N-a}$ distribution under H, where

$$f_1 = \sum_{i=1}^{a} c_{1,i} \overline{Y}_{i\cdot} - d_1, \quad f_2 = \sum_{i=1}^{a} c_{2,i} \overline{Y}_{i\cdot} - d_2,$$

$$g_1 = \sum_{i=1}^{a} c_{1,i}^2/n_i, \quad g_2 = \sum_{i=1}^{a} c_{2,i}^2/n_i, \text{ and}$$

$$g = \sum_{i=1}^{a} c_{1,i} c_{2,i}/n_i.$$

Proof.   The proof of property 1 is a direct consequence of the Gauss-Markov theorem. Property 2 follows immediately (see section 7.3.1). To prove property 3, we see that the restricted least squares estimates $\widehat{\mu}_{i,H}$ of μ_i, $i = 1, \cdots, a$ are obtained by minimizing

$$\sum_{i=1}^{a} \sum_{j=1}^{n_i} (Y_{ij} - \mu_i)^2 + 2\lambda(\sum_{i=1}^{a} c_i \mu_i - d)$$

with respect to μ_i, $i = 1, \cdots, a$ and the Lagrange multiplier λ as

$$\widehat{\mu}_{i,H} = \overline{Y}_{i\cdot} - \widehat{\lambda} c_i/n_i,$$

$$\widehat{\lambda} = \sum_{i=1}^{a}(c_i \overline{Y}_{i\cdot} - d) \Big/ \sum_{i=1}^{a}(c_i^2/n_i).$$

It is easy to verify that

$$SSE_H = SSE + \left[\{\sum_{i=1}^{a} c_i \overline{Y}_{i\cdot} - d\}^2 \Big/ \sum_{i=1}^{a} c_i^2/n_i\right],$$

and (9.2.3) follows. Property 4 corresponds to a *two-part* hypothesis, and its proof is left as an exercise (see Exercise 9.1). ∎

Definition 9.2.3. Two contrasts $\sum_{i=1}^{a} c_{1,i}\mu_i$ and $\sum_{i=1}^{a} c_{2,i}\mu_i$ are said to be orthogonal contrasts when $\sum_{i=1}^{a} c_{1,i}c_{2,i}/n_i = 0$. Their b.l.u.e.'s are respectively $\sum_{i=1}^{a} c_{1,i}\overline{Y}_i$ and $\sum_{i=1}^{a} c_{2,i}\overline{Y}_i$, while the covariance between them is given by $\sigma^2 \sum_{i=1}^{a} c_{1,i}c_{2,i}/n_i = 0$.

9.2.2 Higher-order overparametrized models

In this section, we present inference for additive cross-classified models as well as models with interaction, and for nested or hierarchical models, all in the unbalanced case. Instead of the cell means models (Searle, 1987), we describe the *overparametrized* models.

Two-factor additive models

Suppose an experiment involves Factor A with a levels and Factor B with b levels. A suitable model for unbalanced data is

$$Y_{ijk} = \mu + \tau_i + \beta_j + \varepsilon_{ijk}, \quad k = 1,\cdots,n_{ij}, i = 1,\cdots,a, j = 1,\cdots,b, \quad (9.2.5)$$

where μ is the overall mean effect, τ_i is the effect due to the ith level of Factor A, β_j is the effect due to the jth level of Factor B, and ε_{ijk} are iid $N(0,\sigma^2)$ variables. Let $p = (1+a+b)$ denote the number of model parameters, $n_{i\cdot} = \sum_{j=1}^{b} n_{ij}$, $n_{\cdot j} = \sum_{i=1}^{a} n_{ij}$, $N = \sum_{i=1}^{a}\sum_{j=1}^{b} n_{ij}$, $Y_{i\cdot\cdot} = \sum_{j=1}^{b}\sum_{k=1}^{n_{ij}} Y_{ijk}$, $Y_{\cdot j\cdot} = \sum_{i=1}^{a}\sum_{k=1}^{n_{ij}} Y_{ijk}$, and $Y_{\cdots} = \sum_{i=1}^{a}\sum_{j=1}^{b}\sum_{k=1}^{n_{ij}} Y_{ijk}$. Let $\mathbf{N} = \{n_{ij}\}$ denote the $a \times b$ incidence matrix of cell replications, let $\mathbf{D}_a = \text{diag}(n_{1\cdot},\cdots,n_{a\cdot})$, $\mathbf{D}_b = \text{diag}(n_{\cdot 1},\cdots,n_{\cdot b})$, $\mathbf{U} = \mathbf{D}_a - \mathbf{N}\mathbf{D}_b^{-1}\mathbf{N}'$, $\mathbf{V} = \mathbf{D}_b - \mathbf{N}'\mathbf{D}_a^{-1}\mathbf{N}$, $\mathbf{y}_a = (Y_{1\cdot\cdot},\cdots,Y_{a\cdot\cdot})'$, and $\mathbf{y}_b = (Y_{\cdot 1\cdot},\cdots,Y_{\cdot b\cdot})'$.

The normal equations obtained by minimizing $\sum_{i=1}^{a}\sum_{j=1}^{b}\sum_{k=1}^{n_{ij}} (Y_{ijk} - \mu^0 - \tau_i^0 - \beta_j^0)^2$ with respect to $\mu^0, \tau_i^0, i = 1,\cdots,a$ and $\beta_j^0, j = 1,\cdots,b$ are

$$Y_{\cdots} = N\mu^0 + \sum_i n_{i\cdot}\tau_i^0 + \sum_j n_{\cdot j}\beta_j^0, \quad (9.2.6)$$

$$Y_{i\cdot\cdot} = n_{i\cdot}(\mu^0 + \tau_i^0) + \sum_j n_{ij}\beta_j^0, \quad i = 1,\cdots,a, \quad (9.2.7)$$

$$Y_{\cdot j\cdot} = n_{\cdot j}(\mu^0 + \beta_j^0) + \sum_i n_{ij}\tau_i^0, \quad j = 1,\cdots,b. \quad (9.2.8)$$

Since the set of equations in (9.2.7) add up to (9.2.6), as do the set of equations in (9.2.8), the number of LIN normal equations is at most $r = (a+b-1)$, which is the rank of the matrix $\mathbf{X}'\mathbf{X}$ with the form

$$\mathbf{X}'\mathbf{X} = \begin{pmatrix} N & \mathbf{r}_1 & \mathbf{r}_2 \\ \mathbf{r}_1' & \mathbf{D}_a & \mathbf{N} \\ \mathbf{r}_2' & \mathbf{N}' & \mathbf{D}_b \end{pmatrix},$$

where $\mathbf{r}_1 = (n_1., \cdots, n_a.)$, $\mathbf{r}_2 = (n_{.1}, \cdots, n_{.b})$, and the other terms were defined earlier.

Result 9.2.2.   The following rank conditions hold.

1. $r(\mathbf{X}'\mathbf{X}) = r \begin{pmatrix} \mathbf{D}_a & \mathbf{N} \\ \mathbf{N}' & \mathbf{D}_b \end{pmatrix}.$

2. $r(\mathbf{X}'\mathbf{X}) = r \begin{pmatrix} \mathbf{D}_a & \mathbf{N}' \\ \mathbf{0} & \mathbf{V} \end{pmatrix} = r(\mathbf{V}) + a.$

3. $r(\mathbf{X}'\mathbf{X}) = r \begin{pmatrix} \mathbf{U} & \mathbf{N} \\ \mathbf{0} & \mathbf{D}_b \end{pmatrix} = r(\mathbf{U}) + b.$

Proof.   As we mentioned earlier, the first column of $\mathbf{X}'\mathbf{X}$ is equal to the sum of the next a columns, as well as to the sum of the last b columns. This proves property 1, since deleting the first row and column of the matrix does not alter its rank. Properties 2 and 3 follow because $\mathbf{D}_a$ and $\mathbf{D}_b$ are diagonal,

$$r(\mathbf{X}'\mathbf{X}) = r \begin{pmatrix} \mathbf{I}_a & \mathbf{0} \\ -\mathbf{N}'\mathbf{D}_a^{-1} & \mathbf{I}_b \end{pmatrix} \begin{pmatrix} \mathbf{D}_a & \mathbf{N} \\ \mathbf{N}' & \mathbf{D}_b \end{pmatrix}, \text{ and}$$

$$r(\mathbf{X}'\mathbf{X}) = r \begin{pmatrix} \mathbf{D}_a & \mathbf{N} \\ \mathbf{N}' & \mathbf{D}_b \end{pmatrix} \begin{pmatrix} \mathbf{I}_a & \mathbf{0} \\ -\mathbf{D}_b^{-1}\mathbf{N}' & \mathbf{I}_b \end{pmatrix}. \quad \blacksquare$$

We derive *reduced* normal equations in τ's alone by eliminating the β's, a process which is known in the literature as *absorption* (see Result 3.2.10). When $a < b$, it is easier to eliminate β's from the normal equations, rather than the τ's, in order to obtain least squares solutions of the model parameters.

Result 9.2.3.   Provided the data is connected, i.e., $r(\mathbf{U}) = a - 1$, the least squares solutions are

$$\mu^0 \;=\; 0, \tag{9.2.9}$$

$$\tau_i^0 \;=\; \sum_{i'=1}^{a} U^{ii'} W_i, \quad i = 1, \cdots, a, \text{ and} \tag{9.2.10}$$

$$\beta_j^0 \;=\; Y_{.j}/n_{ij} - \sum_{i=1}^{a} n_{ij}\tau_i^0/n_{.j}, \quad j = 1, \cdots, b, \tag{9.2.11}$$

where $U^{ii'}$ is the (i, i')th element of $\mathbf{U}^-$, a g-inverse of $\mathbf{U}$, and $W_i = Y_{i..} - \sum_{j=1}^{b}\{n_{ij}Y_{.j}/n_{.j}\}$, $i = 1, \cdots, a$.

Proof.   We substitute

$$\mu^0 + \beta_j^0 = Y_{.j}/n_{.j} - \sum_{i=1}^{a} n_{ij}\tau_i^0, \quad j = 1, \cdots, b$$

from (9.2.8) into (9.2.7) and simplify to get

$$Y_{i..} - \sum_{j=1}^{b} n_{ij}Y_{.j.}/n_{.j} = n_{i.}\tau_i^0 - \sum_{i'=1}^{a}\sum_{j=1}^{b} n_{ij}n_{i'j}\tau_{i'}^0/n_{.j}, \quad i = 1, \cdots, a, \text{ i.e.,}$$

$$W_i = \sum_{i'=1}^{a} U_{ii'}\tau_{i'}^0, \text{ say,} \tag{9.2.12}$$

where $U_{ii'}$ are elements of the matrix $\mathbf{U}$ defined by $\mathbf{U} = \mathbf{D}_a - \mathbf{ND}_b^{-1}\mathbf{N}'$. Since $\sum_{i=1}^{a} W_i = 0$, and $\sum_{i'=1}^{a} U_{ii'} = 0$, for $i = 1, \cdots, a$, $r(\mathbf{U}) \leq a - 1$ (see Exercise 9.2), and the a reduced normal equations in (9.2.12) are not LIN. The case when $r(\mathbf{U}) = a - 1$ corresponds to the presence of *connected data*, and exactly one additional constraint on the reduced normal equations is required, such as $\tau_a^0 = 0$, or $\sum_{i=1}^{a} \tau_i^0 = 0$. Subject to this constraint, a solution of (9.2.12) is obtained as (9.2.10). Since $r(\mathbf{X}'\mathbf{X}) = r(\mathbf{U}) + b = a - 1 + b$, we need another constraint to solve the normal equations. Suppose we set $\mu^0 = 0$, which is (9.2.9). Substituting this into the reduced normal equations yields the result in (9.2.11). ∎

If $b < a$, it is simpler to eliminate the τ's from the normal equations, yielding a set of reduced normal equations

$$Z_j = V_{j1}\beta_1^0 + \cdots + V_{jb}\beta_b^0, \quad j = 1, \cdots, b, \tag{9.2.13}$$

where $Z_j = Y_{.j.} - \sum_{i=1}^{a} n_{ij}Y_{i..}/n_{i.}$, $j = 1, \cdots, q$, $\mathbf{z} = (Z_1, \cdots, Z_b)' = (\mathbf{y}_b - \mathbf{N}'\mathbf{D}_a^{-1}\mathbf{y}_a)'$, $V_{jj} = n_{.j} - \sum_{i=1}^{a} n_{ij}^2/n_{i.}$, $V_{jj'} = -\sum_{i=1}^{a} n_{ij}n_{ij'}/n_{i.}$, $j \neq j' = 1, \cdots, b$.

Result 9.2.4.

1. A linear function $\sum_{i=1}^{a} c_i\tau_i$ is estimable if and only if the vector $\mathbf{c} = (c_1, \cdots, c_a)'$ is a linear combination of the row vectors of the matrix $\mathbf{U}$.

2. If the data is connected, all contrasts in τ's and all contrasts in β's are estimable.

3. The b.l.u.e. of a contrast $\mathbf{c}'\tau$ is $\mathbf{c}'\mathbf{U}^-\mathbf{w}$, with variance $\mathbf{c}'\mathbf{C}^-\mathbf{c}\sigma^2$, where $\mathbf{w} = (W_1, \cdots, W_a)'$.

4. The b.l.u.e. of a contrast $\mathbf{d}'\beta$ is $\mathbf{d}'\mathbf{D}_b^{-1}(\mathbf{y}_b - \mathbf{N}'\mathbf{U}^-\mathbf{w})$, with variance $\mathbf{d}'(\mathbf{D}_b^{-1} + \mathbf{D}_b^{-1}\mathbf{N}'\mathbf{U}^-\mathbf{ND}_b^{-1})\mathbf{d}\sigma^2$.

Proof. The proof of property 1 is left as an exercise. From property 1, we can infer that a linear function $\mathbf{c}'\tau$ is estimable if and only if there exists a vector $\mathbf{u} \neq \mathbf{0}$ such that $\mathbf{c} = \mathbf{U}\mathbf{u}$, irrespective of whether the data are connected or not. If the data set is connected, we must have $\mathbf{c}'\mathbf{1} = \mathbf{1}\mathbf{U}\mathbf{u} = 0$, since $\mathbf{1}$ is orthogonal to the rows of $\mathbf{U}$, so that $\mathbf{c}'\tau$ is a contrast, and is estimable. The proof that contrasts in β's are estimable is similar. The form of the b.l.u.e. of $\mathbf{c}'\tau$ follows from (9.2.10) and the Gauss-Markov theorem. Now,

$$
\begin{aligned}
Var(\mathbf{c}'\tau^0) &= Var(\mathbf{u}'\mathbf{U}\tau^0) = Var(\mathbf{u}'\mathbf{w}) \\
&= \mathbf{u}'\mathbf{U}\mathbf{u}\sigma^2 = \mathbf{c}'\mathbf{u}\sigma^2 \\
&= \mathbf{c}'\mathbf{U}^-\mathbf{c}\sigma^2,
\end{aligned}
$$

proving property 3. The proof of property 4 is similar. ■

We next discuss sums of squares that enable tests of hypotheses. Based on the least squares solutions via reduction by eliminating the β's, the model sum of squares is

$$
SS(\mu, \tau, \beta) = \sum_{i=1}^{a} Y_{i\cdot\cdot}\tau_i^0 + \sum_{j=1}^{b} Y_{\cdot j}\{Y_{\cdot j\cdot}/n_{\cdot j} - \sum_{i'=1}^{a} n_{i'j}\tau_{i'}^0\} \quad (9.2.14)
$$

$$
= \sum_{j=1}^{b} Y_{\cdot j}^2/n_{\cdot j} + \sum_{i=1}^{a} \tau_i^0 W_i, \quad (9.2.15)
$$

with $(a+b-1)$ d.f. The quantity $\sum_{i=1}^{a} \tau_i^0 W_i$ is called the SS due to Factor A, adjusted for Factor B. Also, SSE is

$$
\begin{aligned}
SSE &= SST_c - SS_A(\text{adj.}) - SS_B(\text{unadj.}) && (9.2.16) \\
&= \{\sum_{i=1}^{a}\sum_{j=1}^{b}\sum_{k=1}^{n_{ijk}} Y_{ijk}^2 - Y_{\cdots}^2/N\} - \{\sum_{j=1}^{b} Y_{\cdot j}^2/n_{\cdot j} - Y_{\cdots}^2/N\} - \sum_{i=1}^{a} \tau_i^0 W_i.
\end{aligned}
$$
$$
(9.2.17)
$$

The corresponding sums of squares are shown in Table 9.2.2.

Table 9.2.2. ANOVA table after eliminating β effects

Source	d.f.	SS
Factor A (adj.)	$a-1$	$\sum_{i=1}^{a} W_i \tau_i^0$
Factor B (unadj.)	$b-1$	$\sum_{j=1}^{b} Y_{\cdot j}^2/n_{\cdot j} - Y_{\cdots}/N$
Error	$N-a-b+1$	SSE
Corrected Total	$N-1$	SST_c

Note that the sum of squares due to Factor B is *unadjusted*. In order to test τ effects, we use Table 9.2.2. However, the same table cannot be used to test hypotheses on β effects. This situation is peculiar to the unbalanced case. Unlike the balanced case, the unbalanced model is said to be non-orthogonal, i.e., the b.l.u.e.'s of contrasts of τ's and β's are not orthogonal. Table 9.2.3 shows the form of $SS_B(\text{adj.})$, and two tests of hypotheses are shown in Example 9.2.2 for connected data.

Table 9.2.3. ANOVA table after eliminating τ effects

Source	d.f.	SS
Factor A (unadj.)	$a - 1$	$\sum_{i=1}^{a} Y_{i..}^2 - Y_{...}^2/N$
Factor B (adj.)	$b - 1$	$\{\sum_{j=1}^{b} Y_{.j.}/n_{.j} - Y_{...}/N\}$
		$+ \sum_{i=1}^{a} W_i \tau_i^0 - (\sum_{i=1}^{a} Y_{i..}^2 - Y_{...}^2/N)$
Error	$N - a - b + 1$	SSE
Corrected Total	$N - 1$	SST_c

Example 9.2.2.   When the data is connected, the test statistic for the testable hypothesis $H_A : \tau_1 = \cdots = \tau_a$ is

$$F = \{\textstyle\sum_{i=1}^{a} \tau_i^0 W_i/(a - 1)\} / \{SSE/(N - a - b + 1)\}$$

which has an $F_{a-1, N-a-b+1}$ distribution under H_A. Consider a test of $H_B : \beta_1 = \cdots = \beta_b$. The numerator sum of squares in the F-statistic is

$$
\begin{aligned}
SS_B(\text{adj.}) &= SST_c - SS_A(\text{unadj.}) - SSE \\
&= \{\sum_{j=1}^{b} Y_{.j.}/n_{.j} - Y_{...}/N\} + \sum_{i=1}^{a} W_i \tau_i^0 - \{\sum_{i=1}^{a} Y_{i..}^2 - Y_{...}^2/N\}
\end{aligned}
$$

with $(b - 1)$ d.f. The test statistic is

$$F = \{SS_B(\text{adj.})/(b - 1)\} / \{SSE/(N - a - b + 1)\},$$

which follows an $F_{b-1, N-a-b+1}$ distribution under H_B.   □

Numerical Example 9.1.   Fixed-effects two-factor additive model.
Consider the following example (Montgomery, 1991) where a chemical engineer believes that the time of reaction for a chemical process is a function of the type of catalyst employed. For four catalysts under investigation, the experiment consists of selecting a batch of raw material, loading the pilot plant, applying each catalyst in a separate run of the pilot plant and observing the reaction time. Believing that variations in the batches of raw material may affect the performance of the catalysts, the engineer decides to use the batches of raw material as blocks, although each block is large enough to permit only three catalysts to be run. We describe a suitable procedure to compare the treatments in this unbalanced design, i.e., a balanced incomplete block design (BIBD). Information is not available for observation 3 in catalyst 1, observation 1 in catalyst 2, observation 4 in catalyst 3 and observation 2 in catalyst 4. There are only $N = 12$ observations used for this analysis. The ANOVA table and F-test are shown below.

ANOVA table for Numerical Example 9.1.

Source	d.f.	SS	MS	F-value	Pr > F
Model	6	77.750	12.958	19.94	0.0024
Block	3	55.000	18.333	28.21	0.0015
Catalyst	3	32.750	7.583	11.67	0.0107
Error	5	3.250	0.650		
Corrected					
Total	11	81.000			

Both effects due to the catalyst and due to blocks are significant, as evidenced by the F-statistics.   ▲

Two-factor models with interaction

Consider the model

$$Y_{ijk} = \mu + \tau_i + \beta_j + \gamma_{ij} + \varepsilon_{ijk}, \quad i = 1, \cdots, a, j = 1, \cdots, b, \qquad (9.2.18)$$

with $n_{ij} \geq 1$ observations in each of f filled cells ($f \leq ab$); μ is the overall mean effect, τ_i is the effect due to the ith level of Factor A, β_j is the effect due to the jth level of Factor B, γ_{ij} is the effect due to interaction between the ith level of Factor A and the jth level of Factor B, and ε_{ijk} are iid $N(0, \sigma^2)$ variables. The number of model parameters is $p = 1 + a + b + f$ (γ_{ij}'s correspond to the f filled cells), which we attempt to estimate based on f observed cell means $\overline{Y}_{ij.}$.

We use the matrix notation introduced in Chapter 4 and Chapter 7. It may be verified that $r(\mathbf{X}'\mathbf{X})$ for this model is f. In order to solve the p normal equations in the least squares approach, we set $p - f = 1 + a + b$ elements of the overall parameter vector equal to zero. It is simplest to set μ^0, τ_i^0, $i = 1, \cdots, a$, and β_j^0, $j = 1, \cdots, b$ equal to zero to obtain the reduced normal equations $n_{ij}\gamma_{ij}^0 = Y_{ij.}$, with solution $\gamma_{ij}^0 = \overline{Y}_{ij.}$, for the f filled cells. The g-inverse corresponding to this solution is a matrix $\mathbf{G}$ consisting of an $f \times f$ lower block-diagonal matrix $\mathbf{D}\{1/n_{ij}\}$, and zeroes elsewhere. The proof of the next result is left as an exercise.

Result 9.2.5.   Consider a model with some-cells-empty data. The following functions of β are estimable.

1. A cell mean $\mu_{ij} = \mu + \tau_i + \beta_j + \gamma_{ij}$ corresponding to a filled cell, i.e., for $n_{ij} \neq 0$. Its b.l.u.e. is $\widehat{\mu}_{ij} = \gamma_{ij}^0 = \overline{Y}_{ij.}$, with $Var(\widehat{\mu}_{ij}) = \sigma^2/n_{ij}$. Further, $Cov(\widehat{\mu}_{ij}, \widehat{\mu}_{i'j'}) = 0$.

2. Any linear function of estimable μ_{ij}'s is estimable. For example, if the $(1, 2)$th cell and $(2, 2)$th cell are filled, μ_{12} and μ_{22} are estimable, and so is $\mu_{12} - \mu_{22} = \tau_1 - \tau_2 + (\gamma_{12} - \gamma_{22})$.

3. For $i \neq i'$, the function $\tau_i - \tau_{i'} + \sum_{j=1}^{b} c_{ij}(\beta_j + \gamma_{ij}) - \sum_{j=1}^{b} c_{i'j}(\beta_j + \gamma_{i'j})$ is estimable provided $\sum_{j=1}^{b} c_{ij} = \sum_{j=1}^{b} c_{i'j} = 1$, and $c_{ij} = 0$ when $n_{ij} = 0$ and $c_{i'j} = 0$ when $n_{i'j} = 0$. Its b.l.u.e. is $\sum_{j=1}^{b} c_{ij} \overline{Y}_{ij\cdot} - \sum_{j=1}^{b} c_{i'j} \overline{Y}_{i'j\cdot}$ with variance $\sum_{j=1}^{b} (c_{ij}^2/n_{ij} + c_{i'j}^2/n_{i'j})\sigma^2$.

4. For $j \neq j'$, the function $\beta_j - \beta_{j'} + \sum_{i=1}^{a} d_{ij}(\tau_i + \gamma_{ij}) - \sum_{i=1}^{a} d_{ij'}(\tau_i + \gamma_{ij'})$ is estimable provided $\sum_{i=1}^{a} d_{ij} = \sum_{i=1}^{a} d_{ij'} = 1$, and $d_{ij} = 0$ when $n_{ij} = 0$ and $d_{ij'} = 0$ when $n_{ij'} = 0$. Its b.l.u.e. is $\sum_{i=1}^{a} d_{ij} \overline{Y}_{ij\cdot} - \sum_{i=1}^{a} d_{ij'} \overline{Y}_{ij'\cdot}$ with variance $\sum_{i=1}^{a} (d_{ij}^2/n_{ij} + d_{ij'}^2/n_{ij'})\sigma^2$. ∎

It is clear that with some-cells-empty data, the pattern of nonzero n_{ij}'s determines which functions are estimable (see Exercise 9.6). Also, differences such as $\tau_i - \tau_{i'}$, $i \neq i'$, or $\beta_j - \beta_{j'}$, $j \neq j'$ are not estimable. For example, $\mu_{ij} - \mu_{i'j} = (\mu + \tau_i + \beta_j + \gamma_{ij}) - (\mu + \tau_{i'} + \beta_j + \gamma_{i'j}) = \tau_i - \tau_{i'} + \gamma_{ij} - \gamma_{i'j}$, and we cannot eliminate the γ's from the final expression. In other words, no estimable function of μ_{ij}'s is possible which involves only differences such as $\tau_i - \tau_{i'}$ or $\beta_j - \beta_{j'}$, without the γ_{ij}'s. Differences between levels of Factor A can be estimated only in the presence of average effects due to Factor B and the interaction. Any testable hypothesis will involve linear functions of μ_{ij}'s.

Result 9.2.6. Consider a model with all-cells-filled data.

1. For all $i \neq i'$, the test statistic for

$$H : \tau_i - \tau_{i'} + [\sum_{j=1}^{b} \gamma_{ij} - \sum_{j=1}^{b} \gamma_{i'j}]/b = 0 \qquad (9.2.19)$$

is

$$F = \{\sum_{j=1}^{b}(\overline{Y}_{ij\cdot} - \overline{Y}_{i'j\cdot})\}^2 \Big/ \{\sum_{j=1}^{b}(1/n_{ij} + 1/n_{i'j})\hat{\sigma}^2\} \qquad (9.2.20)$$

which has an $F_{1,f-a-b+1}$-distribution under H.

2. The test statistic for

$$H : \tau_i + \sum_{j=1}^{b} \gamma_{ij}/b \text{ equal }, i = 1, \cdots, a \qquad (9.2.21)$$

is

$$F = \frac{1}{(a-1)\hat{\sigma}^2}\left[\sum_{i=1}^{a}(U_i/h_i) - (\sum_{i=1}^{a} V_i/h_i)^2/\sum_{i=1}^{a} 1/h_i\right], \qquad (9.2.22)$$

where $U_i = (\sum_{j=1}^{b} \overline{Y}_{ij\cdot})^2$, $h_i = \sum_{j=1}^{b} 1/n_{ij}$, and $V_i = \sum_{j=1}^{b} \overline{Y}_{ij\cdot}$.

Proof.   Property 1 is a special case of property 3 in Result 9.2.5 with $c_{ij} = c_{i'j} = 1/b$. Its b.l.u.e. is

$$[\textstyle\sum_{j=1}^{b}(\overline{Y}_{ij\cdot} - \overline{Y}_{i'j\cdot})]/b,$$

with variance

$$\sigma^2[1/n_{ij} - 1/n_{i'j}]/b,$$

from which (9.2.20) follows directly. The proof of property 2 is left as an exercise.
∎

Observe that (9.2.20) is also the test statistic for $H : \tau_i - \tau_{i'} = 0$, to which the hypothesis (9.2.19) reduces under the restriction $\sum_{j=1}^{b}\gamma_{ij} = 0$ for all $i = 1, \cdots, a$ in the model. Likewise, the hypothesis (9.2.21) reduces to $H : \tau_1 = \cdots = \tau_a$ under this restriction, and is tested by (9.2.22).

Nested or hierarchical models

We introduced this model in Example 4.2.7, while in Example 7.4.5, we described inference in the balanced case. With unbalanced data, the nested model is written as

$$Y_{ijk} = \mu + \tau_i + \beta_{j(i)} + \varepsilon_{ijk}, \qquad (9.2.23)$$

$k = 1, \cdots, n_{ij}$, $j = 1, \cdots, b_i$, $i = 1, \cdots, a$. The normal equations are derived by minimizing $\sum_{i=1}^{a}\sum_{j=1}^{b}\sum_{k=1}^{n_{ij}}(Y_{ijk} - \mu^0 - \tau_i^0 - \beta_{j(i)}^0)^2$ with respect to the parameters as

$$Y_{\cdots} = N\mu^0 + \sum_{i=1}^{a}n_{i\cdot}\tau_i^0 + \sum_{i=1}^{a}\sum_{j=1}^{b}n_{ij}\beta_{j(i)}^0$$

$$Y_{i\cdots} = n_{i\cdot}\mu^0 + n_{i\cdot}\tau_i^0 + \sum_{j=1}^{b}n_{ij}\beta_{j(i)}^0, \quad i = 1, \cdots, a$$

$$Y_{ij\cdot} = n_{ij}(\mu^0 + \tau_i^0\beta_{j(i)}^0), \quad j = 1, \cdots, b_i, i = 1, \cdots, a,$$

where $n_{i\cdot} = \sum_{j=1}^{b_i}n_{ij}$. By adding the last set of equations over j, we get the second set, and by adding them over i and j, we get the first equation. Let $b_{\cdot} = \sum_{i=1}^{a}b_i$. Only $b_{\cdot}$ of the $1 + a + b_{\cdot}$ normal equations are LIN, on which we impose the constraints $\mu^0 = 0$, and $\tau_i^0 = 0$, $i = 1, \cdots, a$. The solutions to the normal equations subject to these constraints are

$$\beta_{j(i)}^0 = Y_{ij\cdot}/n_{ij} = \overline{Y}_{ij\cdot}, \quad j = 1, \cdots, b_i, i = 1, \cdots, a. \qquad (9.2.24)$$

The corresponding g-inverse is

$$\mathbf{G} = \begin{pmatrix} 0 & 0 \\ 0 & \mathbf{D}\{1/n_{ij}\} \end{pmatrix}.$$

It is routine to verify that $\mu + \tau_i + \beta_{j(i)}$ is estimable with b.l.u.e. $\overline{Y}_{ij\cdot\cdot}$. Functions of the form $\beta_{j(i)} - \beta_{j'(i)}$, $j \neq j'$ are also estimable, with b.l.u.e. $\overline{Y}_{ij\cdot} - \overline{Y}_{ij'\cdot\cdot}$.

In the framework of a nested sequence of hypotheses, we write

$$
\begin{aligned}
\mathcal{S}_{H_0} &= \{Y_{ijk} = \mu + \tau_i + \beta_{j(i)} + \varepsilon_{ijk}, \tau_i^0 = 0, i = 1, \cdots, a, \mu^0 = 0\} \\
\supset \mathcal{S}_{H_1} &= \{Y_{ijk} = \mu + \tau_i + \beta_{j(i)} + \varepsilon_{ijk}, \beta_{j(i)}^0 = 0, \tau_i^0 = 0, \mu^0 = 0\} \\
= \quad &\{Y_{ijk} = \mu + \tau_i + \varepsilon_{ijk}\}, \\
\supset \mathcal{S}_{H_2} &= \{Y_{ijk} = \mu + \tau_i + \beta_{j(i)} + \varepsilon_{ijk}, \tau_i^0 = 0, i = 1, \cdots, a, \mu^0 = 0, \\
&\quad \beta_{j(i)}^0 = 0, \tau_i \text{ equal}, i = 1, \cdots, a\} \\
= \quad &\{Y_{ijk} = \mu + \varepsilon_{ijk}\} \\
\supset \mathcal{S}_{H_3} &\{Y_{ijk} = \varepsilon_{ijk}\}.
\end{aligned}
$$

Here, $\dim(\mathcal{S}_{H_0}) = b.$, $\dim(\mathcal{S}_{H_1}) = a$, $\dim(\mathcal{S}_{H_2}) = 1$, and $\dim(\mathcal{S}_{H_3}) = 0$. The fitted values are $\widehat{Y}_{ijk} = \overline{Y}_{ij\cdot}$, and $SSR(H_0) = \widehat{\mathbf{y}}_{H_0}' \widehat{\mathbf{y}}_{H_0} = \sum_i \sum_j Y_{ij\cdot}^2 / n_{ij}$, $SST = \sum_i \sum_j \sum_k (Y_{ijk} - \overline{Y}_{\cdots})^2$. Let $SSM = N\overline{Y}_{\cdots}^2$. Table 9.2.4 summarizes the sums of squares.

Table 9.2.4. ANOVA table for nested effects model

Source	d.f.	SS
Model	$b. - 1$	$SSR(H_0) - SSM$
Error	$N - b.$	SSE
Corrected Total	$N - 1$	SST_c

9.3   Analysis of covariance

Consider an example where we study the effect of three different diets on the weights of rats. The experiment consists of assigning rats randomly to the diets and maintaining them on the same diet for a period of 2 months. The response variable is the weight of a rat at the end of the two month period. A one-way ANOVA model enables us to study the effect of the treatment (diet) on the weight. Note that it is also reasonable to suppose that the weight of a rat after being on a diet for two months is correlated with its initial weight before the diet application. An analysis of covariance (ANACOVA) model is a combination of ANOVA and regression, which enables us to study the effect of diet on the final weight of the rats, adjusting for their initial weight. Supposing that the initial weight is linearly related to the final weight; the elimination of this linear effect should result in a smaller MSE of fit. We call the initial weight a covariate or a concomitant variable. Note that as an alternative, we could have blocked the rats into different groups based on their initial weight and used a two-way ANOVA model, thereby converting a continuous variable (weight) into a class variable. However, use of the ANACOVA model improves the precision of treatment comparisons. In general, we may use k continuous covariates $X_1, \cdots, X_k$. Analysis of covariance tests for differences in treatment effects, assuming a constant regression relation among groups. Of course, we must first test whether or not the regression coefficients are similar in the different groups. Regression lines will be parallel when there is a single covariate X, and there is no interaction between X and factor levels. Dissimilar coefficients could reflect the presence of an interaction between treatment groups and covariates.

A general formulation of the ANACOVA model is

$$\mathbf{y} = \mathbf{X}\tau + \mathbf{Z}\beta + \varepsilon, \tag{9.3.1}$$

where $\mathbf{y}$ is an N-dimensional vector, $\mathbf{X}$ is an $N \times p$ design matrix with $\text{rank}(\mathbf{X}) = r < p$, τ is a p-dimensional vector of fixed-effects parameters, $\mathbf{Z}$ is an $N \times q$ regression matrix with $\text{rank}(\mathbf{Z}) = q$, β is a q-dimensional vector of regression parameters, the columns of $\mathbf{X}$ are linearly independent of the columns of $\mathbf{Z}$, and ε has an N-variate normal distribution with mean vector $\mathbf{0}$ and covariance matrix $\sigma^2 \mathbf{I}_N$. We can rewrite the model in (9.3.1) as

$$\mathbf{y} = \mathbf{W}\gamma + \varepsilon, \quad \text{where } \mathbf{W} = (\mathbf{X} \quad \mathbf{Z}) \text{ and } \gamma = \begin{pmatrix} \tau \\ \beta \end{pmatrix}. \tag{9.3.2}$$

Result 9.3.1. The least squares solutions for β and τ are

$$\widehat{\beta} = [\mathbf{Z}'(\mathbf{I} - \mathbf{X}(\mathbf{X}'\mathbf{X})^-\mathbf{X}')\mathbf{Z}]^{-1}\mathbf{Z}'(\mathbf{I} - \mathbf{X}(\mathbf{X}'\mathbf{X})^-\mathbf{X}')\mathbf{y} \quad \text{and} \tag{9.3.3}$$

$$\tau^0 = (\mathbf{X}'\mathbf{X})^-\mathbf{X}'\mathbf{y} - (\mathbf{X}'\mathbf{X})^-\mathbf{X}'\mathbf{Z}\widehat{\beta}. \tag{9.3.4}$$

Proof. The normal equations have the form

$$\begin{pmatrix} \mathbf{X}'\mathbf{X} & \mathbf{X}'\mathbf{Z} \\ \mathbf{Z}'\mathbf{X} & \mathbf{Z}'\mathbf{Z} \end{pmatrix} \begin{pmatrix} \tau^0 \\ \beta^0 \end{pmatrix} = \begin{pmatrix} \mathbf{X}'\mathbf{y} \\ \mathbf{Z}'\mathbf{y} \end{pmatrix}$$

Using results on g-inverses of partitioned matrices, we see that

$$\begin{pmatrix} \tau^0 \\ \beta^0 \end{pmatrix} = \begin{pmatrix} \mathbf{X}'\mathbf{X} & \mathbf{X}'\mathbf{Z} \\ \mathbf{Z}'\mathbf{X} & \mathbf{Z}'\mathbf{Z} \end{pmatrix}^- \begin{pmatrix} \mathbf{X}'\mathbf{y} \\ \mathbf{Z}'\mathbf{y} \end{pmatrix},$$

which upon simplification, yields the required result, with $\beta^0 = \widehat{\beta}$ (unique).

For an alternate approach, write the normal equations as

$$\mathbf{X}'\mathbf{X}\tau^0 + \mathbf{X}'\mathbf{Z}\beta^0 = \mathbf{X}'\mathbf{y} \tag{9.3.5}$$

$$\mathbf{Z}'\mathbf{X}\tau^0 + \mathbf{Z}'\mathbf{Z}\beta^0 = \mathbf{Z}'\mathbf{y}. \tag{9.3.6}$$

From (9.3.5), $\tau^0 = (\mathbf{X}'\mathbf{X})^-[\mathbf{X}'\mathbf{y} - \mathbf{X}'\mathbf{Z}\beta^0]$. In a model without the covariate, i.e., $\mathbf{y} = \mathbf{X}\tau + \varepsilon$, let τ^* denote a least squares solution of τ. Then,

$$\tau^0 = \tau^* - (\mathbf{X}'\mathbf{X})^-\mathbf{X}'\mathbf{Z}\beta^0. \tag{9.3.7}$$

Substituting (9.3.7) into (9.3.6) and solving for β^0, we get

$$\beta^0 = \{\mathbf{Z}'(\mathbf{I} - \mathbf{X}(\mathbf{X}'\mathbf{X})^-\mathbf{X}')\mathbf{Z}\}^-\mathbf{Z}'(\mathbf{I} - \mathbf{X}(\mathbf{X}'\mathbf{X})^-\mathbf{X}')\mathbf{y}. \tag{9.3.8}$$

Substituting (9.3.8) back into (9.3.7), we get

$$\tau^0 = (\mathbf{X}'\mathbf{X})^-\mathbf{X}'\mathbf{y} - (\mathbf{X}'\mathbf{X})^-\mathbf{X}'\mathbf{Z}\{\mathbf{Z}'(\mathbf{I} - \mathbf{X}(\mathbf{X}'\mathbf{X})^-\mathbf{X}')\mathbf{Z}\}^-\mathbf{Z}'(\mathbf{I} - \mathbf{X}(\mathbf{X}'\mathbf{X})^-\mathbf{X}')\mathbf{y}.$$

Let $\mathbf{P} = \mathbf{X}(\mathbf{X}'\mathbf{X})^-\mathbf{X}'$ as before, and $\mathbf{Q} = \mathbf{I} - \mathbf{P}$, and recall from Result 3.1.8 that $\mathbf{X}(\mathbf{X}'\mathbf{X})^-\mathbf{X}'$ is invariant to $(\mathbf{X}'\mathbf{X})^-$. Then,

$$\beta^0 = (\mathbf{Z}'\mathbf{Q}\mathbf{Z})^-\mathbf{Z}'\mathbf{Q}\mathbf{y}.$$

Now, $\mathbf{Z}'\mathbf{Q}\mathbf{Z} = \mathbf{Z}'\mathbf{Q}'\mathbf{Q}\mathbf{Z} = (\mathbf{Q}\mathbf{Z})'(\mathbf{Q}\mathbf{Z})$, so that

$$r(\mathbf{Z}'\mathbf{Q}\mathbf{Z}) = r(\mathbf{Q}\mathbf{Z}) = q, \tag{9.3.9}$$

(see Exercise 9.12). Hence, $\mathbf{Z}'\mathbf{Q}\mathbf{Z}$ is nonsingular, and the regression parameter estimate is $\widehat{\beta} = (\mathbf{Z}'\mathbf{Q}\mathbf{Z})^{-1}\mathbf{Z}'\mathbf{Q}\mathbf{y}$. It follows that $\tau^0 = (\mathbf{X}'\mathbf{X})^-\{\mathbf{X}'\mathbf{y} - \mathbf{X}'\mathbf{Z}\widehat{\beta}\}$. ∎

Note that whereas $\widehat{\beta}$ is the unique estimator of β, we can think of τ^0 as one of infinitely many solutions to the normal equations resulting from minimizing the sum of squares in the least squares setup. We next describe inference using the framework of a nested sequence of hypotheses (see section 7.4.1). First, note that $\mathcal{M}(\mathbf{Q}\mathbf{Z}) = \mathcal{M}^\perp(\mathbf{X}) \cap \mathcal{M}(\mathbf{X}, \mathbf{Z})$ (see Exercise 9.17). This is illustrated in Figure 9.3.1.

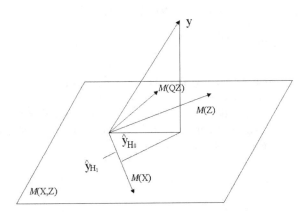

Figure 9.3.1. Geometry of ANACOVA.

We can write the decomposition of the total sum of squares as

$$SST = SS(\mu) + SS(\tau|\mu) + SS(\beta|\tau) + SSE, \tag{9.3.10}$$

where

$$
\begin{aligned}
SST &= \mathbf{y}'\mathbf{y}, \text{ with } N = an \text{ d.f.} \\
SS(\mu) &= N\overline{Y}^2 \text{ with 1 d.f.} \\
SS(\tau|\mu) &= [(\mathbf{X}'\mathbf{X})^-\mathbf{X}'\mathbf{y}]'(\mathbf{X}'\mathbf{X})[(\mathbf{X}'\mathbf{X})^-\mathbf{X}'\mathbf{y}] - N\overline{Y}^2, \text{ with } r-1 \text{ d.f.} \\
SS(\beta|\tau) &= \widehat{\beta}'\mathbf{Z}'(\mathbf{I} - \mathbf{X}(\mathbf{X}'\mathbf{X})^-\mathbf{X}')\mathbf{Z}\widehat{\beta}, \text{ with } q \text{ d.f.} \\
SSE &= \mathbf{y}'\mathbf{y} - SS(\mu) - SS(\tau|\mu) + SS(\beta|\tau), \text{ with } N-r-q \text{ d.f.}
\end{aligned}
$$

To test $H_{0,1} : \mathbf{K}'\tau = \mathbf{m}$, (provided this is a testable hypothesis), we use the test statistic

$$
F = \{Q/r(\mathbf{K}')\}/\{SSE/(N-r-q)\}
$$

which has an $F_{r(\mathbf{K}'),N-r-q}$ under $H_{0,1}$, where

$$
Q = (\mathbf{K}'\widetilde{\gamma} - \mathbf{m})'(\mathbf{K}'\mathbf{G}\mathbf{K})^{-1}(\mathbf{K}'\widetilde{\gamma} - \mathbf{m}), \text{ and}
$$

$$
\widetilde{\gamma} = \begin{pmatrix} \tau^0 \\ \widehat{\beta} \end{pmatrix}, \quad \mathbf{G} = \begin{pmatrix} \mathbf{X}'\mathbf{X} & \mathbf{X}'\mathbf{Z} \\ \mathbf{Z}'\mathbf{X} & \mathbf{Z}'\mathbf{Z} \end{pmatrix}^-.
$$

To test $H_{0,2} : \beta = \mathbf{0}$, we use the test statistic

$$
F = \{SS(\beta|\tau)/q\}/\{SSE/(N-r-q)\},
$$

which has an $F_{q,N-r-q}$ under $H_{0,2}$.

Example 9.3.1. One-factor model with one covariate.   We discuss the statistical analysis for ANACOVA involving one factor, Factor A, and one continuous covariate X. Given data (Y_{ij}, X_{ij}), the experimenter first does some preliminary analysis to verify the equality of the slope of the regression of Y on X in the a groups. If this is indeed so, the model is

$$
Y_{ij} = \mu + \tau_i + \beta(X_{ij} - \overline{X}..) + \varepsilon_{ij}, \quad i = 1, \cdots, a, j = 1, \cdots, n, \qquad (9.3.11)
$$

where β is the common slope parameter and ε_{ij} are iid $N(0, \sigma^2)$ variables. If we assume that τ_i correspond to fixed effects, with $\sum_{i=1}^{a} \tau_i = 0$, and that X_{ij} are unaffected by the treatments, our main interest is in testing for equality of the effects due to the levels of the factor, eliminating the effect of the covariate X on the response. Before we do this, we would like to test whether $\beta = 0$. When $\beta = 0$, the reduction in MSE is likely to be very small, and in this case, the data is better analyzed as a simpler ANOVA model. If we decide that β is significantly different from zero, we would use each of the a regression lines to estimate the mean value of Y for a given treatment level and for a given value of X and also to estimate differences among the τ_i for any value of the covariate.

The following notation is useful.

$$S_{YY} = \sum_{i=1}^{a}\sum_{j=1}^{n}(Y_{ij} - \overline{Y}_{..})^2,$$

$$S_{XX} = \sum_{i=1}^{a}\sum_{j=1}^{n}(X_{ij} - \overline{X}_{..})^2,$$

$$S_{XY} = \sum_{i=1}^{a}\sum_{j=1}^{n}(X_{ij} - \overline{X}_{..})(Y_{ij} - \overline{Y}_{..}),$$

$$T_{YY} = \sum_{i=1}^{a}(\overline{Y}_{i.} - \overline{Y}_{..})^2,$$

$$T_{XX} = \sum_{i=1}^{a}(\overline{X}_{i.} - \overline{X}_{..})^2,$$

$$T_{XY} = \sum_{i=1}^{a}(\overline{X}_{i.} - \overline{X}_{..})(\overline{Y}_{i.} - \overline{Y}_{..}),$$

$$E_{YY} = S_{YY} - T_{YY} = \sum_{i=1}^{a}\sum_{j=1}^{n}(Y_{ij} - \overline{Y}_{i.})^2,$$

$$E_{XX} = S_{XX} - T_{XX} = \sum_{i=1}^{a}\sum_{j=1}^{n}(X_{ij} - \overline{X}_{i.})^2, \text{ and}$$

$$E_{XY} = S_{XY} - T_{XY} = \sum_{i=1}^{a}\sum_{j=1}^{n}(X_{ij} - \overline{X}_{i.})(Y_{ij} - \overline{Y}_{i.}).$$

In the absence of the covariate, we would have $S_{XY} = S_{XX} = E_{XY} = E_{XX} = 0$. In this case, the total sum of squares, treatment sum of squares and error sum of squares would respectively be S_{YY}, T_{YY}, and E_{YY}. In the presence of a covariate however, we must adjust these quantities for the regression of Y on X.

The least squares solutions of the parameters in the *full model* are

$$\mu^0 = \overline{Y}_{..}, \quad \tau_i^0 = (\overline{Y}_{i.} - \overline{Y}_{..}) - \beta^0(\overline{X}_{i.} - \overline{X}_{..}), \quad i = 1, \cdots, a,$$

$$\beta^0 = \frac{E_{XY}}{E_{XX}}, \text{ and } \hat{\sigma}^2 = MSE = \frac{SSE}{a(n-1)-1},$$

where

$$SSE = E_{YY} - (E_{XY})^2/E_{XX}$$

is the "adjusted" error sum of squares with $a(n-1)-1$ d.f.

If there were no effects due to the levels of Factor A, i.e., we reject the null hypothesis $H_0 : \tau_1 = \cdots = \tau_a$, then the *reduced model* is

$$Y_{ij} = \mu + \beta(X_{ij} - \overline{X}_{..}) + \varepsilon_{ij}, \quad i = 1, \cdots, a, \ j = 1, \cdots, n,$$

and the least squares estimates of the parameters in this *reduced model* are

$$\widehat{\mu} = \overline{Y}_{..}, \text{ and } \widehat{\beta} = S_{XY}/S_{XX}.$$

Under this reduced model, the a parallel regression lines coincide. The error sum of squares in this reduced model is

$$SSE' = S_{YY} - (S_{XY})^2/S_{XX} \text{ with } (an-2) \text{ d.f.}$$

Note that $(S_{XY})^2/S_{XX}$ is the reduction in S_{YY} through the regression of Y on X, and is the regression sum of squares with 1 d.f. The difference $SSE' - SSE$ is a reduction in sum of squares due to τ effects, and has $(a-1)$ d.f. Yet another reduced model is

$$Y_{ij} = \mu + \tau_i + \varepsilon_{ij}, \quad i = 1, \cdots, a, \ j = 1, \cdots, n.$$

The least squares estimates of the "adjusted treatment means" $\mu + \tau_i$ under this model are

$$\text{Adj.}\overline{Y}_{i.} = \overline{Y}_{i.} - \widehat{\beta}(\overline{X}_{i.} - \overline{X}_{..}), \quad i = 1, \cdots, a,$$

where $\widehat{\beta} = E_{XY}/E_{XX}$. The standard error of this adjusted treatment mean is

$$s.e.(\text{Adj.}\overline{Y}_{i.}) = [MSE\{1/n + (\overline{X}_{i.} - \overline{X}_{..})^2/E_{XX}\}]^{1/2}.$$

The test statistic for $H_0 : \tau_i$'s equal, $i = 1, \cdots, a$ is

$$F_0 = \{(SSE' - SSE)/(a-1)\}/\{SSE/[a(n-1)-1]\} \sim F_{(a-1),a(n-1)-1}$$

under H_0. We can represent the ANACOVA as an *adjusted ANOVA*, as shown in the following table.

Table 9.3.1. Adjusted ANOVA table for an ANACOVA model

Source	d.f.	SS	MS
Regression	1	$(S_{XY})^2/S_{XX}$	$(S_{XY})^2/S_{XX}$
Treatment	$a-1$	$SSE' - SSE$	$[SSE' - SSE]/(a-1)$
Error	$a(n-1)-1$	SSE	$SSE/[a(n-1)-1]$
Total	$an-1$	S_{YY}	

The F-statistic is $F = \{(SSE' - SSE)/(a-1)\}/MSE$. $\qquad\square$

Numerical Example 9.2. We use data from Littell, Freund and Spector (1991). Four bags, each containing 10 oysters were randomly placed in each of five locations (TRT) in the cooling water canal of a power-generating plant. Two locations are in the intake canal, and two locations are in the discharge canal. In each case, one is at the top and the other at the bottom. One mid-depth location is in the shallow portion. Suppose A and B denote the intake locations, bottom and top respectively; C and D denote the discharge locations, top and bottom; let E denote the mid-depth location. Water in the discharge canal has higher temperature than water in the intake canal, while E is an overall control. The initial weight (X) of the oysters in each bag are recorded, and the final weight (Y) after one month. The results from an ANACOVA analysis with TRT as the fixed-effects factor and X as the continuous covariate are shown below. R^2 was 0.988, and $\hat{\sigma}$ was 0.549.

Least squares estimates for Numerical Example 9.2.

Parameter	Estimate	s.e.	t-value	$\Pr > |t|$
Intercept	2.495	1.028	2.43	0.029
X	1.083	0.048	22.75	0.0001
A	−0.244	0.577	−0.42	0.678
B	−0.280	0.493	−0.57	0.579
C	1.655	0.429	3.85	0.002
D	1.107	0.472	2.35	0.034
E	0.000			

ANOVA Table I

Source	d.f.	SS	MS	F-value	$\Pr > F$
Model	5	354.447	70.889	235.05	0.0001
Error	14	4.222	0.302		
Corrected Total	19	358.670			

ANOVA Table II

Source	d.f.	Unadj. SS	MS	F-value	$\Pr > F$
TRT	4	198.407	49.602	164.47	0.0001
X	1	156.040	156.040	517.38	0.0001
Source	d.f.	Adj. SS	MS	F-value	$\Pr > F$
TRT	4	12.089	3.022	10.02	0.0005
X	1	156.040	156.040	517.38	0.0001

From ANOVA Table II, we see that that the adjusted treatment SS is much smaller than the unadjusted SS. We can argue that the power of the test for treatment differences is increased by the inclusion of X in the model, because most of the error in the analysis is due to variation in X. The next table shows the adjusted treatment means $\overline{Y}_i - \widehat{\beta}(\overline{X}_{i\cdot} - \overline{X}_{\cdot\cdot})$.

Adjusted treatment means

TRT	Unadj. means	Adj. means	s.e.
1	34.475	30.153	0.334
2	31.650	30.117	0.283
3	30.850	32.052	0.280
4	32.225	31.504	0.276
5	25.025	30.398	0.362

The inclusion of initial weight as a covariate adjusts for the biased allocation of oysters of differential weights to the locations.   ▲

9.4   Nonparametric procedures

In this section, we describe nonparametric procedures for carrying out inference in designed experiments, mostly based on the use of the rank transform in classical tests. The use of the rank transform consists of replacing all the observations in a classical test statistic by their ranks in the entire data set (Conover and Iman, 1981). Akritas (1990, 1991, 1993) and Thompson (1991) have argued however that the rank transform procedure is inappropriate for many common hypotheses. Akritas and Arnold (1994) showed in the context of multivariate repeated measures designs that the rank transform procedure is always appropriate for testing fully *nonparametric hypotheses*, which are defined in terms of distribution functions.

Example 9.4.1.   The one-factor robust parametric model has the form

$$Y_{ij} = \mu + \tau_i + \varepsilon_{ij}, \quad \sum_{i=1}^{a} \tau_i = 0, \tag{9.4.1}$$

where ε_{ij}'s have common cdf $F(\varepsilon)$, which could be chosen from a family of distributions in section 5.5.3, say. In general, it may be assumed that Y_{ij} are from a location family of distributions. The hypothesis of interest is $H : \tau_1 = \cdots = \tau_a$. The well known Kruskal-Wallis procedure, which is discussed in section 9.4.1 is a rank test based on the robust parametric model.

Given n_i observations Y_{ij} corresponding to the ith level of Factor A, $i = 1, \cdots , a$, the nonparametric one-factor model only assumes that Y_{ij} has cdf F_i, where $F_i = M(u) + A_i(u)$, with $\sum_i A_i(u) = 0$. For instance, $M(u) = \overline{F}_\cdot(u)$, and $A_i(u) = F_i(u) - \overline{F}_\cdot(u)$, where we compute $\overline{F}_\cdot(u) = \sum_i F_i(u)/a$. In the nonparametric model, the distributional assumption is very general; there is no assumption that Y_{ij} are from a location family. The hypothesis of interest is $A_1 = \cdots = A_a$, i.e., all F_i's are equal. $\square$

Example 9.4.2. Consider an experiment with two factors, Factor A at a levels and Factor B at b levels. The robust parametric model is

$$Y_{ijk} = \mu + \tau_i + \beta_j + \gamma_{ij} + \varepsilon_{ijk}, \qquad (9.4.2)$$

where τ_i, β_j and γ_{ij} satisfy the usual constraints (see Example 4.2.6), and we assume that ε_{ijk} have a common cdf $F(.)$. Friedman's test is a rank test which is widely used in this framework.

The nonparametric model assumes that there are n_{ij} observations Y_{ij} corresponding to the ith level of Factor A and the jth level of Factor B, and that Y_{ij} are distributed with cdf F_{ij}. Let

$$F_{ij} = M(u) + A_i(u) + B_j(u) + C_{ij}(u), \qquad (9.4.3)$$

where $\sum_i A_i(u) = 0$, $\sum_j B_j(u) = 0$, $\sum_i C_{ij}(u) = 0$, and $\sum_j C_{ij}(u) = 0$; let $M(u) = \overline{F}_{..}(u)$, $A_i(u) = \overline{F}_{i.}(u) - \overline{F}_{..}(u)$, $B_j(u) = \overline{F}_{.j}(u) - \overline{F}_{..}(u)$, and $C_{ij}(u) = \overline{F}_{ij}(u) - \overline{F}_{i.}(u) - \overline{F}_{.j}(u) + \overline{F}_{..}(u)$. The hypothesis $C_{ij}(u) = 0$ is the nonparametric hypothesis of no interaction, and is equivalent to hypothesizing that $F_{ij}(u)$ is a mixture of two distributions, one depending on i and the other on j, and having the same mixing parameter for all (i, j). The nonparametric version of the hypothesis for testing whether all the effects due to Factor A are equal (averaged over b levels of interactions) is the test $H : A_i(u) + C_{ij}(u) = 0$, i.e., $F_{ij}(u)$ does not depend on i. $\square$

9.4.1 Kruskal-Wallis procedure

In situations where the normality assumption is not justified, the Kruskal-Wallis test (Kruskal and Wallis, 1952) is used as an alternative to the F-test in the one-way model. This is an extension of the well-known rank sum test to one-factor ANOVA problems. Suppose independent random samples of sizes $n_1, \cdots, n_a$ are drawn from a univariate populations with unknown cdf's F_i, $i = 1, \cdots, a$. We describe a test of the null hypothesis $H : F_1 = \cdots = F_a$ versus alternatives of the form $F_i(x) = F(x - \theta_i)$, for all x, $i = 1, \cdots, a$, with all θ_i's not equal.

The observations Y_{ij}, $j = 1, \cdots, n_i$, $i = 1, \cdots, a$ are first ranked in ascending order, and Y_{ij} is replaced by its rank R_{ij} in the overall sample. If there are ties, i.e., two or more observations are equal, each of the tied observations is given the average of the ranks for which it is tied. Suppose there are G groups of ties. Let t_g be the number of tied observations in group g, $g = 1, \cdots, G$. Let $R_{i.} = \sum_{j=1}^{n_i} R_{ij}$ denote the sum of the ranks in the ith sample, and $\overline{R}_{i.} = R_{i.}/n_i$. Clearly, $\sum_{i=1}^{a} R_{i.} = N(N + 1)/2$.

Result 9.5.1. The Kruskal-Wallis test statistic is

$$KW = \left\{ 12N^{-1}(N + 1)^{-1} \sum_{i=1}^{a} R_{i.}^2/n_i - 3(N + 1) \right\}/A, \qquad (9.4.4)$$

where $N = \sum_{i=1}^{a} n_i$, and

$$A = 1 - \{\sum_{g=1}^{G}(t_g - 1)t_g(t_g + 1)\}/(N^3 - N). \tag{9.4.5}$$

If the a populations are identical, and n_i's are not too small, KW has a χ_{a-1}^2 distribution. With no ties, we set $A = 1$ in (9.4.4).

Proof.   The N-dimensional vector $(R_{11}, \cdots, R_{1n_1}, \cdots, R_{a1}, \cdots, R_{an_a})$ takes as values the $N!$ permutations of $(1, \cdots, N)$ with equal probability under H_0. The test statistic corresponding to the standard analysis of variance (see Example 7.2.7) based on the ranks R_{ij}'s has the form

$$\sum_{i=1}^{a} n_i\{\overline{R}_{i\cdot} - (N + 1)/2\}^2 \Big/ \{\sum_{i=1}^{a}\sum_{j=1}^{n_i}(R_{ij} - \overline{R}_{i\cdot})^2\},$$

and is a monotonically increasing function of

$$\sum_{i=1}^{a} n_i\{\overline{R}_{i\cdot} - (N + 1)/2\}^2 \Big/ \{\sum_{i=1}^{a}\sum_{j=1}^{n_i}(R_{ij} - (N + 1)/2)^2\} . \tag{9.4.6}$$

The denominator in (9.4.6) is a constant because of the use of ranks, and let B denote its numerator. First, we divide B by $(N^2 - 1)/12$, which is the variance of the uniform distribution on the integers $\{1, 2, \cdots, N\}$, and we multiply the resultant expression by the factor $(N - 1)/N$ (to yield $a - 1$ in expectation under H). An algebraic simplification yields the expression in the numerator of (9.4.4). The term A in the denominator is an adjustment for ties.

We show that the statistic has an approximate χ^2 distribution. Suppose $a = 3$. Provided n_i's are not too small, the joint distribution of $\overline{R}_{i\cdot}$ and $\overline{R}_{j\cdot}$ is approximately bivariate normal with

$$\begin{aligned}
\mu_i &= \mu_j = (N + 1)/2, \\
\sigma_i^2 &= (N + 1)(N - n_i)/12n_i, \sigma_j^2 = (N + 1)(N - n_j)/12n_j, \text{ and} \\
\rho &= -\{n_i/(N - n_i)\}^{1/2}\{(n_j/(N - n_j))\}^{1/2}. \tag{9.4.7}
\end{aligned}$$

Note that $\sigma_i^2 = (N + 1)(N - n_i)/12n_i$ is the variance of the mean of n_i numbers drawn at random without replacement from N consecutive integers, while ρ is the correlation between means of samples of sizes n_i and n_j when all $n_i + n_j$ are drawn at random without replacement from a population of N elements. It is well known that -2 times the exponent of this bivariate normal distribution has a χ_2^2 distribution (Mood, 1950, sec. 10.2). Since $n_i + n_j + n_k = N$, and $n_i\overline{R}_i + n_j\overline{R}_j + n_k\overline{R}_k = N(N + 1)/2$, it can be shown that the value of the bivariate normal exponent will be the same whichever pair of samples is used in its computation, and this value will be KW in (9.4.4). In general, with a samples, the mean ranks for any $(a - 1)$ of them have an approximate $(a - 1)$-variate normal distribution, provided that n_i's are not too small. The exponent of this distribution involves means, variances and correlations of the form shown in (9.4.7). It will have the same value irrespective of the set of $(a - 1)$ samples used, and will yield KW when multiplied by -2, and have an approximate χ^2_{a-1} distribution. Kruskal (1952) provides a formal proof of the asymptotic distribution of KW. ∎

If $KW > \chi^2_{a-1,\alpha}$, we reject the null hypothesis at level of significance α. The Kruskal-Wallis test is equivalent to the usual F-test applied to the ranks. It has been suggested that when the normality assumption is suspect, we implement the usual analysis of variance procedure both on Y_{ij} and on R_{ij}. If the results are similar, we would conclude that the assumptions of the usual F-test are satisfied. However, if the results are different, we would suspect that some assumption has been violated and we prefer to use the Kruskal-Wallis test.

9.4.2 Friedman's procedure

This procedure relates to the two-way classification. Consider the two-factor fixed-effects additive model $Y_{ij} = \mu + \tau_i + \beta_j + \varepsilon_{ij}$, $i = 1, \cdots, a$, $j = 1, \cdots, b$. That is, suppose we have balanced data with one observation in each of the ab cells, and $N = ab$. Assume that the errors ε_{ij} are independently distributed random variables from some continuous population. Suppose we wish to test $H : \tau_1 = \cdots = \tau_a$. Within each block, rank the a observations in ascending order. Let $R_{ij} = r(Y_{ij})$. Set $R_i = \sum_{j=1}^{n} R_{ij}$, $R_{i\cdot} = R_i/n$, and $R_{\cdot\cdot} = (a+1)/2$. The test statistic is

$$S = 12n \sum_{i=1}^{a}(R_{i\cdot} - R_{\cdot\cdot})^2 /a(a+1) \qquad (9.4.8)$$

$$= \{12 \sum_{i=1}^{a} R_i^2 /na(a+1)\} - 3n(a+1). \qquad (9.4.9)$$

As $n \to \infty$, we can show that the statistic S has a χ^2_{a-1} distribution, so that critical values from this distribution determine the rejection region. This test arises naturally if we apply the usual F-statistic in the two-factor additive model to ranks instead of the actual responses. For details, see Conover (1980) and Hollander and Wolfe (1973).

We do not discuss nonparametric tests for other designs here. The reader is referred to Akritas and Arnold (1994) and references therein for a discussion of fully nonparametric hypotheses for general factorial designs.

Exercises

9.1. Prove property 4 of Result 9.2.1.

9.2. In the model (9.2.5), show that $\mathbf{U}\mathbf{1}_a = \mathbf{0}$, where $\mathbf{U} = \mathbf{D}_a - \mathbf{N}\mathbf{D}_b^{-1}\mathbf{N}'$. Hence argue that $r(\mathbf{U}) \leq a - 1$.

9.3. (a) Prove property 1 of Result 9.2.4.

(b) In the model (9.2.5), show that a linear function $\sum_{j=1}^{b} d_j \beta_j$ is estimable if and only if the vector $\mathbf{d} = (d_1, \cdots, d_a)'$ is a linear combination of the row vectors of the matrix $\mathbf{V}$. Hence show that if the data is connected, a necessary and sufficient condition for a linear function of β's to be estimable is that it is a contrast in β's.

9.4. In model (9.2.5), show the following.

(a) $Var(\mathbf{y}_a) = \sigma^2 \mathbf{D}_a$, $Var(\mathbf{y}_b) = \sigma^2 \mathbf{D}_b$, and $Cov(\mathbf{y}_a, \mathbf{y}_b) = \sigma^2 \mathbf{N}$.

(b) $Var(\mathbf{w}) = \sigma^2 \mathbf{U}$, $Var(\mathbf{z}) = \sigma^2 \mathbf{V}$, and $Cov(\mathbf{w}, \mathbf{z}) = -\sigma^2 \mathbf{U} \mathbf{D}_a^{-1} \mathbf{N}$.

(c) $Cov(\mathbf{w}, \mathbf{y}_b) = \mathbf{0} = Cov(\mathbf{z}, \mathbf{y}_a)$.

9.5. Prove Result 9.2.5.

9.6. In (9.2.18), verify whether the following functions are estimable.

(a) $[n_{i \cdot} - \sum_{j=1}^{b} n_{ij}^2 / n_{\cdot j}] \tau_i - \sum_{i \neq i'} [\sum_{j=1}^{b} n_{ij} n_{i'j} / n_{\cdot j}] \tau_{i'}$
$+ \sum_{j=1}^{b} [n_{ij} - n_{ij}^2 / n_{\cdot j}] \gamma_{ij} - \sum_{i \neq i'} [\sum_{j=1}^{b} n_{ij} n_{i'j} / n_{\cdot j}] \gamma_{i'j}$, $i = 1, \cdots, a$.

(b) $[n_{\cdot j} - \sum_{i=1}^{a} n_{ij}^2 / n_{i \cdot}] \beta_j - \sum_{j \neq j'} [\sum_{i=1}^{a} n_{ij} n_{ij'} / n_{i \cdot}] \beta_{j'}$
$+ \sum_{i=1}^{a} [n_{ij} - n_{ij}^2 / n_{i \cdot}] \gamma_{ij} - \sum_{j \neq j'} [\sum_{i=1}^{a} n_{ij} n_{ij'} / n_{i \cdot}] \gamma_{ij'}$, $j = 1, \cdots, b$.

9.7. Suppose $a = 3$ and $b = 4$ in (9.2.18), and suppose cells $(1, 2)$, $(2, 3)$, $(2, 4)$ and $(3, 1)$ are empty. Verify whether the following functions are estimable:

(a) $\tau_2 - \tau_3 + \gamma_{22} - \gamma_{32}$,

(b) $\tau_1 - \tau_3 + \gamma_{12} - \gamma_{32}$.

9.8. Prove property 2 of Result 9.2.6.

9.9. In the model $Y_{ijk} = \mu + \tau_i + \beta_j + \gamma_{ij} + \varepsilon_{ijk}$, $k = 1, \cdots, n_{ij}$, $i = 1, \cdots, a$, $j = 1, \cdots, b$, suppose $n_{ij} = n_{i \cdot} n_{\cdot j} / N$. Given that ε_{ijk} are iid $N(0, \sigma^2)$ variables, obtain a statistic for testing $H : \gamma_{ij} = 0 \ \forall \ i, j$.

9.10. In the two-way unbalanced nested model, suppose we impose the restrictions $\mu^0 = 0$ and $\tau_i^0 = 0$, $i = 1, \cdots, a$. Obtain the least squares estimates of $\beta_{j(i)}$ and write down the corresponding g-inverse of $\mathbf{X}'\mathbf{X}$.

9.11. In the two-way unbalanced nested model, show that the function

$$\mu + \tau_i + \sum_{j=1}^{b_i} w_{ij} \beta_{j(i)}, \qquad \sum_j w_{ij} = 1$$

is estimable, with b.l.u.e. given by $\sum_j w_{ij} \overline{Y}_{ij \cdot}$.

9.12. Verify equation (9.3.9).

9.13. Let $Y_{ij} = \mu_i + \gamma_1 Z_{ij} + \gamma_2 W_{ij} + \varepsilon_{ij}$, $i = 1, \cdots, a$, $j = 1, \cdots, b$, and let ε_{ij} be iid $N(0, \sigma^2)$ variables.

(a) Derive the least squares estimate of γ_1, and show that it is unbiased.

(b) Find the variance-covariance matrix of the least squares estimate of $\gamma = (\gamma_1, \gamma_2)'$.

(c) Under what conditions are $\hat{\gamma}_1$ and $\hat{\gamma}_2$ statistically independent?

9.14. Consider the model $Y_{ij} = \mu_i + \gamma_i X_{ij} + \varepsilon_{ij}$, $j = 1, \cdots, b$, $i = 1, 2$, where ε_{ij} are iid $N(0, \sigma^2)$ variables. Set this up as an ANACOVA model, and derive the F-statistic for testing the hypothesis $\gamma_1 = \gamma_2$. Relate this statistic to the usual t-statistic for testing whether two straight lines are parallel.

9.15. Consider the model $Y_{ij} = \mu + \tau_i + \varepsilon_{ij}$, $j = 1, \cdots, n_i$, $i = 1, \cdots, a$, where ε_{ij} are iid $N(0, \sigma^2)$ variables. Suppose we observe a continuous variate Z_i, $i = 1, \cdots, a$ (for each $j = 1, \cdots, n_i$).

(a) Find the sum of squares due to regression, viz., $SS(\beta_0, \beta_1)$ in the model $Y_{ij} = \beta_0 + \beta_1(Z_i - \overline{Z}) + u_{ij}$, where we define $\overline{Z} = (\sum_{i=1}^{a} n_i Z_i)/(\sum_{i=1}^{a} n_i)$.

(b) Compare $SS(\beta_0, \beta_1)$ with $SS(\mu, \tau_1, \cdots, \tau_a)$, which is the "usual" model sum of squares in the one-way fixed-effects ANOVA model.

9.16. Consider the model $Y_{ijk} = \mu_{ij} + \gamma_{ij} Z_{ijk} + \varepsilon_{ijk}$, $i = 1, \cdots, a$, $j = 1, \cdots, b$, and $k = 1, \cdots, c$, where ε_{ijk} are iid $N(0, \sigma^2)$ variables. Obtain a test statistic for $H : \gamma_{ij} = \gamma$, $i = 1, \cdots, a$, $j = 1, \cdots, b$.

9.17. In the ANACOVA setup, show that $\mathcal{M}(\mathbf{QZ}) = \mathcal{M}^{\perp}(\mathbf{X}) \cap \mathcal{M}(\mathbf{X}, \mathbf{Z})$.

9.18. Write down the steps involved in hypothesis testing for the ANACOVA model in the framework of a nested sequence of hypotheses (see section 7.4.1).

Chapter 10

Random-Effects and Mixed-Effects Models

In Chapter 9, we discussed fixed-effects linear models. In many experiments, the levels of the factor of interest are assumed to be randomly drawn from a large population of levels. We then assume that the effects due to this factor are random. The simplest model corresponds to an experiment with a single random factor, Factor A, with a levels. Inference for this model is described in detail in section 10.1. In many practical situations, we find the need to incorporate both fixed effects as well as random effects in order to explain the response variable Y. Such situations are modeled by mixed-effects models, i.e., an additive model involving both fixed effects and random effects. Section 10.2 gives a general description of inference for mixed-effects models, of which the random-effects model is a special case (i.e., there are no fixed effects). Different estimation procedures are described and illustrated on one-factor and two-factor models.

10.1   One-factor random-effects model

In many situations, an experimenter is interested in a factor which has a large number of possible levels. In this case, a of these population levels may be chosen at random for investigation; we then refer to the factor as a random factor. Inference is made not about these randomly selected a levels, but rather about the entire infinite population of factor levels. For example, consider an experiment designed to study the maternal ability of mice using litter weights of ten-day old litters. There are four mothers, each of which has six litters. A single laboratory technician manages the entire experiment. Let Y_{ij} denote the weight of the jth litter corresponding to the ith mouse; a possible model is the one given in (10.1.1), where μ is an overall mean effect, and τ_i denotes the effect due to the ith mouse, $i = 1, \cdots, a$. Since maternal ability is certainly variable across parents, it is unlikely that the experimenter is interested in these four specific female mice. Rather, these mice may be considered to be a random sample from a very large population of mice, and τ_i is a random effect. As another example, suppose that a textile company weaves a fabric with a large number of looms. The process engineer suspects the existence of significant variation between looms in addition to the usual variation in strength of fabric from the same loom. Four looms are selected at random, and four fabric sample strengths are obtained from each. Once again, the loom effect τ_i is treated as a random-effect.

The random-effects model corresponding to a single random Factor A with a levels, and with n replications in each level, is given by

$$Y_{ij} = \mu + \tau_i + \varepsilon_{ij}, \ j = 1, \cdots, n, \ i = 1, \cdots, a, \qquad (10.1.1)$$

where both τ_i and ε_{ij} are random variables, while μ is a constant. We assume that $\tau_i \sim N(0, \sigma_\tau^2)$, and are independent of ε_{ij}, which are assumed to be $N(0, \sigma_\varepsilon^2)$ variables. The quantities σ_τ^2 and σ_ε^2 are called variance components and are unknown parameters that must be estimated along with the overall mean μ, which is a fixed effect. Since $Cov(\tau_i, \tau_k) = 0$, $i \neq k$, and $Cov(\tau_i, \varepsilon_{i'j'}) = 0$, we see that

$$Cov(Y_{ij}, Y_{i'j'}) = \begin{cases} \sigma_\tau^2 + \sigma_\varepsilon^2, & \text{if } i = i', j = j' \\ \sigma_\tau^2, & \text{if } i = i', j \neq j' \\ 0 & \text{if } i = i'. \end{cases}$$

The quantity $\rho = \sigma_\tau^2/(\sigma_\tau^2 + \sigma_\varepsilon^2)$ is called the intra-class correlation, and is the proportion of variance of an observation which is due to the differences between treatments.

Let $N = an$. Equation (10.1.1) can be written in matrix notation, using Kronecker product notation (see section 2.8) as

$$\mathbf{y} = (\mathbf{1}_a \otimes \mathbf{1}_n)\mu + (\mathbf{I}_a \otimes \mathbf{1}_n)\tau + \varepsilon, \qquad (10.1.2)$$

where $\tau = (\tau_1, \cdots, \tau_a)'$, $Cov(\varepsilon) = \sigma_\varepsilon^2 \mathbf{I}_N$, and $Cov(\tau) = \sigma_\tau^2 \mathbf{I}_a$, so that

$$\begin{aligned} Cov(\mathbf{y}) &= (\mathbf{I}_a \otimes \mathbf{1}_n)\sigma_\tau^2 \mathbf{I}_a (\mathbf{I}_a \otimes \mathbf{1}_n)' + \sigma_\varepsilon^2 \mathbf{I}_N \\ &= \sigma_\tau^2 (\mathbf{I}_a \otimes \mathbf{J}_n) + \sigma_\varepsilon^2 (\mathbf{I}_a \otimes \mathbf{I}_n) \\ &= \mathbf{I}_a \otimes (\sigma_\tau^2 \mathbf{J}_n + \sigma_\varepsilon^2 \mathbf{I}_n), \qquad (10.1.3) \end{aligned}$$

and $\mathbf{J}_n$ denotes an $n \times n$ matrix with all elements equal to unity. If $\varepsilon \sim N(\mathbf{0}, \sigma_\varepsilon^2 \mathbf{I}_N)$, it follows that $\mathbf{y} \sim N(\mu \mathbf{1}_N, \mathbf{V})$, where $\mathbf{V} = \mathbf{I}_a \otimes (\sigma_\tau^2 \mathbf{J}_n + \sigma_\varepsilon^2 \mathbf{I}_n)$. Notice that if there are n_i observations in the ith level, $i = 1, \cdots, a$, then the model is unbalanced, and the product formulation in (10.1.2) no longer holds. With $N = \sum_{i=1}^{a} n_i$, we can write the unbalanced random-effects model as

$$\mathbf{y} = \mathbf{1}_N \mu + \{_d \mathbf{1}_{n_i}\}_{i=1}^{a} \tau + \varepsilon, \qquad (10.1.4)$$

where $\{_d\mathbf{1}_{n_i}\}_{i=1}^a$ denotes a block diagonal matrix with diagonal components $\mathbf{1}_{n_1}, \cdots, \mathbf{1}_{n_a}$. Also, $\{_d\mathbf{J}_{n_i}\}_{i=1}^a = \oplus_{i=1}^a \mathbf{J}_{n_i}$. In this case,

$$
\begin{aligned}
Cov(\mathbf{y}) &= \{_d\mathbf{1}_{n_i}\}_{i=1}^a \sigma_\tau^2 \mathbf{I}_a \{_d\mathbf{1}_{n_i}'\}_{i=1}^a + \sigma_\varepsilon^2 \mathbf{I}_N \\
&= \sigma_\tau^2 \{_d\mathbf{J}_{n_i}\}_{i=1}^a + \sigma_\varepsilon^2 \mathbf{I}_N \\
&= \{_d \sigma_\tau^2 \mathbf{J}_{n_i} + \sigma_\varepsilon^2 \mathbf{I}_{n_i}\}_{i=1}^a .
\end{aligned}
\tag{10.1.5}
$$

There are many approaches for estimation of the variance components in a random-effects model. Before we discuss these, we look at estimation of the overall mean μ, which is a fixed effect, and may be estimated using GLS in the model (10.1.4).

Result 10.1.1.   The GLS estimate of μ in the model (10.1.4) is

$$
\widehat{\mu}_{GLS} = \sum_{i=1}^a \frac{n_i \overline{Y}_{i\cdot}}{\sigma_\varepsilon^2 + n_i \sigma_\tau^2} \Bigg/ \sum_{i=1}^a \frac{n_i}{\sigma_\varepsilon^2 + n_i \sigma_\tau^2} .
\tag{10.1.6}
$$

Proof.   The GLS estimate of the vector $\mathbf{1}_N \mu$ is

$$
\mathbf{1}_N (\mathbf{1}_N' \{_d \sigma_\tau^2 \mathbf{J}_{n_i} + \sigma_\varepsilon^2 \mathbf{I}_{n_i}\}^{-1} \mathbf{1}_N)^{-1} \mathbf{1}_N' \{_d \sigma_\tau^2 \mathbf{J}_{n_i} + \sigma_\varepsilon^2 \mathbf{I}_{n_i}\}^{-1} \mathbf{y},
\tag{10.1.7}
$$

so that the GLS estimate of μ is

$$
\widehat{\mu}_{GLS} = \frac{\mathbf{1}_N' \{_d (\sigma_\tau^2 \mathbf{J}_{n_i} + \sigma_\varepsilon^2 \mathbf{I}_{n_i})^{-1}\} \mathbf{y}}{\mathbf{1}_N' \{_d (\sigma_\tau^2 \mathbf{J}_{n_i} + \sigma_\varepsilon^2 \mathbf{I}_{n_i})^{-1}\} \mathbf{1}_N} .
\tag{10.1.8}
$$

Since

$$
(\sigma_\tau^2 \mathbf{J}_{n_i} + \sigma_\varepsilon^2 \mathbf{I}_{n_i})^{-1} = \frac{1}{\sigma_\varepsilon^2} \left(\mathbf{I}_{n_i} - \frac{\sigma_\tau^2}{\sigma_\varepsilon^2 + n_i \sigma_\tau^2} \mathbf{J}_{n_i} \right),
\tag{10.1.9}
$$

it follows that

$$
\begin{aligned}
\widehat{\mu}_{GLS} &= \frac{\sum_{i=1}^a \{Y_{i\cdot} - n_i \sigma_\tau^2 Y_{i\cdot} / (\sigma_\varepsilon^2 + n_i \sigma_\tau^2)\} / \sigma_\varepsilon^2}{\sum_{i=1}^a \{n_i - n_i^2 \sigma_\tau^2 / (\sigma_\varepsilon^2 + n_i \sigma_\tau^2)\} / \sigma_\varepsilon^2} \\[2mm]
&= \frac{\sum_{i=1}^a n_i \overline{Y}_{i\cdot} / (\sigma_\varepsilon^2 + n_i \sigma_\tau^2)}{\sum_{i=1}^a n_i / (\sigma_\varepsilon^2 + n_i \sigma_\tau^2)} \\[2mm]
&= \frac{\sum_{i=1}^a \overline{Y}_{i\cdot} / Var(\overline{Y}_{i\cdot})}{\sum_{i=1}^a 1 / Var(\overline{Y}_{i\cdot})}
\end{aligned}
\tag{10.1.10}
$$

where $Var(\overline{Y}_{i\cdot}) = \sigma_\tau^2 + \sigma_\varepsilon^2 / n_i$. The GLS estimate of μ is the weighted average of the cell means, the weights being the reciprocals of their variances. When

$n_i = n$, $i = 1, \cdots, a$, $\widehat{\mu}_{GLS} = \overline{Y}...$ Note that $\widehat{\mu}_{GLS}$ depends on the unknown variance components which define the variance covariance matrix of $\mathbf{y}$. The final form of the estimate will be obtained by substituting estimates for σ_τ^2 and σ_ε^2 into (10.1.10). ∎

We discuss three methods for the estimation of the variance components – the ANOVA method, method of maximum likelihood and the restricted maximum likelihood (REML) method. The ANOVA method starts from the ANOVA table that we have described in the fixed-effects case, and using the expected mean squares, derives an F-statistic. The likelihood based methods use the assumption that the errors ε_{ij} are normally distributed.

10.1.1 ANOVA method

In the *balanced* random-effects model, we estimate the parameters σ_τ^2 and σ_ε^2 as follows. First, we write down the ANOVA table as if all effects were fixed. In particular, recall the ANOVA decomposition

$$\sum_{i=1}^{a}\sum_{j=1}^{n}(Y_{ij} - \overline{Y}..)^2 = \sum_{i=1}^{a} n(\overline{Y}_{i\cdot} - \overline{Y}..)^2 + \sum_{i=1}^{a}\sum_{j=1}^{n}(Y_{ij} - \overline{Y}_{i\cdot})^2, \text{ i.e. },$$

$$SST_c = SSA + SSE.$$

Result 10.1.2. The ANOVA estimates of the variance components are

$$\widehat{\sigma}_\varepsilon^2 = MSE, \text{ and } \widehat{\sigma}_\tau^2 = \frac{1}{n}(MSA - MSE). \tag{10.1.11}$$

Proof. Let MSA and MSE be the mean squares corresponding to Factor A and the error respectively. Using results in section 5.4, it can be shown that MSA and MSE are distributed independently with $E(MSA) = \sigma_\varepsilon^2 + n\sigma_\tau^2$, and $E(MSE) = \sigma_\varepsilon^2$. It follows that $E(SSA) = (a-1)(n\sigma_\tau^2 + \sigma_\varepsilon^2)$, and $E(SSE) = a(n-1)\sigma_\varepsilon^2$. The ANOVA method of estimation consists of equating the expected sums of squares to the corresponding observed values, i.e.,

$$SSA = (a-1)(n\widehat{\sigma}_\tau^2 + \widehat{\sigma}_\varepsilon^2), \text{ and}$$
$$SSE = a(n-1)\widehat{\sigma}_\varepsilon^2,$$

and solving the resulting equations (which are linear in the variance components) for the expressions in (10.1.11). ∎

This procedure is called the ANOVA method for estimating variance components because it utilizes the components in the usual ANOVA table that we write down in the fixed-effects model. Recall that $\widehat{\mu} = \overline{Y}..$ in the balanced case. These estimators are unbiased for the true parameters, and are computationally simple to obtain. One disadvantage of the ANOVA estimator of σ_τ^2 is that it may be negative, which occurs when $MSA < MSE$. The method itself offers no protection against a negative estimate for σ_τ^2, which may occur with some data. A negative variance component might be interpreted as evidence that σ_τ^2 is in fact equal to zero, and the negative value is a result of sampling variability. This interpretation seems especially sensible when the unbiased estimator $\widehat{\sigma}_\tau^2$ has a large negative value. Then, the model is reduced to $Y_{ij} = \mu + \varepsilon_{ij}$, and the ANOVA estimator of σ_ε^2 is $\widehat{\sigma}_\varepsilon^2 = SST_c/(an - 1)$. Alternatively, a negative $\widehat{\sigma}_\tau^2$ could indicate model misspecification, and we might try to fit a more suitable model to the data. Yet again, it might be an indication of "undersampling", so that collecting more data might yield a positive estimate. In general, we would wish to avoid negative estimates of the variance components.

Result 10.1.3.   Under the normality assumption of the errors,

$$
\frac{(a-1)MSA}{\sigma_\varepsilon^2 + n\sigma_\tau^2} \sim \chi_{a-1}^2,
$$

$$
\frac{a(n-1)MSE}{\sigma_\varepsilon^2} \sim \chi_{N-a}^2
$$

$$
\frac{MSA/(n\sigma_\tau^2 + \sigma_\varepsilon^2)}{MSE/\sigma_\varepsilon^2} \sim F_{a-1,a(n-1)}. \tag{10.1.12}
$$

Proof.   That the distributions of SSA and SSE are chi-square follows directly from results in section 5.4. Also, SSA and SSE are independently distributed. Note that

$$
\widehat{\sigma}_\varepsilon^2 = MSE \sim \{\sigma_\varepsilon^2/a(n-1)\}\chi_{a(n-1)}^2,
$$

i.e., $\widehat{\sigma}_\varepsilon^2$ is distributed as a scaled $\chi_{a(n-1)}^2$ variable, the scale factor being $\sigma_\varepsilon^2/a(n-1)$. Although MSA and MSE are each distributed as a multiple of a χ^2 random variable, and are independently distributed, it does not follow that $(MSA - MSE)$ has a χ^2 distribution, and therefore, neither does $\widehat{\sigma}_\tau^2$; in fact, this estimator does not have a simple closed form distribution. It follows directly from normal distribution theory that

$$
\begin{aligned}
Var(\widehat{\sigma}_\varepsilon^2) &= Var(MSE) = 2\sigma_\varepsilon^4/a(n-1),\\
Var(\widehat{\sigma}_\tau^2) &= Var[(MSA - MSE)/n]\\
&= \frac{2}{n^2}\left\{\frac{(n\sigma_\tau^2 + \sigma_\varepsilon^2)^2}{a-1} + \frac{\sigma_\varepsilon^4}{a(n-1)}\right\}, \text{ and}\\
Cov(\widehat{\sigma}_\varepsilon^2, \widehat{\sigma}_\tau^2) &= -\frac{1}{n}Var(MSE) = \frac{-2\sigma_\varepsilon^4}{an(n-1)}. \tag{10.1.13}
\end{aligned}
$$

Unbiased estimates of these quantities are obtained by replacing σ_ε^2 and σ_τ^2 by $\widehat{\sigma}_\varepsilon^2$ and $\widehat{\sigma}_\tau^2$ respectively, and by replacing $a(n-1)$ by $a(n-1)+2$ in the denominator (i.e., adding 2 to the denominator degrees of freedom) in each formula. Further,

$$
\frac{MSA/(n\sigma_\tau^2 + \sigma_\varepsilon^2)}{MSE/\sigma_\varepsilon^2} \sim F_{a-1,a(n-1)}, \tag{10.1.14}
$$

so that MSA/MSE has a distribution which is a multiple of a central F-distribution, the multiple reducing to 1 when $\sigma_\tau^2 = 0$. ∎

Based on the distribution theory under normality, we can construct *confidence interval* estimates for the variance components. Since

$$P(\chi_{N-a,1-\alpha/2}^2 \le (N-a)MSE/\sigma_\varepsilon^2 \le \chi_{N-a,\alpha/2}^2) = 1 - \alpha,$$

the exact $100(1-\alpha)\%$ confidence interval for σ_ε^2 is

$$\left((N-a)MSE/\chi_{N-a,\alpha/2}^2, (N-a)MSE/\chi_{N-a,1-\alpha/2}^2\right). \tag{10.1.15}$$

There is no exact confidence interval for σ_τ^2. The distribution of $\hat{\sigma}_\tau^2$ is a linear combination of two χ^2 random variables, i.e., $c_1\chi_{a-1}^2 - c_2\chi_{N-a}^2$, where,

$$c_1 = \sigma_\varepsilon^2 + n\sigma_\tau^2/(N-a), \text{ and } c_2 = \sigma_\varepsilon^2/\{n(N-a)\}.$$

Since there is no known closed form expression for this distribution, only an approximate confidence interval for σ_τ^2 can be obtained. It is however, possible to construct exact confidence intervals for functions such as $\rho = \sigma_\tau^2/(\sigma_\varepsilon^2 + \sigma_\tau^2)$, $\sigma_\varepsilon^2/(\sigma_\varepsilon^2 + \sigma_\tau^2)$, and $\sigma_\tau^2/\sigma_\varepsilon^2$. For instance, the confidence interval for ρ is derived using the fact that

$$\{MSA/(\sigma_\varepsilon^2 + n\sigma_\tau^2)\}/\{MSE/\sigma_\varepsilon^2\} \sim F_{a-1,N-a}.$$

Hence,

$$P(F_{a-1,N-a,1-\alpha/2} \le \{MSA/(\sigma_\varepsilon^2 + n\sigma_\tau^2)\}/\{MSE/\sigma_\varepsilon^2\} \le F_{a-1,N-a,\alpha/2}) = 1-\alpha,$$

and after some rearrangement of terms, we obtain the $100(1-\alpha)\%$ confidence interval for $\sigma_\tau^2/\sigma_\varepsilon^2$ as (L, U), where

$$L = \frac{1}{n}\left(\frac{MSA}{(F_{a-1,N-a,\alpha/2})MSE} - 1\right)$$

$$U = \frac{1}{n}\left(\frac{MSA}{(F_{a-1,N-a,1-\alpha/2})MSE} - 1\right).$$

Then, the $100(1-\alpha)\%$ confidence interval for ρ is $\left(\frac{L}{1+L}, \frac{U}{1+U}\right)$. Let us now discuss hypothesis tests. In the random-effects model, it is no longer meaningful to test hypotheses comparing treatment effects τ_i.

Result 10.1.4. Consider a test of

$$H_0 : \sigma_\tau^2 = 0 \text{ versus } H_1 : \sigma_\tau^2 > 0. \tag{10.1.16}$$

The ratio

$$F_0 = MSA/MSE \sim F_{a-1,N-a} \tag{10.1.17}$$

distribution under H_0.

Proof. Under the null hypothesis, all treatments are identical, while treatments are variable under H_1. Under the null hypothesis, we have $SSA/\sigma_\varepsilon^2 \sim \chi_{a-1}^2$, $SSE/\sigma_\varepsilon^2 \sim \chi_{N-a}^2$, and SSA and SSE are distributed independently. Note that under H_0, both MSA and MSE are unbiased estimators of σ_ε^2, while under H_1, we would expect that $E(MSA) > E(MSE)$. The ratio $F_0 = MSA/MSE$ has an $F_{a-1,N-a}$ distribution under H_0, and we would reject H_0 for large values of the test statistic, i.e., if $F_0 > F_{a-1,N-a,\alpha}$, where α is the chosen level of significance. ∎

Under normality, it is possible to compute the probability of a negative estimate for σ_τ^2 as

$$p = P(\hat{\sigma}_\tau^2 < 0) = P(MSA < MSE)$$
$$= P(F_{a-1,N-a} < \frac{\sigma_\varepsilon^2}{\sigma_\varepsilon^2 + n\sigma_\tau^2}) \qquad (10.1.18)$$

for various choices of a and n. Studies indicate that p decreases as either a or n increases. In any experiment, it is more important to have many classes (large a) than it is to have many observations per class (large n). Also, if $\sigma_\tau^2 > \sigma_\varepsilon^2$, p is zero, except for small values of a (say, $a < 4$). If $\sigma_\tau^2 \leq \sigma_\varepsilon^2/10$, then p can be appreciably large (see Searle, Casella and McCulloch, 1992 for more details).

Numerical Example 10.1. Random-effects one-factor model. The process engineer in a textile company suspects that there might be significant variations in strength of a fabric between looms in addition to the usual variation within samples of fabric from the same loom. Four looms are selected at random and four strength determinations are made from fabric on each loom (Montgomery, 1991). We show results from an F-test to see whether the looms are significantly different.

ANOVA table for Numerical Example 10.1.

Source	d.f.	SS	MS	F-value	Pr > F
Model	3	89.188	29.729	15.68	0.0002
Error	12	22.750	1.896		
Corrected					
Total	15	111.938			

From the ANOVA table, we see that the F-statistic is significant at the 5% level of significance, and we reject $H : \sigma_\tau^2 = 0$. ▲

In the *unbalanced* case, the ANOVA decomposition is

$$\sum_{i=1}^{a}\sum_{j=1}^{n_i}(Y_{ij} - \overline{Y}_{..})^2 = \sum_{i=1}^{a} n_i(\overline{Y}_{i.} - \overline{Y}_{..})^2 + \sum_{i=1}^{a}\sum_{j=1}^{n_i}(Y_{ij} - \overline{Y}_{i.})^2, \text{ i.e.,}$$
$$SST_c = SSA + SSE.$$

In this case,

$$E(SSA) \quad = \quad (N - \sum_{i=1}^{a} n_i^2/N)\sigma_\tau^2 + (a-1)\sigma_\varepsilon^2, \text{ and}$$

$$E(SSE) \quad = \quad (N-a)\sigma_\varepsilon^2.$$

By equating the sums of squares to their expected values, as in the balanced case, we obtain estimates of the variance components as

$$\widehat{\sigma}_\varepsilon^2 = MSE, \text{ and } \widehat{\sigma}_\tau^2 = (MSA - MSE)/n^*$$

where

$$n^* = [\sum_{i=1}^{a} n_i - \sum_{i=1}^{a} n_i^2/\sum_{i=1}^{a} n_i]/(a-1).$$

When $n_i = n$ for $i = 1, \cdots, a$, these formulas reduce to those we saw in the balanced case. Once again, there exists the possibility of a negative estimate for σ_τ^2. In this case, we can show that $SSE/\sigma_\varepsilon^2 \sim \chi_{N-a}^2$. However, although SSA and SSE are independently distributed in the unbalanced case, neither SSA nor a multiple of SSA has a χ^2 distribution. This is in contrast to the balanced case with the random-effects model, as well as the balanced and unbalanced cases with the fixed-effects model. After considerable algebra, we can show that

$$Var(\widehat{\sigma}_\varepsilon^2) \quad = \quad Var(MSE) = \frac{2\sigma_\varepsilon^4}{N-a},$$

$$Var(\widehat{\sigma}_\tau^2) \quad = \quad \frac{2N}{(N^2 - \sum_{i=1}^{a} n_i^2)}$$

$$\times \quad [\frac{N(N-1)(a-1)}{(N-a)(N^2 - \sum_{i=1}^{a} n_i^2)}\sigma_\varepsilon^4 + 2\sigma_\varepsilon^2\sigma_\tau^2$$

$$+ \quad \frac{N^2\sum_{i=1}^{a} n_i^2 + (\sum_{i=1}^{a} n_i^2)^2 - 2N\sum_{i=1}^{a} n_i^3}{N(N^2 - \sum_{i=1}^{a} n_i^2)}\sigma_\tau^4],$$

$$Cov(\widehat{\sigma}_\varepsilon^2, \widehat{\sigma}_\tau^2) \quad = \quad \frac{-2(a-1)\sigma_\varepsilon^4}{(N-a)(N - \sum_{i=1}^{a} n_i^2/N)}. \qquad (10.1.19)$$

In the unbalanced random-effects model, MSA/MSE does not even have a distribution which is a multiple of an F-distribution when $\sigma_\tau^2 > 0$. When $\sigma_\tau^2 = 0$, then $SSA \sim \sigma_\varepsilon^2 \chi_{a-1}^2$, and $F = MSA/MSE \sim F_{a-1,N-a}$. We can therefore use the F-test for testing $H_0 : \sigma_\tau^2 = 0$ versus $H_1 : \sigma_\tau^2 > 0$ in the unbalanced case as well.

10.1.2   Maximum likelihood estimation

We describe maximum likelihood estimation of the parameters in the unbalanced model.

Result 10.1.5.   In the unbalanced one-factor random-effects model, the MLE of μ is

$$\widehat{\mu}_{ML} = \dot{\mu} = \left\{ \sum_{i=1}^{a} [n_i/(\widehat{\sigma}^2_{\varepsilon,ML} + n_i\widehat{\sigma}^2_{\tau,ML})] \right\}^{-1} \sum_{i=1}^{a} \{n_i \overline{Y}_{i\cdot}/(\sigma^2_{\varepsilon,ML} + n_i\widehat{\sigma}^2_{\tau,ML})\},$$

(10.1.20)

and the MLE's $\widehat{\sigma}^2_{\varepsilon,ML}$ and $\widehat{\sigma}^2_{\tau,ML}$ are obtained as the solutions $\overset{\cdot}{\sigma}^2_\varepsilon$ and $\overset{\cdot}{\sigma}^2_\tau$ to the equations

$$-\frac{1}{2}\sum_{i=1}^{a} n_i/\dot{\rho}_i + \sum_{i=1}^{a}\{n_i^2(\overline{Y}_{i\cdot} - \dot{\mu})^2\}/2\overset{\cdot}{\rho}^2_i = 0, \text{ and}$$

$$-(N-a)/2\overset{\cdot}{\sigma}^2_\varepsilon - \frac{1}{2}\sum_{i=1}^{a} 1/\dot{\rho}_i + SSE/2\overset{\cdot}{\sigma}^4_\varepsilon + \sum_{i=1}^{a}\{n_i(\overline{Y}_{i\cdot} - \dot{\mu})^2\}/2\overset{\cdot}{\rho}^2_i = 0$$

(10.1.21)

provided the solution $\overset{\cdot}{\sigma}^2_\tau$ in (10.1.21) is positive. However, if this estimate is negative, $\widehat{\sigma}^2_{\tau,ML} = 0$, while $\widehat{\mu}_{ML} = \overline{Y}_{\cdots}$.

Proof.   Since $\mathbf{y} \sim N(\mu\mathbf{1}_N, \mathbf{V})$, where $\mathbf{V} = \{_d\sigma^2_\tau \mathbf{J}_{n_i} + \sigma^2_\varepsilon \mathbf{I}_{n_i}\}$, the likelihood function is defined by

$$L(\mu, \mathbf{V}; \mathbf{y}) = (2\pi)^{-N/2}|\mathbf{V}|^{-1/2}\exp\{-\tfrac{1}{2}(\mathbf{y}-\mu\mathbf{1}_N)'\mathbf{V}^{-1}(\mathbf{y}-\mu\mathbf{1}_N)\}.$$

where,

$$|\mathbf{V}| = \prod_{i=1}^{a}\sigma^{2(n_i-1)}_\varepsilon(\sigma^2_\varepsilon + n_i\sigma^2_\tau), \text{ and } \mathbf{V}^{-1} = \left\{_d\frac{1}{\sigma^2_\varepsilon}\left(\mathbf{I}_{n_i} - \frac{\sigma^2_\tau}{\sigma^2_\varepsilon + n_i\sigma^2_\tau}\mathbf{J}_{n_i}\right)\right\}.$$

We can write the likelihood function as

$$L(\mu, \sigma^2_\tau, \sigma^2_\varepsilon; \mathbf{y}) = (2\pi)^{-N/2}\sigma^{-2[(N-a)/2]}_\varepsilon \prod_{i=1}^{a}(\sigma^2_\varepsilon + n_i\sigma^2_\tau)^{-1/2}$$

$$\times \exp\{-\frac{1}{2\sigma^2_\varepsilon}[\sum_{i=1}^{a}\sum_{j=1}^{n_i}(Y_{ij} - \mu)^2 - \sum_{i=1}^{a}\frac{\sigma^2_\tau}{\sigma^2_\varepsilon + n_i\sigma^2_\tau}(Y_{i\cdot} - n_i\mu)^2]\},$$

and its logarithm is

$$
\begin{aligned}
l(\mu, \sigma_\tau^2, \sigma_\varepsilon^2; \mathbf{y}) &= -\frac{N}{2}\log 2\pi - \frac{(N-a)}{2}\log \sigma_\varepsilon^2 - \frac{1}{2}\sum_{i=1}^{a}\log(\sigma_\varepsilon^2 + n_i\sigma_\tau^2) \\
&\quad -\frac{1}{2\sigma_\varepsilon^2}\sum_{i=1}^{a}\sum_{j=1}^{n_i}(Y_{ij}-\mu)^2 + \frac{1}{2\sigma_\varepsilon^2}\sum_{i=1}^{a}\frac{\sigma_\tau^2}{\sigma_\varepsilon^2 + n_i\sigma_\tau^2}(Y_{i\cdot} - n_i\mu)^2 \\
&= -\frac{N}{2}\log 2\pi - \frac{(N-a)}{2}\log \sigma_\varepsilon^2 - \frac{1}{2}\sum_{i=1}^{a}\log \rho_i - \frac{SSE}{2\sigma_\varepsilon^2} \\
&\quad -\sum_{i=1}^{a}\frac{n_i(\overline{Y}_{i\cdot} - \mu)^2}{2\rho_i},
\end{aligned}
$$

where $\rho_i = \sigma_\varepsilon^2 + n_i\sigma_\tau^2$. Since $\partial\rho_i/\partial\sigma_\varepsilon^2 = 1$, and $\partial\rho_i/\partial\sigma_\tau^2 = n_i$, setting the partial derivatives of the log-likelihood with respect to each parameter equal to zero yields the set of maximum likelihood equations

$$
\frac{\partial l}{\partial \mu} = \sum_{i=1}^{a}\frac{n_i(\overline{Y}_{i\cdot} - \dot\mu)}{\dot\rho_i} = 0,
$$

$$
\frac{\partial l}{\partial \sigma_\tau^2} = -\frac{1}{2}\sum_{i=1}^{a}\frac{n_i}{\dot\rho_i} + \sum_{i=1}^{a}\frac{n_i^2(\overline{Y}_{i\cdot} - \dot\mu)^2}{2\dot\rho_i^2} = 0, \text{ and}
$$

$$
\frac{\partial l}{\partial \sigma_\varepsilon^2} = -\frac{(N-a)}{2\dot\sigma_\varepsilon^2} - \frac{1}{2}\sum_{i=1}^{a}\frac{1}{\dot\rho_i} + \frac{SSE}{2\dot\sigma_\varepsilon^4} + \sum_{i=1}^{a}\frac{n_i(\overline{Y}_{i\cdot} - \dot\mu)^2}{2\dot\rho_i^2} = 0.
$$

Solving $\partial l/\partial \mu = 0$, we obtain the estimate $\dot\mu$ in (10.1.20), which has the form of $\hat\mu_{GLS}$. There are no closed form expressions for $\dot\sigma_\varepsilon^2$, and $\dot\sigma_\tau^2$; they are obtained as numerical solutions to the nonlinear equations $\partial l/\partial \sigma_\tau^2 = 0$ and $\partial l/\partial \sigma_\varepsilon^2 = 0$. These solutions $\dot\mu$, $\dot\sigma_\varepsilon^2$, and $\dot\sigma_\tau^2$ are the maximum likelihood estimates of the corresponding parameters only if they lie within the support of these parameters. Since the likelihood function tends to zero as $\sigma_\varepsilon^2 \to 0$, or $\sigma_\varepsilon^2 \to \infty$, it must attain its maximum at a positive value of σ_ε^2, thereby precluding the possibility of a negative $\hat\sigma_{\varepsilon,ML}^2$. However, it is possible that $\dot\sigma_\tau^2$ is negative. If $0 \le \dot\sigma_\tau^2 < \infty$, $\hat\sigma_{\tau,ML}^2 = \dot\sigma_\tau^2$, $\hat\sigma_{\varepsilon,ML}^2 = \dot\sigma_\varepsilon^2$, and $\hat\mu_{ML} = \dot\mu$; if, on the other hand, $\dot\sigma_\tau^2 < 0$, then, we set $\hat\sigma_{\tau,ML}^2 = 0$, $\hat\sigma_{\varepsilon,ML}^2 = SST_m/N$, and $\hat\mu_{ML} = \overline{Y}_{\cdot\cdot}$; these estimators have asymptotic normal distributions. ∎

In the *balanced* case, the log-likelihood function has the simple form

$$
\begin{aligned}
l(\mu, \sigma_\varepsilon^2, \sigma_\tau^2) &= -\frac{N}{2}\log(2\pi) - \frac{1}{2}a(n-1)\log \sigma_\varepsilon^2 \\
&\quad -\frac{a}{2}\log \lambda - \frac{SSE}{2\sigma_\varepsilon^2} - \frac{SSA}{2\lambda} - \frac{an(\overline{Y}_{\cdot\cdot} - \mu)^2}{2\lambda},
\end{aligned} \tag{10.1.22}
$$

where $\lambda = \sigma_\varepsilon^2 + n\sigma_\tau^2$. Setting the partial derivatives of the log likelihood with respect to μ, σ_ε^2, and σ_τ^2 equal to zero, and solving the resulting equations yields the solutions

$$\overset{.}{\mu} = \overline{Y}_{..}, \quad \overset{.2}{\sigma}_\varepsilon = MSE, \text{ and}$$
$$\overset{.2}{\sigma}_\tau = \frac{(1 - 1/a)MSA - MSE}{n}.$$

Once again, these solutions will be the maximum likelihood estimators if they lie within the support of the parameter space.

10.1.3   Restricted maximum likelihood (REML) estimation

REML is a variation of the method of maximum likelihood in which we maximize just that part of the likelihood function that is *location invariant*. In the one-way random-effects model, this refers to maximizing the portion of the likelihood function that does not involve μ. The restricted likelihood is also referred to as the marginal likelihood of σ_ε^2 and σ_τ^2, and its logarithm has the form

$$\begin{aligned} l_R(\sigma_\varepsilon^2, \sigma_\tau^2 | SS_A, SSE) &= -\frac{1}{2}(an - 1)\log 2\pi - \frac{1}{2}\log an - \frac{1}{2}a(n - 1)\log \sigma_\varepsilon^2 \\ &\quad - \frac{1}{2}(a - 1)\log \lambda - \frac{SSE}{2\sigma_\varepsilon^2} - \frac{SS_A}{2\lambda}. \end{aligned} \quad (10.1.23)$$

The REML estimators are obtained by maximizing (10.1.23) within the parameter space $\sigma_\tau^2 \geq 0$, and $\sigma_\varepsilon^2 > 0$. Equating the partial derivatives

$$\frac{\partial l_R}{\partial \sigma_\varepsilon^2} = \frac{-a(n - 1)}{2\sigma_\varepsilon^2} + \frac{SSE}{2\sigma_\varepsilon^4},$$
$$\frac{\partial l_R}{\partial \lambda} = \frac{-(a - 1)}{2\lambda} + \frac{SS_A}{2\lambda^2}$$

to zero, and solving simultaneously, we get the solutions

$$\overset{.2}{\sigma}_{\varepsilon,R} = \frac{SSE}{a(n - 1)} = MSE,$$
$$\overset{.}{\lambda}_R = \frac{SS_A}{(a - 1)} = MSA, \quad (10.1.24)$$

so that

$$\overset{.2}{\sigma}_{\tau,R} = \frac{1}{n}(MSA - MSE). \quad (10.1.25)$$

These are the REML estimates provided they are nonnegative. Note that these coincide with the ANOVA estimators in the balanced case. The REML solutions are very complicated for the unbalanced case. Westfall (1987) compared the different estimation procedures for the one-way unbalanced random effects model. The conclusion seems to be that REML is favored for estimating σ_τ^2, the ANOVA method for σ_ε^2, while for simultaneous estimation of both σ_τ^2 and σ_ε^2, the ML method is favored.

10.2   Mixed-effects linear models

The linear mixed-effects model underlies analysis of a large number of statistical problems, and has the general form

$$\mathbf{y} = \mathbf{X}\tau + \mathbf{Z}\gamma + \varepsilon, \tag{10.2.1}$$

where $\mathbf{y}$ is an N-dimensional response vector, $\mathbf{X}$ and $\mathbf{Z}$ are known $N \times p$ and $N \times q$ matrices of covariates, $r(\mathbf{X}) = r$, τ is a p-dimensional vector of fixed effects, γ is a q-dimensional vector of random effects, and ε is an N-dimensional vector of random errors which has a $N(\mathbf{0}, \mathbf{R})$ distribution. Assume that $\gamma \sim N(\mathbf{0}, \mathbf{D}_\gamma)$, and $Cov(\gamma, \varepsilon) = \mathbf{0}$. Then, $\mathbf{y} \sim N(\mathbf{X}\tau, \mathbf{V} = \mathbf{R} + \mathbf{Z}\mathbf{D}_\gamma\mathbf{Z}')$. In general, $\mathbf{V}$ need not be p.d. Also, $\mathbf{R}$ and $\mathbf{D}_\gamma$ may be assumed to be diagonal. Let $\theta = (\theta_1, \cdots, \theta_s)'$ denote the unknown parameter vector which represents the variance components in $\mathbf{R}$ and $\mathbf{D}_\gamma$.

Example 10.2.1.   Suppose an experiment involves a fixed factor, Factor A with a levels, and a random factor, Factor B with b levels. Suppose there are n replications of each combination of the levels of Factor A and Factor B. Let $\mathbf{y}$ be an $N = abn$-dimensional response vector, $\mathbf{X}$ be an $N \times a$ known design matrix corresponding to the fixed-effects $\tau = (\tau_1, \cdots, \tau_a)'$, $\mathbf{Z}$ be an $N \times (a+1)b$ known design matrix corresponding to the random main effects and interactions, viz., $\gamma = (\beta_1, \cdots, \beta_b, (\tau\beta)_{11}, \cdots, (\tau\beta)_{ab})'$, and ε be an N-dimensional error vector. The design matrices $\mathbf{X}$ and $\mathbf{Z}$ can be written as

$$\mathbf{X} = \mathbf{I}_a \otimes \mathbf{1}_b \otimes \mathbf{1}_n, \text{ and } \mathbf{Z} = (\mathbf{Z}_1, \mathbf{Z}_2) = (\mathbf{1}_a \otimes \mathbf{I}_b \otimes \mathbf{1}_n, \mathbf{I}_a \otimes \mathbf{I}_b \otimes \mathbf{1}_n).$$

For instance, when $a = 4$, $b = 3$, and $n = 2$,

$$\mathbf{X} = \mathbf{I}_4 \otimes \mathbf{1}_3 \otimes \mathbf{1}_2 = \mathbf{I}_4 \otimes \begin{pmatrix} \mathbf{1}_2 \\ \mathbf{1}_2 \\ \mathbf{1}_2 \end{pmatrix} = \begin{pmatrix} \mathbf{1}_6 & \mathbf{0} & \mathbf{0} & \mathbf{0} \\ \mathbf{0} & \mathbf{1}_6 & \mathbf{0} & \mathbf{0} \\ \mathbf{0} & \mathbf{0} & \mathbf{1}_6 & \mathbf{0} \\ \mathbf{0} & \mathbf{0} & \mathbf{0} & \mathbf{1}_6 \end{pmatrix}.$$

Suppose $Var(\beta_j) = \sigma_\beta^2$, $Var[(\tau\beta)_{jk}] = \sigma_{\tau\beta}^2$, and $Var(\varepsilon_i) = \sigma_\varepsilon^2$, then

$$Var(\gamma) = \begin{pmatrix} \sigma_\beta^2 \mathbf{I}_b & \mathbf{0} \\ \mathbf{0} & \sigma_{\tau\beta}^2 \mathbf{I}_a \otimes \mathbf{I}_b \end{pmatrix} \text{ and } Var(\varepsilon) = \sigma_\varepsilon^2 \mathbf{I}_a \otimes \mathbf{I}_b \otimes \mathbf{I}_n.$$

For Kronecker product algorithms that are useful in constructing sums of squares and covariance matrices in balanced designs of this type, see Moser and Sawyer (1998).   □

In the next section, we discuss an important optimality result for mixed linear models, the extended Gauss-Markov theorem. It is assumed that $\mathbf{V}$ is known. In practice, when $\mathbf{V}$ is unknown, these results may be applied with a suitable estimator of $\mathbf{V}$.

10.2.1 Extended Gauss-Markov theorem

Let $\mathbf{X}^*$ denote an $N \times r$ matrix consisting of (any) r LIN columns of $\mathbf{X}$, and suppose γ^* is a realized, though unobserved value of the vector γ of random effects corresponding to a realized response vector $\mathbf{y}$. Let θ^+ and τ^+ denote the true values of θ and τ. Suppose $\mathbf{c}_1'\tau$ is estimable. Recall that an estimator $t(\mathbf{y})$ of $\mathbf{c}_1'\tau + \mathbf{c}_2'\gamma$ is linear in $\mathbf{y}$ and unbiased if $t(\mathbf{y}) = d_0 + \mathbf{d}'\mathbf{y}$ for some constant d_0, and some N-dimensional vector of constants $\mathbf{d}$, and if $E\{t(\mathbf{y})\} = \mathbf{c}_1'\tau$.

Definition 10.2.1.   The estimator $t(\mathbf{y})$ is called an essentially-unique b.l.u.e. of $\mathbf{c}_1'\tau + \mathbf{c}_2'\gamma^*$ if for any other linear unbiased estimator $d_0 + \mathbf{d}'\mathbf{y}$ of $\mathbf{c}_1'\tau + \mathbf{c}_2'\gamma^*$, $MSE(\mathbf{c}_1'\tau^0 + \mathbf{c}_2'\gamma^{*0}) \leq MSE(d_0 + \mathbf{d}'\mathbf{y})$, with equality holding if and only if $d_0 + \mathbf{d}'\mathbf{y} = \mathbf{c}_1'\tau^0 + \mathbf{c}_2'\gamma^{*0}$ with probability 1.

The following result is called the extended Gauss-Markov theorem for random effects (Harville, 1976, 1977), and states an important optimality result for mixed-effects linear models. When $\mathbf{c}_2 = \mathbf{0}$, Result 10.2.1 reduces to the generalized Gauss-Markov theorem stated in Result 4.5.3. Let τ^0 denote any solution to the general normal equations

$$(\mathbf{X}'\mathbf{V}^\sharp\mathbf{X})\tau^0 = \mathbf{X}'\mathbf{V}^\sharp\mathbf{y}, \qquad (10.2.2)$$

where $\mathbf{V}^\sharp \in \Omega_\mathbf{V}$, a class of g-inverses of $\mathbf{V}$ with certain properties. The notations used here are similar to those used with Result 4.5.3.

Result 10.2.1.   Let $\mathbf{c}_1'\tau^0$ be an essentially-unique b.l.u.e. estimate of the estimable function $\mathbf{c}_1'\tau$ and suppose $\gamma^{*0} = \mathbf{D}_\gamma\mathbf{Z}'\mathbf{V}^-(\mathbf{y} - \mathbf{X}\tau^0)$. Then,

1. the estimator $\mathbf{c}_1'\tau^0 + \mathbf{c}_2'\gamma^{*0}$ is invariant to the choices of $\mathbf{V}^\sharp$, $\mathbf{V}^-$ and the solution to (10.2.2),

2. $\mathbf{c}_1'\tau^0 + \mathbf{c}_2'\gamma^{*0}$ is an essentially-unique b.l.u.e. of $\mathbf{c}_1'\tau + \mathbf{c}_2'\gamma^*$, and

3. when $\mathbf{y}$ has a normal distribution, $\mathbf{c}_1'\tau^0 + \mathbf{c}_2'\gamma^{*0}$ is an essentially-unique best unbiased estimator (b.u.e.) of $\mathbf{c}_1'\tau + \mathbf{c}_2'\gamma^*$.

Proof.   From Exercise 10.4, and Rao and Mitra (1971, Lemma 2.2.6(c)), it follows that for $\mathbf{y} \in \mathcal{C}(\mathbf{X}, \mathbf{V})$, the vector $(\mathbf{y} - \mathbf{X}\tau^0) \in \mathcal{C}(\mathbf{VN})$. Further, for any choice of $\mathbf{V}^-$,

$$\mathbf{D}_\gamma\mathbf{Z}'\mathbf{V}^-\mathbf{V} = \mathbf{D}_\gamma\mathbf{Z}'. \qquad (10.2.3)$$

For $\mathbf{y} \in \mathcal{C}(\mathbf{X}, \mathbf{V})$, property 1 follows directly. To prove property 2, let $u = \mathbf{c}_1'\tau + \mathbf{c}_2'\gamma$, and let $t(\mathbf{y})$ be any estimator with finite second moment. Then,

$$E\{[t(\mathbf{y}) - E(u|\mathbf{y})][E(u|\mathbf{y}) - u]\} = E[E\{[t(\mathbf{y}) - E(u|\mathbf{y})][E(u|\mathbf{y}) - u]|\mathbf{y}\}] = 0,$$

so that

$$E\{t(\mathbf{y}) - u\}^2 = E\{t(\mathbf{y}) - E(u|\mathbf{y})\}^2 + E\{E(u|\mathbf{y}) - u\}^2.$$

Since $t(\mathbf{y})$ is an unbiased estimator of u if and only if $E\{t(\mathbf{y}) - E(u|\mathbf{y})\} = 0$, it follows that $t(\mathbf{y})$ is the b.l.u.e. of u if and only if $t(\mathbf{y}) - \mathbf{c}_2' \mathbf{D}_\gamma \mathbf{Z}' \mathbf{V}^- \mathbf{y}$ is b.l.u.e. for $(\mathbf{c}_1' - \mathbf{c}_2' \mathbf{D}_\gamma \mathbf{Z}' \mathbf{V}^- \mathbf{X})\tau$. From Result 4.5.3, it follows that $t(\mathbf{y})$ is the b.l.u.e. of u if and only if $t(\mathbf{y}) - \mathbf{c}_2' \mathbf{D}_\gamma \mathbf{Z}' \mathbf{V}^- \mathbf{y} = (\mathbf{c}_1' - \mathbf{c}_2' \mathbf{D}_\gamma \mathbf{Z}' \mathbf{V}^- \mathbf{X})\tau$ with probability 1. When $\mathbf{y}$ is normal, replace b.l.u.e. by b.u.e. in this conclusion to obtain property 3 (see Zyskind and Martin, 1969, p. 1200).   ■

The dimension of $\mathbf{V}$ is N, which may result in computational burden. In many applications however, we can assume some structure for $\mathbf{V}$, which reduces the computational effort (see Harville, 1976, section 3). The next result gives the covariance of the essentially-unique b.l.u.e. estimators. In general, suppose $\mathbf{C}_1'\tau$ are s estimable functions of τ, and let $\mathbf{C}_2$ be an arbitrary $q \times s$ matrix.

Result 10.2.2.   For the estimators that are essentially-unique b.l.u.e. as we defined in Result 10.2.1,

$$
\begin{aligned}
Var(\mathbf{C}_1'\tau^0) &= \mathbf{C}_1'(\mathbf{X}'\mathbf{V}^\sharp\mathbf{X})^- \mathbf{X}'\mathbf{V}^\sharp\mathbf{V}(\mathbf{V}^\sharp)'\mathbf{X}\{(\mathbf{X}'\mathbf{V}^\sharp\mathbf{X})^-\}'\mathbf{C}_1 \\
&= \mathbf{C}_1'(\mathbf{X}'\mathbf{V}^\sharp\mathbf{X})^- \mathbf{C}_1, \text{ if } \mathcal{C}(\mathbf{X}) \subset \mathcal{C}(\mathbf{V}), \quad (10.2.4)
\end{aligned}
$$

$$Var(\gamma^{*0} - \gamma) = \mathbf{D}_\gamma - \mathbf{D}_\gamma \mathbf{Z}' \mathbf{V}^- \mathbf{Z} \mathbf{D}_\gamma + \mathbf{D}_\gamma \mathbf{Z}' \mathbf{V}^- \mathbf{X}(\mathbf{X}'\mathbf{V}^\sharp\mathbf{X})^- \mathbf{X}'\mathbf{V}^\sharp\mathbf{Z}\mathbf{D}_\gamma,$$
$$(10.2.5)$$

$$Cov(\mathbf{C}_1'\tau^0, \gamma^{*0} - \gamma) = -Cov(\mathbf{C}_1'\tau^0, \gamma) = -\mathbf{C}_1'(\mathbf{X}'\mathbf{V}^\sharp\mathbf{X})^- \mathbf{X}'\mathbf{V}^\sharp\mathbf{Z}\mathbf{D}_\gamma. \quad (10.2.6)$$

Proof.   Consider

$$
\begin{aligned}
Var\{\mathbf{C}_1'(\tau^0 - \tau) + \mathbf{C}_2'(\gamma^{*0} - \gamma)\} &= Var(\mathbf{C}_1'\tau^0) + \mathbf{C}_2'\{Var(\gamma^{*0} - \gamma)\}\mathbf{C}_2 \\
&+ \{Cov(\mathbf{C}_1'\tau^0, \gamma^{*0} - \gamma)\}\mathbf{C}_2 \\
&+ \mathbf{C}_2'\{Cov(\mathbf{C}_1'\tau^0, \gamma^{*0} - \gamma)\}'.
\end{aligned}
$$

The results follow from (10.2.3), Zyskind and Martin (1969, Theorems 1 and 2) and Rao and Mitra (1971, Lemma 2.2.6 (c)).   ■

10.2.2   Estimation procedures

The ANOVA method is a method of moments type approach, which we illustrated for the one-factor random-effects model in section 10.1. The advantage of the ANOVA method is that estimation does not require any distributional assumption on $\mathbf{y}$, although assumption of normality leads to the usual F-tests of hypotheses. We first give examples of the ANOVA method for two-factor mixed-effects models. In addition to the ANOVA method, there are alternative estimation approaches for the mixed-effects models, which we discuss here. We first describe maximum likelihood estimation under normality. This is followed by the method of restricted maximum likelihood (REML) in the next subsection. We end with a discussion of the minimum norm quadratic unbiased estimation (MINQUE) procedure.

ANOVA method

We have discussed the ANOVA approach in detail in earlier chapters. We give some examples.

Example 10.2.2. Random-effects two-factor nested model. Consider the two-factor model where Factor A has a levels, the b levels of Factor B are *nested* within each of the levels of Factor A, and both factors are random. The two-way nested model is

$$Y_{ijk} = \mu + \tau_i + \beta_{j(i)} + \varepsilon_{ijk},$$

for $i = 1, \cdots, a$, $j = 1, \cdots, b$, $k = 1, \cdots, n$. Suppose τ_i are iid $N(0, \sigma_\tau^2)$ variables, $\beta_{j(i)}$ are iid $N(0, \sigma_\beta^2)$ variables, ε_{ijk} are iid $N(0, \sigma_\varepsilon^2)$ variables which are independent of τ_i and $\beta_{j(i)}$. Similar to the fixed-effects model, the ANOVA decomposition is

$$SST_m = SS_A + SS_{B(A)} + SSE,$$

where the sums of squares were defined in Example 4.2.7. When the effects are random, we can verify that the expected mean squares are

$$
\begin{aligned}
E(MS_A) &= \sigma_\varepsilon^2 + n\sigma_\beta^2 + nb\sigma_\tau^2, \\
E(MS_{B(A)}) &= \sigma_\varepsilon^2 + n\sigma_\beta^2, \text{ and} \\
E(MSE) &= \sigma_\varepsilon^2.
\end{aligned}
\tag{10.2.7}
$$

This list of expected mean squares serves as a guide for the construction of test statistics. Under the $H_0 : \sigma_\beta^2 = 0$, $E(MS_{B(A)}) = \sigma_\varepsilon^2$, and we use the test statistic $F = MS_{B(A)}/MSE$ to test H_0. This statistic has an $F_{a(b-1), ab(n-1)}$ distribution under H_0. Under the hypothesis $H_0 : \sigma_\tau^2 = 0$, we see that $E(MS_A) = \sigma_\varepsilon^2 + n\sigma_\beta^2$, and we reject the null hypothesis at level of significance α if $F = MS_A/MS_{B(A)} > F_{a-1, a(b-1), \alpha}$. $\square$

Example 10.2.3. Random-effects two-factor model. Recall the two-way cross classified model *with interaction* between the two factors (balanced case)

$$Y_{ijk} = \mu + \tau_i + \beta_j + (\tau\beta)_{ij} + \varepsilon_{ijk}, \tag{10.2.8}$$

for $k = 1, \cdots, n$, $i = 1, \cdots, a$, and $j = 1, \cdots, b$. Suppose that the τ, β, and $(\tau\beta)$ effects are all random. Suppose τ_i are iid $N(0, \sigma_\tau^2)$ variables, β_j are iid $N(0, \sigma_\beta^2)$ variables, $(\tau\beta)$ are iid $N(0, \sigma_{\tau\beta}^2)$ variables, $Cov(\tau_i, \beta_j) = 0 = Cov(\tau_i, (\tau\beta)_{ij}) = Cov(\tau_i, \varepsilon_{ijk})$, with similar assumptions about β's and $(\tau\beta)$'s.

Based on the ANOVA table we saw under the fixed-effects case, we can compute the expected mean squares when both Factor A and Factor B are random as

$$
\begin{aligned}
E(MS_A) &= bn\sigma_\tau^2 + n\sigma_{\tau\beta}^2 + \sigma_\varepsilon^2, \\
E(MS_B) &= an\sigma_\beta^2 + n\sigma_{\tau\beta}^2 + \sigma_\varepsilon^2, \\
E(MS_{AB}) &= n\sigma_{\tau\beta}^2 + \sigma_\varepsilon^2, \text{ and} \\
E(MSE) &= \sigma_\varepsilon^2,
\end{aligned}
$$

which are linear combinations of the unknown variance components.

The ANOVA method of estimating variance components from balanced data consists of equating the observed mean squares to these expected mean squares, and solving the resulting equations for $\hat\sigma_\tau^2$, $\hat\sigma_\beta^2$, $\hat\sigma_{\tau\beta}^2$, and $\hat\sigma_\varepsilon^2$. We obtain

$$
\begin{aligned}
\hat\sigma_\varepsilon^2 &= MSE, \\
\hat\sigma_\tau^2 &= \frac{1}{bn}(MS_A - MS_{AB}), \\
\hat\sigma_\beta^2 &= \frac{1}{an}(MS_B - MS_{AB}), \text{ and} \\
\hat\sigma_{\tau\beta}^2 &= \frac{1}{n}(MS_{AB} - MSE).
\end{aligned}
\tag{10.2.9}
$$

Note that once again, there exists a positive probability of negative estimates. In a balanced model, the ANOVA estimators of the variance components are minimum variance, quadratic unbiased estimators (Graybill and Hultquist, 1961), even if normality is not assumed. Under normality, Graybill (1954) showed that the ANOVA estimators are unbiased and have minimum variance.

Under normality, we obtain the following distributions of the sums of squares:

$$
\begin{aligned}
(a-1)MS_A / \{bn\sigma_\tau^2 + n\sigma_{\tau\beta}^2 + \sigma_\varepsilon^2\} &\sim \chi_{a-1}^2, \\
(a-1)(b-1)MS_{AB} / \{n\sigma_{\tau\beta}^2 + \sigma_\varepsilon^2\} &\sim \chi_{(a-1)(b-1)}^2,
\end{aligned}
$$

and these are independently distributed. It follows that the distribution of $\hat\sigma_\tau^2$ is a linear combination of scaled χ^2 variables, i.e.,

$$
\hat\sigma_\tau^2 \sim \frac{bn\sigma_\tau^2 + n\sigma_{\tau\beta}^2 + \sigma_\varepsilon^2}{bn(a-1)}\chi_{a-1}^2 - \frac{n\sigma_{\tau\beta}^2 + \sigma_\varepsilon^2}{bn(a-1)(b-1)}\chi_{(a-1)(b-1)}^2.
$$

However, $\hat\sigma_\varepsilon^2 \sim \{\sigma_\varepsilon^2/ab(n-1)\}\chi_{ab(n-1)}^2$, i.e., MSE always has a scaled χ^2 distribution. The expected mean squares often enable us to determine which mean squares are appropriate in the denominators of test statistics. For instance, in this model, the statistic MS_{AB}/MSE has an $F_{(a-1)(b-1),ab(n-1)}$ distribution under $H_0 : \sigma_{\tau\beta}^2 = 0$. To test $H_0 : \sigma_\tau^2 = 0$, we use the statistic MS_A/MS_{AB}, which has an $F_{a-1,(a-1)(b-1)}$ distribution under this null hypothesis.

To construct confidence intervals, note that the mean squares are distributed independently as multiples of χ^2 variables. Suppose we denote the kth mean square by M_k with corresponding degrees of freedom f_k. Then, an exact $100(1-\alpha)\%$ confidence interval for $E(M_k)$ has the form

$$\{f_k M_k\}/\chi^2_{f_k,U} \le E(M_k) \le \{f_k M_k\}/\chi^2_{f_k,L},$$

where $\chi^2_{f_k,U}$ and $\chi^2_{f_k,L}$ are defined by $P(\chi^2_{f_k,L} \le \chi^2_{f_k} < \chi^2_{f_k,U}) = 1 - \alpha$. $\square$

Example 10.2.4. Mixed-effects two-factor model. In the two-factor cross-classified model, suppose Factor A is fixed, Factor B is random, and we consider interaction between the factors. The expected mean squares are

$$
\begin{aligned}
E(MS_A) &= \sigma^2_\varepsilon + n\sigma^2_{\tau\beta} + nb\sum_{i=1}^{a}\tau_i^2/(a-1) \\
E(MS_B) &= \sigma^2_\varepsilon + an\sigma^2_\beta, \\
E(MS_{AB}) &= \sigma^2_\varepsilon + n\sigma^2_{\tau\beta}, \text{ and} \\
E(MSE) &= \sigma^2_\varepsilon.
\end{aligned}
$$
(10.2.10)

The ANOVA estimators (which are also REML estimators) are

$$
\begin{aligned}
\mu^0 &= \overline{Y}_{...}, \\
\tau_i^0 &= \overline{Y}_{i..} - \overline{Y}_{...}, \quad i=1,\cdots,a, \\
\widehat{\sigma}^2_\beta &= (MS_B - MS_{AB})/an, \\
\widehat{\sigma}^2_{\tau\beta} &= (MS_{AB} - MSE)/n, \text{ and} \\
\widehat{\sigma}^2_\varepsilon &= MSE.
\end{aligned}
$$

Under $H_0 : \sigma^2_{\tau\beta} = 0$, we can show that the test statistic $F_0 = MS_{AB}/MSE$ has an $F_{(a-1)(b-1),ab(n-1)}$ distribution. Under $H_0 : \sigma^2_\beta = 0$, the test statistic $F_0 = MS_B/MS_{AB}$ has an $F_{b-1,(a-1)(b-1)}$ distribution. Under $H_0 : \tau_1 = \cdots = \tau_a$, the test statistic $F_0 = MS_A/MS_{AB}$ has an $F_{a-1,(a-1)(b-1)}$ distribution. $\square$

Method of maximum likelihood

We write the mixed-effects model (10.2.1) as

$$\mathbf{y} = \mathbf{X}\tau + \mathbf{Z}_1\gamma_1 + \cdots + \mathbf{Z}_m\gamma_m + \varepsilon,$$
(10.2.11)

where γ_j is a q_j-dimensional vector of random effects, and $\mathbf{Z}_j$ is the corresponding $N \times q_j$ design matrix, $j = 1,\cdots,m$, ε is the N-dimensional error vector, $\mathbf{X}$ is an $N \times p$ matrix of known regressors, and τ is a p-dimensional vector of fixed effects. We assume that $E(\gamma_j) = \mathbf{0}$, $Var(\gamma_j) = \sigma^2_j\mathbf{I}_{q_j}$, $j = 1,\cdots,m$, $Cov(\gamma_j,\gamma_l) = \mathbf{0}$, $j \ne l$, $Var(\varepsilon) = \sigma^2_\varepsilon\mathbf{I}_N$, and $Cov(\gamma_j,\varepsilon) = \mathbf{0}$, $j = 1,\cdots,m$. Then, $E(\mathbf{y}) = \mathbf{X}\tau$ and

$$\mathbf{V} = Var(\mathbf{y}) = \sum_{j=1}^{m}\sigma^2_j\mathbf{Z}_j\mathbf{Z}'_j + \sigma^2_\varepsilon\mathbf{I}_N.$$

For ease of notation, we set $\varepsilon \equiv \gamma_0$, $N \equiv q_0$, and $\mathbf{Z}_0 \equiv \mathbf{I}_N$.

The likelihood function has the form

$$L(\tau,\mathbf{V}|\mathbf{y}) = (2\pi)^{-N/2}|\mathbf{V}|^{-1/2}\exp\{-\frac{1}{2}(\mathbf{y} - \mathbf{X}\tau)'\mathbf{V}^{-1}(\mathbf{y} - \mathbf{X}\tau)\}.$$
(10.2.12)

Differentiate $\log L(\tau, \mathbf{V}|\mathbf{y})$ with respect to τ and σ_j^2, to yield the likelihood equations

$$\partial \log L / \partial \tau = \mathbf{X}'\mathbf{V}^{-1}\mathbf{y} - \mathbf{X}'\mathbf{V}^{-1}\mathbf{X}\tau = \mathbf{0}, \text{ and} \qquad (10.2.13)$$

$$\partial \log L / \partial \sigma_j^2 = -tr(\mathbf{V}^{-1}\mathbf{Z}_j\mathbf{Z}_j')/2 + (\mathbf{y} - \mathbf{X}\tau)'\mathbf{V}^{-1}\mathbf{Z}_j\mathbf{Z}_j'\mathbf{V}^{-1}(\mathbf{y} - \mathbf{X}\tau) = 0,$$
$$j = 1, \cdots, r. \qquad (10.2.14)$$

The solutions $\dot{\tau}$ and $\dot{\sigma}_j^2$ are obtained by solving (10.2.13) and (10.2.14), the latter being nonlinear functions of the variance components. Usually, closed form solutions do not exist, and moreover, the solutions of the variance components may be negative. Provided $\dot{\sigma}_0^2 > 0$, and $\dot{\sigma}_j^2 \geq 0$, $j = 1, \cdots, m$, they are the MLE's of the variance components, which are otherwise set to zero. The MLE of τ is then obtained by substituting $\dot{\mathbf{V}}$ for $\mathbf{V}$ in (10.2.13). Let us denote the MLE's by $\hat{\tau}_{ML}$, and $\hat{\sigma}_{j,ML}^2$, $j = 0, \cdots, m$. For more details, the reader is referred to chapter 6 of Searle et al. (1992). In Exercise 10.5, we ask the reader to derive the asymptotic variances of these estimators.

Example 10.2.3. (continued). For the two-factor model with interaction, the maximum likelihood estimators do not have a closed form even with balanced data. These must be obtained numerically for each data set. The ML equations are defined by

$$\frac{SS_A}{\dot{\theta}_{11}^2} + \frac{SS_B}{\dot{\theta}_{12}^2} + \frac{SS_{AB}}{\dot{\theta}_1^2} + \frac{SSE}{\dot{\theta}_0^2} = \frac{1}{\dot{\theta}_4} + \frac{a-1}{\dot{\theta}_{11}} + \frac{b-1}{\dot{\theta}_{12}} +$$

$$\frac{(a-1)(b-1)}{\dot{\theta}_1} + \frac{ab(n-1)}{\dot{\theta}_0},$$

$$\frac{SS_A}{\dot{\theta}_{11}^2} = \frac{1}{\dot{\theta}_4} + \frac{a-1}{\dot{\theta}_{11}},$$

$$\frac{SS_B}{\dot{\theta}_{12}^2} = \frac{1}{\dot{\theta}_4} + \frac{b-1}{\dot{\theta}_{12}}, \text{ and}$$

$$\frac{SS_A}{\dot{\theta}_{11}^2} + \frac{SS_B}{\dot{\theta}_{12}^2} + \frac{SS_{AB}}{\dot{\theta}_1^2} = \frac{1}{\dot{\theta}_4} + \frac{a-1}{\dot{\theta}_{11}} + \frac{b-1}{\dot{\theta}_{12}} + \frac{(a-1)(b-1)}{\dot{\theta}_1},$$

where $\theta_0 = \sigma_\varepsilon^2$, $\theta_1 = \sigma_\varepsilon^2 + n\sigma_{\tau\beta}^2$, $\theta_{11} = \sigma_\varepsilon^2 + n\sigma_{\tau\beta}^2 + bn\sigma_\tau^2$, $\theta_{12} = \sigma_\varepsilon^2 + n\sigma_{\tau\beta}^2 + an\sigma_\beta^2$, and $\theta_4 = \theta_{11} + \theta_{12} - \theta_1$. The MLE's are obtained by solving these equations simultaneously. $\square$

REML estimation

The REML procedure was described in section 7.5.4. For a balanced model, the REML estimator coincides with the ANOVA estimator. We show some examples.

Example 10.2.5. Consider the two-factor nested model

$$Y_{ijk} = \mu + \tau_i + \beta_{j(i)} + \varepsilon_{ijk},$$

for $i = 1, \cdots, a$, $j = 1, \cdots, b$ and $k = 1, \cdots, n$. Suppose Factor A is fixed, while Factor B is a random factor whose levels are nested within the levels of Factor A. In this mixed-effects model, we assume that $\sum_{i=1}^{a} \tau_i = 0$, and $\beta_{j(i)}$'s are iid $N(0, \sigma_\beta^2)$ variables , $j = 1, \cdots, b$, $i = 1, \cdots, a$. In this case, μ^0 and τ_i^0 have the same form as in the fixed-effects case, while the estimates of $\hat{\sigma}_\varepsilon^2$ and $\hat{\sigma}_\beta^2$ are given under the random-effects model (see Exercise 10.6). Then,

$$E(MS_A) = \sigma_\varepsilon^2 + n\sigma_\beta^2 + bn\sum_{i=1}^{a} \tau_i^2/(a-1),$$

$$E(MS_{B(A)}) = \sigma_\varepsilon^2 + n\sigma_\beta^2, \text{ and}$$

$$E(MSE) = \sigma_\varepsilon^2.$$

The hypothesis $H_A : \tau_1 = \cdots = \tau_a$ is tested by $F_0 = MS_A/MS_{B(A)}$ which has an $F_{a-1,a(b-1)}$ distribution under H_A. The test statistic for $H_B : \sigma_\beta^2 = 0$ is $F_0 = MS_{B(A)}/MSE$, which has an $F_{a(b-1),ab(n-1)}$ distribution under H_B. □

MINQUE estimation

Consider the model formulation in (10.2.11), with the same moment assumptions on γ_j's and ε. It follows from Rao (1971a, b) that

$$Var(\mathbf{y}) = \sum_{j=1}^{m} \sigma_j^2 \mathbf{Z}_j \mathbf{Z}_j' + \sigma_\varepsilon^2 \mathbf{I}_N = \sigma_\varepsilon^2 \mathbf{T}_0 + \sum_{j=1}^{m} \sigma_j^2 \mathbf{T}_j,$$

where $\mathbf{T}_j = \mathbf{Z}_j \mathbf{Z}_i'$, $j = 1, \cdots, m$, $\mathbf{T}_0 = \mathbf{Z}_0 \mathbf{Z}_0'$, $\mathbf{Z}_0 = \mathbf{I}_N$. For ease of notation, set $\sigma_\varepsilon^2 = \sigma_0^2$. The problem is to estimate a function of the variance components, $F = \sum_{j=0}^{m} f_j \sigma_j^2$, by some quadratic form $\mathbf{y'Ay}$. We require $\mathbf{y'Ay}$ to be

(i) invariant with respect to translation in τ, i.e., if $\tau \to \tau_d = \tau - \tau_0$, we require $\mathbf{y'Ay} = \mathbf{y}_d' \mathbf{Ay}_d$; a condition for this is $\mathbf{Ax} = \mathbf{0}$, and

(ii) we require $E(\mathbf{y'Ay}) = F$, for which we must have

$$E(\mathbf{y'Ay}) = \sum_{j=0}^{m} tr(\mathbf{AT}_j)\sigma_j^2 = F,$$

which in turn requires that $tr(\mathbf{AT}_j) = f_j$, $j = 0, \cdots, m$.

Now, $Var(\gamma_j) = \sigma_j^2 \mathbf{I}_{q_j}$; this implies that if γ_j's are known, a natural estimator of σ_j^2 would be $\gamma_j' \gamma_j/q_j$. If ε were also known, then $\varepsilon'\varepsilon/N$ would be a natural estimate of σ_0^2. In this case, F would be estimated by

$$\hat{F} = \sum_{j=1}^{m} f_j \gamma_j' \gamma_j/q_j + f_0 \varepsilon'\varepsilon/N = \eta' \Delta \eta,$$

say, where,

$$\eta' = (\gamma_1', \cdots, \gamma_m', \varepsilon'), \text{ and}$$
$$\Delta = \text{diag}\{(f_1/q_1)\mathbf{1}_{q_1}, \cdots, (f_m/q_m)\mathbf{1}_{q_m}, (f_0/N)\mathbf{1}_N\}.$$

Since $\mathbf{AX} = \mathbf{0}$, the proposed estimator is

$$\mathbf{y'Ay} = \{\textstyle\sum_{j=1}^m \mathbf{Z}_j\gamma_j + \mathbf{Z}_0\varepsilon\}'\mathbf{A}\{\textstyle\sum_{j=1}^m \mathbf{Z}_j\gamma_j + \mathbf{Z}_0\varepsilon\} = \eta'\mathbf{Z'AZ}\eta,$$

where, $\mathbf{Z} = \{\mathbf{Z}_1, \cdots, \mathbf{Z}_m, \mathbf{Z}_0\}$. Now, $\mathbf{Z}'\Delta\eta$ will be closest to $\mathbf{y'Ay}$ if the term
$\| \mathbf{Z'AZ} - \Delta \|$ is small. The matrix $\mathbf{A}$ is chosen to minimize this norm. Since
$\| \mathbf{Z'AZ} - \Delta \|$ is the sum of squares of elements of $\mathbf{Z'AZ} - \Delta$, we see after some
simplification that

$$\| \mathbf{Z'AZ} - \Delta \| = tr\{(\mathbf{Z'AZ} - \Delta)'(\mathbf{Z'AZ} - \Delta)\}$$
$$= tr(\mathbf{AZZ'})^2 - \sum_{j=1}^m \{f_j^2/q_j + f_0^2/N\}.$$

Let $\mathbf{T} = \sum_{j=0}^m \mathbf{T}_j = \sum_{j=0}^m \mathbf{Z}_i\mathbf{Z}_i' = \mathbf{ZZ'}$. The MINQUE of F is $\mathbf{y'Ay}$, where
$\mathbf{A}$ is such that $tr(\mathbf{AZZ'})^2$, which is equal to $tr(\mathbf{AT})^2$, is minimum subject to
$\mathbf{AX} = \mathbf{0}$, and $tr(\mathbf{AT}_j) = f_j, j = 0, \cdots, m$. Rao (1971) showed that this
minimum occurs when $\mathbf{A} = \sum_{j=0}^m \lambda_j\mathbf{ST}_j\mathbf{S}$, where,

$$\mathbf{S} = \mathbf{T}^{-1} - \mathbf{T}^{-1}\mathbf{X}(\mathbf{X'T}^{-1}\mathbf{X})^{-}\mathbf{X'T}^{-1},$$

and λ_j are solutions of $\sum_{j=0}^m \lambda_j tr\{\mathbf{ST}_j\mathbf{ST}_l\} = f_l, l = 0, \cdots, m$. Hence,
the MINQUE of F is $\mathbf{y'Ay} = \sum_{j=0}^m \lambda_j\mathbf{y'ST}_j\mathbf{Sy} = \sum_{j=0}^m \lambda_j Q_j$, where $Q_j =$
$\mathbf{y'ST}_j\mathbf{Sy}, j = 0, \cdots, m$. To find $\lambda = (\lambda_0, \cdots, \lambda_m)'$, let $w_{jl} = tr(\mathbf{ST}_j\mathbf{ST}_l)$,
$j, l = 0, \cdots, m$, and suppose $\mathbf{W} = \{w_{jl}\}$ is an $(m + 1) \times (m + 1)$ matrix with
these elements. Then, $\sum_{j=0}^m \lambda_j tr\{\mathbf{ST}_j\mathbf{ST}_l\} = f_l, l = 0, \cdots, m$ if and only
if $\mathbf{W}\lambda = \mathbf{f}$, where $\mathbf{f}' = (f_0, \cdots, f_m)$; the solution is $\lambda = \mathbf{W}^{-}\mathbf{f}$. Hence, the
MINQUE of F is

$$\mathbf{y'Ay} = \textstyle\sum_{j=0}^m \lambda_j Q_j = \lambda'\mathbf{Q} = (\mathbf{W}^{-}\mathbf{f})'\mathbf{Q} = \mathbf{f'W}^{-}\mathbf{Q} = \mathbf{f}'\hat{\sigma} = \sum_{j=0}^m f_j\hat{\sigma}_j^2,$$

where $\hat{\sigma} = (\hat{\sigma}_0^2, \cdots, \hat{\sigma}_m^2)' = \mathbf{W}^{-}\mathbf{Q}$.

Exercises

10.1. In the one-way random-effects model, show that

$$Var(\hat{\mu}_{GLS}) = [\sum_{i=1}^a n_i/(n_i\sigma_\tau^2 + \sigma_\varepsilon^2)]^{-1}.$$

10.2 Consider the balanced one-way random-effects model where ε_{ij} are iid
$N(0, \sigma_\varepsilon^2)$ variables, and τ_i are iid $N(0, \sigma_\tau^2)$ variables. Show that the sum
of squares due to the Factor A can be written as $SS_A = \mathbf{y}'(\sum_{i=1}^{a+} \mathbf{J}_n/n - \mathbf{J}_N/N)\mathbf{y}$.

10.3. In the formulation of Exercise 10.2, show that $E(MSA) = n\sigma_\tau^2 + \sigma_\varepsilon^2$. Derive the distributions of $SSA/E(MSA)$ and $SSE/E(MSE)$.

10.4. Show that

(a) $\mathbf{X}(\mathbf{X}'\mathbf{V}^\sharp\mathbf{X})^-\mathbf{X}'\mathbf{V}^\sharp\mathbf{y}$ is invariant to $\mathbf{V}^\sharp$ and $(\mathbf{X}'\mathbf{V}^\sharp\mathbf{X})^-$, and

(b) $\mathcal{C}(\mathbf{X}, \mathbf{V}) = \mathcal{C}(\mathbf{X}, \mathbf{VN})$,

where $\mathbf{N}$ appeared in (4.5.7), and the other quantities appear in Result 10.2.1.

10.5. In the mixed-effects linear model (10.2.11), let $\sigma^2 = (\sigma_0^2, \sigma_1^2, \cdots, \sigma_m^2)'$. Show that, as $N \to \infty$,

1. $Var(\widehat{\tau}_{ML}) \approx (\mathbf{X}'\mathbf{V}^{-1}\mathbf{X})^{-1}$,
2. $Var(\widehat{\sigma}_{ML}^2) = 2\mathbf{S}^{-1}$, where $\mathbf{S} = \{S_{ij}\}$ is an $(m+1) \times (m+1)$ matrix whose (i, j)th element is $S_{ij} \approx 2\{tr(\mathbf{V}^{-1}\mathbf{Z}_i\mathbf{Z}_i'\mathbf{V}^{-1}\mathbf{Z}_j\mathbf{Z}_j')\}$, and
3. $Cov(\widehat{\tau}_{ML}, \widehat{\sigma}_{ML}^2) \to \mathbf{0}$.

10.6. Obtain the ANOVA estimators and maximum likelihood estimators of the variance components in the two-factor (balanced) nested model with random-effects which is described in Example 10.2.2.

10.7. Consider the two-factor additive random-effects model

$$Y_{ijk} = \mu + \tau_i + \beta_j + \varepsilon_{ijk},$$

for $i = 1, \cdots, a$, $j = 1, \cdots, b$, and $k = 1, \cdots, n$. Suppose τ_i are iid $N(0, \sigma_\tau^2)$ variables, β_j are iid $N(0, \sigma_\beta^2)$ variables, ε_{ijk} are iid $N(0, \sigma_\varepsilon^2)$ variables, $Cov(\tau_i, \beta_j) = 0$, $Cov(\tau_i, \varepsilon_{ij}) = 0$, and $Cov(\beta_j, \varepsilon_{ij}) = 0$. Let $N = nab$. Derive the ANOVA, ML and REML estimators of the variance components.

Chapter 11

Special Topics

11.1 Bayesian linear models

We start with a statement of Bayes' theorem, which is a time-honored result dating back to the late eighteenth century. Let $\mathcal{B} = (B_1, B_2, \cdots, B_k)$ denote a partition of a sample space $\mathcal{S}$, and let A denote an event with $P(A) > 0$. By the definition of conditional probability (see Casella and Berger, 1990), we have

$$P(B_j|A) = P(B_j \cap A)/P(A) = P(A|B_j)P(B_j)/P(A).$$

By substituting for $P(A)$ from the law of total probability, i.e.,

$$P(A) = \sum_{i=1}^{k} P(A|B_i)P(B_i),$$

it follows that for any event B_j in $\mathcal{B}$,

$$P(B_j|A) = P(A|B_j)P(B_j) \left/ \sum_{i=1}^{k} P(A|B_i)P(B_i) \right. .$$

When the partition $\mathcal{B}$ represents all possible mutually exclusive states of nature or hypotheses, we refer to $P(B_j)$ as the prior probability of an event B_j. An event A is then observed, and this modifies the probabilities of the events in $\mathcal{B}$. We call $P(B_j|A)$ the posterior probability of B_j.

Now consider the setup in terms of continuous random vectors. Let $\mathbf{x}$ be a k-dimensional random vector with joint pdf $f(\mathbf{x}; \theta)$, where θ is a q-dimensional parameter vector. We assume that θ is also a continuous random vector with pdf $\pi(\theta)$, which we refer to as the *prior* density of θ. Given the likelihood function is $L(\mathbf{x}; \theta) = f(\mathbf{x}; \theta)$, an application of Bayes' theorem gives the posterior density of θ as

$$\pi(\theta|\mathbf{x}) = L(\mathbf{x}; \theta)\pi(\theta) \left/ \int L(\mathbf{x}; \theta)\pi(\theta)d\theta \right. .$$

The following matrix results are useful in combining quadratic forms, and find application in a Bayesian treatment of linear models (Box and Tiao, 1973).

Result 11.1.1.   Let $\mathbf{x}$, $\mathbf{a}$, and $\mathbf{b}$ denote k-dimensional vectors, and let $\mathbf{A}$ and $\mathbf{B}$ be $k \times k$ symmetric matrices such that $(\mathbf{A} + \mathbf{B})^{-1}$ exists. Then,

$$(\mathbf{x} - \mathbf{a})'\mathbf{A}(\mathbf{x} - \mathbf{a}) \quad + \quad (\mathbf{x} - \mathbf{b})'\mathbf{B}(\mathbf{x} - \mathbf{b}) = (\mathbf{x} - \mathbf{c})'(\mathbf{A} + \mathbf{B})(\mathbf{x} - \mathbf{c})$$
$$+ (\mathbf{a} - \mathbf{b})'\mathbf{A}(\mathbf{A} + \mathbf{B})^{-1}\mathbf{B}(\mathbf{a} - \mathbf{b})$$

where $\mathbf{c} = (\mathbf{A} + \mathbf{B})^{-1}(\mathbf{A}\mathbf{a} + \mathbf{B}\mathbf{b})$.

Proof. Clearly,

$$(\mathbf{x} - \mathbf{a})'\mathbf{A}(\mathbf{x} - \mathbf{a}) + (\mathbf{x} - \mathbf{b})'\mathbf{B}(\mathbf{x} - \mathbf{b})$$
$$= \quad \mathbf{x}'(\mathbf{A} + \mathbf{B})\mathbf{x} - 2\mathbf{x}'(\mathbf{A}\mathbf{a} + \mathbf{B}\mathbf{b}) + \mathbf{a}'\mathbf{A}\mathbf{a} + \mathbf{b}'\mathbf{B}\mathbf{b}$$
$$= \quad \mathbf{x}'(\mathbf{A} + \mathbf{B})\mathbf{x} - 2\mathbf{x}'(\mathbf{A} + \mathbf{B})\mathbf{c} + \mathbf{c}'(\mathbf{A} + \mathbf{B})\mathbf{c} + d$$
$$= \quad (\mathbf{x} - \mathbf{c})'(\mathbf{A} + \mathbf{B})(\mathbf{x} - \mathbf{c}) + d$$

where $d = \mathbf{a}'\mathbf{A}\mathbf{a} + \mathbf{b}'\mathbf{B}\mathbf{b} - \mathbf{c}'(\mathbf{A} + \mathbf{B})\mathbf{c}$. The right side is

$$\mathbf{c}'(\mathbf{A} + \mathbf{B})\mathbf{c} \quad = \quad (\mathbf{A}\mathbf{a} + \mathbf{B}\mathbf{b})'(\mathbf{A} + \mathbf{B})^{-1}(\mathbf{A}\mathbf{a} + \mathbf{B}\mathbf{b})$$
$$= \quad [\mathbf{A}(\mathbf{a} - \mathbf{b}) + (\mathbf{A} + \mathbf{B})\mathbf{b}]'(\mathbf{A} + \mathbf{B})^{-1}$$
$$\times \quad [(\mathbf{A} + \mathbf{B})\mathbf{a} - \mathbf{B}(\mathbf{a} - \mathbf{b})]$$
$$= \quad -(\mathbf{a} - \mathbf{b})'\mathbf{A}(\mathbf{A} + \mathbf{B})^{-1}\mathbf{B}(\mathbf{a} - \mathbf{b}) + \mathbf{a}'\mathbf{A}\mathbf{a} + \mathbf{b}'\mathbf{B}\mathbf{b},$$

and the result follows immediately. ■

Result 11.1.2.   Let $\mathbf{x}$, $\mathbf{a}$, and $\mathbf{b}$ denote k-dimensional vectors, and let $\mathbf{A}$ and $\mathbf{B}$ be $k \times k$ p.s.d. symmetric matrices such that $r(\mathbf{A} + \mathbf{B}) = q < k$. Then, subject to the constraints $\mathbf{G}\mathbf{x} = \mathbf{0}$,

$$(\mathbf{x} - \mathbf{a})'\mathbf{A}(\mathbf{x} - \mathbf{a}) \quad + \quad (\mathbf{x} - \mathbf{b})'\mathbf{B}(\mathbf{x} - \mathbf{b}) = (\mathbf{x} - \mathbf{c}^*)'(\mathbf{A} + \mathbf{B} + \mathbf{M})(\mathbf{x} - \mathbf{c}^*)$$
$$+ \quad (\mathbf{a} - \mathbf{b})'\mathbf{A}(\mathbf{A} + \mathbf{B} + \mathbf{M})^{-1}\mathbf{B}(\mathbf{a} - \mathbf{b}),$$

where $\mathbf{G}$ is any $(k - q) \times q$ matrix of rank $(k - q)$ such that the rows of $\mathbf{G}$ are LIN of the rows of the matrix $\mathbf{A} + \mathbf{B}$, $\mathbf{M} = \mathbf{G}'\mathbf{G}$, and

$$\mathbf{c}^* = (\mathbf{A} + \mathbf{B} + \mathbf{M})^{-1}(\mathbf{A}\mathbf{a} + \mathbf{B}\mathbf{b}). \tag{11.1.1}$$

Proof. Since $r(\mathbf{G}) = (k - q)$, there exists a $(k - q) \times q$ matrix $\mathbf{U}$ of rank $(k - q)$ such that $\mathbf{U}\mathbf{G}'$ is nonsingular and $\mathbf{U}(\mathbf{A} + \mathbf{B}) = \mathbf{0}$. Now,

$$\mathbf{U}(\mathbf{A} + \mathbf{B} + \mathbf{M})(\mathbf{A} + \mathbf{B} + \mathbf{M})^{-1} = \mathbf{U}.$$

Since $\mathbf{U}(\mathbf{A} + \mathbf{B}) = \mathbf{0}$, $\mathbf{U}\mathbf{M}(\mathbf{A} + \mathbf{B} + \mathbf{M})^{-1} = \mathbf{U}$. Post multiplying both sides by $\mathbf{A} + \mathbf{B}$, we get $\mathbf{U}\mathbf{M}(\mathbf{A} + \mathbf{B} + \mathbf{M})^{-1}(\mathbf{A} + \mathbf{B}) = \mathbf{0}$. Since $\mathbf{M} = \mathbf{G}'\mathbf{G}$ and $\mathbf{U}\mathbf{G}'$ is nonsingular, this implies that

$$\mathbf{G}(\mathbf{A} + \mathbf{B} + \mathbf{M})^{-1}(\mathbf{A} + \mathbf{B}) \quad = \quad \mathbf{0}, \text{ so that}$$
$$\mathbf{M}(\mathbf{A} + \mathbf{B} + \mathbf{M})^{-1}(\mathbf{A} + \mathbf{B}) \quad = \quad \mathbf{0}.$$

Premultiplying both sides of the last equation by $(\mathbf{A} + \mathbf{B} + \mathbf{M})^{-1}\mathbf{M}$, we obtain

$$\mathbf{M}(\mathbf{A} + \mathbf{B} + \mathbf{M})^{-1}\mathbf{A}(\mathbf{A} + \mathbf{B} + \mathbf{M})^{-1}\mathbf{M}$$
$$+\mathbf{M}(\mathbf{A} + \mathbf{B} + \mathbf{M})^{-1}\mathbf{B}(\mathbf{A} + \mathbf{B} + \mathbf{M})^{-1}\mathbf{M} = \mathbf{0}.$$

Both terms on the left are p.s.d. matrices, which follows from the fact that $\mathbf{A}$ and $\mathbf{B}$ are p.s.d. The above equality therefore implies that each term must be equal to $\mathbf{0}$. For $k \times k$ matrices $\mathbf{C}$ and $\mathbf{D}$, write $\mathbf{A} = \mathbf{C}'\mathbf{C}$ and $\mathbf{B} = \mathbf{D}'\mathbf{D}$. We must then have

$$\mathbf{M}(\mathbf{A} + \mathbf{B} + \mathbf{M})^{-1}\mathbf{C}' = \mathbf{M}(\mathbf{A} + \mathbf{B} + \mathbf{M})^{-1}\mathbf{D}' = \mathbf{0}$$

which implies that

$$\mathbf{M}(\mathbf{A} + \mathbf{B} + \mathbf{M})^{-1}\mathbf{A} = \mathbf{M}(\mathbf{A} + \mathbf{B} + \mathbf{M})^{-1}\mathbf{B} = \mathbf{0}.$$

Since $\mathbf{Mx} = \mathbf{0}$,

$$
\begin{aligned}
(\mathbf{x} - \mathbf{a})'\mathbf{A}(\mathbf{x} - \mathbf{a}) + (\mathbf{x} - \mathbf{b})'\mathbf{B}(\mathbf{x} - \mathbf{b}) &= \mathbf{x}'(\mathbf{A} + \mathbf{B} + \mathbf{M})\mathbf{x} - 2\mathbf{x}'(\mathbf{A} + \mathbf{B} + \mathbf{M})\mathbf{c}^* \\
&\quad + (\mathbf{c}^*)'(\mathbf{A} + \mathbf{B} + \mathbf{M})\mathbf{c}^* + d_1 \\
&= (\mathbf{x} - \mathbf{c}^*)'(\mathbf{A} + \mathbf{B} + \mathbf{M})(\mathbf{x} - \mathbf{c}^*) + d_1
\end{aligned}
$$

where $d_1 = \mathbf{a}'\mathbf{A}\mathbf{a} + \mathbf{b}'\mathbf{B}\mathbf{b} - (\mathbf{c}^*)'(\mathbf{A} + \mathbf{B} + \mathbf{M})\mathbf{c}^*$, and $\mathbf{c}^*$ was defined in (11.1.1). We can now show that

$$(\mathbf{c}^*)'(\mathbf{A} + \mathbf{B} + \mathbf{M})\mathbf{c}^* = -(\mathbf{a} - \mathbf{b})'\mathbf{A}(\mathbf{A} + \mathbf{B} + \mathbf{M})^{-1}\mathbf{B}(\mathbf{a} - \mathbf{b}) + \mathbf{a}'\mathbf{A}\mathbf{a} + \mathbf{a}'\mathbf{A}\mathbf{b}$$

so that

$$d_1 = (\mathbf{a} - \mathbf{b})'\mathbf{A}(\mathbf{A} + \mathbf{B} + \mathbf{M})^{-1}\mathbf{B}(\mathbf{a} - \mathbf{b})$$

which proves the result. ∎

Result 11.1.3. Let $\mathbf{y}$ be an N-dimensional vector, let θ_1 be a k_1-dimensional vector, and suppose that

$$\mathbf{y}|\theta_1 \sim N(\mathbf{A}_1\theta_1, \mathbf{C}_1). \tag{11.1.2}$$

Also, assume that given a k_2-dimensional vector of hyperparameters θ_2,

$$\theta_1|\theta_2 \sim N(\mathbf{A}_2\theta_2, \mathbf{C}_2). \tag{11.1.3}$$

It is assumed that $\mathbf{A}_1, \mathbf{A}_2, \mathbf{C}_1$, and $\mathbf{C}_2$ are known p.d. matrices of appropriate dimensions (Lindley and Smith, 1972).

1. The marginal distribution of $\mathbf{y}$ is given by

$$\mathbf{y} \sim N(\mathbf{A}_1\mathbf{A}_2\theta_2, \mathbf{C}_1 + \mathbf{A}_1\mathbf{C}_2\mathbf{A}_1'). \tag{11.1.4}$$

2. The conditional distribution of θ_1 given $\mathbf{y}$ is $N(\mathbf{Bb}, \mathbf{B})$ where

$$\mathbf{B}^{-1} = \mathbf{A}_1'\mathbf{C}_1^{-1}\mathbf{A}_1 + \mathbf{C}_2^{-1} \tag{11.1.5}$$

and

$$\mathbf{b} = \mathbf{A}_1'\mathbf{C}_1^{-1}\mathbf{y} + \mathbf{C}_2^{-1}\mathbf{A}_2\theta_2. \tag{11.1.6}$$

Proof.   From (11.1.2), we can write $\mathbf{y} = \mathbf{A}_1\theta_1 + \mathbf{u}$, where $\mathbf{u} \sim N(\mathbf{0}, \mathbf{C}_1)$. We can also write (11.1.3) as $\theta_1 = \mathbf{A}_2\theta_2 + \mathbf{v}$, where $\mathbf{v} \sim N(\mathbf{0}, \mathbf{C}_2)$ and $\mathbf{v}$ is independent of $\mathbf{u}$. From these observations, it follows that

$$\mathbf{y} = \mathbf{A}_1\mathbf{A}_2\theta_2 + \mathbf{A}_1\mathbf{v} + \mathbf{u}.$$

By the independence of $\mathbf{u}$ and $\mathbf{v}$, and Result 5.2.6, $\mathbf{A}_1\mathbf{v} + \mathbf{u} \sim N(\mathbf{0}, \mathbf{C}_1 + \mathbf{A}_1\mathbf{C}_2\mathbf{A}_1')$, which leads directly to the proof of property 1. To prove property 2, we see from Bayes' theorem that

$$\pi(\theta_1|\mathbf{y}) \propto L(\mathbf{y}|\theta_1)\pi(\theta_1).$$

By substituting expressions for the respective normal densities in the product on the right side, and simplifying (by completing the square in) the quadratic form in the exponent, we see that the product is $\exp(-Q/2)$, where

$$Q = (\theta_1 - \mathbf{Bb})'\mathbf{B}^{-1}(\theta_1 - \mathbf{Bb}) + [\mathbf{y}'\mathbf{C}_1^{-1}\mathbf{y} + \theta_2'\mathbf{A}_2'\mathbf{C}_2^{-1}\mathbf{A}_2\theta_2 - \mathbf{b}'\mathbf{Bb}]$$

from which property 2 follows. ∎

We give a more general result (Lindley and Smith, 1972) that involves a two-stage hierarchy. The proof is left as an exercise.

Result 11.1.4. Suppose

$$\mathbf{y}|\theta_1 \sim N(\mathbf{A}_1\theta_1, \mathbf{C}_1), \quad \theta_1|\theta_2 \sim N(\mathbf{A}_2\theta_2, \mathbf{C}_2), \quad \text{and} \qquad (11.1.7)$$
$$\theta_2|\theta_3 \sim N(\mathbf{A}_3\theta_3, \mathbf{C}_3)$$

where θ_3 is a known k_3-dimensional vector, and $\mathbf{A}_1, \mathbf{A}_2, \mathbf{A}_3, \mathbf{C}_1, \mathbf{C}_2$ and $\mathbf{C}_3$ are known p.d. matrices of appropriate dimensions. The posterior distribution of θ_1 given $\mathbf{y}$ is $N(\mathbf{Dd}, \mathbf{D})$ where

$$\mathbf{D}^{-1} = \mathbf{A}_1'\mathbf{C}_1^{-1}\mathbf{A}_1 + [\mathbf{C}_2 + \mathbf{A}_2\mathbf{C}_3\mathbf{A}_2']^{-1} \qquad (11.1.8)$$

and

$$\mathbf{d} = \mathbf{A}_1'\mathbf{C}_1^{-1}\mathbf{y} + [\mathbf{C}_2 + \mathbf{A}_2\mathbf{C}_3\mathbf{A}_2']^{-1}\mathbf{A}_2\mathbf{A}_3\theta_3. \qquad (11.1.9)$$

The mean of the posterior distribution is seen to be a weighted average of the least squares estimate $(\mathbf{A}_1'\mathbf{C}_1^{-1}\mathbf{A}_1)^{-1}\mathbf{A}_1'\mathbf{C}_1^{-1}\mathbf{y}$ of θ_1 and its prior mean $\mathbf{A}_2\mathbf{A}_3\theta_3$, and is a point estimate of θ_1. The marginal density (11.1.4) is also called the *predictive* density of $\mathbf{y}$. The three-stage hierarchy can be extended to several stages.

Example 11.1.1.   In the simple linear regression model (4.1.6), suppose a prior on $\beta = (\beta_0, \beta_1)'$ is the noninformative prior $\pi(\beta) = 1$. The OLS estimator $\widehat{\beta}$ is a sufficient statistic for β. The posterior distribution is $\pi(\beta|\mathbf{y}) = \pi(\beta|\widehat{\beta})$, which is a $N_2(\widehat{\beta}, \sigma^2\Sigma)$ distribution, where

$$\Sigma = \frac{1}{SST_c} \begin{pmatrix} \sum_{i=1}^{N} X_i^2 & -\overline{X} \\ -\overline{X} & 1 \end{pmatrix},$$

and SST_c was defined in Table 7.2.2. Also, the joint density of $(\mathbf{y}, \beta)$ given $\mathbf{x}$ is normal. The predictive distribution $p(\mathbf{y}|X^*)$ of $\mathbf{y}$ given a specific preditor value X^* is also normal with mean $\widehat{\beta}_0 + \widehat{\beta}_1 X^*$ and variance $\sigma^2[1 + (1/N) + (\overline{X} - X^*)^2/SST_c]$. □

Example 11.1.2.   Consider the multiple regression model $\mathbf{y} = \mathbf{X}\beta + \varepsilon$, with $\varepsilon \sim N(\mathbf{0}, \sigma^2 \mathbf{I}_N)$. Assume that the components of $\beta = (\beta_0, \cdots, \beta_k)'$ are exchangeable (which may not always be pertinent). Suppose we assume the prior distribution $\beta_j \sim N(\psi, \sigma_\beta^2)$, where we may assume that $\psi = 0$. We consider two cases, one where σ^2 and σ_β^2 are assumed to be known, and the second, and more realistic one in which both the variance parameters are unknown nuisance parameters. In the first case, the posterior mode is

$$\beta^* = \{\mathbf{I}_p + c(\mathbf{X}'\mathbf{X})^{-1}\}^{-1} \widehat{\beta},$$

where $c = \sigma^2/\sigma_\beta^2$ is the ratio of the variances. Note the similarity of this estimate to the ridge regression estimate (see section 8.3.3). In the second case, let us assume that the prior distributions for σ^2 and σ_β^2 are given by

$$\nu\lambda/\sigma^2 \sim \chi_\nu^2, \text{ and } \nu_\beta\lambda_\beta/\sigma_\beta^2 \sim \chi_{\nu_\beta}^2.$$

Then,

$$\pi(\beta, \sigma^2, \sigma_\beta^2) \quad \propto \quad (\sigma^2)^{-(N+\nu-2)/2} \exp\{-[\nu\lambda + (\mathbf{y} - \mathbf{X}\beta)'(\mathbf{y} - \mathbf{X}\beta)]/2\sigma^2\}$$

$$\times \quad (\sigma_\beta^2)^{-(p-\nu_\beta+1)/2} \exp\{-[\nu_\beta\lambda_\beta + \sum_{j=0}^{k}(\beta_j - \widetilde{\beta})^2]/2\sigma_\beta^2\},$$

where $\widetilde{\beta} = \sum_{j=0}^{k} \beta_j/p$. The marginal posterior distributions of β, σ^2 and σ_β^2 may be obtained in closed form, and the posterior modes are obtained from

$$\beta^* = [\mathbf{I}_p + c^*(\mathbf{X}'\mathbf{X})^{-1}(\mathbf{I}_p - p^{-1}\mathbf{J}_p)]^{-1} \widehat{\beta},$$

$$\sigma^{2*} = [\nu\lambda + (\mathbf{y} - \mathbf{X}\beta^*)'(\mathbf{y} - \mathbf{X}\beta^*)]/(N + \nu + 2),$$

$$\sigma_\beta^{2*} = [\nu_\beta\lambda_\beta + \sum_{j=0}^{k}(\beta_j^* - \beta^*)^2]/(p + \nu_\beta + 1),$$

where $c^* = \sigma^{2*}/\sigma_\beta^{2*}$. □

11.2   Dynamic linear models

The general linear model in (4.1.1) describes the relationship between independent responses on N subjects and a set of covariates. In contrast to such cross-sectional data, we frequently encounter situations where the responses and

covariates are observed sequentially over time. It is of interest to develop inference for such problems in the context of a dynamic linear model.

Let $\mathbf{y}_1, \cdots, \mathbf{y}_T$ denote p-dimensional random variables which are available at
times $1, \cdots, T$. Suppose $\mathbf{y}_t$ depends on an unknown q-dimensional *state* vector
θ_t (which may again be scalar or vector-valued) via the *observation equation*

$$\mathbf{y}_t = \mathbf{F}_t \theta_t + \mathbf{v}_t \tag{11.2.1}$$

where $\mathbf{F}_t$ is a known $p \times q$ matrix, and we assume that the observation error
$\mathbf{v}_t \sim N(\mathbf{0}, \mathbf{V}_t)$, with known $\mathbf{V}_t$. The dynamic change in θ_t is represented by the
state equation

$$\theta_t = \mathbf{G}_t \theta_{t-1} + \mathbf{w}_t \tag{11.2.2}$$

where $\mathbf{G}_t$ is a known $q \times q$ state transition matrix, and the state error $\mathbf{w}_t \sim$
$N(\mathbf{0}, \mathbf{W}_t)$, with known $\mathbf{W}_t$. In addition, we suppose that $\mathbf{v}_t$ and $\mathbf{w}_t$ are independently distributed. Note that θ_t is a random vector; let

$$\theta_t | \mathbf{y}_t \sim N(\widehat{\theta}_t, \Sigma_t) \tag{11.2.3}$$

represent the posterior distribution of θ_t. The next two subsections describe
the well-known Kalman filter recursions and Kalman smoother recursions that
enable estimation of the state vector.

11.2.1   Kalman filter equations

The *Kalman filter* is a recursive procedure for determining the posterior distri-
bution of θ_t, and thereby predicting $\mathbf{y}_t$. Let $\mathbf{Y}_{[t]} = (\mathbf{y}_t', \cdots, \mathbf{y}_1')'$ denote all the
observations up to time t and let $\widehat{\theta}_0$ and Σ_0 denote the initial guess about the
mean and variance of the distribution of θ. We assume that $(\theta_{t-1} | \mathbf{Y}_{[t-1]}) \sim$
$N(\widehat{\theta}_{t-1}, \Sigma_{t-1})$. The filter employs Bayes's theorem which describes the state of
knowledge at time t about θ_t:

$$P(\theta_t | \mathbf{Y}_{[t]}) = \frac{P(\mathbf{y}_t | \theta_t, \mathbf{Y}_{[t-1]}) P(\theta_t | \mathbf{Y}_{[t-1]})}{\displaystyle\int_{\text{all } \theta_t} P(\mathbf{y}_t, \theta_t | \mathbf{Y}_{[t-1]}) d\theta_t} \tag{11.2.4}$$

(see Meinhold and Singpurwalla, 1983). Equation (11.2.4) represents the posterior distribution for θ at time t as the product of the likelihood (first term
on the right side) and the prior distribution for θ (second term on the right).
We show how this posterior distribution is derived using the notions of Bayes'
Theorem and the results on multivariate normality from section 5.2.

Result 11.2.1. At time t, the prior distribution of θ is

$$\theta_t | \mathbf{Y}_{[t-1]} \sim N(\mathbf{G}_t \widehat{\theta}_{t-1}, \mathbf{R}_t) \tag{11.2.5}$$

where

$$\mathbf{R}_t = \mathbf{G}_t \Sigma_{t-1} \mathbf{G}_t' + \mathbf{W}_t \qquad (11.2.6)$$

Proof. Prior to observing $\mathbf{y}_t$, the best guess for θ_t is based on (11.2.2) and is $\theta_t = \mathbf{G}_t \theta_{t-1} + \mathbf{w}_t$. Since $(\theta_{t-1}|\mathbf{Y}_{[t-1]}) \sim N(\widehat{\theta}_{t-1}, \Sigma_{t-1})$, we see using Result 5.2.6 that $(\theta_t|\mathbf{Y}_{[t-1]})$ is normal with mean $\mathbf{G}_t \widehat{\theta}_{t-1}$ and covariance $\mathbf{R}_t = \mathbf{G}_t \Sigma_{t-1} \mathbf{G}_t' + \mathbf{W}_t$. ∎

Result 11.2.2. The posterior distribution of θ at time t after observing $\mathbf{y}_t$ is normal with mean

$$\widehat{\theta}_t = \mathbf{G}_t \widehat{\theta}_{t-1} + \mathbf{R}_t \mathbf{F}_t' (\mathbf{V}_t + \mathbf{F}_t \mathbf{R}_t \mathbf{F}_t')^{-1} \mathbf{e}_t \qquad (11.2.7)$$

and covariance matrix

$$\Sigma_t = \mathbf{R}_t - \mathbf{R}_t \mathbf{F}_t' (\mathbf{V}_t + \mathbf{F}_t \mathbf{R}_t \mathbf{F}_t')^{-1} \mathbf{F}_t \mathbf{R}_t \qquad (11.2.8)$$

where

$$\mathbf{e}_t = \mathbf{y}_t - \widehat{\mathbf{y}}_t = \mathbf{y}_t - \mathbf{F}_t \mathbf{G}_t \widehat{\theta}_{t-1}. \qquad (11.2.9)$$

Proof. Let $\widehat{\mathbf{y}}_t$ denote the prediction of $\mathbf{y}_t$ based on $\mathbf{Y}_{[t-1]}$, i.e.,

$$
\begin{aligned}
\widehat{\mathbf{y}}_t &= E(\mathbf{y}_t|\mathbf{Y}_{[t-1]}) \\
&= E[(\mathbf{F}_t \theta_t + \mathbf{v}_t)|\mathbf{Y}_{[t-1]}] \\
&= \mathbf{F}_t \mathbf{G}_t \widehat{\theta}_{t-1}. \qquad (11.2.10)
\end{aligned}
$$

We denote the prediction error by $\mathbf{e}_t = \mathbf{y}_t - \widehat{\mathbf{y}}_t$, which is equal to $\mathbf{y}_t - \mathbf{F}_t \mathbf{G}_t \widehat{\theta}_{t-1}$. We can write (11.2.4) as

$$
\begin{aligned}
P(\theta_t|\mathbf{y}_t, \mathbf{Y}_{[t-1]}) &= P(\theta_t|\mathbf{e}_t, \mathbf{Y}_{[t-1]}) \\
&\propto P(\mathbf{e}_t|\theta_t, \mathbf{Y}_{[t-1]}) P(\theta_t|\mathbf{Y}_{[t-1]})
\end{aligned}
$$

where $P(\mathbf{e}_t|\theta_t, \mathbf{Y}_{[t-1]})$ is equivalent to the likelihood function $L(\theta_t|\mathbf{y}_t)$ by virtue of the fact that observing $\mathbf{y}_t$ is the same as observing $\mathbf{e}_t$, when $\mathbf{F}_t$, $\mathbf{G}_t$, and $\widehat{\theta}_{t-1}$ are known. Using (11.2.1) we can write (11.2.9) as $\mathbf{e}_t = \mathbf{F}_t \left(\theta_t - \mathbf{G}_t \widehat{\theta}_{t-1} \right) + \mathbf{v}_t$, and it follows that

$$E(\mathbf{e}_t|\theta_t, \mathbf{Y}_{[t-1]}) = \mathbf{F}_t \left(\theta_t - \mathbf{G}_t \widehat{\theta}_{t-1} \right), \quad \text{and} \quad Var(\mathbf{e}_t|\theta_t, \mathbf{Y}_{[t-1]}) = \mathbf{V}_t.$$

Again, it follows from Result 5.2.6 that

$$(\mathbf{e}_t|\theta_t, \mathbf{Y}_{[t-1]}) \sim N(\mathbf{F}_t \left(\theta_t - \mathbf{G}_t \widehat{\theta}_{t-1} \right), \mathbf{V}_t). \qquad (11.2.11)$$

An application of (11.2.4) and the equivalence of probabilistic information in $\mathbf{Y}_t$ and $\mathbf{e}_t$ implies

$$P(\theta_t|\mathbf{Y}_{[t]}) = P(\mathbf{e}_t|\theta_t, \mathbf{Y}_{[t-1]})P(\theta_t|\mathbf{Y}_{[t-1]}) \Big/ \int_{\text{all } \theta_t} P(\mathbf{e}_t, \theta_t|\mathbf{Y}_{[t-1]})d\theta_t.$$

It is possible to evaluate $(\theta_t|\mathbf{Y}_{[t]})$ easily by using properties of the multivariate normal distribution that we discussed in section 5.2. Use Result 5.2.11, and let $\mathbf{x}_1$ correspond to $\mathbf{e}_t|\mathbf{Y}_{[t-1]}$, and $\mathbf{x}_2$ correspond to $\theta_t|\mathbf{Y}_{[t-1]}$. From (11.2.5), μ_2 corresponds to $\mathbf{G}_t\widehat{\theta}_{t-1}$, while Σ_{22} corresponds to $\mathbf{R}_t$. From (11.2.11), it follows that $\mu_{1.2} = \mu_1 + \Sigma_{12}\mathbf{R}_t^{-1}(\theta_t - \mathbf{G}_t\widehat{\theta}_{t-1})$ corresponds to $\mathbf{F}_t\left(\theta_t - \mathbf{G}_t\widehat{\theta}_{t-1}\right)$, so that μ_1 corresponds to $\mathbf{0}$, and Σ_{12} to $\mathbf{F}_t\mathbf{R}_t$. Likewise, $\Sigma_{11.2} = \Sigma_{11} - \Sigma_{12}\Sigma_{22}^{-1}\Sigma_{21} = \Sigma_{11} - \mathbf{F}_t\mathbf{R}_t\mathbf{F}_t'$ corresponds to $\mathbf{V}_t$, from which we see that Σ_{11} corresponds to $\mathbf{V}_t + \mathbf{F}_t\mathbf{R}_t\mathbf{F}_t'$. Using the converse relationship discussed following Result 5.2.11, we see that

$$\left[\begin{pmatrix} \theta_t \\ \mathbf{e}_t \end{pmatrix} \Big| \mathbf{Y}_{[t-1]}\right] \sim N\left[\begin{pmatrix} \mathbf{G}_t\widehat{\theta}_{t-1} \\ \mathbf{0} \end{pmatrix}, \begin{pmatrix} \mathbf{R}_t & \mathbf{R}_t\mathbf{F}_t' \\ \mathbf{F}_t\mathbf{R}_t & \mathbf{V}_t + \mathbf{F}_t\mathbf{R}_t\mathbf{F}_t' \end{pmatrix}\right].$$

Now, let the conditioning variable $\mathbf{x}_2$ correspond to $\mathbf{e}_t|\mathbf{Y}_{[t-1]}$, with corresponding mean and covariance equal to $\mathbf{0}$ and $\mathbf{V}_t + \mathbf{F}_t\mathbf{R}_t\mathbf{F}_t'$, we see from Result 5.2.11 that $(\theta_t|\mathbf{e}_t, \mathbf{Y}_{[t-1]})$ has a normal distribution with mean $\widehat{\theta}_t = \mathbf{G}_t\widehat{\theta}_{t-1} + \mathbf{R}_t\mathbf{F}_t'(\mathbf{V}_t + \mathbf{F}_t\mathbf{R}_t\mathbf{F}_t')^{-1}\mathbf{e}_t$ and covariance $\Sigma_t = \mathbf{R}_t - \mathbf{R}_t\mathbf{F}_t'(\mathbf{V}_t + \mathbf{F}_t\mathbf{R}_t\mathbf{F}_t')^{-1}\mathbf{F}_t\mathbf{R}_t$, which are the expressions for the posterior mean and covariance of $\theta_t|\mathbf{Y}_{[t]}$ given in (11.2.7) and (11.2.8). ∎

Example 11.2.1.   Suppose an observed univariate quarterly time series $\{Y_t\}$ is expressed as

$$Y_t = T_t + S_t + v_t,$$

where T_t denotes trend, S_t denotes the seasonal component, and v_t, the error in this structural model (Shumway and Stoffer, 2000, p. 334). Suppose we set

$$\begin{aligned} T_t &= \phi T_{t-1} + w_{t1}, \text{ and} \\ S_t &+ S_{t-1} + S_{t-2} + S_{t-3} = w_{t2}, \end{aligned}$$

where $\phi > 1$, to characterize exponentially increasing trend, and a seasonal component that is expected to sum to zero over 4 quarters. To write this model in the form (11.2.1) and (11.2.2), set the state vector to be $\theta_t = (T_t, S_t, S_{t-1}, S_{t-2})'$. The observation and state equations are

$$Y_t = \begin{pmatrix} 1 & 1 & 0 & 0 \end{pmatrix} \begin{pmatrix} T_t \\ S_t \\ S_{t-1} \\ S_{t-2} \end{pmatrix} + v_t,$$

$$\begin{pmatrix} T_t \\ S_t \\ S_{t-1} \\ S_{t-2} \end{pmatrix} = \begin{pmatrix} \phi & 0 & 0 & 0 \\ 0 & -1 & -1 & -1 \\ 0 & 1 & 0 & 0 \\ 0 & 0 & 1 & 0 \end{pmatrix} \begin{pmatrix} T_{t-1} \\ S_{t-1} \\ S_{t-2} \\ S_{t-3} \end{pmatrix} + \begin{pmatrix} w_{t1} \\ w_{t2} \\ 0 \\ 0 \end{pmatrix},$$

where the observation error variance is V_{11}, and the state error variance is diag$(W_{11}, W_{22}, 0, 0)$. The filter equations follow directly from Result 11.2.1.
□

For convenience, we adopt the following notation (see Shumway and Stoffer, 2000). Let $\theta_t^s = E(\theta_t|\mathbf{Y}_{[s]})$, $\Sigma_{t_1,t_2}^s = E[(\theta_{t_1} - \theta_{t_1}^s)(\theta_{t_2} - \theta_{t_2}^s)']$, and condense $\Sigma_{t,t}^s$ to Σ_t^s. Kalman filter estimates are obtained when $s < t$. The derivations in the next section employ this notation.

11.2.2 Kalman smoothing equations

Estimators of the state vector θ_t based on the entire data $\mathbf{y}_1, \cdots, \mathbf{y}_T$, where $t \leq T$ are called *smoothers* and are denoted by θ_t^T, $t = 1, \cdots, T$. The proof of the next result is along the lines of Rauch, Tung and Streibel (1965).

Result 11.2.3. With initial conditions θ_T^T and Σ_T^T obtained from the filter recursions,

$$\theta_{t-1}^T = \theta_{t-1}^{t-1} + J_{t-1}(\theta_t^T - \theta_t^{t-1}), \text{ and} \tag{11.2.12}$$

$$\Sigma_{t-1}^T = \Sigma_{t-1}^{t-1} + \mathbf{J}_{t-1}(\Sigma_t^T - \Sigma_t^{t-1})\mathbf{J}_{t-1}', \tag{11.2.13}$$

where $\mathbf{J}_{t-1} = \Sigma_{t-1}^{t-1}\mathbf{G}_t'(\Sigma_t^{t-1})^{-1}$.

Proof. Now,

$$
\begin{aligned}
P(\theta_{t-1}, \theta_t|\mathbf{Y}_{[T]}) &\propto P(\theta_{t-1}, \theta_t, \mathbf{Y}_{[T]}) = P(\theta_{t-1}, \theta_t, \mathbf{Y}_{[t-1]}, \mathbf{y}_t, \cdots, \mathbf{y}_T) \\
&= P(\mathbf{Y}_{[t-1]})P(\theta_{t-1}, \theta_t|\mathbf{Y}_{[t-1]})P(\mathbf{y}_t, \cdots, \mathbf{y}_T|\theta_{t-1}, \theta_t, \mathbf{Y}_{[t-1]}),
\end{aligned}
$$

which can be simplified to

$$P(\theta_{t-1}, \theta_t|\mathbf{Y}_{[t-1]}) = \delta_1(\theta_t)P(\theta_{t-1}|\mathbf{Y}_{[t-1]})P(\theta_t|\theta_{t-1}),$$

where $\delta_1(\theta_t)$ does not depend on θ_{t-1}. Clearly,

$$
\begin{aligned}
\theta_{t-1}|\mathbf{Y}_{[t-1]} &\sim N(\theta_{t-1}^{t-1}, \Sigma_{t-1}^{t-1}), \text{ and} \\
\theta_{t-1}|\theta_{t-1} &\sim N(\mathbf{G}_t\theta_{t-1}, \mathbf{W}_t).
\end{aligned}
$$

The smoothers θ_t^T and θ_{t-1}^T are obtained by minimizing

$$
\begin{aligned}
-2\log P(\theta_{t-1}, \theta_t|\mathbf{Y}_{[t-1]}) &\propto (\theta_{t-1} - \theta_{t-1}^{t-1})\{\Sigma_{t-1}^{t-1}\}^{-1}(\theta_{t-1} - \theta_{t-1}^{t-1})' \\
&+ (\theta_t - \mathbf{G}_t\theta_{t-1})\mathbf{W}_t^{-1}(\theta_t - \mathbf{G}_t\theta_{t-1})' + \delta_2(\theta_t),
\end{aligned}
\tag{11.2.14}
$$

where $\delta_2(\theta_t)$ is independent of θ_{t-1}. Substitute the available θ_t^T for θ_t in (11.2.14), and minimize the resulting expression with respect to θ_{t-1} to obtain

$$\theta_{t-1}^T = [\{\Sigma_{t-1}^{t-1}\}^{-1} + \mathbf{G}_t'\mathbf{W}_t^{-1}\mathbf{G}_t]^{-1}[\{\Sigma_{t-1}^{t-1}\}^{-1}\theta_{t-1}^{t-1} + \mathbf{G}_t'\mathbf{W}_t^{-1}\theta_t^T],$$

which yields (11.2.12), on using Exercise 2.28 with $\mathbf{A} = \Sigma_{t-1}^{t-1}$, $\mathbf{B} = \mathbf{W}_t$, and $\mathbf{C} = \mathbf{G}_t$. To derive (11.2.13), we see that from (11.2.12),

$$(\theta_{t-1} - \theta_{t-1}^T) + \mathbf{J}_{t-1}\theta_t^T = (\theta_{t-1} - \theta_{t-1}^{t-1}) + \mathbf{J}_{t-1}\mathbf{G}_t\theta_{t-1}^{t-1},$$

and

$$\Sigma_{t-1}^T + \mathbf{J}_{t-1}E(\theta_t^T\theta_t^{T\prime})\mathbf{J}_{t-1}' = \Sigma_{t-1}^{t-1} + \mathbf{J}_{t-1}\mathbf{G}_t E(\theta_{t-1}^{t-1}\theta_{t-1}^{t-1\prime})\mathbf{G}_t'\mathbf{J}_{t-1}'.$$

Since

$$\begin{aligned}
E(\theta_t^T\theta_t^{T\prime}) &= E(\theta_t\theta_t') - \Sigma_t^T = \mathbf{G}_t E(\theta_{t-1}\theta_{t-1}')\mathbf{G}_t' + \mathbf{W}_t - \Sigma_t^T, \text{ and} \\
E(\theta_{t-1}^{t-1}\theta_{t-1}^{t-1\prime}) &= E(\theta_{t-1}\theta_{t-1}') - \Sigma_{t-1}^{t-1},
\end{aligned}$$

(11.2.13) follows. ■

In practice, the parameters in the model specification, such as elements of $\mathbf{G}_t$, $\mathbf{V}_t$, and $\mathbf{W}_t$ may be unknown, and must be estimated. We refer the reader to Shumway and Stoffer (2000) for details on parameter estimation via maximizing the innovations form of the likelihood or via a variant of the EM algorithm which we described in section 7.5.4. Diagnostics for the dynamic linear model is described in Harrison and West (1991), while West and Harrison (1997) is a good reference for the study of nonnormal dynamic linear models.

11.3   Longitudinal models

In longitudinal studies, measurements on subjects are obtained repeatedly over time. Measurements obtained by following the subjects forward in time are said to be collected prospectively, while extraction of data over time from available records constitutes a retrospective study. Longitudinal studies enable us to estimate changes over time within subjects. In this section, we describe general linear models for longitudinal data on m subjects over several time periods. For example (Diggle, Liang and Zeger, 1994, p. 5), in a study of the effect of ozone pollution on growth of Sitka spruce trees, data for 79 trees over two growing seasons were obtained in normal and ozone-enriched chambers. A total of 54 trees were grown with ozone exposure at 70 ppb, while 25 trees were grown in normal (control) atmospheres. The response variable was $Y = \log(hd^2)$, where h is the height and d, the diameter of a tree.

In general, in longitudinal studies, the natural experimental unit is not the individual measurement Y_{ij}, but the sequence $\mathbf{y}_i$ of repeated measurements over time on a particular subject. Here, replication refers to the number of subjects, and not to the number of individual measurements. A longitudinal study is effective for measuring change. There are two modeling approaches, viz., use of a multivariate model, or use of a two-stage random effects model. We describe both strategies in the next subsections.

11.3.1 Multivariate models

Let

$$Y_{ij} = \beta_0 + \beta_1 X_{ij1} + \beta_2 X_{ij2} + \cdots + \beta_k X_{ijk} + \varepsilon_{ij} = \mathbf{X}'_{ij}\beta + \varepsilon_{ij}, \qquad (11.3.1)$$

where Y_{ij} denotes the response variable, and $\mathbf{X}_{ij}$ is a k-dimensional vector of explanatory variables, all observed at times t_{ij}, for $j = 1, \cdots, n_i$, and for subjects $i = 1, \cdots, m$. In (11.3.1), $\beta = (\beta_0, \beta_1, \cdots, \beta_k)'$ is a p-dimensional vector of unknown regression coefficients and ε_{ij} denotes the random error component with $E\varepsilon_{ij} = 0$, and $Cov(\varepsilon_{ij}, \varepsilon_{ij'}) \neq 0$. In matrix notation, let $\mathbf{y}_i = (Y_{i1}, \cdots, Y_{in_i})'$ denote the n_i-dimensional vector of repeated outcomes on subject i with mean vector $E(\mathbf{y}_i) = \mu_i = (\mu_{i1}, \cdots, \mu_{in_i})'$ and $n_i \times n_i$-dimensional variance-covariance matrix $\sigma^2 \mathbf{V}_i = \sigma^2\{v_{ijk}\}$. Let $\mathbf{y} = (\mathbf{y}'_1, \cdots, \mathbf{y}'_m)'$ denote the N-dimensional response vector, where $N = \sum_{i=1}^{m} n_i$, and let $\sigma^2 \mathbf{V}$ be the block-diagonal matrix with m non-zero blocks representing the covariance structure for each subject. We can write the model (11.3.1) as

$$\mathbf{y}_i = \mathbf{X}_i\beta + \varepsilon_i, \qquad (11.3.2)$$

where $\mathbf{X}_i$ is an $n_i \times p$ matrix with $\mathbf{X}_{ij}$ in the ith row and $\varepsilon_i = (\varepsilon_{i1}, \cdots, \varepsilon_{in_i})$. Clearly, $\mathbf{y} \sim N(\mathbf{X}\beta, \sigma^2\mathbf{V})$, where $\mathbf{X}$ is an $N \times p$ matrix. Although such *multivariate models* for longitudinal data with a general covariance structure are straightforward to implement with balanced data, they may be cumbersome when subjects are measured at arbitrary times, or when the dimension of $\mathbf{V}$ is large. We first show examples with two possible assumptions on the block-diagonal structure of $\sigma^2\mathbf{V}$, each using two parameters. We then describe some estimation approaches for longitudinal models.

Example 11.3.1. Uniform correlation model. For each subject $i = 1, \cdots, m$, we assume that $\mathbf{V}_i = \mathbf{V}_0 = (1 - \rho)\mathbf{I} + \rho\mathbf{J}$, viz., we assume a positive correlation ρ between any two measurements on the same subject. One interpretation of this model is that we introduce a random subject effect U_i, which are mutually independent variables with variance ν^2 between subjects, so that

$$Y_{ij} = \mu_{ij} + U_i + Z_{ij}, \quad j = 1, \cdots, n_i, \, i = 1, \cdots, m,$$

where U_i are $N(0, \nu^2)$ variables, and Z_{ij} are mutually independent $N(0, \tau^2)$ variables, which are independent of U_i. In this case, $\rho = \nu^2/(\nu^2 + \tau^2)$, and $\sigma^2 = \nu^2 + \tau^2$. $\quad\square$

Example 11.3.2. Exponential correlation model. We assume that the correlation between any two measurements on the same subject decays towards zero as the time separation between the measurements increases, i.e., the (j, k)th element of $\mathbf{V}_0$ is

$$Cov(Y_{ij}, Y_{ik}) = \sigma^2 \exp\{-\phi|t_{ij} - t_{ik}|\}.$$

A special case corresponds to equal spacing between observations times; i.e., if $t_{ij} - t_{ik} = d$, for $k = j - 1$, and letting $\rho = \exp(-\phi d)$ denote the correlation between successive responses, we can write $Cov(Y_{ij}, Y_{ik}) = \sigma^2 \rho |j - k|$. One justification for this model is to write

$$Y_{ij} = \mu_{ij} + W_{ij}, \quad j = 1, \cdots, n_i, \, i = 1, \cdots, m,$$

where $W_{ij} = \rho W_{i,j-1} + Z_{ij}$, Z_{ij} are independently distributed as $N(0, \sigma^2\{1 - \rho^2\})$ variables. □

We describe several estimation approaches. We start with the simplest approach, which is weighted least squares (WLS) estimation. We next describe and contrast the method of maximum likelihood and the method of restricted maximum likelihood (REML).

Generalized least squares estimation

We discussed least squares estimation in section 4.5. It follows from (4.5.5) that the weighted least squares estimator of β is

$$\widehat{\beta}_W = (\mathbf{X}'\mathbf{W}\mathbf{X})^{-1}\mathbf{X}'\mathbf{W}\mathbf{y},$$

where $\mathbf{W}$ is a symmetric weight matrix. Note that $\mathbf{W} = \mathbf{I}$ yields the OLS estimate of β, while setting $\mathbf{W} = \mathbf{V}^{-1}$ leads to the most efficient estimator. Implementation of this procedure requires a knowledge of the correlation structure in $\mathbf{y}$. In general, when the parameters in $Cov(\mathbf{y})$ are unknown, a two stage procedure may be used, in which we estimate β and the parameters in $Cov(\mathbf{y})$ in alternate stages, which we iterate to convergence.

Maximum likelihood estimation

The normal log likelihood function for the model (11.3.1) is

$$l(\beta, \sigma^2, \mathbf{V}_0; \mathbf{y}) = \{-N \log(\sigma^2) + m \log(|\mathbf{V}_0|) + \sigma^{-2}(\mathbf{y} - \mathbf{X}\beta)'\mathbf{V}^{-1}(\mathbf{y} - \mathbf{X}\beta)\}/2. \tag{11.3.3}$$

For fixed $\mathbf{V}_0$, the MLE of β corresponds to its generalized least squares estimator $\widehat{\beta}(\mathbf{V}_0)$, which has the form (4.5.5). The corresponding error sum of squares is $SSE(\mathbf{V}_0) = \{\mathbf{y} - \mathbf{X}\widehat{\beta}(\mathbf{V}_0)\}'\mathbf{V}^{-1}\{\mathbf{y} - \mathbf{X}\widehat{\beta}(\mathbf{V}_0)\}$. Substituting $\widehat{\beta}_{GLS}$ into (11.3.3) yields

$$l(\widehat{\beta}(\mathbf{V}_0), \sigma^2, \mathbf{V}_0; \mathbf{y}) = \{-N \log(\sigma^2) + m \log(|\mathbf{V}_0|) + \sigma^{-2}SSE(\mathbf{V}_0)\}/2. \tag{11.3.4}$$

Differentiating (11.3.4) with respect to σ^2 gives

$$\widehat{\sigma}^2(\mathbf{V}_0) = SSE(\mathbf{V}_0)/N. \tag{11.3.5}$$

The reduced log-likelihood function for $\mathbf{V}_0$ is proportional to

$$l_r(\mathbf{V}_0; \mathbf{y}) = l\{\widehat{\beta}(\mathbf{V}_0), \widehat{\sigma}^2(\mathbf{V}0), \mathbf{V}_0\} = -N \log SSE(\mathbf{V}_0)/2 - m \log(|\mathbf{V}_0|)/2. \tag{11.3.6}$$

The estimate $\widehat{\mathbf{V}}_0$ is obtained by numerical maximization of $l_r(\mathbf{V}_0)$ with respect to its distinct elements. The final estimates of β and σ^2 are $\widehat{\beta}(\widehat{\mathbf{V}}_0)$ and $\widehat{\sigma}^2(\widehat{\mathbf{V}}_0)$.

REML estimation

A general description of the REML procedure was given in section 7.5.4. It follows from (10.1.23) that the REML estimator for σ^2 is

$$\widehat{\sigma}^2_{RM}(\mathbf{V}_0) = SSE(\mathbf{V}_0)/(N-p). \tag{11.3.7}$$

The REML estimator of $\mathbf{V}_0$ maximizes the reduced log likelihood function

$$l_{RM}(\mathbf{V}_0; \mathbf{y}) = -N \log SSE(\mathbf{V}_0)/2 - m \log(|\mathbf{V}_0|)/2 - \log(|\mathbf{X}'\mathbf{V}^{-1}\mathbf{X}|)/2. \tag{11.3.8}$$

Substituting the resulting estimator $\widehat{\mathbf{V}}_{0,RM}$ into the form of the GLS estimator of β and (11.3.7) gives the REML estimates of β and σ^2. A comparison of the forms of $l_r(\mathbf{V}_0; \mathbf{y})$ and $l_{RM}(\mathbf{V}_0; \mathbf{y})$ shows that we expect considerable difference between the MLE and REML estimates when p is large (see also Verbyla and Cullis, 1990).

Another approach that is widely used for longitudinal models is the estimation equations approach, which is a multivariate analogue of the quasi-likelihood method that we described in section 7.5.4 (see Diggle, Liang and Zeger, 1994, and references therein).

Example 11.3.3. Repeated measures. Repeated measures designs are used in experiments or surveys where more than one measurement of the same response variable is obtained on each subject, usually taken over time. Examples include systolic blood pressure measurements made once a week for five weeks on subjects who are on a given medication, scores on a spelling test taken four times by each of 20 students with remedial instruction between tests, etc. In such cases, all the subjects may either belong to a single homogeneous population, or to a populations, which we then compare. The simplest repeated measures design is when data is collected as a sequence of equally spaced points in time, i.e., the experimenter assigns treatments to experimental units, and collects data sequentially. The goal of the analysis is to measure (a) how treatment means change over time, and (b) how treatment differences change over time.

The repeated measures model for a single factor experiment is

$$Y_{ij} = \mu + \tau_i + \beta_j + \varepsilon_{ij} \tag{11.3.9}$$

where μ is the overall mean effect, τ_i is the effect of the ith treatment level and β_j is the jth subject effect. The subject effect is treated as random, and we assume that β_j are iid $N(0, \sigma^2_\beta)$. The treatment effect can be either fixed or random; we treat it as a fixed effect here, and assume $\sum_{i=1}^a \tau_i = 0$. A consequence of having the term β_j be common to all a observations on the same subject is that $Cov(Y_{ij}, Y_{i'j})$ is in general nonzero. A simple assumption is one of equal correlation among responses pertaining to the same subject. It is easy to see that

$$Var(Y_{ij}) = \sigma^2_\beta + \sigma^2_\varepsilon = \sigma^2, \text{ say}$$

which is the same for each subject and for each period, and that

$$Cov(Y_{ij}, Y_{lj}) = \sigma_\beta^2.$$

The quantity

$$\rho = \frac{\sigma_\beta^2}{\sigma_\beta^2 + \sigma_\varepsilon^2}$$

denotes the correlation between Y_{ij} and Y_{lj}. Writing in the form $\mathbf{y} \sim N(\mathbf{X}\beta, \Omega)$, where Ω has the intra-class correlation structure, REML estimation is straightforward. In Exercise 11.7, we ask the reader to derive ANOVA type inference for repeated measures in the framework of a split-plot experimental design.   □

11.3.2   Two-stage random-effects models

Laird and Ware (1982) described two-stage random-effects models, which are based on explicit identification of population and individual characteristics. The probability distributions for the response vectors of different subjects are assumed to belong to a single family, but some random-effects parameters vary across subjects, with a distribution specified at the second stage. The two-stage random-effects model for longitudinal data is given below (see (10.2.1)).

1. For each individual $i = 1, \cdots, m$,

$$\mathbf{y}_i = \mathbf{X}_i \tau + \mathbf{Z}_i \gamma_i + \varepsilon_i, \quad i = 1, \cdots, m, \qquad (11.3.10)$$

   where τ is a p-dimensional vector of unknown population parameters, $\mathbf{X}_i$ is an $n_i \times p$ known design matrix, γ_i is a q-dimensional vector of unknown individual effects, and $\mathbf{Z}_i$ is a known $n_i \times q$ design matrix. The errors ε_i are independently distributed as $N(\mathbf{0}, \mathbf{R}_i)$ vectors, while τ and γ_i are fixed parameter vectors.

2. The γ_i are independently distributed as $N(\mathbf{0}, \mathbf{D}_\gamma)$, and $Cov(\gamma_i, \varepsilon_i) = 0$. The population parameters τ are fixed effects.

   Marginally, the $\mathbf{y}_i$ are independent $N(\mathbf{X}_i \tau, \mathbf{V}_i = \mathbf{R}_i + \mathbf{Z}_i \mathbf{D}_\gamma \mathbf{Z}_i')$. Let $\mathbf{W}_i = \mathbf{V}_i^{-1}$. Inference can be based on least squares, maximum likelihood and Bayesian approaches. Let $\theta = (\theta_1, \cdots, \theta_s)'$ denote an s-dimensional vector of "variance components" from $\mathbf{R}_i$, $i = 1, \cdots .m$, and $\mathbf{D}_\gamma$.

Estimation of mean effects

The classical approach to inference derives estimates of τ and θ based on the marginal distribution of $\mathbf{y}' = (\mathbf{y}_1', \cdots, \mathbf{y}_m')$, while an estimate for γ is obtained by use of Harville's (1976) extended Gauss-Markov theorem for mixed-effects models (see Result 10.2.1). Let $\Gamma = (\gamma_1', \cdots, \gamma_m')'$.

Suppose θ is known. Assuming that the necessary matrix inversions exist,

$$\hat{\tau} = \left(\sum_{i=1}^{m} \mathbf{X}_i' \mathbf{W}_i \mathbf{X}_i \right)^{-1} \sum_{i=1}^{m} \mathbf{X}_i' \mathbf{W}_i \mathbf{y}_i, \text{ and} \qquad (11.3.11)$$

$$\hat{\gamma}_i = \mathbf{D}_\gamma \mathbf{Z}_i' \mathbf{W}_i (\mathbf{y}_i - \mathbf{X}_i \hat{\tau}), \qquad (11.3.12)$$

with variances

$$Var(\hat{\tau}) = \left(\sum_{i=1}^{m} \mathbf{X}_i' \mathbf{W}_i \mathbf{X}_i \right)^{-1}, \text{ and} \qquad (11.3.13)$$

$$Var(\hat{\gamma}_i) = \mathbf{D}_\gamma \mathbf{Z}_i' \{ \mathbf{W}_i - \mathbf{W}_i \mathbf{X}_i (\sum_{i=1}^{m} \mathbf{X}_i' \mathbf{W}_i \mathbf{X}_i)^{-1} \mathbf{X}_i' \mathbf{W}_i \} \mathbf{Z}_i \mathbf{D}_\gamma. \qquad (11.3.14)$$

A better assessment of the error of estimation is provided by

$$\begin{aligned} Var(\hat{\gamma}_i - \hat{\gamma}_i) &= \mathbf{D}_\gamma - \mathbf{D}_\gamma \mathbf{Z}_i' \mathbf{W}_i \mathbf{Z}_i \mathbf{D}_\gamma \\ &+ \mathbf{D}_\gamma \mathbf{Z}_i' \mathbf{W}_i \mathbf{X}_i [\sum_{i=1}^{m} \mathbf{X}_i' \mathbf{W}_i \mathbf{X}_i]^{-1} \mathbf{X}_i' \mathbf{W}_i \mathbf{Z}_i \mathbf{D}_\gamma, \quad (11.3.15) \end{aligned}$$

which incorporates the variation in γ_i. Under normality, the estimator $\hat{\tau}$ is the MVUE, and $\hat{\gamma}$ is the essentially-unique MVUE of γ (see Result 10.2.1). The estimate $\hat{\tau}$ also maximizes the likelihood based on the marginal normal distribution of $\mathbf{y}$. We can write

$$\hat{\Gamma} = E(\Gamma | \mathbf{y}, \hat{\tau}, \theta),$$

so that $\hat{\gamma}_i$ is the empirical Bayes estimator of γ_i.

Suppose, as is usually the case in practice, θ is unknown. We estimate τ and θ simultaneously by maximizing their joint likelihood based on the marginal distribution of $\mathbf{y}$. Let $\hat{\theta}$ and $\hat{\tau}(\hat{\theta})$ denote the MLE's of τ and θ respectively. It can be shown that

$$\hat{\tau}(\hat{\theta}) = \left(\sum_{i=1}^{m} \mathbf{X}_i' \widehat{\mathbf{W}}_i \mathbf{X}_i \right)^{-1} \sum_{i=1}^{m} \mathbf{X}_i' \widehat{\mathbf{W}}_i \mathbf{y}_i, \qquad (11.3.16)$$

where $\widehat{\mathbf{W}}_i = \widehat{\mathbf{W}}_i(\hat{\theta})$. The variance of $\hat{\tau}(\hat{\theta})$ follows by replacing $\mathbf{W}_i$ by $\widehat{\mathbf{W}}_i$ in (11.3.13). The corresponding empirical Bayes estimate of Γ in this case is

$$\hat{\Gamma}(\hat{\theta}) = E(\Gamma | \mathbf{y}, \hat{\tau}(\hat{\theta}), \hat{\theta}) = \hat{\mathbf{D}}_\gamma \mathbf{Z}_i' \widehat{\mathbf{W}}_i \{ \mathbf{y}_i - \mathbf{X}_i \hat{\tau}(\hat{\theta}) \}.$$

Estimation of covariance structure

Popular approaches for estimating θ are the method of maximum likelihood and the method of restricted maximum likelihood (REML). In balanced ANOVA models, MLE's of variance components fail to account for the degrees of freedom in estimating the fixed effects τ, and are therefore negatively biased. The REML estimates on the other hand are unbiased. Recall from section 7.5.4 that the REML estimate of θ is obtained by maximizing the likelihood of θ based on any full-rank set of error contrasts, $\mathbf{z} = \mathbf{B}' \mathbf{y}$.

11.4   Generalized linear models

Although linear models are very versatile in many applications, there are some problems: restriction to normality, and the assumption of a linear model function relating the response to the predictors. A motivation for using GLIM is that it permits more general distributions than the normal for the response Y (McCullagh and Nelder, 1991). A link function is used to relate the linear model to the mean of the response variable through a suitable scale. We may think of GLIM's as extensions of the usual normal linear models, which we recall from Chapter 4 and Chapter 7. Let $\mathbf{y}$ be an N-dimensional response vector, with $E(\mathbf{y}) = \mu$, where $\mu \in \mathcal{R}^N$. The *systematic component* of the model specifies μ in terms of a linear function of an unknown p-dimensional parameter vector β, and a given predictor matrix $\mathbf{X}$, i.e., $\mu = \mathbf{X}\beta$ (see (4.1.1)). Since $\mathbf{X}\beta$ also assumes values in a subset of $\mathcal{R}^N$, this is perfectly sensible! The *random component* of the model specification assumes independence, homoscedasticity, and normality of the response random variables on each subject, i.e., $\mathbf{y} \sim N(\mathbf{X}\beta, \sigma^2 \mathbf{I}_N)$. In section 11.4.1, we present a generalization of this specification.

11.4.1   Components of GLIM

There are many situations where $E(\mathbf{y})$ does not assume values in subsets of $\mathcal{R}^N$. For example, suppose we are interested in modeling binary responses, the expectation of Y is the unknown proportion of success π, $0 < \pi < 1$. In order to sensibly "relate" π to the linear predictor, we find the need to introduce a *link function* of the form, say, $\log[\pi/(1-\pi)]$, which assumes values on the real line. As a second example, suppose Y follows a Poisson distribution with mean $\lambda > 0$. The function $\log(\lambda)$ enables us to relate the expected response to the linear predictor in a sensible way. These notions are formalized below.

Note that we may rewrite the systematic component of the linear model as follows: set a linear predictor $\eta = \mathbf{X}\beta$, and set $\eta = g(\mu) = \mu$ (i.e., $g(.)$ denotes the identity function). Further, the random specification in the linear model is generalized to permit a wider class of distributions than the normal, including discrete families of distributions (such as the binomial, Poisson, etc.).

The GLIM specification has the following three components:

1. The **random component** specifies the probability distribution of the response variables. Specifically, it states that the components of $\mathbf{y}$ have pmf or pdf from an exponential family of distributions (see (A22)). Let $E(\mathbf{y}) = \mu$.

2. The **systematic component** specifies a linear predictor $\eta = \mathbf{X}\beta = \sum_{i=1}^{p} \mathbf{x}_j \beta_j$, as a function of explanatory variables $X_1, \cdots, X_k$ and unknown parameters.

3. The **link function** $g(.)$ provides a functional relationship between the systematic component and the expectation of the response in the random component, viz., $\eta = g(\mu)$.

If $g(\mu_i) = \mu_i$, i.e., $\eta_i = \mu_i$, $i = 1, \cdots, N$, we call $g(.)$ the identity link function. As we saw earlier, the usual normal linear model has the identity link function.

Definition 11.4.1. Canonical link. If the pmf or pdf of the response variable Y belongs to the unit dispersion exponential family with $f(y_i; \theta_i) = \exp\{\omega(\theta_i)y_i - b(\theta_i) + c(y_i)\}$, we define the canonical (or natural) link function by $g(\mu_i) = \omega(\theta_i) = \sum_{j=1}^{p} x_{i,j}\beta_j$. For example, the canonical links for the normal, binomial, and Poisson distributions are respectively $\eta = \mu$, $\eta = \log[\pi/(1-\pi)]$, and $\eta = \log(\lambda)$.

For convenience, we write the log likelihood function in terms of the mean-value parameter μ rather than the canonical parameter θ, and denote it by $l(\mu, \phi; \mathbf{y})$.

Example 11.4.1. Models for binary responses. Suppose that for the ith subject, the response Y_i is binary, i.e., it can assume either the value 0, or the value 1. Suppose $P(Y_i = 1) = \pi_i = 1 - P(Y_i = 0)$. Let $\eta_i = \mathbf{x}_i'\beta$ as before, and suppose we choose the logit link function $g_L(\pi_i) = \log[\pi_i/(1-\pi_i)] = \eta_i$. We seek to carry out inference on the unknown vector of proportions $\pi = (\pi_1, \cdots, \pi_N)'$ as a function of the linear predictor η via this link function. The logit link function, which is the canonical link function, maps the unit interval $[0, 1]$ onto $\mathcal{R}$, as do each of the following alternative link functions that are commonly used with binary responses:

1. the probit or inverse Gaussian link function

$$g_{IG}(\pi) = \Phi^{-1}(\pi),$$

 $\Phi(.)$ denoting the cdf of a standard normal variable;

2. the complementary log-log link function

$$g_C(\pi) = \log\{-\log(1 - \pi)\}; \text{ and}$$

3. the log-log link function

$$g_C(\pi) = -\log\{-\log(\pi)\}.$$

The logit function is widely used due to its interpretability as the logarithm of the odds ratio $\pi/(1-\pi)$, and it induces a logistic regression model. In particular, notice that the link function satisfies the condition that $g(\pi) = H^{-1}(\pi)$, where H is the cdf of a given distribution. For instance, the logit link $g_L(\pi)$ corresponds to the cdf $H(\pi) = \exp(\pi)/\{1 + \exp(\pi)\}$, whereas the complementary log-log link is obtained by specifying $H(\pi) = \exp\{-\exp(-\pi)\}$. By considering $H(\pi)$ to be the cdf of an asymmetric distribution, we can develop a skewed link (Stukel, 1988; Chen, Dey and Shao, 1999). If we assume that $Y_i \sim Binomial(m_i, \pi_i)$, $i = 1, \cdots, N$, the variance function is $V(\pi) = \pi(1 - \pi)$. The log-likelihood function, apart from a constant term, has the form

$$l(\pi; \mathbf{y}) = \sum_{i=1}^{N} Y_i \log[\pi_i/(1 - \pi_i)] + m_i \log(1 - \pi_i)$$

which reduces under the logit link to

$$l(\pi(\beta); \mathbf{y}) = l(\beta; \mathbf{y}) = \sum_{i=1}^{N} \sum_{j=1}^{p} Y_i X_{ij} \beta_j - \sum_{i=1}^{N} m_i \log[1 + \exp \sum_{j=1}^{p} X_{ij} \beta_j]. \quad (11.4.1)$$

We return to this example in the next subsection. □

Example 11.4.2. Log-linear model for counts.   Let Y_i denote counts on the ith subject, $i = 1, \cdots, N$, and suppose first that Y_i's are independently distributed as Poisson random variables with mean λ_i. The log-linear GLIM postulates a logarithmic link function $\log(\lambda_i) = \eta_i = \mathbf{x}_i'\beta$, $i = 1, \cdots, N$. The variance function is $V(\lambda) = \lambda$. The logarithm of the likelihood function, apart from a constant is

$$l(\lambda; \mathbf{y}) = \sum_{i=1}^{N} (y_i \log \lambda_i - \lambda_i).$$

Under the log link function, this reduces to

$$l(\lambda(\beta); \mathbf{y}) = l(\beta; \mathbf{y}) = \sum_{i=1}^{N} \sum_{j=1}^{p} Y_i X_{i,j} \beta_j - \sum_{i=1}^{N} \exp(\sum_{j=1}^{p} X_{i,j} \beta_j). \quad (11.4.2)$$

Next, consider the situation where the dispersion of the data exceeds that predicted by the Poisson model, i.e., $Var(Y) > E(Y)$. Without knowledge of the precise mechanism that causes the over (or under) dispersion, it is convenient to assume that $Var(Y) = \phi\lambda$, and carry out inference of ϕ, as well as β.   □

11.4.2   Estimation approaches

Several approaches are useful for estimating parameters in GLIM. In this section, we describe the method of iteratively reweighted least squares (IRLS), and the quasi-likelihood approach.

IRLS estimation

Result 11.4.1.   Let the components of the N-dimensional random vector $\mathbf{y}$ have pdf (or pmf) from the exponential family, let $E(\mathbf{y}) = \mu$ be linked to the linear predictor $\eta = \mathbf{X}\beta$ by $g(\mu) = \eta$. The MLE of $\widehat{\beta}_{ML}$ is obtained as the iteratively reweighted least squares estimate in the linear regression where the response variable is a linearized form of the link function applied to $\mathbf{y}$, and the weights are functions of the fitted vector $\widehat{\mu}$. For large N, $\widehat{\beta}_{ML} \sim N_p(\beta, \Omega)$, where $\Omega = \sum_{i=1}^{N} [(\partial\mu_i/\partial\beta)'V_i^{-1}(\partial\mu_i/\partial\beta)]^{-1}$.

Proof.   Consider the exponential family log likelihood (in canonical) form for a single observation $l(\theta, \phi; Y) = (Y\theta - b(\theta))/a(\phi) + c(Y, \phi)$. Recall that

$b'(\theta) = \mu$, and $b''(\theta) = V(\mu)$. To derive the maximum likelihood equations for β_j, $j = 1, \cdots, p$, we first use the chain rule of differentiation to write

$$\frac{\partial l}{\partial \beta_j} = \frac{\partial l}{\partial \theta} \frac{d\theta}{d\mu} \frac{d\mu}{d\eta} \frac{\partial \eta}{\partial \beta_j}. \tag{11.4.3}$$

Since $d\mu/d\theta = V(\mu)$, and $\partial\eta/\partial\beta_j = X_j$, it follows by letting $W = (d\mu/d\eta)^2/V$ that

$$\begin{aligned}
\frac{\partial l}{\partial \beta_j} &= \frac{(Y - \mu)}{a(\phi)} \frac{1}{V(\mu)} \frac{d\mu}{d\eta} X_j \\
&= \frac{W}{a(\phi)} (Y - \mu) \frac{d\eta}{d\mu} X_j = u_j,
\end{aligned}$$

say, leading to the ML estimating equations

$$\sum_{i=1}^{N} \widetilde{W}_i (Y_i - \mu_i)(d\eta_i/d\mu_i) X_{i,j} = 0, \quad j = 1, \cdots, p.$$

In a GLIM, $\mathbf{u}$ depends only on the mean and variance of Y_i. If the dispersion is constant, i.e., $a(\phi) = \phi$, then $\widetilde{W}_i$ will reduce to W_i. Let

$$\begin{aligned}
A_{rs} &= -E(\partial^2 l/\partial\beta_r \partial\beta_s) = -E(\partial u_r/\partial\beta_s) \\
&= -E \sum_{i=1}^{N} [(Y_i - \mu_i) \frac{\partial}{\partial\beta_s} (\widetilde{W}_i \frac{d\eta_i}{d\mu_i} X_{i,r}) + \widetilde{W}_i \frac{d\eta_i}{d\mu_i} X_{i,r} \frac{\partial}{\partial\beta_s} (Y_i - \mu_i)] \\
&= \sum_{i=1}^{N} \widetilde{W}_i \frac{d\eta_i}{d\mu_i} X_{i,r} \frac{\partial\mu_i}{\partial\beta_s} = \sum_{i=1}^{N} \widetilde{W}_i X_{i,r} X_{i,s}.
\end{aligned}$$

To use Fisher's scoring method set $\mathbf{u} = \partial l/\partial\beta$, and $\mathbf{A} = -E(\partial^2 l/\partial\beta_j \partial\beta_k)$. Given a current estimate $\widehat{\beta}^{(0)}$, we obtain a solution to $\mathbf{A}\delta\widehat{\beta}^{(0)} = \mathbf{u}$, which gives an adjustment $\delta\widehat{\beta}^{(0)}$ to the current estimate. It is easy to verify that the new estimate $\widehat{\beta}^{(1)} = \widehat{\beta}^{(0)} + \delta\widehat{\beta}^{(0)}$ satisfies the equations

$$(\mathbf{A}\widehat{\beta}^{(1)})_r = \sum_{i=1}^{N} \widetilde{W}_i X_{i,r} [\eta_i + (Y_i - \mu_i) \frac{d\eta_i}{d\mu_i}]. \tag{11.4.4}$$

We now show that these equations correspond to the weighted least squares equations.

Let $\widehat{\eta}^{(0)}$ denote an initial estimate of the linear predictor, based on $\widehat{\beta}^{(0)}$, and obtain $\widehat{\mu}^{(0)}$ from $g(\widehat{\mu}^{(0)}) = \widehat{\eta}^{(0)}$. Let $\mathbf{D}^{(0)}$ be the $N \times N$ matrix with (i, j)th element $\partial\eta_i/\partial\mu_j$, evaluated at $\widehat{\mu}^{(0)}$, and let $\mathbf{v}^{(0)}$ denote the variance function vector evaluated at $\widehat{\mu}^{(0)}$. Define the *adjusted dependent variate* by

$$\mathbf{z}^{(0)} = \widehat{\eta}^{(0)} + \mathbf{D}^{(0)}(\mathbf{y} - \widehat{\mu}^{(0)}),$$

and the quadratic weights by the N-dimensional vector $\widetilde{\mathbf{w}}^{(0)}$, with the reciprocal of its ith element given by the ith element of $(\mathbf{D}^{(0)})^2 \mathbf{v}^{(0)} a(\phi)$. Let $\widehat{\beta}^{(1)}$ denote the weighted least squares estimate from the regression of $\mathbf{z}^{(0)}$ on $\mathbf{X}$, with weights $\widetilde{\mathbf{w}}^{(0)}$ (compare with (11.4.4)). The process of creating the adjusted dependent variate and the weights in order to do weighted least squares is iterated to convergence. The final converged estimate $\widehat{\beta}$ is called the iteratively reweighted least squares (IRLS) estimate of β. $\blacksquare$

Example 11.4.3.   The log likelihood function for the binary logit link model was shown in (11.4.1). From (11.4.3), the likelihood equations become

$$\sum_{i=1}^{N} \frac{\partial l}{\partial \beta_r} = \sum_{i=1}^{N} \frac{\partial l}{\partial \pi_i} \frac{d\pi_i}{d\eta_i} \frac{\partial \eta_i}{\partial \beta_r}$$

$$= \sum_{i=1}^{N} \frac{(Y_i - m_i \pi_i)}{\pi_i(1 - \pi_i)} \pi_i(1 - \pi_i) X_{i,r}.$$

Given an initial estimate $\widehat{\beta}^{(0)}$, we compute $\widehat{\pi}^{(0)}$ and $\widehat{\eta}^{(0)}$, based on which we define the adjusted dependent responses

$$Z_i = \widehat{\eta}_i^{(0)} + \{(Y_i - m_i \widehat{\pi}_i^{(0)})/m_i\}\{1/\widehat{\pi}_i^{(0)}(1 - \widehat{\pi}_i^{(0)})\},$$

with a diagonal weight matrix $\mathbf{W} = \mathrm{diag}\{m_i \pi_i(1 - \pi_i)\}$, evaluated at $\widehat{\pi}^{(0)}$. In fact, we can write the maximum likelihood equations in the form $\mathbf{X}'\mathbf{W}\mathbf{X}\widehat{\beta} = \mathbf{X}'\mathbf{W}\mathbf{z}$, from which we can see that $\widehat{\beta}^{(1)} = (\mathbf{X}'\mathbf{W}\mathbf{X})^{-1}\mathbf{X}'\mathbf{W}\mathbf{z}$, all quantities evaluated at $\widehat{\beta}^{(0)}$. $\square$

Example 11.4.2. (continued).   For the log-linear model that we introduced in Example 11.4.2, the likelihood equations follow from (11.4.2) and (11.4.3):

$$\sum_{i=1}^{N} \frac{\partial l}{\partial \beta_r} = \sum_{i=1}^{N} \frac{\partial l}{\partial \lambda_i} \frac{d\lambda_i}{d\eta_i} \frac{\partial \eta_i}{\partial \beta_r}$$

$$= \sum_{i=1}^{N} \lambda_i(Y_i - \lambda_i) X_{i,r}.$$

The IRLS estimation proceeds using the steps in Result 11.4.1. $\square$

Quasi-likelihood estimation

We defined the notion of a quasi-likelihood function in section 7.5.4. Its usefulness for situations where there is insufficient information to construct a likelihood function is well documented in the literature. We first describe the construction of a quasi-likelihood function for problems where the observations are independent and we model $E(\mathbf{y})$. Suppose $E(\mathbf{y}) = \mu$, and $Cov(\mathbf{y}) = \sigma^2 V(\mu)$, where $V(\mu) = \mathrm{diag}\{V_1(\mu), \cdots, V_N(\mu)\}$ is an $N \times N$ matrix of known functions, and σ^2 is unknown. Further, we assume functional independence, i.e.,

$V(\mu) = \text{diag}\{V_1(\mu_1), \cdots, V_N(\mu_N)\}$. The log quasi-likelihood function for $\mathbf{y}$ is defined by

$$Q(\mu, \mathbf{y}) = \sum_{i=1}^{N} Q_i(\mu_i; Y_i), \text{ with}$$

$$Q_i(\mu_i; Y_i) = \int_Y^\mu (Y - t)/\{\sigma^2 V(t)\} dt, \tag{11.4.5}$$

$V(.)$ being the variance function. For many examples, the quasi-likelihood function corresponds to the actual likelihood.

Result 11.4.2.

1. The quasi-likelihood estimator $\widehat{\beta}_{QML}$ is obtained by iterating to convergence the sequence of estimate with the form

$$\widehat{\beta}^{(1)} = \widehat{\beta}^{(0)} + \{\widehat{\mathbf{D}}^{(0)\prime}(\widehat{\mathbf{V}}^{(0)})^{-1}\widehat{\mathbf{D}}^{(0)}\}^{-1}\widehat{\mathbf{D}}^{(0)\prime}(\widehat{\mathbf{V}}^{(0)})^{-1}(\mathbf{y} - \widehat{\mu}^{(0)}), \tag{11.4.6}$$

where $\widehat{\beta}^{(0)}$ is an initial value.

2. $Cov(\widehat{\beta}_{QML}) \approx \sigma^2(\mathbf{D}'\mathbf{V}^{-1}\mathbf{D})^{-1}$.

3. $\widehat{\sigma}^2_{QML} = (\mathbf{y} - \widehat{\mu})'\widehat{\mathbf{V}}^{-1}(\mathbf{y} - \widehat{\mu})/(N - p)$.

Proof.   Consider the function

$$U_i = (Y_i - \mu_i)/\{\sigma^2 V(\mu_i)\}$$

for which

$$E(U_i) = 0, \quad \text{and} \quad Var(U_i) = 1/\{\sigma^2 V(\mu_i)\}.$$

We refer to $\mathbf{U} = (U_1, \cdots, U_N)' = \mathbf{U}(\beta)$ as the quasi-score function. Clearly,

$$E\{\mathbf{U}(\beta)\} = \mathbf{0}, \text{ and}$$
$$Cov\{\mathbf{U}(\beta)\} = -E\{\partial\mathbf{U}(\beta)/\partial\beta\} = \mathbf{D}'\mathbf{V}^{-1}\mathbf{D}/\sigma^2. \tag{11.4.7}$$

Note that $Cov\{\mathbf{U}(\beta)\}$ is similar to the expected Fisher information matrix. The quasi-likelihood estimating equations are obtained by setting equal to zero the first derivatives of the log quasi-likelihood function $Q(\mu, \mathbf{y})$:

$$\mathbf{U}(\widehat{\beta}) = \widehat{\mathbf{D}}\widehat{\mathbf{V}}^{-1}(\mathbf{y} - \mu)/\sigma^2 = \mathbf{0}, \tag{11.4.8}$$

where $\mathbf{D}$ is an $N \times p$ matrix whose (i, j)th element $D_{ij} = \partial\mu_i/\partial\beta_j$. Fisher-scoring yields (11.4.6), and iterating to convergence yields $\widehat{\beta}_{QML}$. To show property 2, note that

$$Cov(\widehat{\beta}_{QML}) \approx \{Cov[\mathbf{U}(\beta)]\}^{-1}.$$

The estimator $\widehat{\sigma}^2_{QML}$ is the method of moments estimator based on the residual vector. ∎

If (i) $\mathbf{U}(\beta)$ is asymptotically normal as $N \to \infty$, and (ii) the eigenvalues of $Cov\{\mathbf{U}(\beta)\}$ tend to infinity for all β in an open neighborhood of the true value β^0, then $\widehat{\beta}_{QML}$ is consistent and has an asymptotic normal distribution.

Example 11.4.5.   For the Poisson model, recall that the variance function is $V(\lambda_i) = \lambda_i$, $i = 1, \cdots, N$. Then,

$$Q_i(\lambda_i; Y_i) = Y_i \log \mu_i - \mu_i.$$

For the binomial model, $V(\pi_i) = \pi_i(1 - \pi_i)$ and

$$Q_i(\pi_i; Y_i) = Y_i \log\{\pi_i/(1 - \pi_i)\} + \log(1 - \pi_i). \quad \square$$

To model dependent observations, we replace the assumption of a diagonal $\mathbf{V}$ matrix by the assumption that $\mathbf{V}$ is an $N \times N$ p.d. matrix of known functions $V_{ij}(\mu)$. In this case too, (11.4.7) holds, the quasi-likelihood estimating equations have the same form as in the independent case, and the form of $Cov(\widehat{\beta}_{QML})$ is the same. However, there are some issues because the matrix of first derivatives of $\mathbf{U}(\beta)$ with respect to β is not necessarily symmetric; the reader is referred to McCullagh and Nelder (1991) for details.

11.4.3   Residuals and model checking

The residuals as well as goodness of fit criteria enable us to assess the adequacy of fit of the GLIM. Let $l(\widehat{\mu}, \phi; \mathbf{y})$ denote the maximized log likelihood function for a fixed value of ϕ, and let $l(\mathbf{y}, \phi; \mathbf{y})$ denote the maximum log likelihood in a *full model* with N parameters. As before, suppose θ denotes the canonical parameter, and suppose that $a_i(\phi) = \phi/w_i$. The discrepancy of fit is proportional to $2[l(\mathbf{y}, \phi; \mathbf{y}) - l(\widehat{\mu}, \phi; \mathbf{y})]$. Let $\widehat{\theta} = \theta(\widehat{\mu})$, and $\widetilde{\theta} = \theta(\mathbf{y})$ denote the estimates of the canonical parameter θ under the fitted and full models respectively. Let

$$d_i = 2w_i[Y_i(\widetilde{\theta}_i - \widehat{\theta}_i) - b(\widetilde{\theta}_i) + b(\widehat{\theta}_i)], \quad i = 1, \cdots, N. \qquad (11.4.9)$$

Definition 11.4.2.   We define three types of residuals.

1. The Pearson residual is defined by

$$r_{i,P} = (Y_i - \widehat{\mu}_i)/\sqrt{V(\widehat{\mu}_i)}, \quad i = 1, \cdots, N. \qquad (11.4.10)$$

2. The Anscombe residual has the general form

$$r_{i,A} = \{A(Y_i) - A(\widehat{\mu}_i)\}/\{A'(\widehat{\mu}_i)\sqrt{V(\widehat{\mu}_i)}\}, \qquad (11.4.11)$$

where the function $A(.)$ is given by

$$A(z) = \int dz/V^{1/3}(z).$$

For the Poisson model,

$$r_{i,A} = 3(Y_i^{2/3} - \widehat{\mu}_i^{2/3})/(2\widehat{\mu}_i^{1/6}).$$

3. The ith deviance residual is defined by

$$r_{i,D} = \text{sign}(Y_i - \widehat{\mu}_i)\sqrt{d_i}, \qquad (11.4.12)$$

where d_i was defined in (11.4.9). For the Poisson model,

$$r_{i,D} = \text{sign}(Y_i - \widehat{\mu}_i)[2(Y_i \log(Y_i/\widehat{\mu}_i) - Y_i + \widehat{\mu}_i)]^{1/2}.$$

For the Poisson model, $\sum_{i=1}^{N} r_{i,P}^2 = X^2$, Pearson's goodness of fit statistic, which led to the construction of $r_{i,P}$. The distribution of $r_{i,P}$ is usually skewed for non-normal response distributions, and the Anscombe residuals may be preferred for this reason. The values of Anscombe residuals and deviance are very similar in most cases (see Pierce and Schafer, 1986 for details). We define two goodness of fit measures, the deviance (and scaled deviance) function, and the generalized Pearson X^2 statistic.

Definition 11.4.3. Deviance function. We define the deviance for the fitted model to be the following function of the data (only):

$$D(\mathbf{y}; \widehat{\mu}) = \sum_{i=1}^{N} 2W_i[Y_i(\widetilde{\theta}_i - \widehat{\theta}_i) - b(\widetilde{\theta}_i) + b(\widehat{\theta}_i)]. \qquad (11.4.13)$$

Definition 11.4.4. Scaled deviance. The scaled deviance function is defined by

$$D^*(\mathbf{y}; \widehat{\mu}) = D(\mathbf{y}; \widehat{\mu})/\phi. \qquad (11.4.14)$$

It is straightforward to compute $D(\mathbf{y}; \widehat{\mu})$ for the normal linear model, the binomial logit model, and the Poisson log-linear model (with intercept) for counts as $\sum_{i=1}^{N}(Y_i - \widehat{\mu}_i)^2$ (which is equal to SSE), $2\sum_{i=1}^{N}[Y_i \log(Y_i/\widehat{\mu}_i) + (m_i - Y_i)\log[(m_i - Y_i)/(m_i - \widehat{\mu}_i)]$, and $2\sum_{i=1}^{N} Y_i \log(Y_i/\widehat{\mu}_i)$. In each case, further inclusion of covariates into the model reduces the deviance. For the normal linear model, we have seen that $D(\mathbf{y}; \widehat{\mu})$ (or SSE) has a χ^2_{N-p} distribution. In the binomial case, the deviance statistic has a limiting χ^2_{N-p} distribution, provided for fixed N, $m_i \to \infty$ for each i, or in fact, $m_i\pi_i(1 - \pi_i) \to \infty$.

The deviance function is most useful for the comparison of nested models, and not so much as an absolute measure of goodness of fit Consider a "full model" and a model reduced by a null hypothesis H_0, by setting some of the β coefficients to zero. Let $\widehat{\mu}_F$ and $\widehat{\mu}_r$ denote the fitted vectors under the full and reduced models. It is easy to see that the deviance difference corresponds to the LRT statistic for testing H_0 versus the alternative of the "full model":

$$D(\mathbf{y};\widehat{\mu}_r) - D(\mathbf{y};\widehat{\mu}_F) = 2l(\widehat{\mu}_F;\mathbf{y}) - 2l(\widehat{\mu}_r;\mathbf{y}).$$

Another criterion that enables us to assess discrepancy in fit is the generalized Pearson X^2 statistic.

Definition 11.4.5. The generalized Pearson X^2 statistic defined by

$$X^2 = \sum_{i=1}^{N}(Y_i - \widehat{\mu}_i)^2/V(\widehat{\mu}_i). \tag{11.4.15}$$

For the normal model, the statistic is SSE, while for the binomial and Poisson models, it is the usual Pearson X^2 statistic.

Model diagnostics similar to those defined in section 8.5 have been studied in the literature (Pregibon, 1981). Diggle, Liang and Zeger (1994) describe generalized linear models for longitudinal data (binary responses, count responses etc.) using (a) marginal models, (b) random effects models, and (c) transition models.

11.4.4 Generalized additive models

Generalized additive models (GAMs) are an extension to the class of GLIMs, where the linear form $\tau + \sum_{j=1}^{p} X_{ij}\beta_j$ is replaced by the sum of component functions, $\tau + \sum_{j=1}^{p} f_j(X_{ij})$. A suitable link function between the predictors and the response which has a general probability distribution is chosen similar to the GLIM setup. Specifically, we assume that the response variable Y has an exponential family density, with mean $\mu = E(Y|X_1, \cdots, X_p)$ which is linked to the predictors via the functional form

$$g(\mu) = \tau + \sum_{j=1}^{p} f_j(X_j). \tag{11.4.16}$$

We estimate $\tau, f_1, \cdots, f_p$ by an algorithm called the local scoring procedure, which is a generalization (using local averaging) of Fisher's scoring procedure that we discussed under the GLIM setup, and has the following steps (for details, see Hastie and Tibsirani, 1990).

(i) Initialization: Set $\tau = g(\sum_{i=1}^{n} Y_i/N)$, and $f_j^0 = 0$, $j = 1, \cdots, p$.

(ii) Update: For $j = 1, \cdots, p$, construct an adjusted dependent variable

$$
\begin{aligned}
z_i &= \eta_i^0 + (y_i - \mu_i^0)\left(\frac{\partial \eta_i}{\partial \mu_i}\right)_0, \\
\eta_i^0 &= \alpha^0 + \sum_{j=1}^{p} f_j^0(x_{ij}), \text{ and} \\
\mu_i^0 &= g^{-1}(\eta_i^0).
\end{aligned}
\tag{11.4.17}
$$

Construct weights

$$w_i = \left(\frac{\partial \eta_i}{\partial \mu_i}\right)_0^2 (V_i^0)^{-1} \tag{11.4.18}$$

where V_i^0 is the variance of Y at μ_i^0. Fit a weighted additive model to z_i, to obtain estimated component functions f_j^1, additive predictor η^1, and fitted values μ_i^1. Compute the convergence criterion

$$\Delta(\eta^1, \eta^0) = \sum_{j=1}^{p} \|f_j^1 - f_j^0\| \bigg/ \sum_{j=1}^{p} \|f_j^0\|, \tag{11.4.19}$$

where, $\|f\|$ may be computed as the length of the vector of evaluations of f at the n sample points.

(iii) Continue (ii), replacing η^0 by η^1, until the convergence criterion $\Delta(\eta^1, \eta^0)$ is smaller than some small value.

Exercises

11.1. Prove Result 11.1.4.

11.2. Suppose $\mathbf{y}_j \sim N(\mu_j \mathbf{1}_{N_j}, \sigma_j^2 \mathbf{I}_{N_j})$, $j = 1, 2$. Also, suppose $\pi(\mu_j, \sigma_j^2) \propto 1/\sigma_j^2$, $j = 1, 2$ and $\pi(\mu_1, \sigma_1^2)$ and $\pi(\mu_2, \sigma_2^2)$ are independent. What is the posterior distribution of $\{S_1^2/S_2^2\}/\{\sigma_1^2/\sigma_2^2\}$?

11.3. Let $\mathbf{y} \sim N(\mu \mathbf{1}_N, \sigma^2 \mathbf{I}_N)$.

   (a) Suppose (μ, σ^2) has a normal-inverse χ^2 prior. Show that the posterior distribution $\pi(\mu, \sigma^2|\mathbf{y})$ also has the normal-inverse χ^2 form and derive its parameters.

   (b) Suppose we use a noninformative prior, i.e., $\pi(\mu, \sigma^2) \propto 1/\sigma^2$. Derive the form of the posterior distribution $\pi(\mu, \sigma^2|\mathbf{y})$. What is the form of the marginal posterior distribution of $\sqrt{N}(\mu - \overline{Y})/S$?

11.4. Let $F(.)$ denote the cdf of $Y|\theta$, and suppose $\pi_j(\theta)$, $j = 1, \cdots, L$ are conjugate prior pdfs for θ. Consider the class $\pi(\theta) = \sum_{j=1}^{L} w_j \pi_j(\theta)$ of finite mixture prior densities, where the weights satisfy $w_j \geq 0$, $j = 1, \cdots, L$ and $\sum_{j=1}^{L} w_j = 1$. Is this also a conjugate class?

11.5. Write a univariate $AR(1)$ model $Y_t = \rho Y_{t-1} + v_t$ as a dynamic linear model and derive the Kalman filter equations.

11.6. Let Z_t be an observed time series at time t, $t = 1, \cdots, T$, which measures a signal with error. Suppose the signal and error terms are additive, and the signal satisfies an AR(1) model. Assuming independent Gaussian errors for the observation and signal processes, derive the Kalman filter recursions.

11.7. For the single factor repeated measures model in (11.3.9), write down the ANOVA table corresponding to the split-plot design framework. What are the forms of the F-test statistics for the treatment effect, the time effect, and the treatment/time interaction ?

11.8. Consider the "conditional-independence model" , i.e., the two-stage random-effects model for longitudinal data in (11.3.10), with $\mathbf{R}_i = \sigma^2 \mathbf{I}$. Obtain the maximum likelihood estimates of the parameters.

11.9. Let $(Y|P = p) \sim Bin(m, p)$, where $P \sim Beta(\alpha, \beta)$, $0 \le p \le 1$. For $\alpha > 0$ and $\beta > 0$, find the marginal distribution of Y, and show that it does not belong to the exponential family. Find $E(Y)$ and $Var(Y)$.

11.10. Assume that Y_t, the number of fatal accidents in a year t is modeled by a Poisson distribution with mean $\lambda_t = \beta_0 + \beta_1 t$. Given data for 20 years, derive the IRLS estimates for β_0 and β_1.

11.11. Let Y_1 denote the number of cars that cross a check-point in one hour, and let Y_2 denote the number of other vehicles (except cars) that cross the point. Consider two models. Under Model 1, assume that Y_1 and Y_2 have independent Poisson distributions with means λ_1 and λ_2 respectively, both unknown. Under Model 2, assume a Binomial specification for Y_1 with unknown probability p and sample size $Y_1 + Y_2$.

  (a) If we define $p = \lambda_1/(\lambda_1 + \lambda_2)$, show that Model 1 and Model 2 have the same likelihood. (Hint: Use Definition 11.4.1).

  (b) What is the relationship between the link canonical functions?

  (c) How can we incorporate a covariate X, which is a highway characteristic, into the modeling?

A Review of Probability Distributions

1. Normal distribution. The pdf of the normal distribution with mean μ and variance σ^2 is given by

$$f(x; \mu, \sigma^2) = \frac{1}{\sqrt{2\pi\sigma^2}} \exp\left\{\frac{-(x-\mu)^2}{2\sigma^2}\right\}, \qquad (A1)$$

where, $-\infty < x < \infty$, $-\infty < \mu < \infty$, and $\sigma^2 > 0$. Note that $E(X) = \mu$, and $Var(X) = \sigma^2$. The random variable $Z = (X - \mu) / \sigma$ is called the standard normal variable with mean $E(Z) = 0$, variance $Var(Z) = 1$, and pdf

$$f(z) = \frac{1}{\sqrt{2\pi}} \exp\left\{\frac{-z^2}{2}\right\}, \qquad -\infty < z < \infty. \qquad (A2)$$

It is easy to verify that

$$\int_{-\infty}^{\infty} f(z)dz = \sqrt{2\pi}. \qquad (A3)$$

The moment generating functions of X and Z are respectively

$$M_X(t) = E[e^{tX}] = \exp\{\mu t + \frac{1}{2}\sigma^2 t^2\} \qquad (A4)$$

and

$$M_Z(t) = E[e^{tZ}] = \exp\{t^2/2\}. \qquad (A5)$$

2. Chi-square χ_k^2 distribution. A random variable U has a chi-square distribution with k degrees of freedom (d.f.) if its pdf is

$$f(u) = \frac{1}{2^{k/2}\Gamma(k/2)} u^{(k/2)-1} e^{-u/2}, \quad 0 < u < \infty. \qquad (A6)$$

The cdf of the distribution is

$$F(u) = P(U \le u) = \begin{cases} 0, & u \le 0 \\ 1 - \exp\{-u/2\}, & u > 0. \end{cases}$$

433

The mean and variance of a χ^2_k random variable are respectively $E(U) = k$, and $Var(U) = 2k$, while its mgf is

$$M_U(t) = (1 - 2t)^{-k/2}, \quad t < 1/2. \tag{A7}$$

The χ^2_k may be derived as a sampling distribution related to a normal random sample. Let $X_1, \cdots, X_{k+1}$ be a random sample of size $(k + 1)$ from a $N(\mu, \sigma^2)$ distribution. Then the random variable $U = kS^2/\sigma^2$ has a chi-square distribution with k degrees of freedom, where $S^2 = \sum_{i=1}^{k+1}(X_i - \overline{X})^2/k$, and $\overline{X} = \sum_{i=1}^{k+1} X_i/(k+1)$.

3. Student's t-distribution.   A random variable T which has a Student's t-distribution with k degrees of freedom has pdf

$$f(t) = \{\Gamma((k+1)/2)/\{\Gamma(k/2)\}(k\pi)^{-1/2}\{1 + t^2/k\}^{(k+1)/2}, \quad -\infty < t < \infty. \tag{A8}$$

Let $X_1, \cdots, X_{k+1}$ be a random sample from a $N(\mu, \sigma^2)$ distribution, and the sample mean and variance respectively be computed as $\overline{X} = \sum_{i=1}^{k+1} X_i/(k+1)$ and $S^2 = \sum_{i=1}^{k+1}(X_i - \overline{X})^2/k$. Then, the random variable $\sqrt{(k+1)}(\overline{X} - \mu)/S$ has a t-distribution with k degrees of freedom with pdf given by the expression in (A8). The moment generating function of T does not exist. Recall that $E(T) = 0$, if $k > 1$, and $Var(T) = k/(k-2)$ if $k > 2$.

4. Snedecor's F-distribution.   A random variable F has Snedecor's F-distribution with numerator degrees of freedom p and denominator degrees of freedom q if its pdf is

$$f(u) = \frac{\Gamma((p+q)/2)}{\Gamma(p/2)\Gamma(q/2)}(p/2)^{p/2}\frac{u^{p/2-1}}{[1 + (p/q)u]^{(p+q)/2}}, \quad 0 < u < \infty. \tag{A9}$$

The mean and variance of the distribution are

$$E(F) = q/(q-2), \quad q > 2$$

$$Var(F) = 2\left(\frac{q}{q-2}\right)^2 \frac{p+q-2}{p(q-4)}, \quad q > 4$$

and the rth raw moment is

$$E(F^r) = \frac{\Gamma((p+2r)/2)\Gamma((q-2r)/2)}{\Gamma(p/2)\Gamma(q/2)}(q/p)^r, \quad r < q/2.$$

The mgf of the distribution does not exist. It can be shown that if

(i) $U \sim F_{p,q}$, then $1/U \sim F_{q,p}$,

(ii) $U \sim t_q$, then $U^2 \sim F_{1,q}$,

(iii) $U \sim F_{p,q}$, then $\frac{(p/q)U}{[1+(p/q)U]} \sim Beta(p/2, q/2)$,

(iv) $U_1 \sim \chi_p^2$, $U_2 \sim \chi_q^2$, U_1 and U_2 are independent, then $U = \left(\frac{U_1}{p}\right) \Big/ \left(\frac{U_2}{q}\right) \sim F_{p,q}$.

The F-distribution is a sampling distribution which may also be derived as follows. Let $X_1, \cdots, X_{n_1}$ be a random sample from a $N(\mu_x, \sigma_x^2)$ population, and let $Y_1, \cdots, Y_{n_2}$ be a random sample from a $N(\mu_y, \sigma_y^2)$ population and suppose the two populations are independent. The random variable

$$F = \frac{S_x^2 / (n_1 - 1)\sigma_x^2}{S_y^2 / (n_2 - 1)\sigma_y^2} \tag{A10}$$

has Snedecor's F-distribution with numerator and denominator degrees of freedom $(n_1 - 1)$ and $(n_2 - 1)$ respectively.

5. Gamma distribution. A random variable X is said to have a Gamma(α, β) distribution if its pdf is

$$f(x; \alpha, \beta) = \frac{1}{\Gamma(\alpha)\beta^\alpha} x^{\alpha-1} \exp\{-x/\beta\}, \quad x > 0, \tag{A11}$$

where $\alpha > 0$ is called the shape parameter, $\beta > 0$ is the scale parameter, and the Gamma function is defined by

$$\Gamma(\alpha) = \int_0^\infty u^{\alpha-1} \exp\{-u\} du. \tag{A12}$$

The mean and variance of the Gamma distribution are respectively

$$E(X) = \alpha\beta, \quad \text{and} \quad Var(X) = \alpha\beta^2.$$

The mgf of X is

$$M_X(t) = [1/(1 - \beta t)]^\alpha, \quad t < 1/\beta.$$

6. Beta distribution. A random variable X is said to have a $Beta(\alpha, \beta)$ distribution of the *first kind* if its pdf is

$$f(x) = \frac{x^{\alpha-1}(1-x)^{\beta-1}}{B(\alpha, \beta)}, \quad 0 \le x < 1, \tag{A13}$$

where $\alpha > 0$, $\beta > 0$, and $B(\alpha, \beta) = \Gamma(\alpha)\Gamma(\beta) / \Gamma(\alpha + \beta)$ is called the Beta function. The mean and variance of X are

$$E(X) = \alpha/(\alpha + \beta), \quad \text{and} \quad Var(X) = \alpha\beta/\{(\alpha + \beta)^2(\alpha + \beta + 1)\}.$$

The mgf of X is

$$M_X(t) = 1 + \sum_{k=1}^\infty \left(\prod_{j=0}^{k-1} (\alpha + j)/(\alpha + \beta + j)\right) \{t^k/k!\},$$

which cannot be simplified further. If $V \sim F_{p,q}$, then

$$X = \frac{(p/q)V}{[1 + (p/q)V]} \sim Beta(p/2, q/2). \tag{A14}$$

A random variable Y is said to have a $Beta(\alpha, \beta)$ distribution of the *second kind* if its pdf is

$$f(y) = \frac{1}{B(\alpha,\beta)} y^{\alpha-1}(1+y)^{-(m+n)}, \quad 0 < y < \infty.$$

Notice that the relation between X and Y is $X = Y/(1+Y)$.

7. Cauchy distribution.   A random variable X is said to have a Cauchy distribution if its pdf is

$$f(x; \mu, \sigma) = \frac{1}{\pi\sigma}\{1 + (x - \mu)/\sigma\}^{-2}, \quad -\infty < x < \infty, \tag{A15}$$

where μ is the location parameter, $-\infty < \mu < \infty$, and $\sigma > 0$ is the scale parameter. The mean and variance of this distribution do not exist and neither does the mgf. Note that if U and V are independent standard normal variables, then $X = U/V$ has a Cauchy distribution with location 0 and unit scale. The Cauchy distribution is a special case of Student's t-distribution with 1 degree of freedom.

8. Double exponential distribution (or Laplace distribution).   A random variable X is said to have a double exponential (or Laplace) distribution if its pdf is

$$f(x; \mu, \sigma) = \frac{1}{2\sigma} \exp\{-\frac{|x - \mu|}{\sigma}\}, \quad -\infty < x < \infty, \tag{A16}$$

where μ is the location parameter, $-\infty < \mu < \infty$, and $\sigma > 0$ is the scale parameter. The pdf attains a maximum value of $(2\sigma)^{-1}$ at $x = 0$, and tails off to zero as $x \to \pm\infty$. The mean and variance of this distribution are

$$E(X) = \mu, \quad Var(X) = 2\sigma^2.$$

The mgf of X is

$$M_X(t) = \exp\{\mu t\}/(1 - \sigma^2 t^2), \quad t < 1/\sigma$$

The standard form of the distribution is obtained by setting $\mu = 0$, and $\sigma = 1$, and has pdf

$$f(z) = \tfrac{1}{2}\exp\{-|z|\}, \quad -\infty < z < \infty.$$

9. Finite mixture distribution.   Let X denote a random variable with pdf

$$f(x) = p_1 f_1(x) + \cdots + p_L f_L(x) \tag{A17}$$

where $p_j > 0$, $j = 1, \cdots, L$, $\sum_{j=1}^{L} p_j = 1$, and $f_j(x)$ are themselves valid pdfs. Then X is said to have a finite mixture distribution with L mixands, and with mixing proportions (or mixing weights) $p_1, \cdots, p_L$. The pdfs $f_j(x)$ are known as the components of the mixture.

10. Mixture of normals distribution. Also referred to as normal mixtures in the literature, these are the most widely studied finite mixture distributions. It is assumed that the jth component of a finite mixture is a univariate normal with mean μ_j and variance σ_j^2. The pdf of a finite normal mixture with mixing proportions $p_1, \cdots, p_L$ is given by

$$f(x) = \frac{1}{\sqrt{2\pi}} \sum_{j=1}^{L} \frac{p_j}{\sigma_j} \exp\left\{ -\frac{1}{2}\left(\frac{x - \mu_j}{\sigma_j} \right)^2 \right\}, \quad -\infty < x < \infty. \quad \text{(A18)}$$

This pdf is determined by $(3L - 1)$ parameters, consisting of μ_j, $j = 1, \cdots, L$, σ_j^2, $j = 1, \cdots, L$, and p_j, $j = 1, \cdots, L$ subject to the constraint $\sum_{j=1}^{L} p_j = 1$. A normal mixture affords a great deal of flexibility for modeling by allowing for multimodality. The expectation and variance of a mixture random variable can be obtained from the means and variances of its components:

$$E(X) = \overline{\mu} = \sum_{j=1}^{L} p_j \mu_j, \quad \text{and} \quad Var(X) = \sum_{j=1}^{L} p_j \sigma_j^2 + \sum_{j=1}^{L} p_j (\mu_j - \overline{\mu})^2. \quad \text{(A19)}$$

11. Scale mixture of normals (SMN) distribution. The distribution of a univariate standardized random variable $X = Z * \lambda$ is said to be a scale mixture of normals (SMN) distribution if Z has a standard normal distribution, and is independent of λ, which itself has either a discrete or a continuous distribution over the positive half of the real line, $\mathcal{R}^+$. The pdf of X has the form

$$f(x; \theta, \sigma) = \int_{\mathcal{R}^+} N(x; \theta, \kappa(\lambda)\sigma^2)\pi(\lambda)d\lambda \quad \text{(A20)}$$

where $\kappa(.)$ is a positive function on $\mathcal{R}^+$, the mixing density $\pi(.)$ is a valid probability function (either discrete or continuous), and λ is called the mixing parameter. In (A20), θ is the location parameter and σ is the scale parameter (Andrews and Mallows, 1974).

12. Stable distribution A random variable X is said to have a four-parameter stable distribution, $S_\alpha(\sigma, \beta, \delta)$ if its characteristic function has the form

$$E[\exp(i\theta X)] = \begin{cases} \exp\{-|\sigma\theta|^\alpha(1 - i\beta \text{sign}(\theta)\tan(\pi\alpha/2) + i\delta\theta\} & \text{if} \quad \alpha \neq 1 \\ \exp\{-|\sigma\theta|(1 + \frac{2}{\pi}i\beta\ln|\theta|\text{sign}(\theta) + i\delta\theta\} & \text{if} \quad \alpha = 1 \end{cases} \quad \text{(A21)}$$

where θ is a real number, and

$$\text{sign}(\theta) = \begin{cases} 1, & \text{if } \theta > 0 \\ 0, & \text{if } \theta = 0 \\ -1, & \text{if } \theta < 0 \end{cases}$$

(Samorodnitsky and Taqqu, 1994). The stability parameter α lies in the range $(0, 2]$, and measures the degree of peakedness of the pdf and the heaviness of its tails. When $\alpha = 2$, the stable distribution reduces to a normal distribution with mean δ and variance $2\sigma^2$. The skewness parameter β, which lies in the range $[-1, 1]$, measures the departure of the distribution from symmetry. The distribution is symmetric when $\beta = 0$, is skewed to the right when $\beta > 0$, and is skewed to the left when $\beta < 0$. The location parameter δ lies in the range $(-\infty, \infty)$, and shifts the distribution to the right or the left. The scale parameter σ lies in the range $(0, \infty)$, and is the parameter in proportion to which the distribution of X around δ is compressed or extended. When $\beta = 1$, $0 < \alpha < 1$, and $\delta = 0$, the distribution is totally skewed to the right, and is referred to as the positive stable distribution. The pdf of this distribution is not available in closed form.

13. Studentized range distribution. Let $X_1, \cdots, X_n$ be independent $N(\mu, \sigma^2)$ random variables. Let $R = \max_i X_i - \min_i X_i = X_{(n)} - X_{(1)}$ denote the range of the n variables. Let S^2 be an unbiased estimate of σ^2 based on ν degrees of freedom, and let $\nu S^2 / \sigma^2 \sim \chi_\nu^2$, independent of $(X_1, \cdots, X_n)$. Then $q = R/S$ has a Studentized range distribution with (n, ν) degrees of freedom.

14. Exponential family of distributions. A family of pmf's or pdf's is called an exponential family if it has the form

$$f(x; \theta, \phi) = \exp\{[\sum_{i=1}^{k} \omega_i(\theta) t_i(x) - b(\theta)]/a(\phi) + c(x, \phi)\}. \qquad \text{(A22)}$$

Here, $\omega_1(\theta), \cdots, \omega_k(\theta)$ are real-valued functions of the possibly vector-valued parameter θ (they may not depend on x), while $t_1(x), \cdots, t_k(x)$ are real-valued functions of x (they may not depend on θ), and $b(\theta)$ is called the cumulant function. If the dispersion parameter ϕ is known, this is a k-parameter exponential family with canonical parameter θ.

For example, the $N(\mu, \sigma^2)$ distribution is a two-parameter exponential family, with $\theta = \mu$, $\phi = \sigma^2$, $a(\phi) = \sigma^2$, $b(\theta) = \mu^2/2$, $c(x, \phi) = -[x^2/\sigma^2 + \log(2\pi\sigma^2)]/2$.

Consider a simple case of (A22)

$$f(x; \theta, \phi) = \exp\{[x\theta - b(\theta)]/a(\phi) + c(x, \phi)\}, \qquad \text{(A23)}$$

and let $l(\theta, \phi; x) = \log f(x; \theta, \phi)$ denote the logarithm of the likelihood function. Since,

$$E(\partial l/\partial \theta) = 0,$$
$$E(\partial^2 l/\partial \theta^2) + E(\partial l/\partial \theta)^2 = 0,$$

and

$$\begin{aligned}
\partial l/\partial\theta &= \{x - b'(\theta)\}/a(\phi), \\
\partial^2 l/\partial\theta^2 &= -b''(\theta)/a(\phi),
\end{aligned}$$

it follows that $E(X) = \mu = b'(\theta)$, and $Var(X) = b''(\theta)a(\phi)$. The function $b''(\theta)$ depends on the canonical parameter, and hence on μ, and is called the variance function, and denoted by $V(\mu)$.

15. Inverse Gamma distribution. A random variable X has an inverse Gamma distribution if

$$f(x|\alpha,\beta) = \{\Gamma(\alpha)\}^{-1}\beta^{-\alpha}x^{-(\alpha+1)}\exp(-1/x\beta), \quad x > 0, \alpha > 0, \beta > 0. \quad \text{(A24)}$$

We can verify that $E(X) = 1/\{\beta(\alpha-1)\}$ if $\alpha > 1$, and $Var(X) = 1/\{\beta^2(\alpha - 1)^2(\alpha-2)\}$ if $\alpha > 2$. Also, the random variable $1/X$ has a *Gamma*(α, β) distribution.

16. p-variate t-distribution. A p-dimensional random vector $\mathbf{x}$ has the p-variate t-distribution with location vector δ, a p.d. scale matrix Ω and degrees of freedom ν if its pdf is

$$\begin{aligned}
f(\mathbf{x}|\delta,\Omega,\nu) &= \{\Gamma[(\nu+p)/2]/\Gamma(\nu/2)\}|\Omega|^{-1/2}(\nu\pi)^{-p/2} \\
&\quad \times \{1 + (\mathbf{x}-\delta)'\Omega^{-1}(\mathbf{x}-\delta)\}^{-(\nu+p)/2}.
\end{aligned}$$

$$\text{(A25)}$$

Then, $(\mathbf{x}-\delta)'\Omega^{-1}(\mathbf{x}-\delta)/p \sim F_{p,\nu}$.

Solutions to Selected Exercises

Chapter 1

1.1. Verify that $|\mathbf{a} \bullet \mathbf{b}| \leq \| \mathbf{a} \| \| \mathbf{b} \|$.

1.3. $a = \pm 1/\sqrt{2}$ and $b = \pm 1/\sqrt{2}$.

1.7. Yes.

1.9. Obtain conditions for $\mathbf{AB} = \mathbf{BA}$.

1.10. $\mathbf{A}^k = \begin{pmatrix} a^k & \beta \\ 0 & 1 \end{pmatrix}$, where, $\beta = b(1 + a + \cdots + a^{k-1})$.

1.11. Show that $\mathbf{C} = \mathbf{A}^{k-1} + \mathbf{A}^{k-2}\mathbf{B} + \cdots + \mathbf{B}^{k-1}$.

1.14. Use property 4 of Result 1.2.8.

1.16. -8.

1.17. $\Delta_n = (1 + a^2 + a^4 + \cdots + a^{2n}) = [1 - a^{2(n+1)}]/[1 - a^4]$.

1.19. $1 + \sum_{i=1}^{n} a_i$.

1.23. For (a), use the definition of orthogonality and Result 1.2.9. For (b), use Definition 1.2.8 and Definition 1.2.21.

1.24. Use properties 1 and 3 of Result 1.2.16.

1.25. The dimension of the column space is 2.

1.27. $r(\mathbf{A}) = 2$.

1.29. The eigenvector corresponding to $\lambda = 3$ is $\mathbf{v} = t(1, 1, 1)'$, for arbitrary t.

1.32. Use the Cauchy-Schwarz inequality.

Chapter 2

2.3. Use Result 2.1.2 to write the determinant of the matrix as $|1||\mathbf{P} - \mathbf{xx}'|$.

2.4. For (a), use Result 1.2.29. For (b), use (a) and property 5 of Result 1.2.12.

2.6. For (a), use Result 2.1.2. To prove (b), let λ be a nonzero eigenvalue of $\mathbf{AB}$, so that we have $P(\lambda) = |\mathbf{AB} - \lambda\mathbf{I}_n| = 0$, where $P(\lambda)$ is the characteristic polynomial of $\mathbf{AB}$; use (a).

2.7. Show that $\mathbf{Aa} = \mathbf{aa}'\mathbf{a} = (\mathbf{a}'\mathbf{a})\mathbf{a}$, and use Definition 1.2.32.

2.8. Write $(\mathbf{A} + \mathbf{BC}) = \mathbf{A}(\mathbf{I}_k + \mathbf{A}^{-1}\mathbf{BC})$, and use Result 2.1.2 on the matrix $\begin{pmatrix} \mathbf{I}_k & -\mathbf{A}^{-1}\mathbf{B} \\ \mathbf{C} & \mathbf{I}_n \end{pmatrix}$.

2.10. Write $(\mathbf{A} + \mathbf{aa}') = \mathbf{A}(\mathbf{I}_k + \mathbf{A}^{-1}\mathbf{aa}')$ and use Result 2.1.2.

2.14. (a) yes; (b) symmetric but not idempotent in general.

2.15. Construct an $n \times (n-k)$ matrix $\mathbf{V}$ such that the columns of $(\mathbf{U}, \mathbf{V})$ form an orthogonal basis for $\mathbf{R}^n$.

2.19. Given that $\mathbf{QAQ}^{-1} = \mathbf{D}$, invert both sides.

2.20. For (a), use the fact that the trace of a matrix is the sum of its eigenvalues. For (b), use Result 2.3.10.

2.21. Suppose on the contrary, that $r(\mathbf{C}) < q$, and use Exercise 2.10 to contradict this assumption.

2.23. $\mathbf{B} = \begin{pmatrix} \sqrt{2} & 0 & 0 \\ -1/\sqrt{2} & 1/\sqrt{2} & 0 \\ -1/\sqrt{2} & 1/\sqrt{2} & \sqrt{3} \end{pmatrix}$.

2.24. $-1/(n-1) < a < 1$.

2.25. Use the simultaneous diagonalization of $\mathbf{A}$ and $\mathbf{B}$ and choose a λ such that $\frac{1}{\lambda} > d > \frac{1}{\lambda} > d_i \ \forall \ i = 1, \cdots, n$, or $1 - \lambda d_i > 0 \ \forall \ i = 1, \cdots, n$.

2.29. For an $n \times n$ nonsingular matrix $\mathbf{P}$ such that $\mathbf{P}^{-1}\mathbf{A}_i\mathbf{P} = \mathbf{D}_i$, $i = 1, \cdots, k$, show that for $j \neq i = 1, \cdots, k$, $\mathbf{P}^{-1}\mathbf{A}_j\mathbf{A}_i\mathbf{P} = \mathbf{P}^{-1}\mathbf{A}_j\mathbf{A}_i\mathbf{P}$.

2.31. Using the properties of Kronecker product and trace, the result follows directly.

2.32. If possible, let $\mathbf{P}_1$ and $\mathbf{P}_1$ be two such matrices. Since $\mathbf{u}$ is unique, $(\mathbf{P}_1 - \mathbf{P}_2)\mathbf{y} = \mathbf{0}$ for all $\mathbf{y} \in \mathcal{R}^n$, so that $\mathbf{P}_1$ must equal $\mathbf{P}_2$.

Chapter 3

3.1. For (a), $r(\mathbf{A}) = 2$, and $\mathbf{A}^- = \begin{pmatrix} -1 & 2 & 0 \\ 1 & -1 & 0 \end{pmatrix}$. For (b), $r(\mathbf{A}) = 2$, and

$$\mathbf{A}^- = \begin{pmatrix} 1/7 & 2/7 & 0 \\ 3/7 & -1/7 & 0 \\ 0 & 0 & 0 \\ 0 & 0 & 0 \end{pmatrix}.$$

3.2. Verify (3.1.1).

3.4. For (a), use property 1 and 2 of Result 3.1.8. For (b), transpose both sides of (a). Use (3.1.7) to obtain (c). For (d), use property 3 of Result 3.1.8.

3.6. Use Definition 3.1.1.

3.10. $\mathbf{AG}_2\mathbf{x} = \mathbf{AG}_2\mathbf{AG}_1\mathbf{x} = \mathbf{AG}_1\mathbf{x} = \mathbf{x}$.

3.12. This follows from property 2 of Result 3.1.8.

3.13. (a) Let $\mathbf{G} = \mathbf{HA}^{-1}$. Then, $\mathbf{ABGAB} = \mathbf{ABHA}^{-1}\mathbf{AB} = \mathbf{ABHB} = \mathbf{AB}$. Conversely, let $\mathbf{ABGAB} = \mathbf{AB}$. That is, $\mathbf{ABGABHB} = \mathbf{ABHB}$, i.e., $\mathbf{GABHB} = \mathbf{HB}$, i.e., $\mathbf{GAB} = \mathbf{HB}$. The solution for (b) is similar.

3.15. Using Result 3.2.2, the system is consistent.

3.16. The unique solution is $(-1, -4, 2, -1)'$.

3.17. This follows directly from Result 3.2.9 (see proof of this result).

3.18. $\mathcal{C}(\mathbf{c}) \subset \mathcal{C}(\mathbf{A})$ and $\mathcal{R}(\mathbf{b}) \subset \mathcal{R}(\mathbf{A})$; use Result 3.2.9.

Chapter4

4.1. Use property 8 of Result 1.2.12 to show that $r(\mathbf{X'X}, \mathbf{X'y}) \geq r(\mathbf{X'X})$. Use properties 4 and 6 of Result 1.2.12 to show that $r(\mathbf{X'X}, \mathbf{X'y}) = r[\mathbf{X'}(\mathbf{X}, \mathbf{y})] \leq \mathbf{X'} = r(\mathbf{X'X})$.

4.3. $\widehat{\theta} = 2\sum_{i=1}^{N} t_i^2 Y_i / \sum_{i=1}^{N} t_i^4$, and $Var(\widehat{\theta}) = 4\sigma^2 / \sum_{i=1}^{N} t_i^4$.

4.4. $\widehat{\nu} = \sum_{i=1}^{N} S_i t_i / \sum_{i=1}^{N} t_i^2$, and $Var(\widehat{\nu}) = \sigma^2 / \sum_{i=1}^{N} t_i^2$.

4.5. $\widehat{\beta} = (0, 3, 1)'$, and $\widehat{\sigma}^2 = 4$.

4.6. $n_1 = 2n_2$.

4.9. (i) $\widehat{\beta}_1 = (Y_2 + Y_4 + Y_6 - Y_1 - Y_3 - Y_5)/6$, with variance $\sigma^2/6$. (ii) $\widehat{\beta}_1 = \{5(Y_2 - Y_5) + 8(Y_4 - Y_3) + 11(Y_6 - Y_1)\}/48$, with variance $420\sigma^2/(48)^2$. The ratio of variances is then $32/35$.

4.10. Argue that there are no d.f. for the error.

4.11. Use (3.1.7).

4.17. For (a), equate (4.5.5) with (4.2.4) and set $\mathbf{y} = \mathbf{Xz}$. (b) follows since $\mathbf{V}^{-1} = (1 - \rho)^{-1}\mathbf{I} - \rho(1 - \rho)^{-1}[1 + (N - 1)\rho]^{-1}\mathbf{J}$, and $\mathbf{1}'\mathbf{y} = 0$.

4.24. $\widehat{\beta} = \mathbf{y}$, and $\widehat{\beta}_r = (\mathbf{I}_N - \mathbf{VC}(\mathbf{C}'\mathbf{VC})^{-1}\mathbf{C}'\mathbf{y}$.

Chapter 5

5.1. (b) $\pi/\sqrt{3}$.

5.2. $a = 19.65$.

5.4. $\mu = \begin{pmatrix} 4 \\ -2 \\ 1 \end{pmatrix}$, and $\Sigma = \begin{pmatrix} 5 & -1 & 2 \\ -1 & 3 & 1 \\ 2 & 1 & 6 \end{pmatrix}$.

5.7. $1/3$.

5.9. From Result 5.2.6, $\mathbf{y} \sim N_k(\mathbf{0}, \sigma^2\mathbf{PP}')$; use the orthogonality of $\mathbf{P}$.

5.13. For(a), $X_2 \sim N(\mu_2, \sigma^2)$ and $X_3 \sim N(\mu_3, \sigma^2)$. For (b) $(X_1|X_2, X_3)$ is normal with mean $\mu_1 + \rho(x_2 - \mu_2)/(1 - \rho^2) - \rho^2(x_3 - \mu_3)/(1 - \rho^2)$ and variance $\sigma^2(1 - 2\rho^2)/(1 - \rho^2)$; it reduces to the marginal distribution of X_1 when $\rho = 0$. For (c), $\rho = -1/2$.

5.21. For (a), by Result 5.4.5, and Result 5.3.4, $E(U) = k + 2\lambda$ and $Var(U) = 2(k + 4\lambda)$. For (b), using Result 5.4.2, $U \sim \chi^2(k, \lambda)$ with $\lambda = \mu'\Sigma^{-1}\mu$. For (c), $\mathbf{x}'\mathbf{Ax} \sim \chi^2(k - 1, \mu'\mathbf{a}\mu/2)$.

5.29. By Result 5.2.5, $\overline{X} \sim (\mu, [1 + (k - 1)\rho]\sigma^2/k)$. Suppose $Q = \mathbf{x}'\mathbf{Ax}$, with $\mathbf{A} = [\mathbf{I} - \mathbf{11}']/\sigma^2(1 - \rho)$. By Result 5.4.5, $Q \sim \chi^2_{k-1}$. By Result 5.4.8, $\overline{X}$ and Q are independent since $\frac{1}{k}\mathbf{1}'[\mathbf{I} - \mathbf{11}'/k] = 0$.

5.31. For (a), use Result 5.4.7. For (b), use Result 5.4.5.

5.32. Verify that $Q_1 = \mathbf{x}'\mathbf{A}_1\mathbf{x}$, and $Q_2 = \mathbf{x}'\mathbf{A}_2\mathbf{x}$, with $\mathbf{A}_1 = \begin{pmatrix} 1 & -1 \\ -1 & 1 \end{pmatrix}$, and $\mathbf{A}_2 = \begin{pmatrix} 1 & 1 \\ 1 & 1 \end{pmatrix}$. Use idempotency of $A_1\Sigma$ and that $\mathbf{A}_1\Sigma\mathbf{A}_2 = \mathbf{0}$.

5.34. The proof follows from Driscoll and Krasnicka (1995).

Chapter 6

6.1. Since $\widehat{\Sigma}_{ML} = \{(N - 1)/N\}\mathbf{S}_N$, $|\widehat{\Sigma}_{ML}|^{N/2} = \left[\frac{N-1}{N}\right]^{kN/2}|\mathbf{S}_N|^{N/2}$; substituting this into the expression (6.1.10),

$$L(\widehat{\mu}_{ML}, \widehat{\Sigma}_{ML}) = \frac{\exp(-\frac{Nk}{2})}{(2\pi)^{Nk/2}\left[\frac{N-1}{N}\right]^{kN/2}|\mathbf{S}_N|^{N/2}}.$$

6.2. The first identity is immediate from the definition of the sample mean, and some algebra. To show the second identity, write

$$
\begin{aligned}
\mathbf{S}_{m+1} &= \sum_{i=1}^{m+1} (\mathbf{x}_i - \overline{\mathbf{x}}_{m+1})(\mathbf{x}_i - \overline{\mathbf{x}}_{m+1})' \\
&= \sum_{i=1}^{m} (\mathbf{x}_i - \overline{\mathbf{x}}_m + \overline{\mathbf{x}}_m - \overline{\mathbf{x}}_{m+1})(\mathbf{x}_i - \overline{\mathbf{x}}_m + \overline{\mathbf{x}}_m - \overline{\mathbf{x}}_{m+1})' \\
&\quad + (\mathbf{x}_{m+1} - \overline{\mathbf{x}}_{m+1})(\mathbf{x}_{m+1} - \overline{\mathbf{x}}_{m+1})' \\
&= \mathbf{S}_m + m(\overline{\mathbf{x}}_m - \overline{\mathbf{x}}_{m+1})(\overline{\mathbf{x}}_m - \overline{\mathbf{x}}_{m+1})' \\
&\quad + (\mathbf{x}_{m+1} - \overline{\mathbf{x}}_{m+1})(\mathbf{x}_{m+1} - \overline{\mathbf{x}}_{m+1})',
\end{aligned}
$$

use the first identity for $\overline{\mathbf{x}}_{m+1}$ and simplify.

6.7. $\widehat{\rho}^2_{0(1,\cdots,k)} = 1 - |\mathbf{S}|/\{S_{00}|\mathbf{S}^{(1)}|\}$.

6.8. Use (6.2.11) and (A14).

Chapter 7

7.1. Property 1 is a direct consequence of Result 5.2.6, while property 2 follows from Result 5.2.7. Property 3 and property 5 are direct consequences of Result 5.4.5, while property 4 follows from the orthogonality of $\mathbf{X}$ and $\mathbf{I} - \mathbf{P}$.

7.2. (c) The test statistic $F_0 = (N-3)Q/SSE \sim F_{1,9}$ under H_0 where $Q = \sum \widehat{\beta}_1 X_i(2\widehat{\beta}_0 + \widehat{\beta}_1 X_i + 2\widehat{\beta}_2 X_i^2)$, and $SSE = \sum (Y_i - \widehat{\beta}_0 - \widehat{\beta}_1 X_i - \widehat{\beta}_2 X_i^2)$.

7.5. Let $N = n_1 + n_2 + n_3$. $SSE_H = \sum_{i=1}^{3} \sum_{j=1}^{n_i} Y_{ij}^2 - \sum_{i=1}^{3} (n_i \overline{Y}_{i.})^2/N$, and $SSE = \sum_{i=1}^{3} \sum_{j=1}^{n_i} Y_{ij}^2 - \sum_{i=1}^{3} Y_{i.}^2/n_i$, so that $F(H) = (N-3)(SSE_H - SSE)/(2SSE) \sim F_{2,N-3}$ under H.

7.7. The MLE is $\widehat{\theta} = [\sum_{t=1}^{N} Y_t Y_{t-1}]/[\sum_{t=1}^{N} Y_t^2]$.

7.8. The 95% C.I. for β_1 is $\widehat{\beta}_1 \pm 4.73\sqrt{11/4}$. For β_2, it is $\widehat{\beta}_2 \pm 4.73\sqrt{3}$. For β_3, it is $\widehat{\beta}_3 \pm 4.73$. For $\beta_1 - \beta_2$, it is $\widehat{\beta}_1 - \widehat{\beta}_2 \pm 4.73\sqrt{59/4}$. For $\beta_1 + \beta_3$, it is $\widehat{\beta}_1 + \widehat{\beta}_3 \pm 4.73\sqrt{27/4}$.

7.9. Scheffe's simultaneous confidence set for $\mathbf{c}'\beta$ has the form $\{\mathbf{c}'\beta^0_{GLS} \pm \widehat{\sigma}_{GLS}[sF_{s,N-r,\alpha}\mathbf{c}'(\mathbf{X}'\mathbf{V}^{-1}\mathbf{X})^{-1}\mathbf{c}]^{1/2}\}$ for all $\mathbf{c} \in \mathcal{L}$, with $\dim(\mathcal{L}) = s$, $r(\mathbf{X}) = r$.

7.14. (a) Let $\beta' = (\lambda_1, \lambda_2)$. Then, $\widehat{\lambda}_1 = [(1+c^2)Y_k - c^3 Y_{k+1} - c^2 Y_{k+2}]/(1+c^2+c^4)$, and $\widehat{\lambda}_2 = [cY_k + Y_{k+1} - c(1+c^2)Y_{k+2}]/(1+c^2+c^4)$, with

$$
Var(\widehat{\beta}) = \frac{\sigma^2}{(1+c^2+c^4)} \begin{pmatrix} 1+c^2 & c \\ c & 1+c^2 \end{pmatrix}.
$$

(b) Under the restriction $\lambda_1 = -\lambda_2 = \lambda$, $\widehat{\lambda} = [Y_k - (1 + c)Y_{k+1} + cY_{k+2}]/2(1 + c + c^2)$, with $Var(\widehat{\lambda}) = \sigma^2/2(1 + c + c^2)$.

(c) $Q/\widehat{\sigma}^2 \sim \chi_1^2$, where $Q = \frac{(1-c+c^2)}{2}\{\frac{1}{(1+c^2+c^4)}[(1+c+c^2)Y_k+(1-c^3)Y_{k+1}- c(1 + c + c^2)Y_{k+2}]\}^2$.

7.15. $F_0 = \{2(Y_1 - Y_2)^2\}/(\sum_{i=1}^4 Y_i)^2$.

7.21. Write $\mathbf{c}_l' = 1/\{l(l+1)\}^{1/2}(0, 1, \cdots, 1, -l, 0, \cdots, 0)$. The 95% marginal C.I. for $\mathbf{c}_l'\beta$ is $\mathbf{c}_l'\beta^0 \pm t_{a(n-1),.025} \times (est.\ s.e.\ \mathbf{c}_l'\beta^0)$.

7.22. Due to orthogonality, the least squares estimates of β_0 and β_1 are unchanged, and equal to $\widehat{\beta}_0 = (Y_1 + Y_2 + Y_3)/3$, and $\widehat{\beta}_1 = (Y_3 - Y_1)/2$.

7.28. $F(H) = (3n-3)Q/SSE \sim F_{1,3n-3}$ under H, where $Q = \frac{2n}{3}[\overline{Y}_{2\cdot} - \frac{1}{2}(\overline{Y}_{1\cdot} + \overline{Y}_{1\cdot})]^2$, and $SSE = \sum_{i=1}^3 \sum_{j=1}^n (Y_{ij} - \overline{Y}_{i\cdot})^2$.

7.30. The mgf of $\mathbf{By}$ is $M_{\mathbf{By}}(\mathbf{t}) = M_{\mathbf{y}}(\mathbf{B't}) = \psi(\mathbf{t'BVB't})\exp\{\mathbf{t'B\mu}\}$. The result follows.

7.31. Differentiating the expression in (7.5.22) twice with respect to θ, and take expectations over the distribution of $\mathbf{y}_{\mathrm{mis}}$ given $\mathbf{y}_{\mathrm{obs}}$ and θ.

Chapter 8

8.1. $Var(\widehat{\beta}_1) = \sigma^2 / \sum_{i=1}^N (X_{i1} - \overline{X}_1)^2(1 - r_{12}^2)$. The width of the 95% confidence interval for β_1 is $2t_{N-3,.025}s.e.(\widehat{\beta}_1)$.

8.2. $F(H) = \frac{Q}{SSE/(N-k-1)} \sim F_{1,N-k-1}$, where $Q = (\widehat{\beta}_j - d)^2/a^{jj}$, a^{jj} being the jth diagonal element of $(\mathbf{X'X})^{-1}$. Also, $s = 1$, and $SSE = \mathbf{y'(I - X(X'X)^{-1}X')y}$ which has a chi-square distribution with $N-k-1$ degrees of freedom.

8.3. $MSE(\widehat{\sigma}^2) = 2\sigma^4/(N - p)$, while $MSE(\mathbf{y'A_1y}) = 2\sigma^4/(N - p + 2)$.

8.6. (a)$\widehat{\alpha}_i = \overline{Y}_i$, $i = 1, 2$, $\widehat{\beta} = [S_{XY}^{(1)} + S_{XY}^{(2)}]/[S_{XX}^{(1)} + S_{XX}^{(2)}]$. The vertical distance between the lines is $D = (\alpha_1 - \alpha_2) + \beta(\overline{X}_1 - \overline{X}_2)$, with $\widehat{D} = (\overline{Y}_1 - \overline{Y}_2) - \widehat{\beta}(\overline{X}_1 - \overline{X}_2)$. Then, $E(\widehat{D}) = D$.

(b) A 95% symmetric C.I. for D is $\widehat{D} \pm \widehat{\sigma}[F_{1,n_1+n_2-3,.05}]^{1/2}s.e.(\widehat{D})$.

8.8. $SSE_{(i)} = SSE - \widehat{\varepsilon}_i^2/(1 - p_{ii}) = SSE - r_i^{*2}\widehat{\sigma}_{(i)}^2$ (see Result 8.5.3), from which the result follows after simplification.

8.9. By Example 2.1.2, $\mathbf{P}_Z = \mathbf{P}_X + \{(\mathbf{I} - \mathbf{P}_X)\mathbf{yy'}(\mathbf{I} - \mathbf{P}_X)\}/\mathbf{y'(I - P}_X)\mathbf{y} = \mathbf{P}_X + \widehat{\varepsilon}\widehat{\varepsilon}'/\widehat{\varepsilon}'\widehat{\varepsilon}$.

8.10. From (8.5.16), $SIC_i = (N - 1)\{T(\widehat{F}_N) - T(\widehat{F}_{(i)})\} = (N - 1)(\widehat{\beta} - \widehat{\beta}_{(i)})$. Simplify using (8.5.24).

8.15. Use Exercise 8.9.

Chapter 9

9.2. $\mathbf{U1}_a = \sum_{j=1}^{a} U_{ij} = U_{ii} + \sum_{j \neq i}^{a} U_{ij} = N_{i \cdot} - \sum_{l=1}^{b} \sum_{j=1}^{a} n_{ij} n_{lj}/N_{\cdot j} = N_{i \cdot} - N_{i \cdot} = 0$, $i = 1, \cdots, a$. This implies $r(\mathbf{U}) \leq a - 1$.

9.3. (b) In (9.2.5), in order that $E(\sum_{i=1}^{a} \sum_{j=1}^{b} c_{ij} Y_{ij}) = \mu \sum_{i=1}^{a} \sum_{j=1}^{b} c_{ij} + \sum_{i=1}^{a} (\sum_{j=1}^{b} c_{ij}) \tau_i + \sum_{j=1}^{b} (\sum_{i=1}^{a} c_{ij}) \beta_j$ is to be function only of β's, we must have $\sum_{i=1}^{a} \sum_{j=1}^{b} c_{ij} = 0$, $\sum_{j=1}^{b} c_{ij} = 0$, $i = 1, \cdots, a$. Then, $RHS = \sum_{j=1}^{b} (\sum_{i=1}^{a} c_{ij}) \beta_j = \sum_{j=1}^{b} d_j \beta_j$, where $\sum_{j=1}^{b} d_j = \sum_{j=1}^{b} \sum_{i=1}^{a} c_{ij} = 0$.

9.7. (a) Yes, (b) No.

9.10. $\beta_{j(i)}^0 = Y_{ij \cdot}/n_{ij} = \overline{Y}_{ij \cdot}$, $j = 1, \cdots, b_i$; $i = 1, \cdots, a$. The corresponding g-inverse is $\mathbf{G} = \begin{pmatrix} \mathbf{0} & \mathbf{0} \\ \mathbf{0} & \mathbf{D} \end{pmatrix}$, where $\mathbf{D} = \text{diag}\{1/n_{ij}\}$.

9.15. (a) $SS(\beta_0, \beta_1) = [Y_{\cdot \cdot}^2/N] + \hat{\beta}_1^2 \sum_i n_i (Z_i - \overline{Z})^2$.
(b) $SS(\mu, \tau_1, \cdots, \tau_a) = \sum_{i=1}^{a} (Y_{i \cdot}^2/n_i) - Y_{\cdot \cdot}^2/N$.
Hence, $SS(\beta_0, \beta_1) - SS(\mu, \tau_1, \cdots, \tau_a) = A/B$, where $A = [\sum_{i=1}^{a} c_i^2 \sum_{i=1}^{a} d_i^2 - (\sum_{i=1}^{a} c_i d_i)^2]$ and $B = [\sum_{i=1}^{a} n_i (Z_i - \overline{Z})^2]$, $c_i = \sqrt{n_i}(\overline{Y}_{i \cdot} - \overline{Y}_{\cdot \cdot})$ and $d_i = \sqrt{n_i}(Z_i - \overline{Z})$. The difference in SS is always nonnegative (by Cauchy-Schwarz inequality), with equality only when $c_i \propto d_i$, $i = 1, \cdots, a$, i.e., only when $\overline{Y}_{i \cdot} - \overline{Y}_{\cdot \cdot} = w(Z_i - \overline{Z})$, where w is a constant.

9.16. $F(H) = (abc - 2ab)(SSE_H - SSE)/(ab - 1)SSE \sim F_{ab-1, abc-2ab}$ under H, where $SSE_H = \sum_i \sum_j \sum_k [Y_{ijk} - \overline{Y}_{ij \cdot} - \hat{\gamma}(Z_{ijk} - \overline{Z}_{ij \cdot})]^2 \sim \chi^2_{abc-(ab+1)}$, and $SSE = \sum_i \sum_j \sum_k [Y_{ijk} - \overline{Y}_{ij \cdot} - \hat{\gamma}_{ij}(Z_{ijk} - \overline{Z}_{ij \cdot})]^2$.

Chapter 10

10.2. Let the $N \times (a+1)$ matrix $\mathbf{X} = (\mathbf{1}_N, \mathbf{x}_1, \cdots, \mathbf{x}_a)$, where the N-dimensional vector $\mathbf{x}_i = (\mathbf{0}, \mathbf{1}_n, \mathbf{0})'$, with the 1's in the ith place. Then, $SSA = \sum_{i=1}^{a} Y_{i \cdot}^2/n - N\overline{Y}_{\cdot \cdot}^2 = \mathbf{y}'\{\frac{1}{n} \sum_i^{a+} \mathbf{x}_i \mathbf{x}_i' - \frac{1}{N} \mathbf{1}_N \mathbf{1}_N'\}\mathbf{y}$, which gives the result.

10.3. Suppose $SSA = \mathbf{y}'\mathbf{M}\mathbf{y}$, then, $E(SSA) = tr(\mathbf{M}\mathbf{V})$, where $\mathbf{V}$ denotes $Cov(\mathbf{y}) = \sigma_\varepsilon^2 \mathbf{I}_N + \sigma_\tau^2 \sum_{i=1}^{a+} \mathbf{J}_n$; simplify.

10.6. Let $SSA = \sum_i nb(\overline{Y}_{i \cdot \cdot} - \overline{Y}_{\cdot \cdot \cdot})^2$, $SSB(A) = \sum_i \sum_j n(\overline{Y}_{ij \cdot} - \overline{Y}_{i \cdot \cdot})^2$, $SSE = \sum_i \sum_j \sum_k (Y_{ijk} - \overline{Y}_{ij \cdot})^2$ with respective d.f. $(a-1)$, $(a(b-1))$ and $ab(n-1)$. The ANOVA estimators are $\hat{\sigma}_\tau^2 = \{MSA - MSB(A)\}/nb$, $\hat{\sigma}_\beta^2 = \{MSB(A) - MSE\}/n$, and $\hat{\sigma}_\varepsilon^2 = MSE$. The ML solutions are $\overset{.2}{\sigma}_\tau = \{(1 - 1/a)MSA - MSB(A)\}/nb$, while $\overset{.2}{\sigma}_\beta$ and $\overset{.2}{\sigma}_\varepsilon$ coincide with their ANOVA estimators.

10.7. The ML equations are

$$\frac{SS_A}{\overset{.2}{\theta}_{11}} + \frac{SS_B}{\overset{.2}{\theta}_{12}} + \frac{SS_{AB} + SSE}{\overset{.2}{\theta}_0} = \frac{1}{\overset{.}{\theta}_4} + \frac{a-1}{\overset{.}{\theta}_{11}} + \frac{b-1}{\overset{.}{\theta}_{12}} + \frac{abn-a-b+1}{\overset{.}{\theta}_0}$$

$$\frac{SS_A}{\overset{.2}{\theta}_{11}} = \frac{1}{\overset{.}{\theta}_4} + \frac{a-1}{\overset{.}{\theta}_{11}}$$

$$\frac{SS_B}{\overset{.2}{\theta}_{12}} = \frac{1}{\overset{.}{\theta}_4} + \frac{b-1}{\overset{.}{\theta}_{12}},$$

where $\theta_0 = \theta_1 = \sigma_\varepsilon^2$, $\theta_{11} = \sigma_\varepsilon^2 + bn\sigma_\tau^2$, $\theta_{12} = \sigma_\varepsilon^2 + an\sigma_\beta^2$, and $\theta_4 = \theta_{11} + \theta_{12} - \theta_0$. The explicit MLE of σ_ε^2 is MSE, while estimates of the remaining variance components must be obtained by numerical solution of these nonlinear equations.

Chapter 11

11.2. F_{N_1-1,N_2-1}.

11.4. Yes.

11.5. The state equation is $x_{t+1} = \rho x_t + w_t$, and the observation equation is $Y_t = x_t$.

11.6. The autoregressive signal-plus-noise model is defined by

$$Z_t = Y_t + v_t$$
$$Y_t = \rho Y_{t-1} + w_t,$$

v_t and w_t are independent error processes, $v_t \sim N(0, \sigma_v^2)$ and $w_t \sim N(0, \sigma_w^2)$. Express this in the form of (11.2.1) and (11.2.2), and the Kalman filter recursions are obtained from (11.2.7)-(11.2.9).

11.8. In the formulas in section 11.3.2, set $\mathbf{V}_i = \sigma^2\mathbf{I} + \mathbf{Z}_i\mathbf{D}_\gamma\mathbf{Z}_i'$.

11.9. Y has a Beta-Binomial distribution with $E(Y) = m\alpha/(\alpha+\beta)$ and $Var(Y) = m\alpha\beta/(\alpha + \beta)^2$.

References

Akaike, H. (1974). A new look at the statistical model identification. *IEEE Trans. Aut. Cont.*, **AC-19**, 716-723.

Akaike, H. (1978). A Bayesian analysis of the minimum AIC procedure. *Ann. Inst. Statist. Math.*, **30**, 9-14.

Akritas, M.G. (1990). The rank transform method in some two-factor designs. *J. Am. Statist. Assoc.*, **85**, 73-78.

Akritas, M.G. (1991). Limitations of the rank transform procedure: a study of repeated measures designs, Part I. *J. Am. Statist. Assoc.*, **86**, 457-460.

Akritas, M.G. (1993). Limitations of the rank transform procedure: a study of repeated measures designs, Part II. *Stat. Prob. Letters*, **17**, 149-156.

Akritas, M.G. and Arnold, S.F. (1994). Fully nonparametric hypotheses for factorial designs I: multivariate repeated measures designs. *J. Am. Statist. Assoc.*, **89**, 336-343.

Anderson, T.W. (1984). *An Introduction to Multivariate Statistical Analysis*, 2nd edition, J. Wiley & Sons, New York.

Anderson, T.W. and Fang, K.T. (1987). Cochran's theorem for elliptically contoured distributions. *Sankhya*, **A49**, 305-315.

Andrews, D.F., Gnanadesikan, R. and Warner, J.L. (1971). Transformations of multivariate data. *Biometrics*, **27**, 825-840.

Andrews, D.F. and Mallows, C.L. (1974). Scale mixtures of normal distributions. *J. R. Statist. Soc.*, **B36**, 99-102.

Andrews, D.F. and Pregibon, D. (1978). Finding outliers that matter. *J. R. Stat. Soc.*, **B40**, 85-93.

Ansley, C.F. (1985). Quick proofs of some regression theorems via the QR algorithm. *Am. Statistician*, **39**, 55-59.

Antoniadis, A., Gregoire, G. and McKeague, I.W. (1994). Wavelet methods for curve estimation. *J. Am. Statist. Assoc.*, **89**, 1340-1353.

Atiqullah, M. (1962). The estimation of residual variance in quadratically balanced least squares problems and the robustness of the F-test. *Biometrika*, **49**, 83-91.

Atkinson, A.C. (1981). Two graphical displays for outlying and influential observations in regression. *Biometrika*, **68**, 13-20.

Atkinson, A.C. (1985). *Plots, Transformations and Regression*. Oxford University Press, UK.

Azzalini, A. and Dalla Valle, A. (1996). The multivariate skew-normal distribution. *Biometrika*, **83**, 715-726.

Bartlett, M.S. (1937). Properties of sufficiency and statistical tests. *Proc. R. Soc.*, **A160**, 268-282.

Bassett, G, and Koenker, R. (1978). Asymptotic theory of least absolute error regression. *J. Am. Statist. Assoc.*, **73**, 618-622.

Basu, D. (1964). Recovery of ancillary information. *Sankhya*, **26**, 3-16.

Beckman, R.J. and Trussel, H.J. (1974). The distribution of an arbitrary studentized residual and the effects of updating in multiple regression. *J. Am. Statist. Assoc.*, **69**, 199-201.

Belsley, D. A., Kuh, E., and Welsch, R.E. (1980). *Regression diagnostics*. John Wiley & Sons, New York.

Belsley, D.A. (1984). Demeaning conditioning diagnostics through centering. *Am. Statistician*, **38**, 73-93.

Belsley, D.A. (1991). *Conditioning Diagnostics, Collinearity and Weak Data in Regression*. John Wiley & Sons, New York.

Berger, J.O. (1980). *Statistical Decision Theory and Bayesian Analysis*. Springer-Verlag, New York.

Bickel, P.J. and Doksum, K.A. (1981). An analysis of transformations revisited. *J. Am. Statist. Assoc.*, **76**, 296-311.

Birkes, D. and Dodge, Y. (1993). *Alternative Methods of Regression.* John Wiley & Sons, New York.

Bishop, C.M. (1995). *Neural Networks for Pattern Recognition.* Oxford University Press, Clarendon.

Bloomfield, P. and Steiger, W.L. (1983). *Least Absolute Deviations.* Birkhauser, Boston.

Box, G.E.P. and Cox, D.R. (1964). An analysis of transformations. *J. R. Stat. Soc.,* **B26**, 211-252.

Box, G.E.P. and Tiao, G.C. (1973). *Bayesian Inference in Statistical Analysis.* Addison-Wesley, Reading, Massachusetts.

Branco, M. and Dey, D.K. (2001). A general class of multivariate skew-elliptical distributions. *J. Mult. Anal.,* **79**, 99-113.

Breusch, T.S. and Pagan, A.R. (1979). A simple test for heteroscedasticity and random coefficient variation. *Econometrica,* **47**, 1287-1294.

Brockwell, P. J. and Davis, R. A. (1987). *Time Series: Theory and Methods.* Springer-Verlag, New York.

Brown, R.L., Durbin, J. and Evans, J.M. (1975). Techniques for testing the constancy of regression relationships (with discussion). *J. Roy. Stat. Soc.,* **B37**, 149-63.

Carroll, R.J. and Ruppert, D. (1988). *Transformations and Weighting in Regression.* Chapman & Hall, London.

Casella, G. and Berger, R.L. (1990). *Statistical Inference.* Wadsworth & Brooks Cole, California.

Charnes, A., Cooper, W.W. and Ferguson, R.O. (1955). Optimal estimation of executive compensation by linear programming. *Mgt. Sci.,* **1**, 138-151.

Chatterjee, S. and Hadi, A.S. (1988). *Sensitivity Analysis in Linear Regression.* John Wiley & Sons, New York.

Chatterjee, S. and Price, B. (1991). *Regression Analysis by Example.* John Wiley & Sons, New York.

Chen, M.-H., Dey, D.K. and Shao, Q.-M. (1999). A new skewed link model for dichotomous quantal response data. *J. Am. Statist. Assoc.,* **94**, 1172-1186.

Cheng, B. and Titterington, D.M. (1994). Neural networks: a review from a statistical prespective. *Stat. Sci.*, **9**, 2-54.

Chmielewski, M.A. (1981). Elliptically symmetric distributions: a review and bibliography. *Inter. Stat. Rev.*, **49**, 67-74.

Cochran, W.G. (1934). The distribution of quadratic forms in a normal system, with applications to the analysis of covariance. *Proc. Camb. Phil. Soc.*, **30**, 178-191.

Cochrane, D. and Orcutt, G.H. (1949). Application of least-squares regressions to relationships containing autocorrelated error terms. *J. Am. Statist. Assoc.*, **44**, 32-61.

Conover, W.J. (1980). *Practical Nonparametric Statistics*. John Wiley & Sons, New York.

Conover, W.J. and Iman, R.L. (1981). Rank transformations as a bridge between parametric and nonparametric statistics (with discussion). *Am. Statistician*, **35**, 124-129.

Cook, R.D. and Weisberg, S. (1980). Characterization of an empirical influence function for detecting influential cases in regression. *Technometrics*, **22**, 495-508.

Cook, R.D. and Weisberg, S. (1982). *Residuals and Influence in Regression*. Chapman & Hall, New York.

Cook, R.D. and Weisberg, S. (1994). *An Introduction to Regression Graphics*. J. Wiley & Sons, New York.

Cox, D.R. and Small, N.J.H. (1978). Testing multivariate normality. *Biometrika*, **65**, 263-272.

Craig, A.T. (1943). Note on the independence of certain quadratic forms. *Ann. Math. Stat.*, **14**, 195-197.

Daniel, C. and Wood, F.S. (1971). *Fitting Equations to Data: Computer Analysis of Multifactor Data*. John Wiley & Sons, New York.

David, F.N. (1938). *Tables of the Correlation Coefficient*. Cambridge University Press, Cambridge, UK.

Dempster, A.P., Laird, N.M. and Rubin, D.B. (1977). Maximum likelihood estimation from incomplete data via the EM algorithm (with discussion). *J. R.*

Stat. Soc., **B39**, 1-38.

Devlin, S.J., Gnanadesikan, R. and Kettenring, J.R. (1976). Some multivariate applications of elliptical distributions. In *Essays in Probability and Statistics* (S. Ikeda, ed.), 365-395, Shinko Tsusho, Tokyo.

Diaconis, P. and Shahshahani, M. (1984). On non-linear functions of linear combinations. *SIAM J. of Scientific and Statistical Computing*, **5**, 175-191.

Diggle, P.J., Liang, K.-Y., and Zeger, S.L. (1994). *Analysis of Longitudinal Data*. Oxford University Press, UK.

Dixon, L.C.W. (1972). *Nonlinear Optimization*. English Universities Press, London.

Dodge, Y. and Jureckova, J. (2000). *Adaptive regression*. Springer-Verlag, New York.

Donoho, D.L. and Johnstone, I.M. (1994). Ideal spatial adaptation by wavelet shrinkage. *Biometrika*, **81**, 425-455.

Draper, N.R. and Smith, H. (1998). *Applied Regression Analysis*. 3rd edition. John Wiley & Sons, New York.

Draper, N.R. and John, J.A. (1981). Influential observations and outliers in regression. *Technometrics*, **23**, 21-26.

Driscoll, M.F. and Krasnicka, B. (1995). An accessible proof of Craig's theorem in the general case. *Am. Statistician*, **49**, 59-62.

Driscoll, M.F. (1999). An improved result relating quadratic forms and chi-square distributions. *Am. Statistician*, **53**, 273-275.

Duncan, D.B. (1955). Multiple range and multiple F-tests. *Biometrics*, **11**, 1-42.

Dunnett, C.W. (1964). New tables for multiple comparisons with a control. *Biometrics*, **20**, 482-491.

Durbin, J. and Watson, G.S. (1950). Testing for serial correlation in least squares regression I. *Biometrika*, **37**, 409-428.

Durbin, J. and Watson, G.S. (1951). Testing for serial correlation in least squares regression II. *Biometrika*, **38**, 159-177.

Dyer, D.D. and Keating, J.P. (1980). On the determination of critical values for Bartlett's test. *J. Am. Statist. Assoc.*, **75**, 313-319.

Ellenberg, J.H. (1973). The joint distribution of the standardized least squares residuals from a general linear regression. *J. Am. Statist. Assoc.*, **68**, 941-943.

Englefield, N. J. (1966). The commuting inverses of a square matrix. *Proc. Camb. Phil. Soc.*, **62**, 667-671.

Fang, K.T. and Anderson, T.W. (1990). *Statistical Inference in Elliptically Contoured and Related Distributions*. Allerton Press Inc., New York.

Fang, K., Kotz, S. and Ng, K. (1990). *Symmetric Multivariate and Related Distributions*. Chapman & Hall, London.

Fisher, R.A. (1921). On the probable error of a coefficient of correlation deduced from a small sample. *Metron*, **1**, 1.

Fraser, D.A.S. and Ng, K.W. (1980). Multivariate regression analysis with spherical error, in *Multivariate Analysis V* (ed. P.R. Krisnaiah). North-Holland, New York, p. 369-386.

Freund, R.J., and Littell, R.C. (1991). SAS System for Regression. SAS Institute Inc.

Friedman, J.H. and Tukey, J.W. (1974). A projection pursuit algorithm for exploratory data analysis. *IEEE Transactions on Computers*, **C23**, 881-890.

Friedman, J.H. and Stuetzle (1981). Projection pursuit regression. *J. Am. Statist. Assoc.*, **76**, 817-823.

Ghosh, M. (1996). Wishart distribution by induction. *Am. Statistician*, **50**, 243-246.

Gnanadesikan, R. (1977). *Methods for Statistical Data Analysis of Multivariate Observations*. John Wiley & Sons, New York.

Goldfeld, S.M. and Quandt, R.E. (1965). Some tests for homoscedasticity. *J. Am. Statist. Assoc.*, **60**, 539-547.

Golub, G.H. and Styan, G.P. (1973). Numerical computations for univariate linear models. *J. Stat. Comput. Simul.*, **2**, 253-274.

Golub, G.H. and Van Loan, C.F. (1989). *Matrix Computations*. 2nd edition. Johns Hopkins University Press, Baltimore.

Golueke, C.G. and McGauhey, P.H. (1970). Comprehensive studies of solid waste management. U.S. Department of Health, Education, and Welfare, Public Health Services Publication No. 2039.

Graybill, F.A. (1954). On quadratic estimates of variance components. *Ann. Math. Stat.*, **25**, 367-372.

Graybill, F.A. (1961). *An Introduction to Linear Statistical Models*. McGraw-Hill, New York.

Graybill, F.A. (1983). *Matrices with Applications in Statistics*. 2nd edition. Wadsworth, Belmont, CA.

Graybill, F.A. and Hultquist, R.A. (1961). Theorems concerning Eisenhart's Model II. *Ann. Math. Stat.*, **32**, 261-269.

Guenther, W.C. (1964). Another derivation of the noncentral chi-square distribution. *J. Am. Statist. Assoc.*, **59**, 957-960.

Gupta, S.S. (1963). Probability integrals of multivariate normal and multivariate t. *Ann. Math. Stat.*, **34**, 792-828.

Gupta, A.K. and Varga, T. (1993). *Elliptically Contoured Models in Statistics*. Kluwer Academic Publishers, Netherlands.

Halmos, P.R. and Savage, L.J. (1949). Applications of the Radon-Nikodym theorem to the theory of sufficient statistics. *Ann. Math. Stat.*, **20**, 225-241.

Hampel, F.R. (1974). The influence curve and its role in robust estimation. *J. Am. Statist. Assoc.*, **62**, 1179-1186.

Harrison, J. and West, M. (1991). Dynamic linear model diagnostics. *Biometrika*, **78**, 797-808.

Harvey, A.C. and Phillips, G.D.A. (1974). A comparison of the power of some tests for heteroscedasticity in the general linear model. *J. Econ.*, **2**, 307-316.

Harville, D.A. (1974). Bayesian inference for variance components using only error contrasts. *Biometrika*, **61**, 383-385.

Harville, D.A. (1976). Extension of the Gauss-Markov theorem to include the estimation of random effects. *Ann. Statist.*, **4**, 384-395.

Harville, D.A. (1977). Maximum likelihood approaches to variance component estimation and to related problems (with discussion). *J. Am. Statist. Assoc.*,

72, 320-340.

Harville, D.A. (1997). *Matrix Algebra From a Statistician's Perspective.* Springer-Verlag, New York.

Hastie, T. J. and Tibsirani, R. J. (1990). *Generalized Additive Models.* Chapman & Hall, London.

Hayes, J.G. (1974). Numerical methods for curve and surface fitting. *J. Inst. Math. Appl.*, **10**, 144-152.

Hayes, K. and Haslett, J. (1999). Simplifying general least squares. *Am. Statistician*, **53**, 376-381.

Hertz, J., Krogh, A. and Palmer, R.G. (1991). *Introduction to the Theory of Neural Computation.* Addison-Wesley, CA.

Heyadat, A. and Robson, D.S. (1970). Independent stepwise residuals for testing homoscedasticity. *J. Am. Statist. Assoc.*, **65**, 1573-1581.

Heyadat, A., Raktoe, B., and Telwar, O. (1977). Examination and analysis of residuals: a test for detecting a monotonic relation between mean and variance in regression through the origin. *Comm. Statist.*, **A6**, 497-506.

Hinkley, D.V. (1975). On power transformation to symmetry. *Biometrika*, **63**, 101-111.

Hoaglin, D.C. and Welsch, R.E. (1978). The hat matrix in regression and ANOVA. *Am. Statistician*, **32**, 17-22.

Hochberg, Y. and Tamhane, A.C. (1987). *Multiple Comparison Procedures.* John Wiley & Sons, New York.

Hoerl, A.E. (1962). Application of ridge analysis to regression problems. *Chemical Engineering Progress*, **58**, 54-59.

Hoerl, A.E. and Kennard, R.W. (1970a). Ridge regression: biased estimation for nonorthogonal problems. *Technometrics*, **12**, 55-67.

Hoerl, A.E. and Kennard, R.W. (1970b). Ridge regression: applications to nonorthogonal problems. *Technometrics*, **12**, 69-82.

Hollander, M. and Wolfe, D.A. (1973). *Nonparametric Statistical Methods.* John Wiley & Sons, New York.

Huber, P. (1964). Robust estimation of a location parameter. *Ann. Math. Statist.*, **35**, 73-101.

Huber, P. (1981). *Robust Statistics*. John Wiley & Sons, New York.

James, G.S. (1952). Notes on a theorem of Cochran. *Proc. Camb. Phil. Soc.*, **48**, 443.

John, J.A. and Draper, N.R. (1980). An alternate family of transformation. *Appl. Statist.*, **29**, 190-197.

Johnson, N.L. and Kotz, S. (1972). *Distributions in Statistics: Continuous Multivariate Distributions*. John Wiley & Sons, New York.

Johnson, R.A. and Wichern, D.W. (1988). *Applied Multivariate Statistical Analysis*. 2nd edition. Prentice-Hall, Englewood Cliffs, NJ.

Judge, G.G., Griffiths, W.E., Hill, R. C., Lutkepohl, H. and Lee, T.-C. (1985). *The Theory and Practice of Econometrics*. John Wiley & Sons, New York.

Judge, G.G., Griffiths, W.E., Hill, R. C., Lutkepohl, H. and Lee, T.-C. (1988). *Introduction to the Theory and Practice of Econometrics*. John Wiley & Sons, New York.

Kelker, D. (1970). Distribution theory of spherical distributions and a location-scale parameter generalization. *Sankhya*, **A32**, 419-430.

Kendall, M. G. and Stuart, A. (1958). *The Advanced Theory of Statistics, Vol. 1*. Hafner Publishing Co., New York.

Kendall, M.G. and Stuart, A. (1963). *The Advanced Theory of Statistics, Vol. 2*. Hafner Publishing Co., New York.

Keuls, M. (1954). Testing differences between means in an analysis of variance. *Biometrics*, **10**, 167-168.

Khuri, A. I. (1999). A necessary condition for a quadratic form to have a chi-squared distribution: an accessible proof. *Int. J. Math. EDuc. Sci. Technol.*, **30**, 335-339.

Kruskal, W.H. (1952). A nonparametric test fo the several sample problem. *Ann. Math. Stat.*, **23**, 525-540.

Kruskal, W. (1968). When are Gauss-Markov and least squares estimators identical? A coordinate-free approach. *Ann. Math. Stat.*, **39**, 70-75.

Kruskal, W.H. and Wallis, W.A. (1952). Use of ranks in one-criterion variance analysis. *J. Am. Statist. Assoc.*, **47**, 583-621.

Laha, R.G. (1956). On the stochastic independence of two second-degree polynomial statistics in normally distributed variables. *Ann. Math. Stat.*, **27**, 790-796.

Laird, N.M. and Ware, J.H. (1982). Random-effects models for longitudinal data. *Biometrics*, **38**, 963-974.

Larsen, W.A. and McCleary, S.A. (1972). The use of partial residual plots in regression analysis. *Technometrics*, **14**, 781-790.

Levene, H. (1960). In *Contributions to Probability and Statistics.* Stanford University Press, Stanford, CA., p. 278.

Liang, K.-Y. and Zeger, S.L. (1986). Longitudinal data analysis using generalized linear models. *Biometrika*, **73**, 13-22.

Lindley, D. V. and Smith, A.F.M. (1972). Bayes estimates for the linear model. *J. R. Stat. Soc.*, **B34**, 1-41.

Littell, R.C., Freund, R.J. and Spector, P.C. (1991). *SAS System for Linear Models.* SAS Institute Inc., Cary, NC, USA.

Little, R.J.A. and Rubin, D.B. (1987). *Statistical Analysis with Missing Data.* John Wiley & Sons, New York.

Lucas, H.L. (1962). Unpublished lecture notes on the linear model and its analysis. Univ. North Carolina, Raleigh.

McCullagh, P. and Nelder, J.A. (1991). *Generalized Linear Models.* Chapman & Hall, London.

McElroy, F.W. (1967). A necessary and sufficient condition that ordinary least-squares estimators be best linear unbiased. *J. Am. Statist. Assoc.*, **62**, 1302-1304.

Magnus, J.R. and Neudecker, H. (1988). *Matrix Differential Calculus with Applications in Statistics and Econometrics.* John Wiley & Sons, New York.

Mallows, C.L. (1973). Some comments on C_p. *Technometrics*, **15**, 661-675.

Mallows, C.L. (1995). More comments on C_p. *Technometrics*, **37**, 362-372.

Manly, B.F. (1976). Exponential data transformation. *The Statistician*, **25**, 37-42.

Mardia, K.V. (1970). Measures of multivariate skewness and kurtosis with applications. *Biometrika*, **57**, 519-530.

Mardia, K.V. (1975). Assessment of multinormality and the robustness of Hotelling's T^2 test. *Appl. Statist.*, **24**, 163-171.

Mardia, K.V., Kent, J.T. and Bibby, J.M. (1979). *Multivariate Analysis*. Academic Press, London.

Mathew, T. and Nordstrom, K. (1997). An inequality for a measure of deviation in linear models. *Am. Statistician*, **51**, 344-349.

Meinhold, R.J. and Singpurwalla, N. D. (1983). Understanding the Kalman filter. *Am. Statistician*, **37**, 123-127.

Miller, R.G. (1981). *Simultaneous Statistical Inference*. Springer-Verlag, New York.

Montgomery, D.C. (1991). *The Design and Analysis of Experiments*. John Wiley & Sons, New York.

Mood, A. M. (1950). *Introduction to the Theory of Statistics*. McGraw-Hill, New York.

Moser, B.K. and Sawyer, J.K. (1998). Algorithms for sums of squares and covariance matrices using Kronecker products. *Am. Statistician*, **52**, 54-57.

Mosteller, F. and Tukey, J.W. (1977). *Data analysis and Regression*. Addison Wesley, Reading, MA.

Muirhead, R.J. (1982). *Aspects of Multivariate Statistical Theory*. John Wiley & Sons, New York.

Mukhopadhyay, N. (2000). *Probability and Statistical Inference*. Marcel Dekker, Inc., New York.

Myers, R.H. (1971). *Response Surface Methodology*. Allyn & Bacon, Inc., Boston.

Nadaraya, E.A. (1964). On estimating regression. *Theory Probab. Appl.*, **9**, 141-142.

Newman, D. (1939). The distribution of the range in samples from a normal population, expressed in terms of an independent estimate of standard deviation. *Biometrika*, **31**, 20-30.

Ogasawara, T. and Takahashi, M. (1951). Independence of quadratic forms in normal system. *J. Sci. Hiroshima University*, **15**, 1-9.

Ogawa, J. (1950). On the independence of quadratic forms in a noncentral normal system. *Osaka Mathematical Journal*, **2**, 151-159.

Ogawa, J. (1993). A history of the development of Craig-Sakamoto's theorem viewed from Japanese standpoint (in Japanese and English). *Proc. Inst. Statist. Math.*, **41**, 47-59.

Patterson, H.D. and Thompson, R. (1971). Recovery of intra-block information when block sizes are unequal. *Biometrika*, **58**, 545-554.

Pearson, E.A.S. and Hartley, H.O. (1970). *Biometrika Tables for Statisticians*, Vol. 1 and Vol. 2. Cambridge University Press, UK.

Phillips, G.D.A. and Harvey, A.C. (1974). A simple test for serial correlation in regression analysis. *J. Am. Statist. Assoc.*, **69**, 935-939.

Pierce, D.A. and Schafer, D.W. (1986). Residuals in generalized linear models. *J. Am. Statist. Assoc.*, **81**, 977-986.

Powell, J.L. (1984). Least absolute deviations estimation for the censored regression model. *J. Econ.*, **25**, 303-325.

Pregibon, D. (1981). Logistic regression diagnostics. *Ann. Statist.*, **9**, 705-724.

Pringle, R.M. and Rayner, A.A. (1971). *Generalized Inverse Matrices with Applications to Statistics*. Griffin, London.

Rao, C.R. (1952). Some theorems on minimum variance estimation. *Sankhya*, **12**, 27-42.

Rao, C.R. (1971a). Estimation of variance and covariance components-MINQUE theory. *J. Mult. Anal.*, **1**, 257-275.

Rao, C.R. (1971b). Minimum variance quadratic unbiased estimation of variance components. *J. Mult. Anal.*, **1**, 445-456.

Rao, C.R. (1973a). *Linear Statistical Inference and its Applications*. 2nd edition. John Wiley & Sons, New York.

Rao, C.R. (1973b). Representations of best linear unbiased estimators in the Gauss-Markoff model with a singular dispersion matrix. *J. Mult. Anal.*, **3**, 276-292.

Rao, C.R. (1988). Methodology based on the L_1-norm in statistical inference. *Sankhyã*, **A50**, 289-313.

Rao, C.R. and Mitra, S.K. (1971). *Generalized Inverse of Matrices and its Applications*. John Wiley & Sons, New York.

Rao, C.R. and Toutenberg, H. (1995). *Linear Models: Least Squares and Alternatives*. Springer-Verlag, New York.

Rao, C.R. and Zhao, L.C. (1993). Asymptotic normality of LAD estimator in censored regression models. *Mathematical Methods of Statistics*, **2**, 228-239.

Rauch, H.E., Tung, F. and Streibel, C.T. (1965). Maximum likelihood estimation of linear dynamic systems. *J. AIAA*, **3**, 1445-1450.

Reid, J.G. and Driscoll, M.F. (1988). An accessible proof of Craig's theorem in the noncentral case. *Am. Statistician*, **42**, 139-142.

Rodgers, J.L. and Nicewander, W.A. (1988). Thirteen ways to look at the correlation coefficient. *Am. Statistician*, **42**, 59-66.

Rumelhart, D.E., Hinton, G.E., and Williams, R.J. (1986). Learning internal representation by back-propagation errors. *Nature* **323**, 533-536.

Ruppert, D. and Carroll, R.J. (1980). Trimmed least squares estimation in the linear model. *J. Am. Statist. Assoc.*, **75**, 828-838.

Samorodnitsky, G. and Taqqu, M.S. (1994). *Stable Non-Gaussian Random Processes: Stochastic Models with Infinite Variance*. Chapman & Hall, New York.

Saxena, K.M. and Alam, K. (1982). Estimation of the noncentrality parameter of a chi-squared distribution. *Ann. Stat.*, **10**, 1012-1016.

Scheffe, H. (1953). A method for judging all contrasts in the Analysis of Variance. *Biometrika*, **40**, 87-104.

Scheffe, H. (1959). *The Analysis of Variance*. John Wiley & Sons, New York.

Schwarz, G. (1978). Estimating the dimension of a model. *Ann. Statist.*, **6**, 461-464.

Searle, S. R. (1971). *Linear Models.* John Wiley & Sons, New York.

Searle, S.R. (1982). *Matrix Algebra Useful for Statistics.* John Wiley & Sons, New York.

Searle, S.R. (1987). *Linear Models for Unbalanced Data.* John Wiley & Sons, New York.

Searle, S.R., Casella, G. and McCulloch, C.E. (1992). *Variance Components.* John Wiley & Sons, New York.

Seber, G.A.F. (1977). *Linear Regression Analysis.* John Wiley & Sons, New York.

Seber, G.A.F. (1984). *Multivariate Observations.* John Wiley & Sons, New York.

Seber, G. A. F. and Wild, C.J. (1989). *Nonlinear Regression.* John Wiley & Sons, New York.

Seely, J.F., Birkes, D., and Lee, Y. (1997). Characterizing sums of squares by their distributions. *Am. Statistician*, **51**, 55-58.

Shanbhag, D. N. (1966). On the independence of quadratic forms. *J. R. Stat. Soc.*, **B28**, 582-583.

Shapiro, S.S. and Wilk, M.B. (1965). An analysis of variance test for normality (complete samples). *Biometrika*, **52**, 591-611.

Shumway, R.H. and Stoffer, D.S. (2000). *Time Series Analysis and its Applications.* Springer Verlag, New York.

Solomon, P.J. (1985). Transformations for components of variance and covariance. *Biometrika*, **72**, 233-239.

Sprent, P. (1961). Some hypotheses concerning two phase regression lines. *Biometrics*, **17**, 634-645.

Stukel, T. (1988). Generalized logistic models. *J. Am. Statist. Assoc.*, **83**, 426-431.

Stewart, G.W. (1973). *Introduction to Matrix Computations.* Academic Press, New York.

Tang, P.C. (1938). Power function of the analysis of variance tests with tables and illustrations of their use. *Statistical Research Memoirs*, **2**, p.126.

Theil, H. (1965). The analysis of disturbances in regression analysis. *J. Am. Statist. Assoc.*, **60**, 1067-1079.

Thisted, R.A. (1988). *Elements of Statistical Computing: Numerical Computation.* Chapman & Hall, New York.

Thompson, G.L. (1991). A unified approach to rank tests for multivariate and repeated measures designs. *J. Am. Statist. Assoc.*, **86**, 410-419.

Tukey, J.W. (1957). The comparative anatomy of transformations. *Ann. Math. Stat.*, **28**, 602-632.

Velleman, P.F. and Welsch, R.E. (1981). Efficient computing of regression diagnostics. *Am. Statistician*, **35**, 234-242.

Verbyla, A.P. and Cullis, B.R. (1990). Modeling in repeated measures experiments. *Appl. Statist.*, **39**, 341-356.

Vidakovic, B. (1999). *Statistical Modeling by Wavelets.* John Wiley & Sons, New York.

Wang, Y. (1995). Jump and sharp cusp detection by wavelets. *Biometrika*, **82**, 385-397.

Warner, B. and Misra, M. (1996). Understanding neural networks as statistical tools. *Am. Statistician*, **50**, 284-293.

Watson, G.S. (1964). Smooth regression analysis. *Sankhya*, **A26**, 359-372.

Wedderburn, R.W.M. (1974). Quasi-likelihood functions, generalized linear models, and the Gauss-Newton method. *Biometrika*, **61**, 439-447.

Weeks, D.L. and Williams, D.R. (1964). A note on the determination of connectedness in an N-way cross classification. *Technometrics*, **6**, 319-324.

West, M. and Harrison, J. (1997). *Bayesian Forecasting and Dynamic Models.* Springer-Verlag, New York.

Westfall, P.H. (1987). A comparison of variance components estimates for arbitrary underlying distributions. *J. Am. Statist. Assoc.*, **82**, 866-874.

White, H. (1980). A heteroscedasticity-consistent covariance matrix estimator with a direct test for heteroscedasticity. *Econometrica*, **48**, 817-838.

Williams, E.J. (1959). *Regression Analysis.* John Wiley & Sons, New York.

Wood, F.S. (1973). The use of individual effects and residuals in fitting equations to data. *Technometrics* **15**, 677-695.

Woods, H., Steinour, H.H., and Starke, H.R. (1932). Effect of composition of Portland cement on heat evolved during hardening. *Industrial and Engineering Chemistry*, **24**, 1207-1214.

Wu, L.S.-Y., Hosking, J.R.M. and Ravishanker, N. (1993). Reallocation outliers in time series. *Appl. Statist.*, **42**, 301-313.

Zyskind, G. and Martin, F. B. (1969). On best linear estimation and a general Gauss-Markov theorem in linear models with arbitrary nonnegative covariance structure. *SIAM J. Appl. Math.*, **17**, 1190-1202.

Author Index

Subject Index